Manual of Neurologic Therapeutics

S0-AKD-072

Manual of Neurologic Therapeutics

Fifth Edition

Edited by

Martin A. Samuels, M.D.

Professor of Neurology,
Harvard Medical School;
Neurologist-in-Chief,
Brigham and Women's Hospital;
Director, Harvard Longwood
Neurology Training Program, Boston

Little, Brown and Company
Boston New York Toronto London

Library of Congress Cataloging-in-Publication Data

Manual of neurologic therapeutics /
    edited by Martin A. Samuels.—5th ed.
      p.   cm.
    Rev. ed. of: Manual of neurology. 4th ed. c1991.
    Includes bibliographical references and index.
    ISBN 0-316-77004-3
    1. Neurology—Handbooks, manuals, etc.   I. Samuels, Martin A.,
  1945–   .   II. Manual of neurology.
      [DNLM: 1. Nervous System Diseases—diagnosis—outlines.
    2. Nervous System Diseases—therapy—outlines.   WL 18 M294   1994]
    RC355.M36   1994
    616.8—dc20
    DNLM/DLC
    for Library of Congress   94-11939
                                                              CIP

Printed in the United States of America

SEM

Editorial: Nancy Megley
Production Editor: Cathleen Cote
Copyeditor: Debra Corman
Indexer: Dorothy Hoffman
Production Supervisor: Cate Rickard
Cover Designers: Linda Dana Willis and Patrick Newbury

Third Printing

Cover: Tremor study of a patient with essential tremor in which the movements are very regular and EMG bursts occur simultaneously in antagonistic muscle groups. This type of tremor was first successfully treated with propranolol based on an observation made by Gerald F. Winkler and Robert R. Young. (Winkler, GF, Young, RR. The control of essential tremor by propranolol. *Trans Am Neurol Assoc* 96:66–68, 1971. Winkler, GF, Young, RR. Efficacy of chronic propranolol therapy in action tremors of the familial, senile or essential varieties. *N Engl J Med* 290:984–988, 1974.)

This manual is dedicated to Robert R. Young, M.D., Professor and Vice Chair, Department of Neurology, University of California, Irvine, and Chief, Neurology Service, Department of Veterans Affairs Medical Center, Long Beach, California. Prior to his recent move to California, Dr. Young was Professor of Neurology at Harvard Medical School and Chief of the Spinal Cord Injury Service at the Department of Veterans Affairs Medical Center, Brockton–West Roxbury. He is world renowned for his clarification of the pathophysiology of numerous movement disorders, most notably essential tremor, and the development of new and creative approaches for the application of electromyography to the elucidation of the causes of movement disorders.

We remember Bob in another way. During our neurology residency, he was the Director of the Clinical Neurophysiology Laboratory at the Massachusetts General Hospital and as such was our mentor in EEG, EMG, and the clinical aspects of peripheral neurology. His lectures on the usually arcane details of electrophysiology were remarkable for their clarity. His own profound understanding of the basic physiologic principles translated into extraordinarily lucid and seemingly simple ways of unraveling complex problems. This uncanny ability to demystify difficult problems was carried to the bedside. Bob was known as a master clinician well beyond the limits of peripheral neurology. Residents competed for the opportunity to be on the service during his months of attending. To this day we find ourselves trying to emulate his ability to cut to the core of the problem to unearth what is usually a simple solution to an apparently confounding clinical presentation. All of us among the contributors were privileged to be exposed to Bob during our training and are pleased to dedicate this fifth edition of the *Manual of Neurologic Therapeutics* to him.

Previous editions of this manual were dedicated to Raymond D. Adams, M.D., C. Miller Fisher, M.D., Edward P. Richardson, Jr., M.D., and David C. Poskanzer, M.D.

Contents

Contributing Authors

Telmo M. Aquino, M.D.

Chief of Neurology, Hospital de Clinicas, Asuncion, Paraguay

Raymond J. Fernandez, M.D.

Associate Professor of Pediatrics, University of South Florida College of Medicine; Active Staff, Tampa General Hospital, Tampa, Florida

Robert D. Helme, Ph.D.

Professor of Geriatric Medicine, University of Melbourne; Director, National Aging Research Institute, Melbourne, Australia

Daniel B. Hier, M.D.

Chairman and Professor of Neurology, University of Illinois College of Medicine; Chief of Neurology Service, University of Illinois Hospital, Chicago

Richard C. Hinton, M.D.

Assistant Professor of Neurology, University of Texas Southwestern Medical School at Dallas; Attending Neurologist, Presbyterian Hospital of Dallas, Dallas

Robert L. Martuza, M.D.

Professor and Chairman, Department of Neurosurgery, Georgetown University Medical Center, Washington, D.C.

Dawn McGuire, M.D.

Special Consultant to the Fifth Edition Assistant Professor of Neurology, University of California, San Francisco, School of Medicine; Director, AIDS Neurology Clinics, The Medical Center at the University of California, San Francisco, and San Francisco General Hospital, San Francisco

George B. Murray, M.D.

Associate Professor of Psychiatry, Harvard Medical School; Chief, Psychiatric Consultation Service, Massachusetts General Hospital, Boston

Mark R. Proctor, M.D.

Special Consultant to the Fifth Edition Resident in Neurosurgery, Georgetown University School of Medicine and Georgetown University Hospital, Washington, D.C.

Stephen M. Sagar, M.D.

Professor of Neurology, University of California, San Francisco, School of Medicine; Assistant Chief of Neurology, San Francisco Veterans Affairs Medical Center, San Francisco

Martin A. Samuels, M.D.

Professor of Neurology, Harvard Medical School; Neurologist-in-Chief, Brigham and Women's Hospital; Director, Harvard Longwood Neurology Training Program, Boston

Thomas M. Walshe III, M.D.

Assistant Professor of Neurology, Harvard Medical School, Boston; Associate Chief, Neurology Service, Brockton-West Roxbury Veterans Affairs Medical Center, Brockton, Massachusetts

Howard D. Weiss, M.D.

Assistant Professor of Neurology, Johns Hopkins University School of Medicine; Attending Neurologist, Sinai Hospital, Baltimore

Preface to the Fifth Edition

Since publication of the fourth edition of the *Manual of Neurologic Therapeutics,* (entitled *Manual of Neurology: Diagnosis and Therapy*), major changes have begun to occur in the way medical care is delivered. It is clear that we are facing a mini-revolution with a dramatic reduction in specialists and a concomitant increase in the number of generalists in the offing. Neurology, long considered a rather arcane corner of medicine and left to the expertise of neurologists, will now fall mainly under the purview of general internists, family physicians, and general practitioners.

With this in mind, the fifth edition of the *Manual* has been sculpted to be a useful tool for the non-neurologist who must face and deal with many common neurologic problems as part of the general practice of medicine. Subspecialty consultations will become increasingly difficult to obtain, so it will be important for the generalist to be confident in diagnosing and treating common problems such as headache, dizziness, altered mental status, seizures, stroke, and a panoply of ubiquitous patient complaints referable to nervous system disease.

We have aimed to provide a compact source of state-of-the-art treatments that are cost-effective and can be applied by well-informed generalists. The *Manual* contains enough diagnostic information to assist the well-trained physician in making the correct diagnosis. Therapeutic information provides the physician a clear, stepwise course of therapeutic action.

A great deal has happened since the fourth edition was published in 1991. Some of the highlights included in the fifth edition are the introduction of two new anticonvulsants (felbamate and gabapentin) with two more close behind (vigabatrin and lamotrigine); the use of a short-acting barbiturate (midazolam) in the management of status epilepticus; the widespread use of botulinum toxin in the treatment of many common movement disorders; the expansion of the number of molecularly based diagnostic tests (e.g., the CSF polymerase chain reaction for the diagnosis of herpes simplex encephalitis); the approval of the first drug aimed at stemming the progression of Alzheimer's disease (tacrine); the use of a new, less Parkinson-inducing antipsychotic drug (clozapine); and many others.

We again wish to thank all of our colleagues and families who advised us in the preparation of the manuscript.

M. A. S.

Preface to the First Edition

Until very recently the neurologist's primary task was to categorize and organize the structure and pathologic alterations of the nervous system. In fact, neurology has long been known as a discipline with elegantly precise and specific diagnostic capabilities but little or no therapeutic potentiality. Further, many surgeons, pediatricians, and internists have traditionally thought of the neurologist as an impractical intellectual who spends countless hours painstakingly localizing lesions while ignoring pragmatic considerations of treatment. Perhaps this conception is largely attributable to the peculiar complexity of the nervous system and the consequent relative naivete of physicians in their understanding of its functions.

Many of the classic descriptions of disease states in other medical disciplines were completed in the last century; in neurology, these have only been described in the past generation, and only in the last ten years has neurology begun to be characterized by subcellular mechanistic concepts of disease. This maturity has meant that the neurologist is now as much involved in the therapeutic aspects of his specialty of medicine as any of his colleagues. Certain neurologic diseases, such as epilepsy, have been treatable for relatively long periods of time, but understanding of the subcellular mechanisms of other diseases has led to newer, more effective forms of therapy.

An example of this is the enlarged understanding we now have of the biochemical alterations in Parkinson's disease, and the resultant therapeutic implications. Now, much as the endocrinologist treats diabetes with insulin and the cardiologist treats congestive heart failure with digitalis, the neurologist treats Parkinson's disease with L-dopa. In all these situations, the underlying condition is not cured; rather, an attempt is made to alter the pathophysiologic processes by utilizing a scientific understanding of the function of the diseased system.

This manual embodies a practical, logical approach to the treatment of neurologic problems, based on accurate diagnosis, that should prove useful to both clinician and student. No attempt is made to reiterate the details of the neurologic examination; it is assumed that the reader is competent to examine the patient—although particularly important or difficult differential diagnostic points are mentioned when appropriate. In this regard, it should be emphasized that this manual is only a guide to diagnosis and therapy, and each patient must be treated individually. The manual is organized to best meet the needs of the clinician facing therapeutic problems. Thus, the first seven chapters are concerned with symptoms, such as dizziness and headache, while the last ten consider common diseases, such as stroke and neoplasms.

I thank the many colleagues and friends whose criticism and comments were useful in the preparation of this book, in particular Drs. G. Robert DeLong, C. Miller Fisher, George Kleinman, James B. Lehrich, Steven W. Parker, Henry C. Powell, E. P. Richardson, Jr., Maria Salam, Bagwan T. Shahani, Peter Weller, James G. Wepsic, and Robert R. Young. In addition I am indebted to Sara Nugent and Helen Hyland for their assistance in the preparation of the many manuscripts, and to Diana Odell Potter, formerly of Little, Brown and

Company, for her editorial skills. Jane Sandiford, formerly of Little, Brown, and Kathleen O'Brien and Carmen Thomas of Little, Brown provided invaluable assistance in the final preparation of this material. Deep appreciation goes to Lin Richter, Editor in Chief of the Medical Division, Little, Brown and Company, for her support throughout this effort. I further thank Jon Paul Davidson, also formerly of Little, Brown, for his valuable encouragement and help early in the course of this project. Much support and encouragement was derived from my new colleagues in the Peter Bent Brigham Hospital Neurology Section, The Longwood Avenue Neurology Program, and the West Roxbury Veterans Administration Hospital. A great deal of inspiration came from the birth of my daughter Marilyn, and my deepest thanks go to my wife, Linda, who provided constant encouragement, editorial skill, and infinite patience.

M.A.S.

Neurologic Symptoms

Coma and Other Alterations in Consciousness

Telmo M. Aquino and
Martin A. Samuels

I. **General principles.** When confronted with a patient with impaired consciousness, the clinician proceeds in an orderly, systematic manner. He or she gathers information while performing specific therapeutic maneuvers aimed at maintaining vital functions and avoiding further neurologic damage.

Impairment of consciousness may derive from a variety of causes. The first priority is to define and treat, as expeditiously as possible, those causes that are potentially reversible (see sec. **V**).

II. **Pathophysiology.** Consciousness consists of two components: **awareness** and **arousal** (or wakefulness). **Awareness** refers to the higher-level integration of multiple sensory inputs that permit meaningful understanding of self and environment. The mechanisms of awareness reside diffusely in the cerebral cortex. **Arousal** refers to a more primitive set of responses, the structures for which are located entirely within the brainstem and diencephalon and which are synchronized by a diffuse network of nuclei and interconnecting tracts. The ascending reticular activating system (ARAS) mediates such responses as eye opening to painful stimuli, which is one clinical expression of intact arousal mechanisms. Other testable aspects of ARAS functioning include corneal reflexes, pupillary reactions, and ocular motility, either spontaneous or reflex (e.g., oculocephalic and vestibuloocular reflexes). Via thalamic relay nuclei, the ARAS projects diffusely to the cerebral cortex, acting thus as a "switch" for the cortical awareness system. In normal circumstances, it is the cycling of this system that accounts for the sleep-wake cycles and the corresponding EEG findings.

With these simple anatomic and physiologic points in mind, one can conceive of three mechanisms by which consciousness may be impaired:

A. **Bilateral diffuse cerebral cortex failure,** leading to a state of impaired awareness with intact arousal mechanisms (the so-called vegetative state). This circumstance most commonly results from a diffuse anoxic or ischemic insult such as cardiac arrest or the end stage of degenerative diseases.

B. **Brainstem failure,** leading to a state of impaired arousal. In such cases, awareness is untestable, since the ARAS "switch" is shut off and would produce, in effect, a state of pathologic sleep. In clinical practice, a state of brainstem failure could be due to either

1. **Primary brainstem pathology,** such as midbrain and/or diencephalic hemorrhage or infarction.

2. **Secondary brainstem injury** due to compression from masses that are normally situated in other compartments; examples of this are transtentorial (uncal) or cerebellar herniations due to a mass in the temporal lobe or the cerebellum, respectively. Such compressing masses can cause permanent brain lesions (e.g., Duret hemorrhages) by distorting the brainstem's vascular supply through stretch or torque.

C. **Combined bilateral cortical and brainstem failure** is seen most commonly in cases of metabolic encephalopathy and intoxications in which the relative participation of brainstem, as opposed to cortical, dysfunction varies, depending on the toxin involved and the type and severity of the metabolic derangement.

III. **Diagnosis**

A. **History.** Frequently, no information is available. Whenever possible, family, friends, ambulance personnel, and physicians who have previously treated the patient should be contacted. **Important features** of the history are trauma, previous illnesses, medications, use of drugs or alcohol, and psychiatric disorders.

B. General physical examination
1. **Vital signs:** airway patency, circulatory and ventilatory status, and fever.
2. **Skin:** signs of trauma, stigmata of liver disease, needle marks, and infective or embolic phenomena.
3. **Head:** Battle's sign (i.e., hematoma over the mastoid process), localized tenderness, and crepitus and/or hemorrhage from ears or nostrils indicate basilar skull fracture.
4. **Neck stiffness** may be indicative of infection, trauma, or subarachnoid bleeding. **(Do not manipulate the neck if there is suspicion of cervical spine fracture.)**
5. **Chest, abdomen, heart, and extremities** must be examined routinely. **Rectal and pelvic** examinations plus a stool test for blood should also be performed.
6. **Breath** may suggest liver failure (fetor hepaticus, "liver breath"), ketoacidosis, alcohol ingestion, or uremia.

C. A neurologic examination is performed in all patients and recorded. Aiming to define presence, location, and nature of the causal process, special emphasis is placed on the following:
1. **Observation of the patient**
   a. If the patient **lies in a natural, comfortable position,** as though in natural sleep, coma is probably not very deep. Yawning and sneezing have the same significance, although other automatisms such as coughing, swallowing, or hiccuping do not necessarily reflect light coma.
   b. **Jaw and lid tone** also indicates the severity of unconsciousness. Open lids and hanging jaw bespeak deep coma.
2. **Level of unconsciousness.** Abnormalities of consciousness comprise a continuum, ranging from mild confusion to total unresponsiveness. It is useful in clinical practice to categorize patients with abnormal consciousness according to stages of progressive unresponsiveness. Given the confusion surrounding the meanings of terms describing levels of consciousness, it is good practice to describe in detail on the record the responses of the patient to various stimuli. Use of terms such as *lethargy, somnolence,* or *obtundation* should be substantiated by a brief descriptive paragraph in the history.
   a. **Confusion** (or encephalopathy) is defined as the inability to maintain a coherent stream of thought or action. The neurologic substrate for confusion is inattention. **Attention** is difficult to define, but it refers to the ability of the individual to sort out and stratify the many sensory inputs and potential motor outputs so that a particular thought or action may be completed in an organized and logical fashion. It is evident from the concept that the mechanisms for attention must involve both arousal and awareness. Thus, confusion may be seen in states of cortical and/or ARAS dysfunction. The most common cause of confusion is metabolic or toxic derangement, although it may be seen with certain focal cortical lesions, particularly those of the right parietal lobe. Confusion is evident clinically when the apparently awake patient fails tasks requiring sustained attention, such as the serial 7s test. Such patients may also show very disturbed writing.
   Delirium is a confusional state plus excess sympathetic activity. The term *delirium* applies when the confused patient also has tachycardia, diaphoresis, tremor, mydriasis, and hypertension. In general, pure confusion is seen in most metabolic encephalopathies including mild intoxication with sedative drugs, whereas delirium is caused by disorders that lead to increased levels of circulating catecholamines, such as intoxication with stimulant drugs (e.g., phencyclidine, amphetamines), high fever, and withdrawal from alcohol or sedative drugs (e.g., benzodiazepines, barbiturates).
   b. **Drowsiness** is characterized by ready arousal, ability to respond verbally, and fending-off movements induced by verbal stimuli.
   c. **Stupor** is characterized by incomplete arousal to painful stimuli. There is no or little response to verbal commands. No verbal response or moaning is elicited. The motor responses are still of the purposeful, fending-off type.

   d. **Light coma** is characterized by primitive and disorganized motor responses to painful stimuli. There is no response to attempts at arousal.
   e. **Deep coma** is characterized by absence of response to even the most painful stimuli.
   f. When there is a question of **psychogenic unresponsiveness,** try to obtain a forced conscious response, for example, by letting the patient's hand fall toward the face. Do not apply noxious stimuli to eyes, testicles, breasts, or other sensitive areas.
3. **Respiration.** The respiratory pattern is helpful in localizing and, in certain instances, determining the nature of the process.
   a. **Cheyne-Stokes respiration** is characterized by periods of hyperventilation that gradually diminish to apnea of variable duration; breathing then resumes and gradually builds up again to hyperventilation. Cheyne-Stokes breathing indicates bilateral deep hemispheric and basal ganglionic dysfunction. The upper brainstem also may be involved.
      Note: Cheyne-Stokes respiration is most commonly observed in nonneurologic conditions, such as congestive heart failure.
   b. **Central neurogenic hyperventilation** refers to continuous rapid, regular, and deep respirations at a rate of about 25/minute. It has no segmental localizing significance. Regularity is an unfavorable prognostic sign, since increasing regularity correlates with increasing depth of coma.
      Systemic acidosis (e.g., diabetic ketoacidosis, lactic acidosis) and hypoxemia should be excluded (two partial pressure of oxygen [PO_2] determinations over 70 mm Hg in 24 hours is considered adequate for this purpose) before it is concluded that hyperventilation is of neurogenic origin.
   c. **Apneustic breathing** consists of a prolonged inspiratory phase followed by apnea (the inspiratory cramp). It may be followed by **cluster breathing,** which consists of closely grouped respirations followed by apnea. Either pattern implies pontine damage.
   d. **Ataxic breathing** and **gasping breathing** (Biot's respirations) imply damage to the medullary respiratory centers. In ataxic breathing, respirations are chaotic. Gasping breathing is characterized by gasps followed by apnea of variable duration. Both are agonal events and usually precede respiratory arrest.
   e. **Depressed breathing** consists of shallow, slow, and ineffective breathing caused by medullary depression, usually produced by drugs.
   f. **Coma with hyperventilation** is seen frequently in metabolic disorders.
      (1) **Metabolic acidosis** (e.g., diabetic ketoacidosis, uremia, ingestion of organic acids, lactic acidosis).
      (2) **Respiratory alkalosis** (e.g., hepatic encephalopathy, salicylate poisoning).
4. **Position of the head and eyes.** The normal cerebral hemisphere tends to move both head and eyes conjugately toward the opposite side. In hemispheric lesions, the healthy hemisphere becomes unopposed, deviating the head and eyes toward the lesion and away from the hemiparesis. The reverse occurs in pontine lesions, in which the eyes deviate toward the hemiparesis and away from the lesion.
5. **Visual fields and funduscopy**
   a. In patients who are not completely unresponsive, visual fields should be tested with threatening movements, which normally evoke a blink. Asymmetry of the blink response suggests hemianopia (in the absence of blindness or optic nerve damage). Air movement in the eyes can produce a false-positive response.
   b. Funduscopy may reveal papilledema suggestive of increased intracranial pressure. A **subhyaloid hemorrhage** — a rounded, well-defined clot on the retinal surface — is commonly associated with ruptured aneurysms.
6. **Pupils.** Note size, roundness, and equality to light reaction, both directly and consensually.
   a. **Midposition (3–5 mm) nonreactive pupils** are evidence of midbrain damage.
   b. **Reactive pupils** indicate midbrain intactness. In the presence of unresponsiveness and absent extraocular movements and corneal reflexes, reactive

pupils suggest metabolic abnormality (e.g., hypoglycemia) or drug ingestion (e.g., barbiturate).

c. **A unilaterally dilated and unreactive pupil** in a comatose patient (Hutchinson's pupil) may be a sign of third-nerve compression due to temporal lobe herniation. Other components of third-nerve dysfunction (e.g., drooping of the eyelid and abduction of the eye as the result of unopposed action of the lateral rectus muscle) may be concomitant with or follow pupillary dilatation. Less frequently, direct or compressive midbrain damage is expressed by a dilated, nonreactive pupil.

Note: A fixed and/or dilated pupil in an alert patient is *not* a sign of brain herniation. This finding may be due to essential anisocoria, old injury to the iris, migraine, a posterior communicating artery aneurysm, Adie's syndrome, or a mydriatic agent that was inadvertently or purposefully instilled in the eye. One or two drops of 1% pilocarpine (a parasympathetic agonist) instilled into the eye will result in miosis in patients in whom the oculomotor nerve is compressed (e.g., aneurysm) but will fail to do so if parasympathetic receptors in the iris are occupied by a mydriatic drug (e.g., scopolamine).

d. **Small but reactive pupils** signify pontine damage, as in infarction or hemorrhage. Opiates and pilocarpine also produce pinpoint reactive pupils. A magnifying glass may be necessary to appreciate the pupillary reaction.

e. **Dilatation** of the pupils in response to a painful stimulus in the neck (the normal ciliospinal reflex) indicates lower brainstem integrity.

7. **Extraocular movements (EOMs).** If the patient is responsive enough to follow commands, saccadic and pursuit eye movements should be tested. A large number of ocular and gaze palsies may be present. In unresponsive patients, a great deal of information may be obtained by testing the vestibuloocular reflex (VOR), which is mediated by pathways that traverse the brainstem from the vestibular nuclei in the medulla to the oculomotor nuclei in the midbrain. **The most useful tests of the VOR** are as follows:

a. **Doll's-head maneuver, passive head turning** or **oculocephalic reflex (do not perform this maneuver when there is a question of cervical spine injury),** is performed by turning the patient's head with quick lateral and vertical displacements. In unconscious patients, **the reflex is normal or preserved** if the eyes move in the orbits in the direction opposite to the rotating head, maintaining their position in relation to the environment. **Abnormal response** (no movement of the eyes in the orbits, or asymmetry of movements) is suggestive of a destructive lesion at the pontine-midbrain level. Barbiturate poisoning also may abolish the reflex. In conscious (or partially conscious) patients, the VOR is suppressed (or partially suppressed). In this circumstance, the integrity of the pathways mediating the VOR may be tested by asking the patient to look at a fixed visual stimulus while the head is turned passively by the examiner.

b. **Ice water calorics** are reflex eye movements in response to irrigation of the tympanic membrane with cold water. The ice water calorics test the integrity of the VOR.

(1) **Position the head** 30 degrees with respect to the horizontal. Make certain that the external auditory canal is not occluded with cerumen and that the tympanic membrane is intact. **Instill** 30 ml of ice water into the external auditory canal of one ear, and observe the eyes. Repeat the procedure in the opposite ear after 3–5 minutes.

(2) The **normal response in a conscious patient** is nystagmus, which consists of tonic deviation of the eyes toward the ice water infusion (slow phase), followed by a quick corrective movement toward the opposite side (fast phase). The **slow phase** of the nystagmus is mediated by brainstem pathways extending from the vestibular nuclei in the medulla to the oculomotor nuclei in the midbrain. The **fast phase** is a corrective movement generated from the frontal lobe contralateral to the direction of the fast phase. It requires integrity of the frontal cortex, the descending

frontopontine fibers, and the brainstem eye movement pathways extending from the medulla to the midbrain. The fast phase can be present only when a slow phase occurs. Thus, the VOR is extremely useful in evaluating comatose patients, since it provides information about both brainstem function (the slow phase of the nystagmus) and cerebral hemisphere function (the fast phase of the nystagmus). Several responses are possible in performing the VOR test on a comatose patient.

    (a) Slow phases may be defective in one or both directions (fast phases, of course, will be absent as well), suggesting brainstem failure as a cause of the coma.

    (b) Slow phases will be normal bilaterally, but no fast phases are noted in either direction; this suggests bilateral cerebral hemisphere dysfunction as the cause of the coma.

    (c) Slow and fast phases are normal bilaterally (i.e., a normal response). This finding exonerates both the cerebral hemispheres and brainstem and suggests that the unresponsive state is not true coma but a conversion reaction (i.e., "hysterical" coma).

  (3) An abnormal VOR helps to **localize** the abnormality causing the coma. The **nature** of the abnormality may be structural or functional. This distinction requires historical data or other tests to clarify.

8. Motor responses may be spontaneous, induced, or reflexive.

  a. Spontaneous

    (1) Seizures may be focal, in which case they have some localizing value. Generalized seizures do not help in localizing the lesion but are a somewhat favorable sign, since they indicate some degree of integrity of the motor system from its origin in the frontal cortex to its termination in the muscle. Multifocal seizures are suggestive of a metabolic process.

    (2) Myoclonic jerks also point to metabolic encephalopathies (e.g., hypoxia, hepatic failure uremia). **Asterixis** has the same significance.

    (3) Absence of movements on one side of the body, or asymmetry of movements, suggests hemiparesis.

  b. Induced movements (e.g., fending-off or other complex, purposeful movements, such as scratching the nose in response to tickling of the nostril) require integrity of the corresponding corticospinal tract. Poorly organized, incomplete movements, especially when unilateral, suggests corticospinal tract dysfunction or damage.

  c. Reflex movements are always elicited by a stimulus and have a certain time relationship between stimulus and response.

    (1) Decerebrate movements consist of extension, adduction, and internal rotation of the arms and extension of the legs. The lesion is in the upper brainstem, between the red nucleus and the vestibular nuclei.

    (2) Decorticate movements consist of flexion and adduction of the arms and extension of the legs. The lesion is deep hemispheric or just above the midbrain.

    (3) Abduction of a limb usually indicates relative intactness of the motor system. Such a limb usually will regain full function if the underlying cause of the coma can be managed successfully.

9. Sensory system. In drowsy or obtunded patients, the response to pain may be asymmetric, evidencing a hemisensory defect in the absence of paralysis. Facial and corneal sensation should be tested, since they also may be asymmetric.

IV. Pseudocoma states

  A. Psychogenic unresponsiveness. The patient appears unresponsive but is physiologically awake. The neurologic examination is otherwise normal, and there may be active opposition to attempts at eye opening by the examiner. With ice water calorics, there will be slow and quick components of nystagmus. The EEG is normal or may show only drowsiness.

  B. In **the locked-in syndrome,** a destructive process (usually basilar artery occlusion with brainstem infarction) interrupts the descending corticobulbar and corticospinal tracts, sparing only the fibers controlling blinking and vertical eye movements. The patient is able to communicate by means of blinks or vertical eye movements but otherwise is completely paralyzed.

C. Severe bilateral prefrontal lobe disease may produce profound apathy **(abulia),** which may be severe enough to result in a state of akinetic mutism. Such patients appear awake but are mute and either fail to respond to stimuli or respond only after very long delays.

D. Nonconvulsive status epilepticus simulating coma is extremely rare. Usually there are some telltale signs of seizure activity such as rhythmic blinking of the eyelids or conjugate jerking of the eyes. Nearly all such patients are known epileptics. If this diagnosis is considered, a small test dose of intravenous benzodiazepine (e.g., lorazepam, 1–4 mg) should result in improvement. The EEG is diagnostic of continuous seizure activity, and the definitive therapy is usually valproic acid or benzodiazepines.

V. Etiology. Causes of impaired consciousness are multiple, many of which are not primarily neurologic. Consequently, a detailed history derived from all available sources, thorough physical and neurologic examinations, and extensive laboratory screening often are needed. Causes of impaired consciousness can be categorized as follows:

A. Coma due to primary brain injury or disease is usually associated with a demonstrable structural lesion.
   1. Trauma
      a. Concussion.
      b. Contusion.
      c. Laceration or traumatic intracerebral hemorrhage.
      d. Subdural hematoma.
      e. Epidural hematoma.
   2. Vascular disease
      a. Intracerebral hemorrhage
         (1) Hypertensive (putaminal, thalamic, pontine, cerebellar, or lobar).
         (2) Ruptured aneurysm with intraparenchymatous hematoma.
         (3) Arteriovenous malformation.
         (4) Miscellaneous (e.g., bleeding disorders, intratumoral hemorrhages, congophilic angiopathy).
      b. Subarachnoid hemorrhage
         (1) Ruptured aneurysm.
         (2) Arteriovenous malformation.
         (3) Secondary to trauma (e.g., contusion, laceration).
      c. Infarct
         (1) Thrombosis of intracranial and extracranial vessels.
         (2) Embolism.
         (3) Vasculitis.
         (4) Malaria.
   3. Infections
      a. Meningitis.
      b. Encephalitis.
      c. Abscess.
   4. Neoplasms
      a. Primary intracranial.
      b. Metastatic.
      c. Nonmetastatic complications of malignancy (e.g., progressive multifocal leukoencephalopathy).
   5. Seizures (status epilepticus).
B. Coma due to systemic causes (affecting the brain secondarily)
   1. Metabolic encephalopathies
      a. Hypoglycemia.
      b. Diabetic ketoacidosis.
      c. Hyperglycemic nonketotic hyperosmolar states.
      d. Uremia.

      e. Hepatic encephalopathy.

      f. Hyponatremia.

      g. Myxedema.

      h. Hypercalcemia and hypocalcemia.

  2. Hypoxic encephalopathies

      a. Severe congestive heart failure.

      b. Chronic obstructive pulmonary disease with decompensation.

      c. Hypertensive encephalopathy.

  3. Toxicity

      a. Heavy metals.

      b. Carbon monoxide.

      c. Drugs (e.g., opiates, barbiturates, cocaine).

      d. Alcohol.

  4. Physical causes

      a. Heat stroke.

      b. Hypothermia.

  5. Deficiency states (e.g., Wernicke's encephalopathy).

VI. Laboratory screening

  A. Routine. CBC, urinalysis, electrolytes, BUN, creatinine, blood sugar, calcium, phosphate, liver function studies, enzymes, osmolality, ECG, and chest x ray.

  B. Toxic screen should be obtained, when clinically indicated, in blood, urine, and gastric aspirate, and should include screening for opiates, barbiturates, sedatives, antidepressants, cocaine, and alcohol.

  C. Special studies

    1. Skull x rays.

    2. CT scan (see sec. **VI.C.6**).

    3. MRI (see sec. **VI.C.6**).

    4. EEG.

    5. Angiography.

    6. Lumbar puncture should be done if there is suspicion of intracranial infection (e.g., meningitis, encephalitis). Keep in mind the possibility of temporal lobe or cerebellar herniation in patients with increased intracranial pressure. The advent of CT scanning and MRI has made it possible to diagnose intracranial hemorrhage without resorting to lumbar puncture in the majority of patients. When the hemorrhage is small enough to escape undetected by CT scanning or MRI, lumbar puncture is safe and will determine whether angiography is needed.

VII. Management

  A. Immediate therapeutic measures are initiated promptly in all comatose patients to forestall further neurologic damage.

    1. Establish a good airway. Intubation and artificial ventilation may be necessary. Do not manipulate the head and neck until it is known for certain that there was no neck trauma. Nasotracheal intubation is preferred over the orotracheal method for this reason.

    2. Insert a large-bore IV catheter.

    3. Draw blood for routine studies and toxic screen if indicated (see sec. **VI**).

    4. In possible **Wernicke's encephalopathy,** give **thiamine** (100 mg IV) to prevent acute deficiency due to the administration of dextrose.

    5. Give 25–50 ml of **50%** dextrose in water **(D/W)** IV.

    6. If there is some evidence that coma results from **opiate overdose,** give **naloxone,** 0.4 mg IV q5–10min, until consciousness returns. In patients with opiate addiction, this might provoke an acute withdrawal state requiring narcotic therapy. The duration of action of naloxone is shorter than that of methadone, so repeat doses may be necessary.

  B. Management of the specific processes (e.g., trauma, infections, tumor) is covered in the corresponding chapters.

  C. Nursing care of the comatose patient is crucial in management. Fastidious nursing care is essential to prevent the multiple complications of the unresponsive state.

    1. Circulation. Give **fluids** to maintain blood pressure at sufficient levels to ensure adequate cerebral, myocardial, and renal perfusion. In the initial stages, at least, **cardiac monitoring** is useful.

2. **Ventilation. Adequate oxygenation** and **prevention of infection, aspiration,** and **hypercapnia** are the goals.

   a. Remove dentures.

   b. Insert and tape a short oropharyngeal airway of a size adequate to prevent the tongue from obstructing airflow.

   c. Prevent aspiration by suction of secretions.

      (1) Suction the nasopharynx and mouth frequently.

      (2) Place the patient in the lateral decubitus position, with the neck slightly extended and the face turned toward the mattress. If there are no contraindications (e.g., raised intracranial pressure), Trendelenburg's position is helpful for drainage of tracheobronchial secretions.

   d. If ventilation is unsatisfactory or secretions are uncontrollable, insert a cuffed endotracheal tube. If intubation is necessary for longer than 3 days, consider tracheostomy.

   e. Insert a nasogastric tube and evacuate gastric contents to improve ventilation and prevent aspiration.

   f. Obtain arterial blood gases as often as necessary to make sure ventilation is adequate.

3. **Skin.** Turn the patient q1–2h. Keep sheets tightly drawn. Pad bony prominences to prevent formation of sores.

4. **Nutrition** should be provided initially by IV solutions. Later, when the situation is stable, tube feedings are started. Vitamin supplements are used.

5. **Bowel care.** Diarrhea may result from the tube feedings, antacids given concomitantly with steroids, and fecal impaction. Frequent rectal examinations for impaction are necessary.

6. **Bladder care**

   a. A condom catheter may be used for male patients. Penile maceration should be avoided.

   b. If an indwelling catheter becomes necessary, a three-way catheter should be used, with continuous irrigation with 0.25% acetic acid. This acidifies the urine and prevents stone formation.

   c. Clamp the catheter intermittently to maintain bladder tone. Release q3–4h.

7. **Eyes.** Avert corneal injury by taping the eyelids closed or by using methylcellulose eye drops, two drops in each eye bid or tid.

8. **Restlessness and agitation.** In the recovery phase of many metabolic processes, head trauma, and drug intoxications, agitation and restlessness may occur. Avoid unnecessary sedation. If heavy sedation becomes necessary due to excessive severity or duration of agitation, a short-acting benzodiazepine (e.g., lorazepam, 1–2 mg q12h) may be indicated. A potent neuroleptic (e.g., haloperidol, 1–5 mg IM q12h) may also be used.

D. **Management of cerebral edema and increased intracranial pressure.** A number of processes (e.g., trauma, hemorrhage, large infarcts, tumors) may result in cerebral edema and a consequent rise in intracranial pressure. When focal masses are present, increased intracranial pressure may lead to herniation of brain from one compartment to another (e.g., temporal lobe [uncal] herniation from the supratentorial to infratentorial compartment, across the rigid dural tentorium cerebelli). When the increased pressure is generalized, systemic blood pressure rises reflexively as if in an effort to maintain cerebral perfusion pressures at adequate levels. If the baroreceptor reflex arc is intact, this systemic hypertension will result in a reflex bradycardia. The combination of hypertension and bradycardia (Cushing's reflex) is a sign of critically increased intracranial pressure. When intracranial pressure rises beyond the ability of systemic blood pressure to compensate, cerebral perfusion pressures fall, leading to global cerebral ischemic anoxia.

In many patients, neurologic deterioration is caused by increased intracranial pressure, which may be reversible. Treatment of increased intracranial pressure may be lifesaving until definitive therapy aimed at correcting the specific pathologic process can be carried out.

1. **General measures** are important in managing patients with increased intracranial pressure. Patients should be placed in bed with the head elevated 45 degrees and in the midline. Stimulation by family and staff (e.g., turning the head, suctioning) should be kept to a minimum.
2. **Avoid hypotonic IV solutions** or fluids that contain large amounts of free water (e.g., 5% D/W). **Restrict fluids** to 1000 ml of normal saline/sq m body surface area/day, and monitor blood pressure, serum osmolality, and urine output. In children, initially restrict fluids to one-half to one-third of maintenance, using 0.20–0.45% saline in 5% D/W.
3. **Hyperventilation** produces hypocapnia and respiratory alkalosis, decreasing cerebral blood flow and effectively reducing intracranial pressure. Its effects are immediate. The partial pressure of carbon dioxide (PCO_2) should be lowered to 25 mm Hg.
4. **Hyperosmolar agents.** Mannitol 20% may be given in a dose of 1.0 g/kg IV over 10–30 minutes, according to the severity of the situation. The usual dose for a normal adult is 500 ml of the 20% solution or 100 g of mannitol. A dose of 25 g may be repeated q4h. In children, 0.25–1.00 g/kg may be given over 10–30 minutes and repeated q4h as necessary. The effect starts within minutes and lasts several hours. An indwelling bladder catheter is necessary. Monitor vital signs, electrolytes, BUN, and osmolality frequently, aiming for a serum osmolality of 300–320 mOsm/liter.
5. **Steroids.** Dexamethasone (Decadron) may be administered, 10 mg, by rapid IV infusion followed by 4–6 mg IV q6h. In infants and children, the initial dose of dexamethasone is 0.15 mg/kg, followed by 0.25 mg/kg/day, divided into 4 doses. The effect begins in 4–6 hours and peaks at 24 hours. The effect of steroids is greater on vasogenic cerebral edema (e.g., that associated with brain tumors) than on cytotoxic cerebral edema (e.g., that associated with anoxia). Occasionally, much higher doses (e.g., up to 100 mg of dexamethasone) will provide additional benefit. Steroids are rarely, if ever, used when stroke or head trauma is the cause for the increased intracranial pressure, but are quite useful to treat brain tumor–related edema or acute disseminated encephalomyelopathy.
6. **Barbiturate coma.** When other methods of controlling increased intracranial pressure fail and when adequately experienced personnel and facilities are available, intravenous barbiturates may be used to control increased intracranial pressure. Although there is no definite evidence that this technique reduces the morbidity and mortality of coma from any cause, there is some indication that it may be useful in some situations (e.g., severe Reye's syndrome — see Chap. 14, sec. **I.E.5.d**). When barbiturates are used, the following guidelines should be followed:
   a. The patient should be placed in a neurologic or neurosurgical intensive care unit or in an intensive care unit with personnel experienced in the techniques of intracranial pressure monitoring.
   b. An intracranial pressure monitoring device should be placed by a neurosurgeon or experienced critical care physician. The specific device varies from center to center, but a subarachnoid bolt, intraventricular catheter, or Camino catheter frequently is used.
   c. An arterial monitoring line is placed.
   d. The mean cerebral perfusion pressure ($\overline{CPP}$) is calculated using the following formula:

$$\overline{CPP} \text{ (mm Hg)} = \text{mean arterial pressure (mm Hg)}$$
$$- \text{ mean intracranial pressure (mm Hg)}$$

$$\left[\begin{array}{l} \text{Mean intracranial pressure (mm Hg)} \\ \qquad = \dfrac{\text{mean intracranial pressure (cm } H_2O)}{1.3} \end{array} \right.$$

   e. The goal of therapy is to maintain a $\overline{CPP}$ of greater than 50 mm Hg.
   f. If the conventional methods as listed in sec. **VII.D.1–5** have failed, pentobarbital, 3–5 mg/kg, is administered by rapid IV infusion.

g. Pentobarbital, 1–2 mg/kg/hr, is administered, aiming for
   (1) Pentobarbital serum level of 2–4 mg/dl.
   (2) CPP greater than 50 mm Hg.
   (3) Mean arterial blood pressure of 60–90 mm Hg.
7. **Surgery.** When all else has failed, large bifrontal craniectomies have been performed to decompress the intracranial contents under conditions of massively increased and medically unresponsive intracranial pressures. Such procedures may be lifesaving, but patients in this dire circumstance are nearly all left with severe permanent neurologic disability.
E. **Seizures** should be vigorously treated (see Chap. 6 for details).
F. **Subsequent management** depends on the nature of the underlying disorder. The strategies of diagnosis and management are parallel and are based on the basic pathophysiologic principles outlined in sec. **II**. A decision-tree protocol for the management of the comatose patient is summarized in Fig. 1-1, which emphasizes the interaction between diagnostic maneuvers aimed at determining the site and nature of the underlying disorder and the selection of therapy.

VIII. **Persistent coma.** Patients who are chronically unresponsive with preserved brainstem function are said to be in a persistent vegetative state (see also Chap. 7, sec. **II**). In a general hospital, many patients are chronically comatose secondary to hypoxic-ischemic encephalopathy (e.g., after cardiac arrest), and it is important to be able to prognosticate about the likelihood of a favorable outcome. Figure 1-2 summarizes the results of a large cooperative study of such patients, showing that simple bedside tests (e.g., eye movements, motor responses) can be used to predict statistically the ultimate outcome. It should be emphasized that this study applies to patients with nontraumatic, non–drug-induced and non–degenerative disease–induced coma. In other words, only patients known to be comatose from a hypoxic-ischemic insult can be analyzed using the data summarized in Fig. 1-2.

IX. **Sleep disorders**
A. **Physiology of sleep.**
   1. There are two types of normal sleep. Non-rapid eye movement (Non-REM) sleep is characterized by four levels, defined by EEG patterns, corresponding roughly to the depth of sleep (I being the lightest; IV, the deepest). During non-REM sleep, body tone is maintained, and the person shifts postures frequently. The other variety, REM sleep, is characterized by total loss of tone in all muscles except the extraocular muscles and some muscles of the nasopharynx. An electromyograph (EMG) placed on these muscles will document this fact.
   2. The EEG taken during REM sleep shows light sleep, which can be distinguished from stage I non-REM sleep only by placing EMG and electronystagmograph (ENG) leads over the extraocular muscles to document the characteristic rapid conjugate movement of the eyes.
   3. Normally, when a person goes to sleep, he or she passes through at least one cycle of non-REM sleep (I through IV) before entering REM sleep. The relation between REM and non-REM portions of sleep changes with age. In infants, a large proportion of time is spent in REM sleep, but this decreases with age; in adults, only about 20% of the night is spent in REM sleep. It is during this portion that dreaming is thought to occur.
   4. It is believed that control of the relation between the waking state with REM and non-REM sleep is mediated in part by the reticular activating system in the brainstem.
B. **Categories of sleep disorders.** There are a large number of sleep disorders, which have been traditionally divided into four major categories: disorders of initiating and maintaining sleep (DOIMS) or insomnias, disorders of excessive somnolence (DOES) or hypersomnias, disorders of the sleep-wake schedule, and dysfunction associated with sleep, sleep stages, or partial arousal (parasomnias). This classification was revised in 1990, as the International Classification of Sleep Disorders (ICSD) and is based on pathophysiologic mechanisms rather than presentive symptoms.
   1. **Dyssomnias**
      a. **Intrinsic sleep disorders**
         (1) Psychophysiologic insomnia.

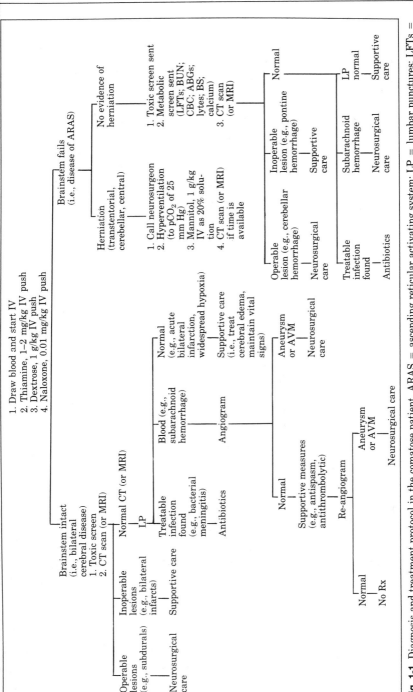

Fig. 1-1. Diagnosis and treatment protocol in the comatose patient. ARAS = ascending reticular activating system; LP = lumbar punctures; LFTs = liver function tests; ABGs = arterial blood gases; BS = blood sugar; AVM = arteriovenous malformation.

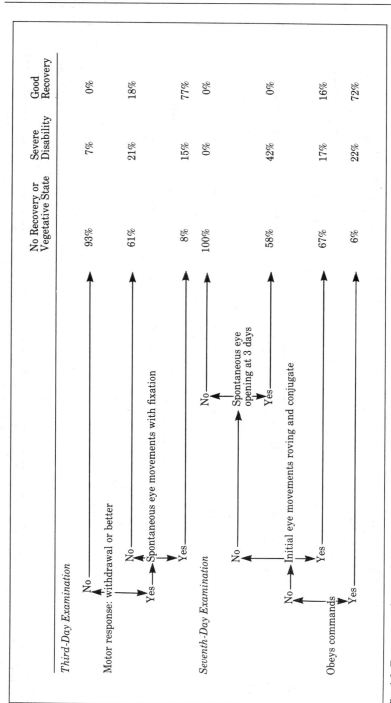

Fig. 1-2. Features predictive of neurologic recovery in hypoxic-ischemic coma patients in accordance with their best functional state within the first year. Residual anesthetics, anticonvulsants, or metabolic derangements may be confounding. (Modified from D. E. Levy et al., Predicting outcome from hypoxic-ischemic coma. *J.A.M.A.* 253:1420, 1985.)

      (2) Sleep state misperception.
      (3) Idiopathic insomnia.
      (4) Narcolepsy.
      (5) Recurrent hypersomnia.
      (6) Idiopathic hypersomnia.
      (7) Posttraumatic hypersomnia.
      (8) Obstructive sleep apnea syndrome.
      (9) Central sleep apnea syndrome.
   (10) Central alveolar hypoventilation syndrome.
   (11) Periodic limb movement disorder.
   (12) Restless legs syndrome.
   (13) Intrinsic sleep disorder not otherwise specified (NOS).
  b. Extrinsic sleep disorders
      (1) Inadequate sleep hygiene.
      (2) Environmental sleep disorder.
      (3) Altitude insomnia.
      (4) Adjustment sleep disorder.
      (5) Insufficient sleep syndrome.
      (6) Limit-setting sleep disorder.
      (7) Sleep-onset association disorder.
      (8) Food allergy insomnia.
      (9) Nocturnal eating (drinking) syndrome.
   (10) Hypnotic-dependent sleep disorder.
   (11) Stimulant-dependent sleep disorder.
   (12) Alcohol-dependent sleep disorder.
   (13) Toxin-induced sleep disorder.
   (14) Extrinsic sleep disorder NOS.
  c. Circadian rhythm sleep disorders
      (1) Time zone change (jet lag) syndrome.
      (2) Shift work sleep disorder.
      (3) Irregular sleep-wake pattern.
      (4) Delayed sleep phase syndrome.
      (5) Advanced sleep phase syndrome.
      (6) Non–24-hour sleep-wake disorder.
      (7) Circadian rhythm sleep disorder NOS.
2. Parasomnias
  a. Arousal disorders
      (1) Confusional arousals.
      (2) Sleepwalking.
      (3) Sleep terrors.
  b. Sleep-wake transition disorders
      (1) Rhythmic movement disorder.
      (2) Sleep starts.
      (3) Sleep talking.
      (4) Nocturnal leg cramps.
  c. Parasomnias usually associated with REM sleep
      (1) Nightmares.
      (2) Sleep paralysis.
      (3) Impaired sleep-related penile erections.
      (4) Sleep-related painful erections.
      (5) REM sleep-related sinus arrest.
      (6) REM sleep behavior disorder.
  d. Other parasomnias
      (1) Sleep bruxism.
      (2) Sleep enuresis.
      (3) Sleep-related abnormal swallowing syndrome.
      (4) Nocturnal paroxysmal dystonia.
      (5) Sudden unexplained nocturnal death syndrome.
      (6) Primary snoring.

(7) Infant sleep apnea.
(8) Congenital central hypoventilation syndrome.
(9) Sudden infant death syndrome.
(10) Benign neonatal sleep myoclonus.
(11) Other parasomnia NOS.
3. Sleep disorders associated with medical/psychiatric disorders
  a. Associated with mental disorders
    (1) Psychoses.
    (2) Mood disorders.
    (3) Anxiety disorders.
    (4) Panic disorders.
    (5) Alcoholism.
  b. Associated with neurologic disorders.
    (1) Cerebral degenerative disorders.
    (2) Dementia.
    (3) Parkinsonism.
    (4) Fatal familial insomnia.
    (5) Sleep-related epilepsy.
    (6) Electrical status epilepticus of sleep.
    (7) Sleep-related headaches.
  c. Associated with other medical disorders
    (1) Sleeping sickness.
    (2) Nocturnal cardiac ischemia.
    (3) Chronic obstructive pulmonary disease.
    (4) Sleep-related asthma.
    (5) Sleep-related gastroesophageal reflux.
    (6) Peptic ulcer disease.
    (7) Fibrositis syndrome.
4. Proposed sleep disorders
  a. Short sleeper.
  b. Long sleeper.
  c. Subwakefulness syndrome.
  d. Fragmentary myoclonus.
  e. Sleep hyperhidrosis.
  f. Menstrual-associated sleep disorder.
  g. Pregnancy-associated sleep disorder.
  h. Terrifying hypnagogic hallucinations.
  i. Sleep-related neurogenic tachypnea.
  j. Sleep-related laryngospasm.
  k. Sleep choking syndrome.
C. Treatment of the most common sleep disorders
  1. Sleep apnea syndromes
    a. Obstructive
      (1) Weight loss.
      (2) Tracheostomy.
      (3) Surgical correction of anatomically narrowed airway (e.g., adenoid removal, tonsillectomy).
    b. Central
      (1) Theophylline or caffeine.
      (2) Progesterone.
      (3) Electrical pacing of the diaphragm.
  2. Narcolepsy (see Chap. 6, sec. **X.A** for details of treatment)
    a. Sleep attacks and excessive daytime sleepiness
      (1) Methylphenidate.
      (2) Pemoline.
      (3) Amphetamines.
      (4) Caffeine.
    b. Cataplexy
      (1) Tricyclic antidepressants (especially clomipramine and protriptyline).

  (2) Monoamine oxidase inhibitors.
  c. Sleep paralysis usually responds to stimulants.
  d. Hypnagogic hallucinations usually respond to stimulants.
3. Depression
  a. Psychotherapy.
  b. Antidepressant drugs.
4. Periodic movements of sleep and restless legs syndrome
  a. Benzodiazepines (diazepam, lorazepam, clonazepam).
  b. Anticonvulsants.
  c. L-Dopa–carbidopa.
  d. Bromocriptine.
5. Drug and alcohol dependency
  a. Psychotherapy.
  b. Behavior modification.

Selected Readings

Anch, A., Browman, C. P., and Mitler, M. M. *Sleep: A Scientific Perspective*. Englewood Cliffs, NJ: Prentice Hall, 1988.

Bates, D. The management of medical coma. *J. Neurol. Neurosurg. Psychiatry* 56:589, 1993.

Diagnostic Classification Steering Committee. ICSD—International Classification of Sleep Disorders: Diagnostic and Coding Manual. Rochester, MN: American Sleep Disorders Association, 1990.

Easton, J. D. Coma and Related Disorders. In J. H. Stein (ed.), *Internal Medicine* (4th ed.). St. Louis: Mosby, 1993. Pp. 1014–1020.

Fisher, C. M. The neurological evaluation of the comatose patient. *Acta Neurol. Scand.* [*Suppl. 36*] 1:56, 1969.

Fishman, R. A. Brain edema. *N. Engl. J. Med.* 293:706, 1975.

Levy, D. E., et al. Predicting outcome from hypoxic-ischemic coma. *J.A.M.A.* 253:1420, 1985.

Matheson, J. K. Sleep and Its Disorders. In J. H. Stein (ed.), *Internal Medicine* (4th ed.). St. Louis: Mosby, 1993. Pp. 1003–1014.

Plum, F., and Posner, J. B. *Diagnosis of Stupor and Coma* (3rd ed.). Philadelphia: Davis, 1980.

Ropper, A. H. (ed.). *Neurological and Neurosurgical Intensive Care* (3rd ed.). New York: Raven, 1993.

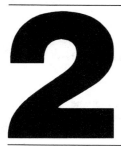

Headache

Daniel B. Hier

Headache is one of the most frequent complaints heard in the offices of internists and neurologists. Most people accept that an occasional headache is normal. Patients come to physicians because of unusual headache severity or frequency. Patients seek medical attention for headaches that have changed in character, become more severe, or become more frequent. A few patients seek attention for headaches that are of explosive onset or relentless progression. Most chronic or recurrent headaches are either migraine headaches, cluster headaches, or psychogenic headaches. Acute severe headaches carry a more ominous prognosis and may reflect serious underlying disease.

I. **Evaluation of the patient with headache**
   A. **History.** A careful history provides both the data necessary for correct diagnosis and the therapeutic rapport necessary for successful treatment of most headaches. **Special inquiry** should be made into the quality of the head pain, its frequency, its duration, its location, and any associated symptoms (Table 2-1). The family's history of headache and the patient's psychosocial history also are essential to the evaluation.
   B. **Physical examination.** Each patient with a complaint of headache should undergo careful neurologic and general physical examination. Occasionally the examination will yield clues as to the etiology of the headache (Table 2-2), but generally it will serve to reassure both patient and physician that nothing serious is causing the pain.
   C. **Ancillary tests**
      1. Any headache patient in whom **neurologic examination discloses an abnormality** should undergo further studies.
      2. When the **neurologic examination is normal,** no further studies are indicated **except** when
         a. An element of the history suggests a specific diagnosis (e.g., epilepsy or brain tumor).
         b. The headaches have developed a new quality, are more severe, or have become intractable to treatment.
         c. The headaches are atypical (e.g., trigeminal neuralgia in a patient under age 30).

II. **Migraine headache**
   A. **Description.** Migraine is a recurrent, throbbing headache. Although the headache is usually unilateral, opposite sides of the head may be affected during different attacks. In children, the headache is often bifrontal rather than unilateral. People with migraine have a greater than expected prevalence of infantile colic, motion sickness, and episodic abdominal pains in childhood.
      1. In **classic migraine,** a visual aura precedes the throbbing headache by 10–20 minutes. Commonly, this prodrome consists of scintillations, migrating scotomata, or waviness and blurriness of vision. The prodrome is followed by a unilateral throbbing headache that intensifies over 1–6 hours. The headache usually abates in 6–24 hours but occasionally lasts longer. Vomiting, nausea, photophobia (light sensitivity), phonophobia (sound sensitivity), irritability, and malaise are common.

      Most patients experience their first migraine headache between the ages of 10 and 30 years, although about 25% will recall childhood vomiting attacks or

Table 2-1. Important features of the pain in the evaluation of chronic recurrent headaches

Headache	Quality	Location	Duration	Frequency	Associated symptoms
Common migraine	Throbbing	Unilateral head or bilateral head	6–48 hours	Sporadic (often several times monthly)	Nausea, vomiting, malaise, photophobia
Classic migraine	Throbbing	Unilateral head	3–12 hours	Sporadic (often several times monthly)	Visual prodrome, vomiting, nausea, malaise, photophobia
Cluster	Boring, sharp	Unilateral head (especially orbit)	15–120 minutes	Closely bunched clusters with long remissions	Ipsilateral tearing, facial flushing, nasal stuffiness, Horner's syndrome
Psychogenic	Dull, pressure	Diffuse, bilateral	Often unremitting	May be constant	Depression, anxiety
Trigeminal neuralgia	Lancinating	Fifth nerve distribution	Brief (15–60 seconds)	Many times daily	Identifiable trigger zone
Atypical facial pain	Dull	Unilateral or bilateral face	Often unremitting	May be constant	Often depression, occasionally psychosis
Lower-half headache	Dull or throbbing	Unilateral face	6–48 hours	Sporadic	Nausea, vomiting
Sinus headache	Dull or sharp	Unilateral or bilateral over sinuses	Variable	Sporadic or constant	Nasal discharge

Table 2-2. Important physical findings in the evaluation of headache

Physical finding	Possible etiology
Optic atrophy, papilledema	Mass lesion, hydrocephalus, benign intracranial hypertension
Focal neurologic abnormality (hemiparesis, aphasia)	Mass lesion
Stiff neck	Subarachnoid hemorrhage, meningitis, cervical arthritis
Retinal hemorrhages	Ruptured aneurysm, malignant hypertension
Cranial bruit	Arteriovenous malformation
Thickened, tender temporal arteries	Temporal arteritis
Trigger point for pain	Trigeminal neuralgia
Lid ptosis, third nerve palsy, dilated pupil	Cerebral aneurysm

motion sickness. About 60–75% of patients are women. In women, migraine headaches commonly occur premenstrually.

2. **Migraine variants**
   a. In **common migraine,** the characteristic throbbing headache occurs without the visual prodrome of classic migraine. Common migraine usually has a slightly longer course than classic migraine.
   b. In **migraine associée,** the headache is accompanied by a transient neurologic deficit. Examples of migraine associée are ophthalmoplegic migraine, hemiplegic migraine, and migraine with aphasia. The neurologic deficit usually precedes the headache but may follow it or even occur in the absence of headache **(migraine dissociée).**
   c. Rarely, these neurologic deficits persist, suggesting that cerebral infarction has occurred **(complicated migraine).** In these patients, vasoconstrictors (e.g., ergotamine) should be used with caution or not at all, because of the danger of exacerbating cerebral infarction.
   d. **"Lower-half"** headaches are unilateral facial pains affecting the nose, palate, cheek, and ear. These pains, believed to represent attacks of atypical migraine, may be associated with nausea and vomiting. Lower-half headaches also may respond to treatment with ergotamine, beta blockers, or tricyclic antidepressants.
   e. Occasionally attacks of migraine may last days without remission. Some attacks are associated with severe continuing pain as well as persistent nausea and vomiting complicated by dehydration. This unremitting form of migraine has been termed **status migrainosus.** Status migrainosus may require treatment with intravenous hydration and either sumatriptan or dihydroergotamine. Sometimes a course of intravenous or oral corticosteroids is required to halt an attack of status migrainosus.
   f. Some patients with migraine develop a syndrome of nearly continuous headaches known as **chronic daily headaches.** Chronic daily headaches are duller and less well localized than acute migraine headaches; nausea and vomiting are often absent. In some migraine headache patients, chronic daily headaches simply reflect the natural history of the disorder; in others, chronic daily headaches signal overuse of sedative medication, narcotics, barbiturates, or ergotamines. In patients overusing these drugs, chronic daily headaches are best treated by carefully supervised drug withdrawal.

B. **Treatment of migraine**
   1. **General measures**
      a. In many patients, **inciting factors** can be identified and partially controlled. Some patients report an increase in the frequency and severity of their

migraine attacks in relation to smoking, alcohol ingestion, lack of sleep, stress, fatigue, or the ingestion of certain foods, especially chocolate and tyramine-containing cheeses. Vasodilators (e.g., nitroglycerin, dipyridamole) may elicit migraine headaches in some individuals.

b. **Anxiety** and **depression** should be treated with appropriate psychotherapy and medication.

c. In about one-third of women with migraine who are taking **oral contraceptives,** the incidence of headaches is increased. Discontinuation of oral contraceptives in these women for a trial period may be worthwhile. On the other hand, some women with migraine who start on oral contraceptives experience improvement in their headaches.

d. **Cerebral arteriography** is usually contraindicated during an attack of migraine, since vasospasm and cerebral infarction have been reported to occur as rare complications during acute attacks. The incidence of migraine in patients with either saccular aneurysms or arteriovenous malformations is not much higher than in the general population, so migraine alone is not an indication for neuroradiologic procedures. However, when migraine is accompanied by permanent neurologic deficits, seizures, or a history suggestive of subarachnoid hemorrhage, neuroimaging and sometimes cerebral arteriography are warranted.

2. **Abortive therapy** should be initiated as early as possible. The patient with classic migraine can begin therapy at the onset of the prodrome, while the patient with common migraine must await the onset of headache. Some authorities recommend awaiting the onset of headache in either case, since some migrainous prodromes will not be followed by headache.

Both **ergotamine** and **isometheptene** have proved superior to placebo in aborting migraine attacks. Placebo alone ameliorates the course of about one-third of migraine attacks.

a. **Ergotamine** may be administered alone or in combination with antiemetics, analgesics, or sedatives. Many preparations contain caffeine (Cafergot, Wigraine), which also is capable of producing cerebral vasoconstriction and is known to potentiate the action of ergotamine. When the oral route is unsatisfactory because of nausea or vomiting, ergotamine may be administered rectally, sublingually, or by inhalation (Table 2-3).

Ergotamine preparations are contraindicated in the presence of peripheral artery or coronary artery disease, hepatic or renal disease, hypertension, or pregnancy (Table 2-4). Side effects of ergotamine include nausea, vomiting, and cramps. Rare cases of ergotism with mental changes and gangrene have been reported even at therapeutic dosages.

The usual oral dosage is 1 mg at onset, followed by 1 mg q30min, to a maximum of 5 mg/attack or 10 mg/wk (see Table 2-3).

b. **Isometheptene** either alone (Octin) or in combination with other agents (Midrin) is somewhat less effective than ergotamine but has fewer contraindications and adverse reactions (see Table 2-4). The usual dosage is two capsules at onset, followed by one capsule each hour, to a maximum of five per attack, or until the headache is relieved (see Table 2-3).

c. **Dihydroergotamine (DHE)** is available for parenteral administration (SC, IM, or IV). To abort acute migraine headaches, it is recommended to administer 1.0 mg of DHE IV over 2–3 minutes preceded by 5 mg of prochlorperazine to reduce nausea. If the headache does not subside within 30 minutes, another 0.5 mg of DHE is given IV. Side effects include diarrhea, leg cramps, and abdominal discomfort. Rare instances of coronary artery spasm and peripheral arterial spasm have been reported. Idiosyncratic hypersensitivity reactions may occur. DHE should be administered by individuals familiar with its use.

d. **Sumatriptan** (Imitrex) is an effective agent in aborting migraine headaches. It is given subcutaneously by an autoinjector. Sumatriptan has been shown to be effective in ending migraine headaches regardless of whether it is given at the onset of migraine or later in the attack. Sumatriptan is also effective in relieving the nausea associated with migraine. The usual dose is 6 mg SC,

Table 2-3. Drugs useful in the abortive therapy of migraine headaches

Drug	Dosage
Dihydroergotamine (DHE)	1 mg IV at onset preceded by 5 mg IV of prochlorperazine
Ergotamine, 1-mg (Gynergen) tablets	1 tablet PO immediately; repeat q30min to maximum of 5 mg/attack or 10 mg/wk
Ergotamine, 1-mg/caffeine, 100 mg (Cafergot) tablets	1 or 2 tablets PO immediately; repeat to maximum of 5/attack or 10/wk
Ergotamine, 1-mg/belladonna, 0.1-mg/caffeine, 100-mg/phenacetin, 130-mg (Wigraine) tablets	1 tablet PO immediately; repeat q30min to maximum of 5/attack or 10/wk
Ergotamine, 2 mg sublingual (Ergomar)	1 tablet SL; repeat in 30 min if necessary, to maximum of 3 tablets/d
Ergotamine/caffeine (Cafergot) suppositories	1 suppository immediately; repeat in 1 hr if necessary
Ergotamine/caffeine/phenacetin/belladonna (Wigraine) suppositories	1 suppository immediately; repeat in 1 hr if necessary
Ergotamine inhaler (Medihaler Ergotamine)	1 inhalation immediately; repeat in 5 min if necessary, to maximum of 6 inhalations/d
Isometheptene, 130 mg (Octin)	1 tablet immediately, then 1 qh to maximum of 5/d or 10/wk
Isometheptene, 65-mg/acetaminophen, 325-mg/dichloralphenazone, 100-mg (Midrin) capsules	2 capsules immediately, then 1 qh to maximum of 5/d as needed or 10/wk
Sumatriptan (Imitrex)	6 mg SC at onset; may repeat in 1 hr if necessary; not to exceed 2 mg/d

which may be repeated in 1 hour if necessary (not to exceed 12 mg in any 24-hour period). Side effects are usually mild and include local skin reactions, flushing, heat, tingling, and neck pain. Chest discomfort of uncertain origin occurs in 3–5% of patients. Sumatriptan is contraindicated in patients with angina, coronary artery disease, hypertension, or concomitant use of ergotamines or other vasoconstrictors.

3. **Preventive therapy** should be considered only in patients with frequent or disabling attacks of migraine that have failed to respond to abortive therapy (Table 2-5). Preventive therapy for migraine is contraindicated during pregnancy or in women attempting to become pregnant.

   Classes of drugs useful in prevention of migraine include beta blockers, tricyclic antidepressants, antiserotonin drugs, and nonsteroidal anti-inflammatory drugs. Limited evidence supports the use of chronic therapy with anticonvulsants, ergotamines, or calcium channel blockers for migraine prevention. In general, preventive therapy should be initiated with either a **beta blocker** or a **tricyclic antidepressant**.

   a. **Beta blockers** are often effective in preventing migraine headaches.
      (1) The most experience has been with **propranolol** (Inderal), but other beta blockers such as nadolol (Corgard), 40–240 mg/day, and atenolol (Tenormin), 50–200 mg/day, are probably equally effective in migraine prophylaxis. Their mechanism of action in migraine is unknown. The usual effective dosage of propranolol is between 80 and 160 mg in divided doses. A **time-released** form (Inderal LA) makes once-a-day dosing possible. Propranolol should not be used in patients with asthma or congestive heart failure.

Table 2-4. Adverse reactions and contraindications for drugs used in treatment of headache

Drug	Indications	Adverse reactions	Contraindications*
Ergotamine preparations (Cafergot, Wigraine, Gynergen, Ergomar)	Migraine	Nausea; vomiting; angina; numbness and tingling; cramps	Renal and hepatic failure; coronary artery and peripheral vascular disease; pregnancy; hypertension
Methysergide (Sansert)	Migraine, cluster	Retroperitoneal, valvular, and pulmonary fibrosis; vasoconstriction; nausea; vomiting; drowsiness; neutropenia	Pregnancy; fibrotic and collagen diseases; renal, valvular, pulmonary, and hepatic disease; hypertension; coronary artery and peripheral vascular disease
Isometheptene preparations (Midrin, Octin)	Migraine	Dizziness	Glaucoma; severe cardiac, renal, or hepatic disease
Tricyclic antidepressants (Elavil, Tofranil)	Psychogenic, migraine	Dry mouth; tremor; urinary retention; glaucoma; arrhythmias; agitation	Coronary artery disease; MAO inhibitors
Propranolol (Inderal)	Migraine, cluster	Bronchospasm; heart failure; bradycardia; hypotension; drowsiness; depression	Heart failure; asthma; bradycardia; MAO inhibitors
Cyproheptadine (Periactin)	Cluster, migraine	Drowsiness; dry mouth	MAO inhibitors; glaucoma
Carbamazepine (Tegretol)	Trigeminal neuralgia	Bone marrow depression; hepatic dysfunction; ataxia; drowsiness; nausea; vomiting	MAO inhibitors; bone marrow depression; hepatic disease
Phenytoin (Dilantin)	Trigeminal neuralgia, migraine	Gingivitis; rash; ataxia; macrocytic anemia	
Verapamil (Calan)	Migraine, cluster	Headache, fatigue; hypotension; constipation; heart block	Heart failure, sick sinus; heart block
Sumatriptan (Imitrex)	Migraine	Skin reaction, dizziness, chest discomfort	Hypertension, angina, coronary artery disease, use of ergotamines

Key: MAO = monoamine oxidase.
* All drugs cited are contraindicated in the presence of allergy or hypersensitivity.

Table 2-5. Drugs useful in the preventive therapy of migraine

Drug	Dosage
Methysergide (Sansert)	4–8 mg/d in divided doses (do not continue drug for longer than 6 mo at a time)
Ergotamine (Gynergen)	1 mg bid, not to exceed 10 mg/wk (2 days/wk must be skipped)
Ergotamine/belladonna/phenobarbital (Bellergal)	2–4 tablets/d
Propranolol (Inderal)	10–40 mg qid
Cyproheptadine (Periactin)	2–4 mg qid
Amitriptyline (Elavil)	50–75 mg/d in divided doses
Phenytoin (Dilantin)	200–400 mg/d
Verapamil (Calan)	80 mg tid or qid
Valproate (Depakote)	250–500 mg bid or tid
Atenolol (Tenormin)	25–100 mg qd

(2) If the patient is already under treatment for hypertension, it is often useful to substitute a beta blocker for one of the patient's antihypertensive drugs. Excessive drowsiness and depression occur in some patients on beta blockers. These side effects may be less with some of the more selective beta blockers such as nadolol or atenolol.
b. Tricyclic antidepressants have been shown to be effective in migraine prophylaxis.
  (1) Amitriptyline (Elavil) or **imipramine** (Tofranil), 50–75 mg in divided doses or at bedtime, provides effective migraine prophylaxis for some patients.
  (2) Other tricyclic antidepressants are probably equally effective, and some have fewer side effects. Their action against migraine appears to be independent of their antidepressant action. Nervousness, tremor, and anticholinergic side effects can be troublesome in certain patients.
c. Anti-inflammatory drugs are sometimes of benefit in preventing migraine. Some patients may benefit from the daily use of **aspirin. Indomethacin** (Indocin), 25 mg tid, or **ibuprofen** (Motrin), 400 mg tid, may be effective migraine prophylaxis in some patients. Other nonsteroidal anti-inflammatory drugs appear to have comparable efficacy.
d. Chronic use of **ergotamines** often leads to undesirable side effects. **Ergotamine** (Gynergen) in a dosage of 1 mg bid will sometimes abolish recurrent attacks of migraine. No more than 10 mg should be given weekly. Rarely, prolonged usage of ergotamine leads to ischemic complications. **Bellergal** (ergotamine, 0.3 mg/belladonna, 0.1 mg/phenobarbital, 20 mg combination), two to four tablets daily, is of benefit to some patients.
e. Anti-serotonin drugs have long been used for migraine prophylaxis.
  (1) Methysergide (Sansert). About three-fourths of patients respond favorably to methysergide (4–8 mg daily in divided doses). Although this drug has been implicated as a rare cause of retroperitoneal, cardiac valvular, and pulmonary fibrosis, in most patients the fibrosis is reversible if the drug is discontinued. Methysergide should be prescribed with utmost caution. Its use is contraindicated during pregnancy or in the presence of cardiac valvular, collagen vascular, coronary artery, peripheral vascular, pulmonary, or fibrotic disease. No patient should be continued on the drug for longer than 6 months at a time, and patients should be monitored for the appearance of azotemia, dyspnea, or cardiac murmurs. A 1-month "vacation" from the drug for every 6 months of use is usually adequate to avert serious complications.

(2) **Cyproheptadine** (Periactin), 8–16 mg daily in divided doses, is an antihistamine that, like methysergide, has antiserotonin properties; fibrotic complications have not been reported. This drug lacks the effectiveness of methysergide. Drowsiness, especially at higher dosages, is bothersome to some patients.

f. **Anticonvulsants**

(1) **Phenytoin** (Dilantin). Some patients with migraine benefit from phenytoin (200–400 mg daily). Certain of these patients probably have headaches as seizure equivalents. The existence of "migrainous epilepsy" as a distinct entity is controversial, and this drug should not be considered as a standard treatment for migraine. However, phenytoin (5 mg/kg/day) seems to be of benefit in children with migraine.

(2) **Valproic acid** (Depakote). Valproic acid (250–500 mg PO bid) has been shown to reduce migraine headache frequency in one controlled study. Its mechanism of action is unknown.

g. **Calcium channel blockers** are sometimes used as second-line prophylaxis for migraine when beta blockers or tricyclics are ineffective. **Verapamil** (Isoptin, Calan), 80 mg tid or qid, may be tried. This drug is contraindicated in sick sinus syndrome, second- or third-degree heart block, and congestive heart failure. Side effects include edema, hypotension, fatigue, dizziness, headache, constipation, and atrioventricular heart block.

4. **Symptomatic therapy**

a. Many patients obtain adequate relief of **occasional migraine headaches** with aspirin or acetaminophen. Some patients get better relief when a small amount of barbiturate is added (e.g., Fiorinal, Esgic). Propoxyphene (Darvon) may be useful when aspirin is poorly tolerated.

b. **Severe headaches** should be treated with codeine, 30–60 mg, or morphine, 4–8 mg, q3–4h.

c. **Nausea and vomiting** may be produced by the headache itself, by ergotamine, or by narcotics. Vomiting can be controlled with promethazine (Phenergan), 25–50 mg, or prochlorperazine (Compazine), 5–10 mg.

d. Allowing the patient to sleep by administering a hypnotic, such as flurazepam (Dalmane), 15–60 mg, is generally an effective way of ending the migraine.

e. Extensive use of drugs that contain barbiturates, caffeine, and opiates should be avoided, since these drugs may themselves lead to withdrawal headaches.

III. **Cluster headache**

A. **Description.** Cluster headache (histamine cephalalgia, Horton's headache) is a periodic, paroxysmal headache disorder. Excruciating unilateral head pain (often localized to the orbit) occurs in brief episodes (15 minutes to 2 hours) without prodrome. The headaches are distributed into clusters, occurring daily for 3 weeks to 3 months, then remitting entirely for months or years. The pain is sharp, boring, and piercing and unaccompanied by either nausea or vomiting. Headaches are most common late at night or early in the morning. This is one of the few headaches that awaken patients from their sleep. Some patients experience facial flushing, Horner's syndrome, nasal stuffiness, or eye tearing ipsilateral to the headache. Men are affected 5 times as frequently as women, and most patients have their first attack between the ages of 20 and 40. Exacerbation of the headaches due to alcohol consumption is common. The mechanism underlying cluster headache is not well understood but is believed to be vascular.

B. **Treatment**

1. **Ergotamine.** The lack of aura and the short duration of cluster headaches make abortive therapy of these headaches difficult. Occasionally, a patient can successfully end a cluster headache by promptly taking an ergotamine preparation (e.g., Cafergot, Ergomar). Other patients may improve with ergotamine prophylaxis during an attack of cluster headaches (Gynergen), 1 mg bid or 2 mg at bedtime.

2. **Methysergide.** About 50–80% of patients improve substantially with methysergide (4–8 mg daily in divided doses). Caution must be exercised in the use of this drug (see Table 2-4), but a bout of cluster headaches is self-limited, and it is rarely necessary to continue the drug for longer than 3 months.

3. **Cyproheptadine.** If methysergide is contraindicated, poorly tolerated, or ineffective, cyproheptadine (8–16 mg daily in divided doses) is sometimes of benefit.
4. **Propranolol.** Uncontrolled studies indicate that propranolol (40–160 mg daily in divided doses) is effective in certain patients.
5. **Prednisone.** Some authors recommend a short course of prednisone (20–40 mg daily, followed by a gradual tapering) for refractory cases of cluster headaches.
6. **Lithium carbonate,** 300 mg tid or qid, has been suggested as treatment when methysergide is ineffective or poorly tolerated. Serum levels should be kept below 1.2 mg/dl to avert toxic effects.
7. **Oxygen inhalation** at a flow rate of 7 liters/min for 10 minutes, is said to abort about 80% of cluster headaches.
8. **Indomethacin** (Indocin) in a dosage of 25–50 mg tid may be effective for some cluster headaches.
9. **Histamine desensitization** is of historic interest but rarely indicated.
10. **Narcotics.** Symptomatic relief of cluster headaches may require narcotic agents (e.g., codeine, 30–60 mg q3–4h).
11. **Calcium channel blockers** such as verapamil (80 mg PO tid) may benefit some patients with cluster headaches.
12. **Intravenous DHE** may abort cluster headaches in some patients.
13. **Lidocaine.** Intranasal instillation of 1 ml of 4% topical lidocaine may abort cluster headaches in some patients.

IV. **Psychogenic headaches**
   A. **Description**
   1. The term *psychogenic headache* encompasses several entities, including **tension headache, muscle contraction headache,** and the headaches of **anxiety** and **depression.** The individual with sporadic headaches that are relieved by aspirin or acetaminophen, or with occasional neck and scalp muscle tightness that is relieved by massage, rarely consults a physician. In contrast, most patients with psychogenic headaches who seek medical attention have had daily or unremitting headaches for months or years that are not relieved by simple analgesics or even narcotics (unlike the headaches of intracranial masses).
   2. In our experience, the great majority of these patients are depressed; **signs of depression,** including tearfulness, hopelessness, insomnia, anorexia, and an inability to enjoy life, are often prominent.
   3. These patients describe ill-defined, diffuse aching or pressure sensation. The **pain** may be occipital, temporal, or frontal in distribution, but it is almost invariably bilateral. The unilateral throbbing pain characteristic of migraine is uncommon.
   B. **Treatment**
   1. **General measures**
      a. Initiation of **therapeutic rapport** between physician and patient is very often the first step toward improvement. Some patients respond positively to the physician's forceful reassurance that nothing is physically wrong inside their brain or head, thus dispelling fears of brain tumor or other intracranial disease.
      b. An assessment should be made as to whether **anxiety** or **depression** is present. Some patients accept the suggestion that their headaches are related to depression and welcome a therapeutic program directed against it, while other patients will be uncomfortable with this diagnosis, even though it is indicated. For the latter, emphasis is better left on treating the headache. Depression and anxiety sometimes can be controlled by examination and modification of the life events contributing to these emotions. When the depression is severe, refractory to treatment, or complicated by threats of suicide, the patient should be referred to a psychiatrist.
   2. **Tricyclic antidepressants.** Aspirin or acetaminophen may be of value for some patients with psychogenic headaches, but when depression is prominent the use of analgesics is usually futile, and sedating tranquilizers may deepen the depression. Several controlled studies have shown tricyclic antidepressants to be superior to analgesics or minor tranquilizers in the treatment of these headaches. A variety of polycyclic antidepressants are now available (see Chap. 9). These

drugs differ somewhat in their sedative and anticholinergic properties. When administered in a single bedtime dose, their sedating effects may help to correct the sleep disturbance of certain depressed patients.

3. **Benzodiazepines.** In the smaller group of patients in whom muscle contraction and anxiety predominate, treatment with **diazepam** (Valium), 5–30 mg daily, **chlordiazepoxide** (Librium), 10–75 mg daily, or **oxazepam** (Serax), 30–90 mg daily, in conjunction with aspirin or acetaminophen, is useful. **Alprazolam** (Xanax) is a benzodiazepine drug that appears to have both antianxiety and antidepressant actions. The usual dosage is 0.25–0.50 mg tid.

4. **Relaxation techniques.** The value of hypnosis, biofeedback, meditation, and other relaxation techniques in the treatment of psychogenic headaches has not been established.

V. **Trigeminal neuralgia**

A. **Description.** Trigeminal neuralgia (tic douloureux) is characterized by brief, lancinating paroxysms of pain (lasting for seconds or minutes) in the distribution of the fifth cranial nerve. The third and second divisions of the trigeminal nerve are affected more frequently than the first, and **trigger points** can often be found on the face. Attacks occur spontaneously or during toothbrushing, shaving, chewing, yawning, or swallowing.

In over 90% of patients with trigeminal neuralgia, onset occurs after age 40, and women are affected somewhat more frequently than men. In most patients, no etiology for trigeminal neuralgia can be found. When it is associated with **hypesthesia** in the distribution of the fifth cranial nerve, with **other cranial nerve palsies,** or with **onset before the age of 40,** so-called symptomatic, or atypical, trigeminal neuralgia should be suspected. Further investigation may reveal multiple sclerosis, a trigeminal nerve tumor, or other posterior fossa tumor.

B. **Treatment**

1. **Phenytoin.** Many patients get relief from phenytoin alone (200–400 mg daily).

2. **Carbamazepine** (Tegretol). About 80% of patients with trigeminal neuralgia respond to initial treatment with carbamazepine (400–1200 mg daily). Response to carbamazepine is helpful in differentiating trigeminal neuralgia from certain cases of atypical facial pain (see sec. **VI.A**). Both phenytoin and carbamazepine can produce troublesome ataxia (especially when used concurrently). Rare complications of carbamazepine are leukopenia, thrombocytopenia, and liver function abnormalities, so its use requires periodic monitoring of WBC count, platelet count, and liver function. After initial improvement, many patients develop **recurrent pain** despite adequate blood levels of one or both of these drugs.

3. **Baclofen** (Lioresal) may provide relief in some patients. Baclofen may be given alone or in combination with either **phenytoin** or **carbamazepine.** The usual initial dosage is 5–10 mg tid, with gradual increases as needed, up to 20 mg qid.

4. Anecdotal reports suggest that **clonazepam** (Klonopin) 0.5–1.0 mg PO tid may be effective in some patients with trigeminal neuralgia.

5. **Surgery.** Three surgical procedures are commonly used in the treatment of trigeminal neuralgia:

   a. **Radiofrequency selective thermal rhizotomy** of the trigeminal ganglion or rootlets can be performed percutaneously with local anesthesia in conjunction with short-acting barbiturates. Selective destruction of pain fibers with relative sparing of tactile-related fibers minimizes the possibility of corneal anesthesia with subsequent abrasions and the possibility of anesthesia dolorosa. However, some patients find the numbness unpleasant, and procedures for first-division pain carry a higher incidence of corneal problems. Other methods for destruction of pain fibers in the trigeminal nerve include **cryosurgery** and **balloon inflation** in Meckel's cave.

   b. **Glycerol injection into the trigeminal cistern** (Meckel's cave) can be done percutaneously. This may produce pain relief with minimal sensory loss on the face.

   c. For many patients, particularly those who are younger, **suboccipital craniectomy** with **microsurgical repositioning of a blood vessel** cross-compressing the trigeminal nerve at the root entry zone offers a relatively safe alternative without sensory loss.

VI. Atypical facial pain

A. Description. Atypical facial pain must be distinguished from trigeminal neuralgia and lower-half headaches. Commonly it is seen in young or middle-aged patients as a unilateral, boring, or aching facial pain that lacks both the paroxysmal quality and the well-defined anatomic distribution characteristic of trigeminal neuralgia. The etiology of atypical facial pain is unknown.

B. Treatment. Patients are unimproved by either phenytoin or carbamazepine. Surgical procedures on the trigeminal nerve are not indicated, since they do not relieve the pain and may produce analgesia algera. Most patients should have a trial at antidepressant therapy. Encouraging results have been reported with the tricyclic antidepressants. When the pain has a delusional quality, a major tranquilizer may be of benefit. Many cases prove difficult to treat.

VII. Temporal arteritis (giant-cell arteritis)

A. Description. Temporal arteritis, a systemic illness of elderly patients, is characterized by inflammatory infiltrates of lymphocytes and giant cells in cranial arteries. It manifests itself variously in temporal headache, visual loss, or generalized malaise. **When visual loss is present, it should be considered a medical emergency.** It is estimated that only about one-half of patients complain of headache or have tender temporal arteries, although nearly all patients have some systemic symptoms, including low-grade fever, weight loss, anorexia, or weakness. The erythrocyte sedimentation rate (ESR) is elevated in all patients, usually between 60 and 120 mm/hour. Onset before age 50 is uncommon. **Jaw claudication** is a useful diagnostic clue to the presence of temporal arteritis. Visual loss occurs in 10–40% of untreated patients.

The relationship of temporal arteritis to **polymyalgia rheumatica** is controversial. There appears to be considerable overlap between the two illnesses, and some patients with polymyalgia rheumatica exhibit giant-cell arteritis on temporal artery biopsy.

B. Diagnosis

1. The diagnosis should be confirmed by **temporal artery biopsy,** since this procedure can be performed easily under local anesthesia, even in debilitated patients. Rarely, the biopsy will be normal in the presence of active arteritis because of patchy involvement of the temporal artery.

2. Angiography often will confirm the presence of arteritis in equivocal cases.

C. Treatment

1. High-dose **corticosteroids** should be initiated immediately to avert visual loss. When the diagnosis is suspected, initiation of therapy should not await the pathology report of the temporal artery biopsy. **Prednisone** (60 mg daily) will abolish systemic symptoms and normalize the ESR within 4 weeks in most patients. The dosage can then be gradually reduced to 5–10 mg daily over a period of several months.

2. A rise in ESR or a **recrudescence of systemic symptoms** sometimes necessitates a temporary increase in corticosteroid dosage.

3. Temporal arteritis is **self-limited,** and corticosteroids can usually be discontinued within 6 months to 2 years.

4. Patients must be observed for **complications** of high-dose corticosteroid therapy, including psychosis, osteoporosis, vertebral body collapse, and gastrointestinal hemorrhage.

VIII. Postconcussion syndrome

A. Description. Following cerebral concussion, patients may complain of decreased concentration, vague headaches, dizziness, fatigue, and photophobia. The forcefulness of these complaints does not correlate with either the severity of the concussion or any objective finding, except that the complaint of **dizziness** is sometimes correlated with the finding of **nystagmus.** The postconcussion syndrome usually remits spontaneously, but it occasionally follows a protracted course over a period of years (especially if litigation is pending). The **etiology** of this syndrome is largely psychogenic; fear that cerebral damage has been suffered plays a role in some cases.

However, CT scan of the brain may reveal unsuspected brain lesions in a small minority of patients with postconcussion syndrome.

B. **Treatment**
   1. **Anxiety** should be allayed with repeated assurances that nothing is amiss. Benzodiazepine tranquilizers may be given if necessary.
   2. **Depressive symptoms** may require short-term psychotherapy or a brief course of antidepressants.
   3. The management of **dizziness** is discussed in Chap. 4.
   4. Some cerebral concussion patients describe **headaches** that are migrainous in nature and that respond to migraine headache therapy. Propranolol, 20–40 mg qid, may be especially effective in controlling certain throbbing headaches that follow head injury. When litigation is pending, all forms of therapy may prove futile.

IX. **Idiopathic intracranial hypertension (IIH)**
   A. **Description.** Idiopathic intracranial hypertension (also known as **pseudotumor cerebri** or **benign intracranial hypertension)** is a syndrome of increased intracranial pressure without evidence of mass lesion or hydrocephalus. **Headache** and **papilledema** are usually present. Rarely, IIH occurs with headache but not papilledema. About 90% of the patients are both obese and female. Occurrence after age 45 is rare. The **etiology** of most cases is unknown, although vitamin A intoxication, tetracycline use, corticosteroid use or withdrawal, and dural sinus thrombosis occasionally have been implicated. About 5% of the patients experience a **decrease in visual acuity** associated with the papilledema; this loss may be permanent if increased intracranial pressure persists unrelieved. **Localizing neurologic signs** do not occur, although unilateral or bilateral sixth nerve palsies may occasionally produce diplopia.
   B. **Diagnosis**
      1. **Headache** and **papilledema** should always prompt a thorough investigation for mass lesions or hydrocephalus.
      2. The **CT scan** delineates most supratentorial lesions as well as many infratentorial lesions capable of producing papilledema. Special attention should be paid to the patency of the venous sinuses. The ventricles are either diminished in size (slitlike) or normal in configuration. Enlarged ventricles cast great doubt on the diagnosis of IIH and suggest hydrocephalus.
      3. The **MRI scan** is especially useful in detecting **venous sinus occlusions** that can be confused with the syndrome of IIH.
      4. When these preliminary tests are **normal** and localizing signs are absent, **lumbar puncture** can be safely performed in the presence of papilledema. The diagnosis of benign IIH is confirmed by the finding of normal cerebrospinal fluid (CSF) under increased pressure (usually 250–500 mm H_2O). Any abnormality of the CSF (cytology, protein, sugar) should prompt further investigation.
      5. When the CT scan or MRI is **abnormal,** extreme care should be exercised before proceeding to lumbar puncture.
   C. **Treatment**
      1. About one-third of these patients have spontaneous remission after the first lumbar puncture. Most other patients can be successfully managed by repeated lumbar punctures, daily at first, then every third day, weekly, or even monthly, as needed. Sufficient CSF (up to about 30 ml) should be removed at each lumbar puncture to reduce the CSF pressure to less than 180 mm H_2O.
      2. Patients **who do not respond** to repeated lumbar punctures may be tried on **prednisone** (40–60 mg daily) or **dexamethasone** (6–12 mg daily). Response to corticosteroids generally occurs within 1 week. Refractory cases may require repeated lumbar punctures, acetazolamide (250–500 mg tid), or furosemide (40–80 mg daily).
      3. Visual fields and visual acuity need to be monitored carefully in all patients with IIH. When visual loss is progressing despite medical therapy, **surgical therapy** should be considered. Current practice is to perform **optic nerve sheath decompression** for patients with progressive visual loss due to IIH.
      4. Although most cases of benign IIH resolve in 6–12 months, a few cases will require repeated intervention over the course of several years.

X. Other headache syndromes

A. Headache in association with **fever** and **stiff neck** (with or without mental changes) can be due to **encephalitis** or **meningitis** (see Chap. 8).

B. The **violent onset** of headache (with or without loss of consciousness) followed by stiff neck suggests **subarachnoid hemorrhage** (see Chap. 10). The headache is often described in dramatic terms, such as "the worst headache of my life" or "a headache like something snapped in my head." Photophobia and malaise may be present. Funduscopy may reveal preretinal (subhyaloid) hemorrhages. The headache of ruptured saccular aneurysm is generally more severe than that of leaking arteriovenous malformations. A **dull unremitting headache** that persists for days following a subarachnoid hemorrhage is sometimes due to the increased intracranial pressure of **communicating hydrocephalus** (see Chap. 3). The headache may be relieved by lumbar puncture. Occasionally, a shunting procedure is necessary to control the hydrocephalus.

C. Headache occurs with a variety of **intracranial mass lesions** such as subdural hematoma (Chap. 12), brain tumor (Chap. 11), and brain abscess (Chap. 8). The headache of **brain tumors** is usually paroxysmal at first (often worse early in the morning, on arising). Later, the headaches become unremitting and may be complicated by vomiting. The initial side of the headache may reflect the side of the tumor, but this is not a highly reliable sign. Headache is the first symptom of about 80% of posterior fossa tumors and 30% of supratentorial tumors.

D. The headache of **increased intracranial pressure** (Chap. 11) may be intensified by coughing, sneezing, or bending over. **Cough headache** also exists as a benign entity without known intracranial pathology.

E. **Occipital headache** associated with pain on movement of the neck may be due to **cervical arthritis.** Arthritic changes can be confirmed by plain x-ray examinations of the cervical spine. A trial of aspirin in combination with diazepam, 5–30 mg daily, gives relief to some patients. Cervical collars and cervical traction are occasionally of benefit. Nonsteroidal anti-inflammatory drugs (e.g., ibuprofen, 400 mg tid) benefit some patients. Other patients may benefit from the epidural injection of steroids.

When signs of **radiculopathy** (radicular pain in an extremity, weakness, hyporeflexia) or **myelopathy** (hyperreflexia, Babinski's signs, weakness, spasticity) are present, neuroimaging with either CT or MRI may reveal spinal cord or nerve root compression by a spondylitic bar or herniated disk. An electromyogram is useful in cases of suspected radiculopathy. When radiculopathy or myelopathy is present, surgical management is often indicated.

F. The headache that occurs **after lumbar puncture** is exacerbated by standing and relieved by lying down. These headaches appear to be due to persistent leakage of CSF from the subarachnoid space; most can be prevented by use of a small-bore needle (20- or 22-gauge). Post–lumbar puncture headaches usually can be managed by a combination of bed rest, analgesics, and hydration. When conservative measures fail, an epidural patch with autologous blood usually provides relief.

G. Tumors of the **foramen magnum** produce an occipital headache that worsens on recumbency and is relieved by standing.

H. Nasal stuffiness or discharge associated with pain or percussion over the sinuses suggests that the headache may be due to **acute sinusitis.**

I. Headache in association with a red painful eye can be produced by **acute closed-angle glaucoma.** Open-angle glaucoma (which is more common) does not produce headache.

J. There is no correlation between headache and moderate elevations of blood pressure. An occasional patient with **hypertension** has relief from early morning headaches with control of blood pressure, but hypertension should not be considered a common cause of headache.

K. Head pain due to **temporomandibular joint syndrome** is characterized by pain on chewing or jaw use, temporomandibular joint clicking and crepitation, and jaw restriction.

L. Sudden severe headaches that are maximal at their onset **(thunderclap headaches)** may occur in patients known to have migraine headaches. These sudden, severe head pains may occur in certain known contexts (e.g., orgasmic headache, exercise-induced headache) or may appear without obvious precipitants. The ominous diagnosis of subarachnoid hemorrhage should be rigorously excluded using CT, MRI, or lumbar puncture before the more benign diagnosis of thunderclap headache is made. Migraine headache patients may also experience benign brief stabs of cranial pain known as **ice-pick pains.**

Selected Readings

GENERAL

Dalessio, D. J., and Silberstein, S. D. *Wolff's Headache and Other Head Pain* (6th ed.). New York: Oxford University Press, 1993.

Diamond, S. Headache. *Med. Clin. North Am.* 75:521, 1991.

Lance, J. W. *The Mechanism and Management of Headache* (5th ed.). London: Butterworth, 1993.

Raskin, N. H. *Headache* (2nd ed.). New York: Churchill-Livingstone, 1988.

MIGRAINE AND CLUSTER HEADACHES

Cady, R. K., et al. Treatment of acute migraine with subcutaneous sumatriptan. *J.A.M.A.* 265:2831, 1991.

Feniuk, W., et al. Rationale for the use of 5HT-like agonists in the treatment of migraine. *Neurology* 238:s57, 1991.

Greenberg, D. A. Calcium channel antagonists and their treatment of migraine. *Clin. Neuropharmacol.* 9:311, 1986.

Raskin, N. H. Repetitive intravenous dihydroergotamine as therapy for intractable migraine. *Neurology* 36:995, 1986.

Rosen, J. A. Observations on the efficacy of propranolol for the prophylaxis of migraine. *Ann. Neurol.* 13:92, 1983.

Sorensen, K. J. Valproate: A new drug for migraine prophylaxis. *Acta Neurol. Scand.* 78:346, 1988.

Tfelt-Hansen, P., et al. Timolol vs. propranolol vs. placebo in common migraine prophylaxis: A double-blind multicenter trial. *Acta Neurol. Scand.* 69:1, 1984.

Weber, R. B., and Reinmuth, O. M. The treatment of migraine with propranolol. *Neurology* 21:404, 1971.

Welch, K. M. A. The therapeutics of migraine. *Curr. Opinion Neurol. Neurosurg.* 6:264, 1993.

PSYCHOGENIC HEADACHE

Budzynski, T. H., et al. EMG biofeedback and tension headache: A controlled outcome study. *Psychosom. Med.* 35:484, 1973.

Lance, J. W., and Curran, D. A. Treatment of chronic tension headache. *Lancet* 1:1236, 1964.

Loh, L., et al. Acupuncture versus medical treatment of migraine and muscle tension headache. *J. Neurol. Neurosurg. Psychiatry* 47:333, 1984.

Okasha, A., Ghaleb, H. A., and Sadek, A. A double-blind trial for the clinical management of psychogenic headaches. *Br. J. Psychol.* 122:181, 1973.

Weatherhead, A. D. Headache associated with psychiatric disorders: Classification and etiology. *Psychosomatics* 21:832, 1980.

TRIGEMINAL NEURALGIA AND ATYPICAL FACIAL PAIN

Dalessio, D. J. Medical treatment of the major neuralgias. *Semin. Neurol.* 8:286, 1988.

Delaney, J. F. Atypical facial pain as a defense against psychosis. *Am. J. Psychol.* 133:10, 1976.

Fromm, G. H., Terrence, G. F., and Chatta, A. S. Baclofen in the treatment of refractory trigeminal neuralgia. *Neurology* 29:550, 1979.

Hankanson, S. Trigeminal neuralgia treated by injection of glycerol into trigeminal cistern. *Neurosurgery* 9:638, 1981.

Jannetta, P. J. Treatment of trigeminal neuralgia by suboccipital and transtentorial cranial operations. *Clin. Neurosurg.* 24:538, 1977.

Killian, J. M., and Fromm, G. H. Carbamazepine in the treatment of neuralgia. *Arch. Neurol.* 19:129, 1968.

Solomon, S., and Lipton, R. B. Atypical facial pain: A review. *Semin. Neurol.* 8:332, 1988.

Sweet, W. H. Percutaneous methods for the treatment of trigeminal neuralgia and other faciocephalic pain: Comparison with microvascular decompression. *Semin. Neurol.* 8:272, 1988.

Zakrzewska, J. M., and Thomas, D. G. T. Patient assessment of outcome after 3 surgical procedures for the management of trigeminal neuralgia. *Acta Neurochir.* (Wien) 122:225, 1993.

TEMPORAL ARTERITIS

Aiello, P. D., et al. Visual prognosis in giant cell arteritis. *Ophthalmology* 100:550, 1993.

Allison, M. C., and Gallagher, P. J. Temporal artery biopsy and corticosteroid treatment. *Ann. Rheum. Dis.* 43:416, 1984.

Bengtsson, B. A., and Malmvall, B. E. Prognosis in giant cell arteritis including temporal arteritis and polymyalgia rheumatica: A follow-up study on ninety patients treated with corticosteroids. *Acta Med. Scand.* 209:337, 1981.

Buchbinder, R., and Detsky, A. S. Management of suspected giant cell arteritis: A decision analysis. *J. Rheumatol.* 19:1120, 1992.

Chmelewski, W. L. et al. Presenting features and outcomes in patients undergoing temporal artery biopsy: A review of 98 patients. *Arch. Intern. Med.* 152:1690, 1992.

Genereau, T., and Cabane, J. Benefits of corticosteroids in the treatment of temporal arteritis and polymyalgia rheumatica: Advantages and disadvantages—a meta-analysis. *Rev. Med. Interne* 13:387, 1992.

Hunder, G. G., et al. Daily and alternate-day corticosteroid regimens in treatment of giant cell arteritis: Comparison in a prospective study. *Ann. Intern. Med.* 82:613, 1975.

BENIGN INTRACRANIAL HYPERTENSION

Corbett, J. J. Idiopathic Intracranial Hypertension (Pseudotumor Cerebri). In R. T. Johnson and J. W. Griffin (eds.), *Current Therapy in Neurologic Disease* (4th ed.). St. Louis: Mosby–Year Book, 1993.

Corbett, J. J., and Thompson, H. S. The rational management of idiopathic intracranial hypertension. *Arch. Neurol.* 46:1049, 1989.

Corbett, J. J., et al. Visual loss in pseudotumor cerebri: Follow-up of 57 patients from five to 41 years and a profile of 14 patients with permanent severe visual loss. *Arch. Neurol.* 39:461, 1982.

Kilpatrick, C. J., et al. Optic nerve decompression in benign intracranial hypertension. *Clin. Exp. Neurol.* 18:161, 1981.

Johnston P. K., Corbett, J. J., and Maxner, C. E. Cerebrospinal fluid protein and opening pressure in idiopathic intracranial hypertension (pseudotumor cerebri). *Neurology* 41:1040, 1991.

Marcelis, J., and Silberstein, S. D. Idiopathic intracranial hypertension without papilledema. *Arch. Neurol.* 48:392, 1991.

Wall, M., and George, D. Idiopathic intracranial hypertension: A prospective study of 50 patients. *Brain* 114:155, 1991.

OTHER HEADACHE SYNDROMES

Carbatt, P. A. T., and van Crevel, H. Lumbar puncture headache: Controlled study of the preventive effect of 24 hours' bed rest. *Lancet* 2:1133, 1981.

Lidvall, H. F., Linderoth, B., and Norlin, V. Causes of the postconcussional syndrome. *Acta Neurol. Scand.* [*Suppl.*] 56:3, 1974.

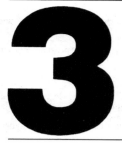

Intellectual Dysfunction: Mental Retardation and Dementia

Raymond J. Fernandez and
Martin A. Samuels

Intelligence refers to the ability to comprehend ideas and their relationships and to reason about them. This extremely complex function consists, in neurologic terms, of multiple capacities, including those for general knowledge, memory, acquisition of new knowledge, attention, comprehension, judgment, abstract thinking, language, understanding of mathematical concepts, orientation, perception, and association.

Mental retardation is defined as subnormal intellectual capacity with associated deficits in at least 2 or 10 areas of adaptive behavior. The 10 areas of adaptive behavior that should be analyzed are communication, self-care, home living skills, social skills, leisure, health and safety, self-direction, functional academics, community use, and work. To determine this, it is necessary to understand better the mentally retarded individual in the framework of his or her environment and how he or she will best function in the home and community. The term implies a static process, the onset of which occurs prenatally or early in life.

Dementia is defined as loss of previously acquired intellectual function. It may be a static or progressive disorder with onset at any age. The term generally excludes acute confusion, delirium, and abnormalities in level of consciousness. Psychiatric illnesses in particular are excluded from the category of dementia (see sec. III). Isolated abnormalities of one cortical function (e.g., isolated aphasias) are not generally considered dementias, despite their ability to produce impairment of intellect.

I. **Measurement of intelligence.** Attempts to quantify intelligence and developmental level have been made using many psychological testing methods, the most common of which are the following:

   A. The **Wechsler Adult Intelligence Scale Revised (WAIS-R)** provides a verbal, nonverbal, and overall intelligence quotient (IQ) and is appropriate for testing people over the age of 16.

   B. The **Wechsler Intelligence Scale for Children Revised (WISC-R)** is designed for testing children of 6–16 years of age; it also yields verbal, nonverbal (performance), and full-scale IQ measurements. A discrepancy between verbal IQ and performance IQ often provides a clue to perceptual handicaps.

   C. The **Stanford-Binet** test (4th edition) is appropriate for people aged 2 years to adulthood and yields mental age (MA) and IQ values. It is heavily weighted toward verbal performance and thus may underestimate the intelligence of children with specific communication disorders or from environments that have not stimulated their verbal capacity.

   D. The **Denver II** measures four areas of behavior: gross motor, fine motor, language, and personal-social and is a screening instrument for developmental assessment in infancy and preschool years. It is not an IQ test.

   E. The **Early Language Milestone Scale (ELM)** and the **Central Linguistic Auditory Milestones Scale (CLAMS)** are easily administered screening instruments that are sensitive indicators of delay in expressive and receptive language up to the age of 3 years.

   F. Individuals with **mental retardation** may then be classified according to their intellectual capacity as mildly, moderately, or profoundly retarded.

      1. **The mildly retarded** (educable) have IQ scores of 55–70. This group constitutes approximately 75% of the retarded population. They may never attain more than third- or fourth-grade educational skills but, after reaching adulthood, should be able to function in the community with some degree of supervision.

2. **The moderately retarded** (trainable) have IQs between 45 and 55. Most are capable of learning self-care skills but will never display significant academic achievement. Individuals in this group may live at home and attend sheltered workshops. Those who do not live at home will require a considerable amount of supervision in a group setting. They compose approximately 20% of the retarded population.

3. **The severely retarded** (IQ 25–45) and **profoundly retarded** (IQ < 25) are totally dependent. Some are bedridden and never achieve any degree of socialization. This group comprises only approximately 5% of the retarded population.

4. While the above classification according to intellectual capacity has been used for many years and is useful in certain situations, more recently it has been proposed that mentally retarded individuals be classified into one of two groups:

   a. Mild mental retardation—IQ 50–70.

   b. Severe mental retardation—IQ below 50.

G. **Limitations of testing.** These tests are of varying reliability; all suffer from poor reproducibility, especially in young subjects, and all fail to correct successfully for the known effects of cultural and educational background, interest, motivation, and effort on intelligence test scores. Furthermore, certain psychiatric disorders—particularly depression and schizophrenia—may lower IQ. Whether this occurs because of actual lowering of intelligence or because of impaired motivation in these conditions is unknown.

Despite these drawbacks, psychological testing is presently the only scientific method of estimating intelligence, and it can be useful in evaluating and following patients with intellectual dysfunction—as long as the limitations of the tests are clearly understood by the physician.

II. **Evaluation of the patient with intellectual dysfunction**

A. **History.** A careful history of the **onset and course of the intellectual dysfunction** is obtained.

1. In **children,** one must attempt to discern whether the problem is one of mental retardation or dementia, since the further evaluation of the patient depends heavily on this distinction.

2. Exact descriptions of the abnormal behavior may help in ascertaining the **cortical distribution** of the dysfunction (i.e., frontal, parietal, temporal, or occipital).

3. The **course of the illness** deserves special consideration, and one should note particularly whether it occurred in steps or gradually; the former onset suggests strokes, and the latter a degenerative process.

4. History of possible **intracranial hemorrhage** strongly suggests **occult hydrocephalus.**

5. **A general medical history** is taken, with particular emphasis placed on the following factors:

   a. Prior gastric surgery (predisposing the patient to vitamin B_{12} deficiency).

   b. Thyroid disease.

   c. Use of drugs or ingestion of toxins, such as bromide-containing drugs.

   d. **Family history** of other neurologic or psychiatric illness.

6. In children, a careful history of the **pregnancy and condition perinatally** is particularly important.

B. **Physical examination**

1. The **general physical examination** is aimed at excluding any medical illness that may underlie the intellectual dysfunction, such as

   a. Uremia.

   b. Liver failure.

   c. Anemia.

   d. Hypertension.

   e. Malignancy.

2. In **children,** the condition underlying the intellectual dysfunction may be obvious on physical examination (e.g., Down's syndrome).

3. The **mental status examination** helps to define the extent and precise type of dysfunction. Functions to be tested include

   a. Attention.
   b. Orientation.
   c. Alertness.
   d. Speech.
   e. Comprehension.
   f. Memory.
   g. Naming.
   h. Repetition.
   i. Reading.
   j. Writing.
   k. Calculations.
   l. Right-left discrimination.
   m. Praxis.
   n. Developmental level in children.
   4. The **neurologic examination** excludes signs of focal brain disease, such as
   a. Hemiparesis.
   b. Primary modality sensory loss.
   c. Hemianopia.
   d. Cranial nerve abnormalities.
   5. In **children,** particular attention is paid to head size and rate of head growth.
   6. In **infants** under 18 months of age, transillumination of the skull is routinely done to detect a fluid-filled structure such as a subdural effusion, porencephalic cyst, or massive hydrocephalus.

III. Conditions with intellectual dysfunction as a major manifestation

A. Degenerative diseases

   1. Alzheimer's disease and **Pick's disease** (presenile dementia and senile dementia of the Alzheimer-type)

   a. Description. Alzheimer's disease is a common cause of dementia. The older concept of presenile (before age 65) and senile (after age 65) dementias now has little clinical relevance, since the **pathology** (i.e., decreasing number of cortical neurons with accumulation of lipofuscin in neurons and the presence of neurofibrillary degeneration of neurons and senile plaques containing the amyloid beta protein; deepening cortical sulci; and increasing ventricular size with progressive decrease in brain weight and amyloid infiltration of small pial vessels [congophilic angiopathy]) and the **clinical course** of Alzheimer's disease are known to be the same in all age groups.

   (1) Symptoms and signs of dysfunction. Since the cortical degeneration is widespread, one might expect nearly every part of the cerebral cortex to show dysfunction. In practice, most patients begin to have difficulty in parietal and temporal lobe function, with memory loss and spatial disorientation. As the disease progresses, signs of frontal lobe dysfunction appear, with loss of social inhibitions and concomitant incontinence and abulia (loss of spontaneity). Aphasia and apraxia are common and may occur at any point in the course of the disease. However, this sequence of events is not always seen, and some patients will have extensive frontal lobe difficulty long before temporal and parietal lobe functions are disturbed. Many patients with Alzheimer's disease show a variety of movement disorders including akinesia, dystonias, and myoclonus; therefore, these findings do not necessarily imply a different diagnosis.

   In a less common degenerative dementia, **Pick's lobar atrophy,** only frontal and temporal pole degeneration is seen. Despite this difference in pathology, there is no reliable method clinically to separate Alzheimer's from Pick's disease. In both Alzheimer's and Pick's diseases, **it is exceedingly rare to see signs of pyramidal tract dysfunction** (i.e., hemiparesis, hyperreflexia, or Babinski's signs) or **loss of primary sensory modalities.** Such findings should raise suspicion that a space-occupying lesion or areas of encephalomalacia account for the dementia.

   (2) Patient behavior and prognosis. Patients with Alzheimer's disease can be extremely difficult to manage. Such patients are commonly incontinent of urine and feces, may wander away from home and be unable to find their way back, may be agitated and confused intermittently (particularly at night), and may use embarrassingly inappropriate language and actions. Early in the course of the illness, depression may be a major problem.

The disease is progressive, inevitably terminating in complete incapacity and death. The course is extremely variable, but most patients die within 4–10 years of the time of diagnosis.

b. Etiology. The cause of Alzheimer's disease is still unknown, but various theories are being investigated and may have important implications for diagnosis and treatment.

(1) Genetic. Approximately 15% of Alzheimer's disease cases are autosomal dominantly inherited, and patients with three copies of chromosome 21 (i.e., Down's syndrome) develop the pathologic changes characteristic of Alzheimer's disease. Genetic linkage analysis has detected DNA markers on the long arm of chromosome 21 that segregate with the familial Alzheimer's disease trait in some families. Some other families have been found to have a disorder localized to other chromosomes. Furthermore, it has been found that the risk for Alzheimer's disease segregates with the gene for isotype 4 of apoprotein E in white people. In the nonwhite population a similar, but weaker, association has been found with isotype 2 of apoprotein E. It is possible, but unproved, that the absence of the normal apoprotein E, isotype 3, may be related to the development of Alzheimer's disease. At the moment, the mechanism of this association is unknown.

(2) Amyoid. A great deal of evidence has accumulated suggesting that the amyloid protein, which is deposited in the center of senile plaques and in cerebral vessels of patients with Alzheimer's disease, may be pathogenetic in some or all cases of Alzheimer's disease. The precursor protein for the amyloid protein is also located on chromosome 21. Strategies aimed at preventing the accumulation of amyloid protein may form the rationale of some future treatment.

(3) Toxins such as aluminum are not considered likely candidates for the cause of Alzheimer's disease.

(4) Prions, which are known to cause some other rare neurodegenerative diseases (e.g., Gerstmann-Straussler, fatal familial insomnia), have *not* been demonstrated to be a cause of Alzheimer's disease.

(5) Viruses have never been consistently found in the brains of patients with Alzheimer's disease, and the disease has not been transmitted to other animals.

(6) Excitotoxins such as glutamate may have some role in the cell death in many neurodegenerative diseases including Alzheimer's disease. Glutamate receptor blockers may have some role in future treatment strategies.

(7) Endogenously produced toxins, analogous to 1-methyl-4-phenyl-1236-tetrahydropyridine (MPTP), a toxic cause of parkinsonism, have not been demonstrated in the brains of patients with Alzheimer's disease, but the use of deprenyl, a monoamine oxidase inhibitor (which works to prevent the toxicity of MPTP), may have a future role in the treatment of Alzheimer's disease.

c. Treatment. There is no specific therapy aimed at reversing or arresting the underlying pathologic changes of Alzheimer's disease. However, several maneuvers are often useful palliatively.

(1) Abulia and inattention

(a) Methylphenidate (Ritalin), 10–60 mg PO daily, divided into two or three doses.

(b) Dextroamphetamine sulfate (Dexedrine), 10–60 mg PO daily, divided into two or three doses.

(2) Depression

(a) Imipramine (Tofranil), 75–300 mg PO, once a day at bedtime.

(b) Amitriptyline (Elavil), 75–300 mg PO, once a day at bedtime.

(c) **Desipramine** (Norpramin), 75–300 mg PO, once a day at bedtime.

(3) Agitation and confusion

(a) Avert periods of **decreased sensory stimulation** by keeping the lights on in the patient's room at night if nighttime confusion and agitation ("sundowning") are a problem.

(b) **Short-acting benzodiazepines** (e.g., lorazepam [Ativan], 1–2 mg PO or IM at bedtime) are often effective in providing behavior control without the long-term dangers of neuroleptic drugs.

(c) **Haloperidol** (Haldol), 1–6 mg PO daily, divided into two or three doses.

(4) Cholinergic therapy with choline or lecithin in doses up to several grams per day has been tried in an attempt to treat the underlying memory disorder. This is based on the observation that cholinergic neuronal systems may be selectively diminished in the brains of patients dying with Alzheimer's disease. There is some evidence that cholinergic therapy is capable of improving memory in selected patients with Alzheimer's disease, but this effect is not dramatic.

(5) Anticholinesterase therapy is based on the observation that blocking the enzyme that normally degrades acetylcholine (i.e., acetycholinesterase) may lead to an increase in cortical acetylcholine, thereby reversing the depletion of acetylcholine that occurs in Alzheimer's disease, presumably due to the degeneration of neurons in the basal forebrain (i.e., the basal nucleus of Meinert and the diagonal band of Broca). The only currently approved anticholinesterase drug is 1,2,3,4-tetrahydro-9-acridinamine monohydrochloride monohydrate (tacrine hydrochloride [Cognex]), which may have a modest beneficial effect on the course of Alzheimer's disease. The drug is hepatotoxic in a large number of patients, so liver function tests must be monitored closely during drug administration. The current recommendation for administration of tacrine, supplied in 10-, 20-, 30-, and 40-mg tablets, is 10 mg PO qid for 6 weeks, monitoring serum ALT (formerly known as SGPT) once per week. If ALT remains equal to or less than 3 times the upper limit of normal, raise the dosage to 80 mg/day for 6 more weeks. If ALT remains equal to or less than 3 times the upper limit of normal, raise the dosage to 120 mg/day for 6 more weeks. If ALT remains equal to or less than 3 times the upper limit of normal, raise the dosage to 160 mg/day. If, at any point during the dosage escalation, the ALT rises to greater than 3 times but equal to or less than 5 times the upper limit of normal, then reduce the dosage by 40 mg/day and resume the dosage titration when the ALT falls to equal or less than 3 times the upper limit of normal. **If, at any point during the dosage escalation, the ALT rises to greater than 5 times the upper limit of normal, then discontinue tacrine treatment immediately.** Patients who develop asymptomatic elevations in the ALT may be rechallenged with tacrine once the level returns to normal, **but patients who develop clinical jaundice confirmed by a significant elevation in total bilirubin (> 3 mg/dl) should permanently discontinue tacrine and not be rechallenged.**

2. Progressive supranuclear palsy (Steele-Richardson-Olszewski syndrome)

a. Description. Progressive supranuclear palsy is a degenerative disease in which there is neurofibrillary and granular degeneration of neurons, chiefly in the nuclear structures of the reticular formation of the midbrain, pretectal regions, substantia nigra, globus pallidus, subthalamic nuclei, and dentate nuclei of the cerebellum. These lesions account for the **clinical picture** of progressive hypertonia, supranuclear ocular palsies (particularly conjugate downward gaze), and disturbances of wakefulness. The dementia found in progressive supranuclear palsy tends to be characterized by slowness and abulia (the so-called subcortial dementia) rather than the multiple cognitive deficits as seen in Alzheimer's disease.

b. Treatment. There is no specific treatment for the dementia or the movement disorder. Idazoxan, a selective alpha-2 presynaptic inhibitor, has been shown to have a modest beneficial effect on some aspects of motor function in this disease, but the drug is not currently available in the United States. Palliative measures as outlined in sec. **III.A.1.c** may be useful.

3. Parkinson's disease

a. Description

(1) The triad of **tremor, rigidity,** and **akinesia** that characterizes Parkinson's disease is discussed in detail in Chap. 15.

(2) There is an **increased incidence of dementia** in parkinsonian patients. This is sometimes difficult to recognize for two reasons:

(a) These patients are often extremely **difficult to test,** since their movement disorder may be so severe that it interferes with their ability to respond appropriately in the test situation.

(b) **Alzheimer's disease is common** in the age group affected by Parkinson's disease, so undoubtedly some of the dementia seen in parkinsonian patients is due only to the coexistence of these two relatively common conditions.

(3) It is generally agreed, however, that Parkinson's disease itself is a dementing illness. Some patients develop a dementia similar to that seen in Alzheimer's disease, while others show a more subcortical picture, as described under progressive supranuclear palsy (see sec. **III.A.2**).

There is a disorder seen in the Marianas Islands, known as **Parkinson's dementia complex,** in which dementia is regularly seen with Parkinson's disease. Many patients with this disease develop a motor neuron disease that is clinically indistinguishable from amyotrophic lateral sclerosis. The pathology of both conditions is characterized by prominent neurofibrillary and granulovacuolar neuronal degeneration and suggests that these syndromes may be linked by a common pathophysiology.

b. Treatment. The treatment for the movement disorder of Parkinson's disease is discussed in Chap. 15. There is no specific therapy for the dementia, and it is unlikely to respond to standard antiparkinsonian drug therapy. Palliative measures as noted in sec. **III.A.1.c** may be useful.

4. Huntington's disease (Huntington's chorea)

a. Description. Huntington's disease is an autosomal dominantly inherited disorder with variable expressivity. Pathologically, it is characterized by degeneration of the basal ganglia (particularly the neostriatum) and cerebral cortex. Clinically, it is characterized by progressive movement disorder and dementia. The treatment of the movement disorder is discussed in Chap. 15. The onset of the dementia often precedes the movement disorder, but dementia may masquerade for many years as an apparent psychiatric disorder characterized by immaturity, impulsivity, and sometimes depression. As it progresses, it takes on a "frontal lobe" character, with apathy and emotional liability; it finally becomes global, affecting all cognitive functions.

b. Treatment

(1) Presymptomatic diagnosis. Recently, the mutation responsible for Huntington's disease was discovered to consist of an expanded segment of the gene due to insertion of trinucleotide repeat sequences (CAG) at 4p16.3. At the time of this writing, this is the latest example of an unstable DNA segment that is responsible for a neurologic disease; other examples include myotonic dystrophy, fragile X syndrome, and Kennedy's syndrome (X-linked spinal-bulbar atrophy). This has led to presymptomatic and even prenatal diagnosis of Huntington's disease. Furthermore, understanding the nature of the gene defect could lead to rational therapies for the disease.

The diagnosis of presymptomatic (including prenatal) Huntington's disease can be made using DNA linkage analysis with accuracy as high as 99%, depending on the number of markers employed. Despite the high degree of accuracy, testing should only be performed after detailed counseling has been provided the family, and long-term follow-up must also be available.

(2) **Medical treatment.** No medical treatment has been proved effective for the dementia of Huntington's disease, but several treatment modalities **may be** of benefit.

(a) **Antidopamine therapy** with haloperidol (see Chap. 15 for details).

(b) **Cholinergic therapy** with choline or lecithin, up to several grams per day (precise dosage is unknown).

B. Multi-infarct dementia and Binswanger's disease

1. **Description.** The syndrome of **multiple strokes** is a cause of dementia. The precise clinical picture depends on the locations of the infarctions or hemorrhages.

a. **When multiple lacunar infarctions** have occurred in the basal ganglia, internal capsule, and pons, a lacunar state (état lacunaire) may develop that is characterized by rigidity, hyperreflexia, pseudobulbar palsy, and dementia. The dementia in this condition is primarily a subcortical type, with prominent abulia and apathy. The reason for the development of this particular type of dementia is unknown.

b. **Dementia due to multiple strokes** often may be distinguished from a degenerative disease on the basis of its history, which may show a stepwise development of symptoms, rather than the insidious, smoothly progressing course of a degenerative disease. Furthermore, multi-infarct dementia tends to be characterized more by inattention (i.e., chronic confusion) rather than the amnestic, aphasic, and apraxic syndrome that is more commonly seen in Alzheimer's disease.

c. The presence of **hypertension** in a patient with a progressive dementing illness and signs of bilateral pyramidal tract disease, including pseudobulbar palsy, may suggest the lacunar state, although bilateral cerebral infarctions or hemorrhages could present a similar clinical picture. CT scanning or MRI often will reveal cerebral infarctions or hemorrhages but are less likely to show small lacunar infarctions, either supratentorially or infratentorially. These small infarctions must be suspected on clinical grounds alone.

In some hypertensive patients, a similar clinical state is seen in which there are very few or no discrete infarctions, but rather a diffuse loss of white matter in the centrum semiovale. This is thought to be due to chronic ischemia in the distribution of cerebral arterioles due to the hypertensive cerebrovascular disease, arteriolar sclerosis; it is known as **Binswanger's subcortical leukoencephalopathy.**

d. The loss of tensile strength of the ventricular walls caused by multiple deep infarctions combined with the effects of systemic hypertension transmitted through the ventricular fluid may produce an association between multi-infarct dementia and occult hydrocephalus. If this occurs, treatment of the hydrocephalus may be indicated (see sec. **III.C**).

2. **Treatment.** There is no specific treatment for the dementia of multiple strokes once it has developed, but it may be possible to influence the development or progression of this illness by treating the risk factors for stroke, particularly **hypertension** and sources of **emboli** (see Chap. 10). Palliative treatment as outlined in sec. **III.A.l.c** may be useful. The treatment of occult hydrocephalus may occasionally be valuable, as noted in sec. **III.C**.

C. Chronic hydrocephalus

1. **Terminology.** Chronic hydrocephalus may produce dementia or mental retardation. (The syndrome of acute hydrocephalus is a neurologic emergency and does not manifest itself as a dementia [see Chap. 11].) The terminology of chronic hydrocephalus is summarized as follows:

a. **Nonobstructive** (ex vacuo)

(1) Alzheimer's disease.

(2) Pick's disease.

(3) Multiple cerebral infarctions.

(4) Huntington's disease.

b. **Obstructive**

(1) **Communicating** (normal pressure, low pressure, tension)

(a) Postsubarachnoid hemorrhage.
(b) Postmeningitis.
(c) Idiopathic.
(2) Noncommunicating (internal)
(a) Aqueductal stenosis.
(b) Masses compressing the fourth ventricle (e.g., cerebellar tumors).
(c) Malformations at the foramen magnum (e.g., Arnold-Chiari and Dandy-Walker malformations).

2. Description

a. Nonobstructive, or ex vacuo, hydrocephalus is due to degeneration or destruction of cerebral tissue with secondary increase in ventricular size.

b. Obstructive hydrocephalus is divided clinically according to the site of cerebrospinal fluid (CSF) blockage: If the blockage is within the ventricular system, the term **noncommunicating hydrocephalus** applies; if the blockage is outside the ventricular system, the term **communicating hydrocephalus** is appropriate. It should be emphasized that, in cases of obstructive hydrocephalus that present as dementia, the blockage is never complete, since a total block of CSF flow would result in acute hydrocephalus, massively increased intracranial pressure, and death within a few hours (see Chap. 11).

(1) In **children,** a common site of obstruction is within the ventricular system (noncommunicating hydrocephalus), due either to aqueductal stenosis or to incomplete development of the foramina of Magendie and Luschka. This type of abnormality, often only one manifestation of a generalized maldevelopment of the nervous system, is associated with such abnormalities as microgyria, macrogyria, porencephaly, agenesis of the corpus callosum, fusion of the cerebral hemispheres, agenesis of the cerebellar vermis, spina bifida, meningocele, encephalocele, syringomyelia, hydromyelia, and the Arnold-Chiari malformation. Children may also develop communicating hydrocephalus due to adhesions in the subarachnoid space at the base of the brain. These adhesions may be produced by perinatal subarachnoid or intraventricular hemorrhages.

(2) In **adults,** chronic hydrocephalus is usually communicating, with the block in the subarachnoid space. Rarely, noncommunicating hydrocephalus due to aqueductal stenosis is seen in adults.

3. Diagnosis. The diagnosis of hydrocephalus is suspected in **children** whose head circumference enlarges too rapidly and in **adults** who have a subcortical type of dementia (prominent abulia, incontinence, and gait disturbance with the intellectual deterioration) of unclear etiology. It should be remembered that ventricular dilatation precedes an increase in head growth. A history of intracranial hemorrhage or meningitis further raises the suspicion of chronic hydrocephalus. Although a **CT scan** will reliably and safely reveal the presence of hydrocephalus, **MRI** provides better anatomic detail and, while not necessarily recommended as the initial or screening study, should eventually be performed in all patients with hydrocephalus. Although the pattern of ventricular enlargement on CT or MRI gives clues to the site of blockage, a CSF flow study (with either radioiodinated serum albumin [RISA] or radioactive indium) may be required in determining the exact site of the obstruction (if this information is deemed necessary). Cranial ultrasound will reliably demonstrate ventricular enlargement, provided that the anterior fontanelle is open.

4. Treatment

a. Surgery

(1) Rationale. Theoretically, chronic hydrocephalus may be relieved by the **shunting of CSF** around the blockage. This will lower the pressure in the ventricular system proximal to the block and thereby prevent further damage to brain tissue. However, **shunting must be done before excessive irreversible loss of brain tissue has taken place.** This can be done easily in children before the sutures and fontanelles have closed, since the diagnosis of hydrocephalus can be made relatively early in the course of the illness because of excessive head growth, which is readily apparent and often precedes decompensation due to increased intracranial pressure. However, many, if not all, patients will have significant ventricular dilatation prior to excessive increase in head circumference. Once the sutures have closed irreversibly, head measurements are of no value in the diagnosis of hydrocephalus.

(2) **When to shunt.** It is not known how long a period can elapse prior to shunting before irreversible damage has occurred, but it appears that **the likelihood of a good result from shunting is inversely proportional to the length of time from the onset of symptoms to the time of diagnosis.** No specific time limit can be set beyond which surgery can be said to be of no benefit, but most studies in adults have shown much better results in patients who have had symptoms for less than 6 months. However, it should be emphasized that many patients with longer-term illness have improved with shunting. Candidates for shunting should undergo a lumbar puncture with lowering of CSF pressure to below 100 mm H_2O. If gait improves with this procedure, shunting is more likely to confer a long-term benefit.

In children, the width of the cortical mantle does not necessarily correlate with the ultimate intellectual outcome, so all should be evaluated for shunting. However, in some early mild cases in children (usually a communicating hydrocephalus with a known etiology, such as intraventricular hemorrhage or postmeningitis), the patient may be observed carefully, with frequent serial head measurements, ultrasound, and CT scans or MRI, in the hope that the process will arrest spontaneously and thereby render a shunting procedure unnecessary.

(3) **Cortical atrophy**

(a) Since Alzheimer's disease is a common cause of dementia in adults, one should always be sure to rule out cerebral atrophy (hydrocephalus ex vacuo) as either the sole or partial cause of the dementia because this aspect of the hydrocephalus will not respond to shunting procedures, since there is no obstruction to CSF flow.

(b) A radionuclide **CSF flow study** should show persistent activity in the lateral ventricles and no activity over the cerebral convexities in pure-communicating hydrocephalus. Some activity seen over the convexities, even as late as 72 hours after injection, suggests a mixed (i.e., ex vacuo plus obstructive) form of hydrocephalus, which is less likely to respond to surgery.

(c) **When a significant degree of cerebral atrophy is demonstrated by CT scan or MRI, even if there is a component of obstructive hydrocephalus, shunting procedures are unlikely to show good results.**

(4) **Indications for shunting.** Patients who should have shunting procedures include

(a) **Children** in whom the diagnosis of chronic progressive hydrocephalus has been made and in whom the likelihood of spontaneous arrest has been ruled out.

(b) **Adults** who have a relatively recent onset of dementia, who show a purely obstructive hydrocephalus by CT scan, MRI, or CSF flow studies, and who respond to lowering CSF pressure by lumbar puncture.

(5) **Procedures.** Many shunting operations are available, but the one most commonly employed is the **ventriculoperitoneal** shunt.

(6) **Complications of shunting.** Even in the ideal case, with good initial response to shunting, one must remain vigilant for complications of the shunt. These include

(a) Infection. If the shunt becomes infected, it must be removed and the infection treated as outlined in Chap. 8.

(b) Mechanical malfunction.

(c) Movement of the cannula and consequent inadequate draining of the ventricles.

(d) Emboli and endocarditis (with ventriculoatrial shunts).

(e) Ascites, peritonitis, and ruptured viscus (with ventriculoperitoneal shunts).

(f) Subdural hematoma.

(7) Any deterioration in mental functioning is an indication for reevaluation of ventricular size, preferably by CT scanning.

b. **Medical treatment** of chronic obstructive hydrocephalus is relatively ineffective and should be used only when surgery is not possible. Occasionally, in children in whom the diagnosis of mild hydrocephalus has been made, medical therapy may be used pending a decision about surgery. The rationale for medical management of chronic obstructive hydrocephalus is based on the observation that acetazolamide (Diamox) may decrease the rate of CSF production by the choroid plexus. The dosage of acetazolamide is 10–25 mg/kg/day PO divided into three doses in children and 250 mg PO tid in adults. Serial lumbar punctures and intermittent ventricular drainage may be used as a means of postponing a shunt procedure in premature infants unable to tolerate the operation.

D. **Spongiform encephalopathies**
1. These rare diseases, which include kuru and Jakob-Creutzfeldt disease, are characterized by diffuse cerebral, basal ganglion, and spinal cord neuronal degeneration; glial proliferation; and spongy appearance of the cortex. They are characterized by a rapidly progressive, subacute dementia similar to Alzheimer's disease but usually accompanied by striking myoclonus and sometimes by cerebellar signs, rigidity, and weakness (see also Chap. 8). There is usually an associated characteristic EEG pattern consisting of high-voltage, periodic sharp activity superimposed on a slow background.
2. **Treatment.** There is no specific therapy for the disease itself. Palliative measures as noted in sec. **III.A.1.c** are sometimes useful. In addition, the myoclonus may respond to the use of one of the benzodiazepine derivatives such as
   a. **Clonazepam** (Klonopin), 1.5–2.0 mg PO daily, divided into three doses.
   b. **Diazepam** (Valium), 15–30 mg PO daily, divided into three doses.

E. **Viral encephalitides** (see also Chap. 8)
1. **Description.** Many of the viral encephalitides may result in dementia due to destruction of the cerebral cortex. Any of these diseases may be incriminated: arbovirus infections (eastern, western, St. Louis, Venezuelan, and California equine encephalitides), herpes simplex encephalitis, subacute sclerosing panencephalitis, and human immunosuppression virus (HIV). The critical factor in the development of dementia is presumably the amount of brain destroyed by the infection. However, the encephalitis itself may be inapparent, only presenting with the late onset of dementia. This is particularly true of HIV and herpes simplex encephalitis. In some patients, only memory loss is seen, but in many others there is widespread higher cortical dysfunction.
2. **Treatment.** There is no specific treatment for the viral encephalitides, with the exception of herpes simplex encephalitis (see Chap. 8). If dementia develops, the palliative maneuvers noted in sec. **III.A.1.c** may be beneficial.

F. **Neurosyphilis** (see also Chap. 8)
1. **Description.** In the late stages of neurosyphilis in adults, one may see the syndrome of **dementia paralytica,** or **general paresis of the insane.** The mental changes take many forms, including frank psychosis, memory deficit, impairment of judgment, excessive liability of mood, and others. Usually, patients who have congenital paretic syphilis have been known to be defective physically and mentally from birth. Between the ages of 6 and 21 years, the affected child often begins to function less well in school and has associated irritability and inattention. Psychometric tests show a decrease in IQ. Neurologic examination may or may not be abnormal but often shows pupillary abnormalities, choreiform movements, incoordination, spasticity, optic atrophy, or deafness.
2. **Treatment.** The treatment of neurosyphilis is outlined in Chap. 8. The dementia often does not respond well to treatment, although the further progression of dementia is arrested in most treated patients. About one-third of adult patients have complete remission of symptoms, and another 25% show a partial improve-

ment. The degree of improvement depends on the stage of the disease at which it is treated. Children with congenital syphilis have an even poorer prognosis for recovery of normal function than do adults.

G. Posttraumatic encephalopathies
  1. **Description.** Some patients who suffer head trauma fail to recover their full premorbid mental capacities. This is more common in patients who lose consciousness, particularly as a result of massive head trauma, than in trivial head injuries, but it may be seen in either situation. Older patients are more likely than younger ones to develop this posttraumatic dementia. If the patient appears to recover completely from the head trauma and subsequently begins to show a dementing illness, one must suspect development of either a communicating hydrocephalus, precipitated by blood in the subarachnoid space, or chronic subdural hematoma. Both of these conditions may require neurosurgical treatment. If the patient never fully regains normal mentation, various components of the so-called posttraumatic or postconcussion syndrome also may be seen, including headache, dizziness, insomnia, irritability, inability to concentrate, and personality changes. It is not known whether these symptoms are directly related to brain damage or are psychological in origin. Many of these symptoms resemble those of depression, and their resolution is often delayed when litigation is pending.
  2. **Treatment**
     a. **Insomnia, irritability, restlessness, personality change, loss of ability to concentrate**
        (1) Imipramine (Tofranil), 75–150 mg PO daily.
        (2) Amitriptyline (Elavil), 75–150 mg PO daily.
        (3) Desipramine (Norpramin), 75–150 mg PO daily
     b. **Headache**
        (1) Aspirin, 600 mg PO q4h or as needed for pain.
        (2) Polycyclic antidepressants as in sec. **III.G.2.a** may also be useful if aspirin is not effective.
     c. **Dementia.** No specific therapy is available aside from those measures listed above. Reassurance is important because most patients show steady improvement even though recovery may take several years. In a minority of patients (usually elderly patients who have survived massive head trauma), severe permanent intellectual dysfunction may require institutionalization and treatment as outlined in sec. **III.A.1.c.**

H. Congenital and early-acquired disorders
  1. **Definitions and classification.** Disorders resulting in intellectual dysfunction that originate prenatally or during infancy or childhood may result in mental retardation or dementia. Differential diagnosis, diagnostic studies, and outcome will depend on this basic distinction, which is of primary importance. A useful method of classification is based on the time at which the illness is determined.
     a. **Prenatally determined**
        (1) Chromosomal abnormalities.
        (2) Hereditary syndromes with multiple anomalies, but without identifiable chromosomal abnormalities.
        (3) Multifactorial inheritance (polygenic and environmental factors).
        (4) Major malformations of uncertain etiology.
        (5) Congenital infections.
        (6) Maternal and environmental factors.
        (7) Metabolic and degenerative disorders.
            (a) Amino acid abnormalities.
            (b) Lysosomal storage diseases.
            (c) Mitochondrial diseases (e.g., Leigh's disease due to cytochrome oxidase deficiency).
            (d) Peroxisomal diseases (e.g., adrenoleukodystrophy).
     b. **Perinatally determined**
        (1) Complications of prematurity.

    (2) Hypoxic-ischemic encephalopathy—uncommon in the full-term infant.

    (3) Infections.

    (4) Metabolic abnormalities.

  c. Postnatally determined

    (1) Infections.

    (2) Trauma.

    (3) Hypoxic-ischemic insults.

    (4) Toxic-metabolic disorders.

    (5) Neoplasms.

2. Clinical and laboratory approach

  a. An appropriately detailed history and physical examination will usually allow the clinician to place the patient within one of the above categories, and, at times, a specific diagnosis may be made.

  b. If further diagnostic study is needed, as is often the case, biochemical, radiologic, electrophysiologic, and genetic studies should be obtained as indicated by the history and physical examination. A battery of routine studies is rarely, if ever, warranted in the child with unexplained intellectual dysfunction. Exceptions include thyroid and amino acid studies because one may be dealing with a rare, but treatable, condition.

3. Causes of mental retardation

  a. Chromosomal abnormalities. Identifiable chromosomal abnormalities may often be diagnosed on clinical grounds alone and include trisomies 13, 18, and 21; Klinefelter's syndrome; and other less common disorders. Chromosome studies are indicated if these disorders are suspected and also in patients with unexplained mental retardation.

    Fragile X syndrome is a common identifiable cause of mental retardation, with a prevalence rate of 1 in 1250 males and 1 in 2500 females. The clinical diagnosis of fragile X syndrome is often not made because the phenotype varies in relation to puberty and includes a wide variety of nonspecific findings. The classic features of large ears, a long face, prominent jaw, and large testes are usually not present until after puberty. Behavioral and developmental syndromes, including hyperactivity and autism, are often earlier manifestations. Direct DNA testing is now available that will demonstrate the genetic abnormality in the majority of affected individuals and carriers. The abnormality consists of an expanded segment of the FMR-1 gene, in band Xq27.3, due to insertion of trinucleotide repeat sequences (CGG). The syndrome becomes clinically manifest when the gene is expanded to contain at least 200 trinucleotide repeat sequences. Direct DNA testing is the preferred method over the previously available cytogenetic test that can demonstrate the fragile X site. If the direct DNA test does not demonstrate the abnormality and the diagnosis remains suspect, cytogenetic analysis should then be performed. Because findings are nonspecific, fragile X testing is recommended in all boys in whom mental retardation is unexplained, even in the absence of classic dysmorphic features. While X-linked, the syndrome is dominantly inherited and can be seen in females. Testing, therefore, should be considered in girls with unexplained mental retardation.

  b. Multiple anomalies. Hereditary syndromes with multiple anomalies but without identifiable chromosomal abnormalities are varied, and individual description is beyond the scope of this text. These disorders may be classified according to associated defects; several atlases are available that may aid in establishing a diagnosis (see Smith in the Selected Readings).

  c. Multifactorially determined conditions. Conditions caused by multifactorial inheritances are found in a large percentage of mildly retarded persons and are heavily represented within socially disadvantaged groups. The inheritance of multiple genes from both parents is compounded by substandard environmental factors that further impair learning. Usually no specific abnormalities are found in these individuals.

  d. Isolated malformations. Other isolated major malformations of diverse etiologies include primary and secondary microcephaly and various anomalies associated with hydrocephalus. Radiographic studies, including MRI and CT scanning, may be indicated for defining the exact nature and extent of the anomaly.

e. **Amino acid disorders** and related conditions (organic acid and urea cycle disorders) are a complex group of diseases that are difficult to distinguish from each other and from other degenerative diseases of the nervous system. After a variable period of normal development (at times extremely short, as in maple syrup urine disease), signs of diffuse involvement of the nervous system may become manifest; such signs include delay or deterioration in intellectual or motor development, lethargy (at times proceeding to coma), seizures, ataxia, and alterations of muscle tone. Several disorders may be associated with fairly consistent physical features and unusual odors, such as light pigmentation and eczema in phenylketonuria and the characteristic smell of the urine in maple syrup urine disease. Early diagnosis is essential, since several of these disorders are treatable by exclusion or addition of dietary substances (Table 3-1). Blood and urine amino acid and organic acid analyses are essential for the diagnosis.

f. **Lysosomal storage diseases.** The lysosomal storage disorders are a group of genetic diseases in which storage of certain metabolites occurs within lysosomes, due to a specific enzyme deficiency. Table 3-2 lists lysosomal storage diseases with known enzyme deficiencies and the major accumulating metabolites. Disorders that primarily involve gray matter (e.g., ganglioside storage diseases) result in dementia and seizures early in their course. As a rule, ataxia and spasticity appear early in the course of primary white matter degenerative disease, with seizures and dementia appearing later.

g. **Mitochondrial diseases.** Involvement of brain, spinal cord, muscle, peripheral nerve, and other organs may occur in a variety of mitochondrial diseases with or without known enzyme deficiency.

   (1) Cytochrome c oxidase and pyruvate dehydrogenase deficiency, for example, are causes of **Leigh's disease.** Age of onset is usually within the first 2 years of life; signs and symptoms include developmental delay, failure to thrive, hypotonia, weakness, ataxia, ophthalmoplegia, and irregular respirations. Characteristic signal abnormality may be seen on MRI within basal ganglia and brainstem nuclei. Levels of lactate and pyruvate are usually elevated in blood and CSF.

   (2) **The MERRF syndrome** (myoclonic epilepsy with ragged red fibers) is associated with a point mutation in mitochondrial DNA at nucleotide pair 8,344. Clinical and laboratory features include myoclonus, ataxia, weakness, dementia, short stature, hearing loss, lactic acidosis, and ragged red fibers are seen on muscle biopsy.

   (3) **The MELAS syndrome** (mitochondrial encelphalomyopathy, lactic acidosis, and strokelike episodes) is associated with a point mutation at position 3,243 of mitochondrial DNA. Features include short stature, seizures, recurrent vomiting, recurrent headaches, recurrent strokelike episodes, dementia, lactic acidosis, and ragged red fibers in muscle.

   (4) Dementia is a feature of **Kearns-Sayre syndrome,** along with progressive external ophthalmoplegia, ataxia, weakness, retinal degeneration, heart block, lactic acidosis, elevated CSF protein, and ragged red fibers, due to a deletion of mitochondrial DNA.

   (5) **Alper's disease,** characterized by early onset of seizures, dementia, spasticity, blindness, and liver dysfunction, has been shown to be due to deficiency of complex I of the respiratory chain. Complex I deficiency has been associated with other mitochondrial disorders discussed in this section so that it appears to be nonspecific.

h. **Peroxisomal diseases**

   (1) **Disorders of peroxisomal biogenes with deficiency of multiple peroxisomal enzymes.** Included in this category are Zellweger's syndrome with characteristic dysmorphic features and absence of peroxisomes in various tissues; neonatal adrenoleukodystrophy, inherited in an autosomal reces-

Table 3-1. Metabolic diseases associated with mental retardation that may be treatable by dietary restriction or supplementation

Disease	Restrict	Supplement
Phenylketonuria	Phenylalanine	
Maple syrup urine disease	Branched-chain amino acids	Thiamine (rarely), carnitine
Tyrosinemia (tyrosine transaminase deficiency)	Tyrosine and phenylalanine	
Tryptophanuria		Nicotinamide
Hyperornithinemia	Protein	
Beta-alaninemia	Protein	Pyridoxine
Hemocystinuria		
Type I	Methionine	Pyridoxine
Type II	Methionine	Vitamin B_{12}
Type III	Methionine	Folic acid
Methionine malabsorption	Methionine	
Urea cycle disorders	Protein	Varying combinations of benzoate, phenylacetate, arginine, and citrulline
Methylmalonic aciduria	Protein	Vitamin B_{12}, carnitine
Propionic acidemia	Protein	Biotin, carnitine
Isovaleric acidemia	Protein	Glycine, carnitine
Multiple carboxylase deficiency		Biotin
Biotinidase deficiency		Biotin
Galactosemia	Eliminate galactose	
Pyruvate dehydrogenase deficiency	Carbohydrate, protein	Thiamine, biotin, lipoic acid, fat (ketonemia without exacerbation of acidosis)
Pyruvate carboxylase deficiency	Carbohydrate, protein	Thiamine, biotin, lipoic acid, fat (ketonemia without exacerbation of acidosis)
Pyridoxine-dependent seizures		Pyridoxine
Maternal phenylketonuria[a]	Phenylalanine	
Carnitine deficiency: primary—systemic, myopathic; secondary[b]		L-Carnitine
Glutaric aciduria I	Protein, lysine, tryptophan	Riboflavin, L-carnitine
Glutaric aciduria II	Protein, fat	Riboflavin, L-carnitine
Medium-chain acetylcoenzyme A dehydrogenase deficiency		Carbohydrate, avoid fasting, L-carnitine
Glycerol kinase deficiency	Glycerol	Avoid fasting
Hereditary fructose intolerance	Fructose	
Glucose transporter protein deficiency		Ketogenic diet

[a] Pregnant women with phenylketonuria should be treated to prevent fetal brain damage.
[b] Secondary carnitine deficiency occurs in a number of metabolic diseases, some of which are included in this table.

Table 3-2. Lysosomal storage diseases

Disease	Approximate age of onset (yr)	Enzyme deficiency	Major accumulating metabolites
Glycogenoses			
Type 2—Pompe's disease			
Infantile	1	α-Glucosidase	Glycogen
Adult	> 20	α-Glucosidase	Glycogen
Sphingolipidoses			
G_{M1} gangliosidosis			
Type 1—infantile generalized	1	β-Galactosidase	G_{M1} ganglioside, oligosaccharide
Type 2—juvenile	1–2	β-Galactosidase	G_{M1} ganglioside, oligosaccharide
G_{M2} gangliosidosis			
Tay-Sachs disease	1	Hexosaminidase A	G_{M2} ganglioside
Sandhoff's disease	1	Hexosaminidases A and B	G_{M2} ganglioside, globoside, oligosaccharide
AB variant	1	G_{M2} activator factor	G_{M2} ganglioside
Juvenile Tay-Sachs disease	> 2	Hexosaminidase A	G_{M2} ganglioside
Juvenile Sandhoff's disease	> 2	Hexosaminidases A and B	G_{M2} ganglioside, globoside
Adult Tay-Sachs disease	> 15	Hexosaminidase A	G_{M2} ganglioside
Sulfatidoses			
Metachromatic leukodystrophy			
Late-infantile	1–3	Arylsulfatase A	Sulfatide
Juvenile	4–15	Arylsulfatase A	Sulfatide
Adult	> 16	Arylsulfatase A	Sulfatide
Activator factor deficiency	1–2	Cerebroside sulfate sulfatase activator factor	Sulfatide
Mucosulfatidosis	1	Arylsulfatases A, B, C, steroid sulfatase, iduronide-sulfate sulfatase, heparan-N-acetylgalactosamine-6-sulfate sulfatase, N-acetylglucosamine-6-sulfate sulfatase	Sulfatide, steroid sulfate, heparan sulfate, dermatan sulfate

Disease	Age of onset	Enzyme deficiency	Stored material
Krabbe's disease			
Infantile	1	Galactocerebrosidase	Galactocerebroside
Juvenile	4	Galactocerebrosidase	Galactocerebroside
Fabry's disease	> 10	α-Galactosidase A	Ceramide trihexoside
Gaucher's disease			
Type 1—adult form	1–70	β-Glucosidase	Glucocerebroside
Type 2—infantile form	1	β-Glucosidase	Glucocerebroside
Type 3—juvenile form	> 10	β-Glucosidase	Glucocerebroside
Niemann-Pick disease			
Type A—late-infantile, neuropathic	1	Sphingomyelinase	Sphingomyelin
Type B—juvenile, nonneuropathic	2	Sphingomyelinase	Sphingomyelin
Type C—without sphingomyelinase deficiency	1–2	Activating factor	Sphingomyelin
Type D—Nova Scotia type	Childhood	Unknown	Sphingomyelin
Farber's disease	1	Ceramidase	Ceramide
Mucopolysaccharidoses			
Hurler's syndrome	1	α-Iduronidase	Dermatan and heparan sulfate
Hurler-Scheie complex	1–2	α-Iduronidase	Dermatan and heparan sulfate
Scheie's syndrome	Childhood	α-Iduronidase	Dermatan and heparan sulfate
Hunter's syndrome			
Severe	1	Iduronate sulfatase	Dermatan and heparan sulfate
Mild	Childhood	Iduronate sulfatase	Dermatan and heparan sulfate
Sanfilippo's syndrome			
Type A	1	Heparan-N-sulfamidase	Heparan sulfate
Type B	1	α-N-Acetylglucosaminidase	Heparan sulfate
Type C	1	Heparan-N-acetyltransferase	Heparan sulfate
Type D	1	α-N-Glucosamine-6-sulfatase	Heparan sulfate
Morquio's disease			
Type A	Childhood	N-Acetylgalactosamine-6-sulfate sulfatase	Keratan sulfate
Type B	Childhood	β-Galactosidase	Keratan sulfate
Maroteaux-Lamy syndrome			
Severe	2	Arylsulfatase B	Dermatan sulfate
Intermediate	Childhood	Arylsulfatase B	Dermatan sulfate
Mild	Adulthood	Arylsulfatase B	Dermatan sulfate

Table 3-2 (continued).

Disease	Approximate age of onset (yr)	Enzyme deficiency	Major accumulating metabolites
β-Glucuronidase deficiency (Sly's disease)	Childhood	β-Glucuronidase	Dermatan and heparan sulfate
Oligosaccharidoses			
Fucosidosis			
Late-infantile	1	α-Fucosidase	Fucosyl-sphingolipids, oligo-saccharides, and glycopeptides
Juvenile	Childhood	α-Fucosidase	Fucosyl-glycoconjugates as in late-infantile type
Mannosidosis	Childhood	α-Mannosidase	Mannosyl-oligosaccharides
Aspartylglucosaminuria	Childhood	Aspartylglucosamine amide hydrolase	Aspartyl-2-deoxy-2 acetamidoglucosylamine
Sialidosis			
Type 1	< 1	α-Neuraminidase	Sialyloliposaccharides
Type 2			
Congenital	< 1	α-Neuraminidase	Sialyloliposaccharides
Infantile	1	α-Neuraminidase (primary) plus β-galactosidase (secondary)	Sialyloliposaccharides
Juvenile	Childhood		
I-cell disease	1	Uridine diphosphate-N-acetylglucosamine-1-phosphate transferase	Various glycoconjugates
Mucolipidosis III	2	Uridine diphosphate-N-acetylglucosamine-1-phosphate transferase	Various glycoconjugates
Mucolipidosis IV	1	Ganglioside α-neuraminidase	$G_{M3} + G_{D3}$
Others			
Wolman's disease	1	Acid lipase	Cholesterol esters, triglycerides
Acid-phosphatase deficiency	1	Lysosomal acid phosphatase	Phosphate esters

Source: Adapted from E. H. Kolodny and W. J. L. Cable, Inborn errors of metabolism. *Ann. Neurol.* 11:221, 1982.

sive manner and associated with accumulation of very long–chain fatty acids; and infantile Refsum's disease with elevated plasma phytanic acid levels and hyperpipecolic acidemia that resembles Zellweger's syndrome.

(2) Disorders with deficiency of a single peroxisomal enxyme. X-linked adrenoleukodystrophy usually becomes manifest in childhood, but sometimes not until adolescence or adulthood. It is characterized by changes in behavior and personality followed by progressive neurologic deterioration and signs of adrenal insufficiency. Evidence of white matter disease is seen on CT or MRI, and there is accumulation of very long–chain fatty acids in various tissues, usually measured in plasma.

i. Congenital infections. Patients with mental retardation due to the recognizable congenital infections (e.g., herpesvirus, rubella, *Toxoplasma,* cytomegalovirus) usually have additional abnormalities; these include intrauterine growth retardation, neonatal jaundice, petechiae, hepatosplenomegaly, microcephaly or hydrocephalus, and intracranial calcifications. Patients with the congenital rubella syndrome frequently have cataracts and congenital heart lesions. Valuable laboratory studies during the neonatal period include attempted viral isolation in urine and total and specific IgM antibody determinations if available (if not, serial IgG titers must be obtained to differentiate passive transfer from active antibody production by the infant).

j. Prenatal insults. Prenatal maternal and environmental factors associated with mental retardation include chronic placental insufficiency, toxemia, diabetes, malnutrition, alcoholism, ingestion of certain drugs, and exposure to radiation.

k. Perinatal insults to the developing brain may occur during labor, delivery, or the first several days of life. These may include hypoxic-ischemic injuries (often accompanied by intraventricular [periventricular] and/or subarachnoid hemorrhages), trauma, infections, and toxic-metabolic disturbances. All perinatal injuries, with the possible exception of mechanical trauma, are more commonly seen in premature infants.

(1) Periventricular (germinal matrix) hemorrhage with intraventricular and subarachnoid extension is essentially a disease of the premature infant. This is a common disorder that can be documented by CT or ultrasonic scan in 40–50% of premature infants weighing less than 1500 g, many of whom are apparently asymptomatic. Many infants with large hemorrhages die or are left with serious sequelae. The majority of infants with smaller hemorrhages survive, and although many develop normally, hydrocephalus and nonprogressive intellectual and motor deficits may result. Spastic diplegia with normal intelligence is a common finding in these infants.

(2) Subarachnoid hemorrhage is also associated with hypoxic insults, and although it is more common in premature infants, it occurs with significant frequency in full-term neonates as well. The immediate and long-term outlooks are variable.

(3) Acute subdural hemorrhage is uncommon in newborns but does occur in full-term infants, often following traumatic instrument-assisted deliveries. Subdural tap is indicated if this disorder is suspected.

(4) Other important causes of permanent neurologic disability with onset during the perinatal period include meningitis, symptomatic hypoglycemia, and kernicterus.

l. Inherited metabolic diseases without enzyme deficiencies. A large number of inherited nervous system diseases occur for which no specific enzyme deficiency is yet known.

(1) Neuronal ceroid lipofuscinoses (also known as Batten's disease) are characterized by accumulation in neurons of autofluorescent lipopigment with consequent intellectual failure, seizures, extrapyramidal syndromes, and blindness. These disorders are subtyped by age of onset into infantile (Haltia-Santavouri), late infantile (Bielschowsky-Jansky), juvenile (Spielmeyer-Vogt), and adult (Kufs') disease. The diagnosis is suspected clinically. Urinary dolichol levels may be elevated; characteristic intracellular inclusions are seen on skin biopsy.

(2) **Hereditary ataxias** include diseases allied clinically to Friedreich's ataxia.

m. **Postnatal factors** in mental retardation include head trauma, CNS infections, hypoxic-ischemic insults, CNS neoplasms, and toxic-metabolic disturbances.

n. **Cerebral palsy.** Chronic, nonprogressive motor disability, often associated with seizures and mental retardation, is commonly referred to as cerebral palsy. This group of disorders may be classified by their neurologic signs into **spastic, choreoathetotic, ataxic,** and **mixed** varieties. Motor findings may evolve and not become manifest until the second year of life, making differentiation from a progressive neurologic disorder extremely difficult. With regard to **etiology,** prematurity and its complications are important factors. In the child born at term, cerebral palsy is usually prenatally determined, and perinatal events are usually not of primary importance. Before concluding that perinatal asphyxia is causally related to cerebral palsy, there should be evidence of severe and prolonged intrapartum asphyxia, moderate to severe hypoxic-ischemic encephalopathy during the immediate perinatal period, evidence of injury to multiple organs, and exclusion of other conditions that could also explain the clinical syndrome.

I. **Demyelinating diseases**
 1. **Description.** Demyelinating diseases, of which the most common is **multiple sclerosis,** are discussed in detail in Chap. 13. When the disease becomes advanced, multiple lesions in the subcortical white matter may produce personality change, inappropriate emotional reactions, and intellectual deterioration. It is exceedingly rare, however, for multiple sclerosis to manifest itself as a dementia with no other associated abnormalities. Schilder's disease may be considered a variant of multiple sclerosis; this disease, with prominent involvement of cerebral white matter, occurs in children who may prove to have adrenoleukodystrophy.

 Progressive multifocal leukoencephalopathy (PML), adrenoleukodystrophy, Krabbe's disease, metachromatic leukodystrophy, Alexander's disease, Canavan's disease, and **Pelizaeus-Merzbacher disease** are relatively rare diseases of myelin, all of which may include dementia as a prominent feature. PML is usually associated with an underlying malignancy (most often lymphoma) or AIDS.

 2. **Treatment** is outlined in Chap. 13. A dramatic reversal of the dementia in advanced demyelinating disease is unusual.

J. **Intracranial space-occupying lesions**
 1. **Description.** Masses within the cranial cavity may produce dementia by directly destroying or compressing the brain, by producing increased intracranial pressure, or by producing hydrocephalus. Intracranial masses are found in some patients with dementia. Any mass within the cranial cavity may produce dementia, but the most common masses are primary brain tumors, brain abscesses, and chronic subdural hematomas. The specific clinical picture of each of these conditions is covered elsewhere in this book, but all should be diagnosable by using the combination of history, physical examination, and CT scan.

 2. **Treatment** varies according to the underlying condition, but in general, improvement of the dementia depends on surgical removal of the mass.

IV. **Systemic diseases with cerebral pathology**
 A. **Nutritional diseases**
  1. **Pellagra**
   a. **Description.** Pellagra is caused by nicotinamide (niacin) deficiency, although, as in most B-vitamin deficiency states, it is usually accompanied by signs of other B-vitamin deficiency diseases. It is seen in association with chronic alcoholism, dietary peculiarities, hyperthyroidism, pregnancy, and the stress of injury or surgical procedure. In the advanced state, it is characterized by the classic "three Ds"—dermatitis, diarrhea, and dementia. Its earliest symptoms are often referable to the nervous system and include irritability,

insomnia, weakness, memory loss, and paresthesias. Some patients may show a true dementia, but most show a confusional state. Irreversible intellectual deterioration may occur in untreated patients.

   b. **Treatment** consists of nicotinamide (niacin), 500 mg PO daily for 7–10 days and then 50–100 mg PO daily until symptoms have ameliorated. The minimum daily requirement to prevent disease is 5–10 mg, depending on the patient's age.

2. **Wernicke-Korsakoff syndrome**

   a. **Description.** Thiamine (vitamin B_1) deficiency, usually caused by chronic alcoholism but also occasionally by starvation states, may produce two syndromes that are often seen together.

   (1) **Wernicke's encephalopathy** is an acute, life-threatening disease, covered in detail in Chap. 14.

   (2) **Korsakoff's psychosis** may be caused by many disorders, including encephalitis, posterior cerebral artery strokes, and head trauma, but it is often the result of chronic or recurrent thiamine deficiency in alcoholics. It is characterized by poor memory, disorientation, and tendency to confabulate.

   b. **Treatment.** The Wernicke-Korsakoff syndrome is treated with thiamine (see Chap. 14 for details). However, once severe Korsakoff's psychosis is well established, a dramatic response to thiamine therapy is not to be expected.

3. **Vitamin B_{12} deficiency**

   a. **Description.** The neurologic implications of vitamin B_{12} deficiency are complex and are covered in more detail in Chap. 14. Rarely, vitamin B_{12} deficiency may produce a subcortical type of dementia before it produces any hematologic or spinal cord abnormalities. For this reason, all patients being evaluated for dementia should have a serum vitamin B_{12} determination as part of the initial laboratory work.

   b. **Treatment.** Vitamin B_{12}, 1000 μg IM daily for 5 days; then 1000 μg IM monthly.

B. **Chronic metabolic insults**

1. **Description.** The major syndromes of chronic metabolic insults that may lead to intellectual dysfunction include hypoglycemia, hypoxia, uremia, and hepatic failure. The acute neurologic syndromes associated with these abnormalities are described in Chap. 14. The degree of chronic intellectual loss is related to the degree of cerebral damage induced by the metabolic insult. Once metabolic derangement has been corrected, the patient may be left with a permanent intellectual deficit.

   a. **Hypoglycemia and hypoxemia.** A history of repeated episodes of transient neurologic deficits, often with seizures, suggests recurrent attacks of hypoglycemia or hypoxemia. Hypoglycemia is most often seen in insulin-dependent diabetics or occasionally in patients on oral hypoglycemic agents, while hypoxemia may be due to a number of conditions including ischemic anoxia (e.g., cardiac arrest), anoxemic anoxia (e.g., pulmonary insufficiency, carbon monoxide poisoning), or cytotoxic anoxia (e.g., cyanide poisoning). In the chronic state, hypoxemic and hypoglycemic encaphalopathy are difficult to distinguish from one another, since both consist of varying degrees of focal neurologic deficits (e.g., hemipareses, aphasias, apraxias, hemianopsias) and dementia.

   In a significant proportion of patients who have undergone surgery requiring extracorporeal circulation, there is a residual, nonprogressive disorder of intellectual function characterized by poor memory, inability to concentrate, and change in mood, with an affect reminiscent of depression. This is probably due to widespread, multifocal hypoxic cerebral damage related in some way to the cardiopulmonary bypass process.

   b. **Uremia and hepatic failure.** The neurologic impairments in uremia and liver failure are similar, consisting of various mixtures of confusion, irritability, convulsions, tremor, asterixis, myoclonus, and peripheral neuropathy. In rare patients on chronic hemodialysis, a progressive dementia (dialysis dementia or dialysis encephalopathy) may develop, characterized by progressive dysarthria, myoclonus, and dementia. The EEG may show periodic sharp activity. The EEG abnormality and dysarthria may initially respond to intravenous diazepam, but there is no proven long-term treatment.

2. **Treatment.** There is no effective treatment for the dementia of any of these metabolic abnormalities once it is established. The acute confusional state may be treated by administering the appropriate agent (e.g., glucose, oxygen) or treating the underlying condition (e.g., renal failure, hepatic failure) as outlined in Chap. 14. The aim is to prevent recurrent or prolonged periods of metabolic insult and thus prevent the development or progression of intellectual dysfunction.

C. **Endocrine disorders**
  1. **Hypothyroidism**
   a. **Description.** Hypothyroidism can occur at any age and can be either primary (thyroid failure) or secondary (anterior pituitary failure). Congenital hypothyroidism ranges from mild to severe. The fully developed syndrome is known as **cretinism.** Secondary hypothyroidism can occur at any age due to thyroid-stimulating hormone (TSH) deficiency as a result of anterior pituitary failure.
    (1) **Cretinism** may be evident at birth, but more commonly hypothyroidism becomes obvious in the first several months of life. The infant shows the characteristic facies (broad, flat nose with widely spaced eyes, coarse features, thick lips, and protruding tongue), a hoarse cry, and an umbilical hernia. Early diagnosis is vital, since the degree of intellectual impairment is related to the age at which therapy is initiated. Although rare, cretinism is an important treatable cause of mental retardation and should be considered in every evaluation of a mentally retarded child, even if the physical stigmata mentioned previously are absent.
    (2) **Adult hypothyroidism.** In the older child and adult, hypothyroidism is manifested by puffy eyelids; alopecia of the outer third of the eyebrows; dry, rough skin; brittle, dry hair; induration and doughiness of the subcutaneous tissues; slurred speech and hoarse voice; constipation; anemia; increased sensitivity to cold; cerebellar ataxia; muscle weakness and slowed deep tendon reflexes; and intellectual dysfunction. This intellectual impairment may represent any one of a wide range of syndromes, including hallucinations, disorientation, agitation and confusion ("myxedema madness"), and true dementia (memory loss, incontinence, and lowered IQ).

      Myxedema coma is a medical emergency not appropriately covered in this discussion. However, milder forms of hypothyroidism may manifest themselves as a dementia, so every patient initially evaluated for intellectual dysfunction should have a serum thyroxine measurement. A serum TSH level is often useful when the thyroxine is in the low borderline range, since it is usually elevated in primary hypothyroidism. Furthermore, a very low TSH in the presence of a clearly low thyroxine suggests secondary hypothyroidism. Such patients should be referred to an endocrinologist for further evaluation of anterior pituitary function and treatment.

  b. **Treatment of primary hypothyroidism**
   (1) **Cretinism**
    (a) Sodium levothyroxine (Synthroid), 0.025 mg/day, increased at weekly or biweekly intervals to 0.3–0.4 mg/day, **or**
    (b) Thyroid (USP), 15 mg PO daily, gradually increased at weekly or biweekly intervals to about 90–180 mg/day.
   (2) **Adult hypothyroidism**
    (a) Sodium levothyroxine (Synthroid), 0.025 mg/day, increasing at weekly intervals to 0.1–0.2 mg/day, **or**
    (b) Thyroid (USP), 15 mg PO daily, gradually increased at weekly or biweekly intervals until the euthyroid state is achieved (usually about 90–180 mg/day).

      c. Treatment of secondary and tertiary hypothyroidism depends on detailed endocrine evaluation of pituitary and hypothalamic function, which is beyond the scope of this manual.

D. Toxic disorders

    1. Heavy metal poisoning. Several varieties of chronic heavy metal poisoning may be manifested with dementia, including poisoning by lead, mercury, arsenic, manganese, and thallium. The diagnosis and treatment of these conditions are discussed in Chap. 14.

    2. Drug intoxications

      a. Alcohol. Marchiafava-Bignami disease is a rare complication of alcohol abuse characterized pathologically by degeneration of the corpus callosum. The disease is indistinguishable clinically from the Alzheimer-Pick–type dementia. There is no specific therapy, but discontinuation of alcohol use is recommended to prevent further progression of the process.

      b. Medications. Many drugs are capable of producing mental deterioration suggestive of dementia. Most, however, produce a **toxic confusional state** easily distinguished from true dementia by such signs and symptoms as hallucinations, tachycardia, changes in blood pressure, diaphoresis, dysarthria, and nystagmus. Any patient with apparent dementia in whom drug use is suspected should have toxic screening of the urine and blood, depending on the agents suspected. Treatment of the common drug intoxications is discussed in Chap. 14.

V. Psychiatric diseases. A number of psychiatric illnesses may result in intellectual dysfunction caused by either interference with motivation or actual impairment of intellect, or both.

A. Depression may simulate dementia in many respects, including inability to carry out tests of intellectual function. A therapeutic trial of antidepressant medication is of little value diagnostically, since many patients with Alzheimer's disease may be depressed early in the course of the illness. A slight response to antidepressant therapy does not exclude the diagnosis of a degenerative dementing disease. On the other hand, a patient with an apparent dementia who actually is suffering only from depression may benefit greatly from the therapy and has a much better prognosis than the patient with a degenerative disease. It is often difficult clinically to distinguish depression from dementia, but some guidelines are valuable.

    1. Unlike most demented patients, depressed patients usually have insight that they are functioning poorly.

    2. Aphasias and apraxias often are seen in dementias but rarely in primary depression.

    3. Careful testing reveals no memory impairment in primary depression, in contrast to dementia.

    4. Incontinence is more common in dementia, although it may be seen in very severe depression as well.

B. Schizophrenia was originally called **dementia praecox** by Kraepelin, and it can, in fact, result in a dementing illness similar in many respects to Alzheimer's disease. Some guidelines for distinguishing between schizophrenia and Alzheimer's disease are:

    1. The **age of the patient** is of considerable value in making this distinction, but Alzheimer's disease does occur rarely in younger patients in the age group at risk for schizophrenia.

    2. Apraxias and aphasias, common components of Alzheimer's disease, are not seen in schizophrenia, but when these are absent the distinction may be more difficult than it initially seems.

    3. The **course of the illness** should help to make the distinction; the schizophrenia will wax and wane over many years, with only very slow deterioration of intellect, whereas Alzheimer's disease progresses inexorably, with development of unmistakable features within a few years.

Selected Readings

DEMENTIA

Bartus, R. T., et al. The Cholinergic Hypothesis: A Historical Overview, Current Perspective and Future Directions. In C. Olton, E. Gamzu, and S. Corkin (eds.), *Memory Dysfunctions: Integration of Animal and Human Research from Clinical and Preclinical Perspectives.* New York: New York Academy of Science, 1985. Pp. 332–358.

Black, P. M. Idiopathic normal pressure hydrocephalus: Results of shunting in 62 patients. *J. Neurosurg.* 52:371, 1980.

Borgesen, S. E., and Gjerris, F. The predictive value of conductance to outflow of CSF in normal pressure hydrocephalus. *Brain* 105:65, 1982.

Caplan, L. R., and Schoene, W. C. Clinical features of subcortical arteriosclerotic encephalopathy (Biswanger's disease). *Neurology* 28:1206, 1978.

Chedru, F., and Geschwind, N. Disorders of higher cortical function in acute confusional states. *Cortex* 8:395, 1972.

Cummings, J. L., and Benson, D. F. *Dementia: A Clinical Approach* (2nd ed.). Boston: Butterworth, 1992.

Davis, K. L., et al. A double-blind placebo-controlled multicenter study of tacrine for Alzheimer's disease. *N. Engl. J. Med.* 327:1253, 1992.

Drachman, D. A., et al. Memory decline in the aged: Treatment with lecithin and physostigmine. *Neurology* 32:944, 1982.

Ghikar, J., et al. Idazoxan treatment in progressive supranuclear palsy. *Neurology* 4:986, 1991.

Growdon, J. H., and Corkin, S. Neurochemical Approaches to the Treatment of Senile Dementia. In J. O. Cole and J. E. Barretts (eds.), *Psychopathology in the Aged.* New York: Raven, 1980. Pp. 281–296.

Hachinski, V. C., Lassen, N. A., and Marshall, J. Multi-infarct dementia: A cause of mental deterioration in the elderly. *Lancet* 2:207, 1974.

Hier, D. B., and Caplan, L. R. Drugs for senile dementia. *Drugs* 20:74, 1980.

Joachim, C. L., Morris, J. H., and Selkoe, D. J. Clinically diagnosed Alzheimer's disease: Autopsy results in 150 cases. *Ann. Neurol.* 24:50, 1988.

Katzman, R. Alzheimer's disease. *N. Engl. J. Med.* 314:964, 1986.

Martin, J. B., and Gusella, J. F. Huntington's disease: Pathogenesis and management. *N. Engl. J. Med.* 315:1267, 1986.

Meyer, J. S., et al. Pathogenesis of normal pressure hydrocephalus: Preliminary observations. *Surg. Neurol.* 23:121, 1985.

Risse, S. C., and Barnes, R. Pharmacologic treatment of agitation associated with dementia. *J. Am. Geriatr. Soc.* 34:368, 1986.

MENTAL RETARDATION

Barlow, C. F. *Mental Retardation and Related Disorders.* Philadelphia: Davis, 1978.

Breningstall, G. Approach to diagnosis of oxidative metabolism disorders. *Pediatr. Neurol.* 9:81, 1993.

Capute, A. J., et al. The Clinical Linguistic and Auditory Milestone Scale (CLAMS). *Am. J. Dis. Child.* 140:694, 1986.

Coplan, J. *ELM Scale: The Early Language Milestone Scale, Revised.* Austin, TX: Pro-Ed., 1987.

DeVivo, D. C., et al. Defective glucose transport across the blood-brain barrier as a cause of persistent hypoglycorrhachia, seizures and developmental delay. *N. Engl. J. Med.* 325:703, 1991.

Frankenburg, W. K., et al. The Denver II: A major revision and restandardization of the Denver Development Screening Test. *Pediatrics* 89:91, 1992.

Freeman, J. M., and Nelson, K. B. Intrapartum asphyxia and cerebral palsy. *Pediatrics* 84:240, 1988.

The Huntington's Disease Collaborative Research Group. A novel gene containing a trinucleotide repeat that is expanded and unstable on Huntington's disease chromosomes. *Cell* 72:971, 1993.

Kolodny, E. H., and Cable, W. J. L. Inborn errors of metabolism. *Ann. Neurol.* 11:221, 1982.

Luckasson, R. (ed.). *Mental Retardation: Definition, Classification and Systems of Support* (9th ed.). Washington, DC: American Association on Mental Retardation, 1992.

Naidu, S., and Moser, H. W. Peroxisomal disorders. *Neurol. Clin.* 8(3):507, 1990.

Schaefer, G. S., and Bodensteiner, J. B. Evaluation of the child with idiopathic mental retardation. *Pediatr. Clin. North Am.* 39(4):929, 1992.

Scriver, C. (ed.). *The Metabolic Basis of Inherited Disease* (6th ed.). New York: McGraw-Hill, 1989.

Smith, D. W. *Recognizable Patterns of Human Malformations*. Philadelphia: Saunders, 1982.

Tarleton, J. C., and Saul, R. A. Molecular genetic advances in fragile-X syndrome. *J. Pediatr.* 122:169, 1993.

Tulinias, M. H., et al. Mitochondrial encephalomyopathies in childhood: I. Biochemical and morphologic investigations. *J. Pediatr.* 119:242, 1991.

Tulinias, M. H., et al. Mitochondrial encephalomyopathies in childhood: II. Clinical manifestations and syndromes. *J. Pediatr.* 119:251, 1991.

Wappner, R. S. Biochemical diagnosis of genetic diseases. *Pediatr. Ann.* 22:282, 1993.

Dizziness

Howard D. Weiss

Dizziness is one of the most common complaints for which people seek medical attention. Yet, many physicians are uncomfortable and distraught when they learn that their next patient is complaining of dizziness. This attitude reflects the bewildering variety of disorders in the realms of neurology, otology, cardiology, ophthalmology, psychiatry, and medicine that cause "dizziness." The logical evaluation of the dizzy patient and treatment of the disorders that cause dizziness will be reviewed in this chapter (Figs. 4-1 and 4-2).

I. **Definitions. Dizziness** is an ambiguous term that patients use to describe several entirely different subjective states. Therefore, the first step in differential diagnosis is to obtain an accurate description of the patient's subjective experience using words more descriptive than *dizzy*. The complaint of dizziness generally can be divided into one of four categories:

A. **Vertigo** is defined as an **illusion of movement** of the patient or the patient's surroundings. The vertiginous sensation may be described as **rotating, spinning, tilting,** or **swaying.** Acute vertigo is often accompanied by autonomic symptoms (e.g., nausea, vomiting, diaphoresis, apprehension), disequilibrium (imbalance), and nystagmus (which may cause blurred vision). The presence of vertigo implies a disturbance in the peripheral or CNS pathways of the vestibular system.

B. **Syncope** or **presyncope** implies a sense of **impending loss of consciousness** or fainting. This is often accompanied by diaphoresis, nausea, apprehension, and transient bilateral visual loss. Syncope occurs when cerebral perfusion falls below the level required to supply adequate oxygen and glucose to the brain. Syncope or presyncope generally implies hypotension, autonomic reflex, or cardiac dysfunction (see Fig. 4-1) and has entirely different implications than vertigo.

C. **Disequilibrium** is a sense of imbalance, unsteadiness, or "drunkenness" *without* vertigo which occurs in patients who have a mismatch of inputs from the systems subserving spatial orientation. Patients with vestibular, proprioceptive, cerebellar, visual, or extrapyramidal system disorders often will refer to their sense of disequilibrium as dizziness.

D. **Ill-defined dizziness** occurs in patients suffering from various **emotional disorders,** including hyperventilation syndrome, anxiety neurosis, hysterical neurosis, and depression. The complaint is usually of a vague light-headedness, giddiness, or fear of falling that is distinct from the vertigo, presyncope, or disequilibrium described above. However, it is important to realize that all forms of dizziness may provoke considerable patient anxiety and that anxiety itself is *not* the sine qua non of psychogenic dizziness.

E. Some patients have difficulty in adequately describing their dizzy sensation. In this group, it is useful to put the patient through a series of maneuvers that can trigger various types of dizziness.

1. Some of the **standard dizziness simulation tests** include
   a. Checking for orthostatic hypotension.
   b. Vigorous hyperventilation for 3 minutes.
   c. Sudden turns when walking or spinning the patient while standing.
   d. The Nylen-Bárány test for positional vertigo, which can trigger acute attacks of vertigo and nystagmus (see sec. **III.B**).
   e. Valsalva maneuvers, which can exacerbate vertigo associated with craniover-

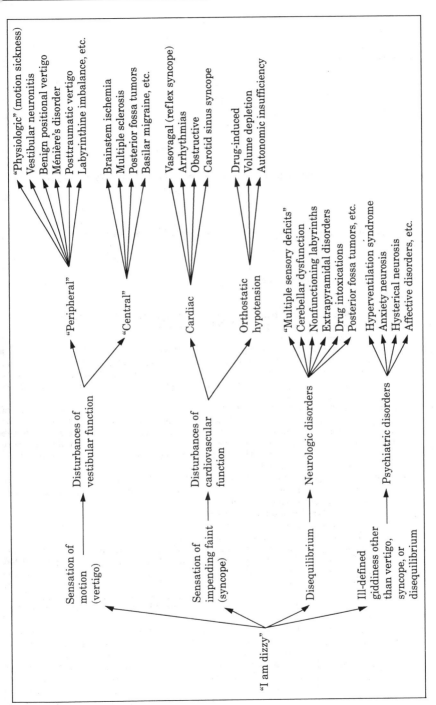

Fig. 4-1. Clinical spectrum of dizziness.

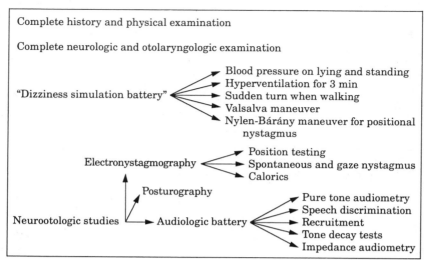

Fig. 4-2. Clinical evaluation of the dizzy patient.

tebral junction anomalies (e.g., Chiari malformation) or perilymph fistula as well as induce presyncopal light-headedness in patients with cardiovascular disease.

2. **After each maneuver,** the patient is asked whether the sensation of dizziness (if any) matches the spontaneous complaint. In cases of orthostatic hypotension, hyperventilation syndrome, positional vertigo, and related vestibular disorders, the patient's symptom may be reproduced, thereby providing important diagnostic information.

II. **Clinical evaluation of patients with vertigo.** Evaluation requires an understanding of vestibular system interactions with the oculomotor, auditory, and spinocerebellar systems. There are two basic vestibular system reflexes. The **vestibulooocular reflexes** stabilize the position of the eye with respect to space so that images remain stationary on the retina for best acuity. The **vestibulospinal reflexes** stabilize head and body position for motor control and for remaining upright.

A. **Nystagmus** is a useful indicator of vestibular malfunction in patients with vertigo. Review of a few simple physiologic principles will help reduce the mystique that often clouds the interpretation of nystagmus.

1. **Semicircular canal-ocular reflexes.** Each semicircular canal is connected via neuronal circuitry in the brainstem to the eye muscles in such a way that inhibition of a canal results in eye movement toward the plane of that canal. Conversely, excitation of the canal results in eye movement away from the plane of that canal. The semicircular canals and otolith organs in the right and left inner ears normally send continuous equal and opposite messages to the brainstem. However, a sudden inequality in the vestibulooocular pathway input will result in a slow vestibular-induced eye deviation that is interrupted by a quick cortically controlled corrective movement in the opposite direction **(nystagmus).**

2. **Labyrinthine disorders** generally produce inhibition of one or more semicircular canals. Consequently, acute *unilateral* peripheral vestibular disorders produce unidirectional nystagmus, with the slow phase moving toward the affected ear, and the rapid phase beating away from the affected ear. The nystagmus is rotary or horizontal; it increases in intensity as the eyes are deviated in the direction of the rapid component (i.e., toward the normal ear). Patients are often uncertain regarding the direction of their vertiginous illusion. It is often helpful to evaluate

the perceived direction of rotation with the patient's eyes closed. Patients with acute vestibular disorders experience vertigo as a sensation that the environment is spinning in the direction of the fast component of the nystagmus or that their bodies are spinning in the direction of the slow component. They tend to past point and veer in the direction of the slow phase of their nystagmus (i.e., toward the malfunctioning ear).

   3. **Central nystagmus.** Multidirectional nystagmus (nystagmus that changes direction with different directions of gaze) is more common with drug intoxications or brainstem-posterior fossa disorders. Vertical nystagmus (upbeat or downbeat) is almost pathognomonic of brainstem or midline cerebellar disorders.

B. **Caloric stimulation.** Normal physiologic stimuli always affect both vestibular organs at the same time. Caloric stimulation is a convenient clinical method of investigating the function of each labyrinth separately. The test is performed with the patient recumbent with the head flexed 30 degrees. Cool water induces a flow of endolymph that inhibits the neural impulses from the horizontal canal on that side. This normally results in nausea and vertigo accompanied by horizontal nystagmus, with the slow component toward the side of cool-water stimulation and the fast component in the opposite direction. These manifestations of cold-water irrigation are identical to the effects of unilateral vestibular hypofunction (e.g., vestibular neuronitis and labyrinthitis).

   The direction, duration, and amplitude of the nystagmus should be observed carefully. A reduced response in one ear implies a disorder in the vestibular labyrinths, vestibular nerve, or the vestibular nuclei on that side. The test should not be performed unless the tympanic membranes are intact.

C. **Electronystagmography.** The retina is electronegative to the cornea; thus, eye movements cause changing electric fields and currents. Electronystagmography (ENG) involves placing, on the skin around the eyes, electrodes that can detect these changes and provide a means for objectively recording eye movements. The ENG provides quantitative data regarding direction, velocity, and duration of the eye movements in nystagmus. **Vestibular function tests** use ENG to record spontaneous nystagmus, positional nystagmus, rotation-induced nystagmus, and caloric-induced nystagmus. ENG can also record nystagmus when the eyes are closed. Since ocular fixation often tends to suppress nystagmus, ENG recording with the eyes closed sometimes provides additional information that is not available on routine clinical examination.

D. **Hearing loss or tinnitus** can occur in disorders of the peripheral vestibular system (inner ear and eighth nerve) due to coinvolvement of the auditory apparatus. Auditory symptoms seldom accompany CNS disorders. Audiologic testing often provides useful diagnostic information in patients with vertigo.

   1. **Pure tone audiometry** measures the listener's threshold of hearing as a function of the frequency and intensity of a sound stimulus. The threshold by **air conduction** is compared with that by **bone conduction** to distinguish conductive versus sensorineural hearing loss.

   2. Additional evaluations that contribute to complete audiologic assessment include a speech discrimination, speech reception, recruitment, and tone decay (Table 4-1).

E. **Moving platform posturography tests** measure the automatic postural responses that are used to prevent falls and quantify the ability of patients to use various sensory cues to maintain balance.

F. Vestibular function tests, ENG, and posturography are expensive procedures. These tests do not replace the careful clinical examination of patients with vertigo and are *not* necessary to arrive at a diagnosis or treatment strategy in the vast majority of patients with dizziness.

III. **Diagnosis and treatment of diseases causing vertigo** (Table 4-2). Vestibular neuronitis and benign positional vertigo are the two most common causes of acute vertigo and account for the majority of cases of vertigo seen in clinical practice.

A. **Vestibular neuronitis** (also known as acute peripheral vestibulopathy or vestibular neuritis)

   1. **Description.** Vestibular neuronitis is characterized by a sudden prolonged attack of **vertigo**, often accompanied by nausea, vomiting, disequilibrium, and appre-

Table 4-1. Audiologic evaluation of cochlear and retrocochlear disorders

Test	Cochlear lesions	Retrocochlear (eighth nerve) lesions
Pure tone audiometry	Sensorineural hearing loss	Sensorineural hearing loss
Speech discrimination	Good	Poor
Recruitment	Yes	No
Stapedial reflex	Normal	Impaired
Tone decay	No	Yes
Clinical examples	Ménière's syndrome	Acoustic schwannoma

hension. The symptoms are exacerbated by head movement or changes in position. Patients feel severely ill and prefer to stay motionless in bed. Spontaneous **nystagmus** occurs, with the slow phase toward the abnormal ear, and there is reduced caloric excitability in the diseased ear. Positional nystagmus is present in many patients. **Tinnitus** or a sensation of fullness in the ear occurs in some patients. Hearing remains unimpaired, and audiologic tests are normal. Except for unsteadiness, there are no neurologic signs (e.g., focal weakness, diplopia, dysarthria, sensory loss) to suggest brainstem disease. The disorder affects adults of any age. The acute vertigo usually resolves spontaneously over several hours but may recur over the ensuing days or weeks. Some patients experience residual impairment of vestibular function, which produces a state of chronic disequilibrium that is most noticeable when the patient is moving. Follow-up studies reveal that about half the patients will have recurrent episodes of vertigo months to years later. The cause of vestibular neuronitis remains unknown. A viral etiology (similar to that producing Bell's palsy) has been postulated, but this has not been proved. This disorder is a clinical syndrome rather than a well-defined disease. Careful neurologic and neurootologic examination, as outlined, indicates a peripheral disorder in patients with vestibular neuronitis and rules out the more ominous central disorders.

   2. Treatment
      a. Drugs. Since vestibular neuronitis is a self-limited illness of unknown cause, treatment is directed at suppressing the symptoms. The drugs listed in Table 4-3 have some effectiveness in suppressing vertigo due to vestibular neuronitis, motion sickness, or other vestibular disorders. When nausea is a severe problem, the antivertigo drugs can be administered by suppository or parenterally. Hospitalization may be necessary for patients with profound disequilibrium or intractable vomiting requiring intravenous rehydration.

Table 4-2. Common disorders producing acute attacks of vertigo

Vestibular etiology
   "Physiologic" (e.g., motion sickness, height vertigo)
   Vestibular neuronitis (acute peripheral vestibulopathy)
   Labyrinthitis
   Benign positional vertigo
   Ménière's syndrome
   Labyrinthine imbalance
   Posttraumatic vertigo
   Perilymphatic fistula
Central etiology
   Brainstem transient ischemic attacks
   Multiple sclerosis
   Basilar artery migraine
   Posterior fossa tumors

Table 4-3. Drugs useful in the symptomatic treatment of vertigo

Generic name	Trade name	Duration of activity (hr)	Usual oral adult dosage	Relative levels of sedation	Other modes of administration
Cyclizine	Marezine	4–6	50 mg q6h	+	IM
Dimenhydrinate	Dramamine	4–6	25–50 mg q6h	+ +	Rectal, IM, IV
Diphenhydramine	Benadryl	4–6	25–50 mg q6h	+ +	IM, IV
Meclizine	Bonine, Antivert	12–24	12.5–25.0 mg q8–12h	+	
Promethazine	Phenergan	4–6	25 mg q6h	+ +	Rectal, IM, IV
Scopolamine	Transderm Scōp	72 (transdermal)	0.5 mg	+	PO, SC, IV
Hydroxyzine	Vistaril	4–6	25–100 mg tid	+ +	IM
Ephedrine		4–6	25 mg q6h	0	IM

(1) Antihistamines

    (a) Mechanism of action. Suppression of vertigo is not a general property of all antihistamines and does not seem to correlate with their peripheral potency as histamine antagonists. The activity of those antihistamines that do counteract vertigo (dimenhydrinate, diphenhydramine, meclizine, and cyclizine) seems specific and not simply a matter of suppression of the brainstem vomiting center; in fact, many commonly used antiemetics are of little value in relieving patients with vertigo. The antivertigo antihistamines also exert anticholinergic activity in the CNS. The central anticholinergic property may be the underlying biochemical mechanism of antivertigo activity.

    (b) Side effects. The major side effect of these agents is **sedation.** The ability to induce somnolence is somewhat more pronounced during therapy with dimenhydrinate or diphenhydramine. In severely vertiginous patients, sedation may be a desirable side effect. However, for patients who do not desire as much sedation, meclizine or cyclizine is preferable.

    Anticholinergic side effects, such as **dry mouth** or **blurred vision,** occasionally occur with these drugs. The relatively long half-life of meclizine enables the patient to take medication only once or twice per day, compared with 3 or more times per day with other drugs.

(2) Anticholinergic drugs that are centrally active suppress vestibular system activity and can be useful in reducing vertigo. An adhesive unit containing **scopolamine** for **transdermal** administration is available. This drug delivery system is programmed to release 0.5 mg of scopolamine directly into the bloodstream through the skin over a period of 72 hours. This small amount of drug is effective against motion sickness and may help in the symptomatic treatment of vestibular neuronitis and other vertiginous conditions. The combination of scopolamine with promethazine or ephedrine may have useful synergistic effects. The **side effects** (parasympathetic blockade) and contraindications for scopolamine therapy are similar to those for other belladonna alkaloids. Scopolamine should be used with great caution in elderly patients for fear of triggering mental confusion or bladder outlet obstruction.

(3) Phenothiazines comprise a large group of drugs with antiemetic effects. Not all antiemetics are effective antimotion sickness or antivertigo agents. For example, chlorpromazine (Thorazine) and prochlorperazine (Compazine) are highly effective against chemically induced nausea but are much less effective against motion sickness and vertigo. However, one widely used phenothiazine derivative, **promethazine** (Phenergan), also has significant antihistaminic properties. Promethazine has been the most effective phenothiazine for treating vertigo and motion sickness, ranking with the other antihistamines listed in Table 4-3. **Drowsiness** is the major limiting side effect of promethazine; it is much less likely to induce acute dystonias or other extrapyramidal reactions than the other phenothiazines.

(4) Sympathomimetic agents also suppress vertigo.

    (a) Amphetamine has been used in combination with promethazine or scopolamine to prevent vertigo and motion sickness in astronauts. However, amphetamine is a controlled substance due to its great drug-abuse potential and cannot be prescribed to patients with vestibular neuronitis.

    (b) Ephedrine is another sympathomimetic agent that has synergistic action when combined with other antivertigo drugs. The stimulant effects of ephedrine may combat the sedative effects of other drugs but can also cause insomnia, nervousness, and palpitations.

(5) Mild tranquilizers such as diazepam or lorazepam are helpful in alleviating the acute **anxiety** that often accompanies vertigo. Hydroxyzine is a tranquilizer that also has antihistaminic and antiemetic properties, giving it therapeutic value against vertigo. The usual adult dosage of hydroxyzine is 25–100 mg tid–qid.

(6) The duration of treatment is variable. In most patients, medications can be discontinued when the nausea and vertigo have subsided. Experimentally, the vestibular sedative medications retard central compensatory mechanisms, so that prolonged use of these drugs may be counterproductive. Nevertheless, there are some patients who require small doses of medication on a chronic basis to remain comfortable. Patients who do not experience symptomatic relief with one antivertigo medication may respond well to a different medication. The number of medications available is indicative of the fact that none is completely satisfactory. Combinations of medications from different classes (e.g., an anticholinergic with a sympathomimetic) may have synergistic effects in suppressing vertigo.

b. Other measures. The patient can perform simple maneuvers to lessen the sensation of vertigo.

(1) Since head motion aggravates vertigo, the patient should be allowed to lie still in a darkened room for the first day or two.

(2) Visual fixation tends to inhibit nystagmus and diminish the subjective feeling of vertigo in patients with peripheral vestibular disorders, such as vestibular neuronitis. Patients may find that fixing their gaze on a nearby object, such as a picture or outstretched finger, is preferable to lying with closed eyes.

(3) Since intellectual activity or mental concentration may facilitate vertigo, the discomfort is best minimized by **mental relaxation** coupled with intense visual fixation.

(4) When nausea and vomiting are severe, intravenous fluids should be administered to prevent dehydration.

(5) When vertigo is not relieved. Many patients with acute peripheral vestibular disorders will not have dramatic symptomatic improvement in the first day or two. The patient feels acutely ill and may become extremely fearful of future attacks. An important aspect of therapy in this situation is a firm statement of **reassurance** that vestibular neuronitis and most of the other acute vestibular disorders are **benign and self-limited conditions.** The physician can tell the patient that the nervous system eventually adapts to an imbalance between the two vestibular end organs, and the vertigo ultimately stops. Even in disorders that permanently destroy one vestibular apparatus, the vertigo will diminish after several days as the brain begins to adapt. Such assurances greatly alleviate the patient's apprehension.

(6) Vestibular exercises can be initiated several days after the acute symptoms have subsided. These exercises enhance CNS compensatory mechanisms for acute vestibular disturbances (see sec. III.L.2).

B. Benign positional vertigo (benign paroxysmal positional vertigo)

1. Description. Benign positional vertigo is probably the most common vestibular syndrome seen in clinical practice. Patients with this disorder do not have vertigo while sitting or standing still but find that attacks are precipitated by movement or position change in the head or body. This is particularly true if the movements are in the pitch (forward-backward) plane. This commonly occurs when the patient lays back in bed and rolls over into the vulnerable position, at which time the "room begins to spin." The vertigo usually lasts only a few seconds. Observant patients can often identify a head position that reproducibly triggers the symptoms.

Changes in head position aggravate vertigo in vestibular neuronitis and many other peripheral or central vestibular disorders. However, patients with benign positional vertigo develop symptoms *only* after the appropriate head movement and not at other times.

2. Distinction from positional vertigo of central disorders. Positional vertigo can also occur in a variety of conditions, including serious **brainstem disorders** (e.g., multiple sclerosis, infarct, tumors).

a. The **Nylen-Bárány maneuvers** help distinguish benign positional nystagmus from more ominous central conditions and is an important part of the clinical examination of the vertiginous patient. The test is performed by moving the patient from the sitting position to a lying position with the head extended 45 degrees backward. This maneuver is repeated with the head extended and turned to the right and then to the left. The patient is observed for the development of nystagmus and vertigo.

b. The **latency, duration, direction,** and **fatigability** of the nystagmus reveal important diagnostic information (Table 4-4). In benign positional vertigo there is a latency period of several seconds before the vertigo and nystagmus appear. Rotary nystagmus is seen, with the rapid phase beating toward the undermost ear. The nystagmus and vertigo are transitory (< 30 seconds) and disappear on repetition of the provocative maneuver ("fatigue").

The Nylen Bárány maneuvers can confirm the diagnosis of benign positional vertigo. A "negative" test does not exclude the diagnosis, since the symptoms can be intermittent and do not necessarily recur every time the head is placed in the vulnerable position.

3. **Etiology.** Some cases of benign positional vertigo follow **head trauma, viral illnesses,** middle ear infection, or stapedectomy. Positional nystagmus is also common in intoxications (alcohol, barbiturates). Most spontaneous cases of benign positional vertigo are attributed to **cupulolithiasis**: degenerated otoconial deposits that settle on the cupula of the posterior semicircular canal. This makes the canal very sensitive to the changes in gravity associated with different head positions.

4. **Course.** The course of benign positional vertigo is quite variable. In many patients, the symptoms spontaneously subside in a few weeks, only to recur months or years later. Some patients suffer only a single transient attack. Only seldom do patients retain a persistent susceptibility to positional vertigo that does not abate.

5. **Treatment.** Symptomatic treatment with one of the vestibular sedative drugs (see Table 4-3) is seldom of great benefit. Deliberately carrying out those movements that provoke vertigo will eventually "fatigue" the symptomatic response. Some physicians suggest that a remission of symptoms in benign positional vertigo can be accelerated by **head exercises** of this type. Patients are instructed to tilt their head into the position that triggers vertigo for 30 seconds. This is repeated 5 times every few hours. This simple physical approach will relieve the majority of cases.

Table 4-4. Nylen-Bárány maneuver for positional nystagmus

Sign	Peripheral (vestibular) disorder	Brainstem–posterior fossa disorder
Latent period before onset of positional nystagmus	2–20 sec.	None
Duration of nystagmus	< 30 sec	> 30 sec
Fatigability	Nystagmus disappears with repetition of maneuver	Nystagmus recurs on repeating the maneuver
Direction of nystagmus in one head position	One direction	May change direction in a given head position
Intensity of vertigo	Severe	Slight or none
Head position	A single critical head position elicits vertigo	More than one position
Clinical examples	Benign positional vertigo	Acoustic neuroma, vertebrobasilar ischemia, multiple sclerosis

within several weeks. Some patients who find the head exercises too unpleasant may experience symptomatic improvement by wearing a soft cervical collar; presumably the collar limits head movement so that the patient will be less likely to place his or her head in the provocative posture. As with vestibular neuronitis, often the most important aspect of therapy is **reassuring the patient** that the condition is self-limited and, although extremely unpleasant, does not represent a life-threatening illness. Surgical sectioning of the ampullary nerve from the posterior semicircular canal on the diseased side has been palliative for the very rare case of refractory severe positional vertigo.

C. **Posttraumatic vertigo.** Although protected by a bony capsule, the delicate labyrinthine membranes are susceptible to trauma. Uncomplicated concussions are followed by vertigo in over 20% of patients. (It should be remembered that transient autonomic disturbances, such as palpitations, flushing, and sweating, also occur after head trauma and can produce light-headed and dizzy sensations other than vertigo.) The posttraumatic vertigo syndromes fall into two main categories.

1. **Acute posttraumatic vertigo. Vertigo, nausea,** and **vomiting** may begin acutely after head injury, due to sudden unilateral vestibular paresis **(labyrinthine concussion).** Laceration of the tympanic membrane with blood in the external auditory canal or hemotympanum suggests a longitudinal or transverse fracture of the temporal bone, respectively. However, most cases of acute posttraumatic vertigo are not associated with temporal bone fracture.

   a. **Symptoms.** The vertigo is persistent. There is spontaneous **nystagmus** with the rapid component beating away from the affected side, loss of balance, and past pointing toward the affected side. The symptoms and signs are aggravated by rapid head motion and worsened with the affected side down.

   b. **Treatment.** One of the **vestibular sedative drugs** (see Table 4-3) is often effective in diminishing the unpleasant symptoms. For the acute episode, **scopolamine** is often most efficacious. For long-term oral therapy, both **meclizine** and **dimenhydrinate** have been widely used. The symptoms spontaneously improve over the first few days and then more gradually over the ensuing weeks. In most patients, the symptoms resolve within 1–3 months.

2. **Posttraumatic positional vertigo.** Several days or weeks after the injury, the patient may experience recurrent brief attacks of vertigo triggered by changes in head position.

   a. **Symptoms.** The symptoms are identical to those outlined for benign positional vertigo. The patient develops sudden **brief attacks of vertigo** and **nausea** precipitated by changing head position.

   b. **Prognosis.** The prognosis in posttraumatic positional vertigo is usually very good, and most patients undergo spontaneous remission within 2 months, and almost all within 2 years of the injury.

3. **Perilymph fistula.** The perilymph space surrounds the endolymph-filled membranous labyrinth. Head trauma can produce a tear in the region of the oval or round window, causing a perilymph fistula. When a fistula is present, changes in middle ear pressure will directly affect the inner ear.

   a. **Symptoms.** Patients with this problem will experience **intermittent vertigo** or **positional vertigo,** fluctuating sensorineural **hearing loss,** or both. Most patients with a fistula find that their symptoms are exacerbated by changes in altitude (e.g., rapid ascent in an elevator) or with activities that induce a Valsalva maneuver (e.g., straining, weight lifting). Some patients will experience vertigo on exposure to loud sounds (the Tullio phenomenon). In fact, straining, sneezing, coughing, and diving **(barometric trauma)** are other potential causes of perilymphatic fistulas.

   b. The **diagnosis** is suggested by the history of vestibular or auditory symptoms following trauma. The signs and symptoms of perilymph fistula can be highly variable and can be confused with other disorders (e.g., Ménière's syndrome, benign positional vertigo, abnormalities at the craniovertebral junction). Tests monitoring the response to external pressure changes, ENG, and posturography do not generally reveal pathognomonic abnormalities. Perilymph fistula may account for many cases of vertigo of unknown etiology.

   c. Treatment. Perilymph fistulas usually heal spontaneously, and as a conse quence, the symptoms resolve. Surgical exploration through tympanotomy t find and repair a perilymphatic fistula of the oval or round window may b indicated in refractory cases where a fistula is strongly suspected. If a fistul is found at surgery, it can be patched. Surgical interventions are more likely to reduce vestibular symptoms than improve hearing loss.

D. Ménière's syndrome (Ménière's disease)

  1. Description. Ménière's syndrome commonly has its onset in the third or fourth decade of life. The patient experiences spontaneous **bouts of intense vertig** lasting for minutes to hours. Fullness or **pressure in the ear, tinnitus, an** fluctuating **hearing loss** usually precede, but may follow, the episodes of vertigo A state of **chronic disequilibrium** that is particularly noticeable when the patient is in motion can persist between acute attacks.

  2. The **course** of the disease is characterized by **remissions** and **relapses.** Early in the disease, there are often sporadic episodes of low-tone sensorineural hearing loss, with hearing returning to normal between attacks. As a result of multiple attacks, hearing loss becomes progressively worse, with some spontaneous fluctuations.

  3. Pathophysiology. The main pathologic finding in patients with Ménière's syndrome is a **distention** and increase in the volume of endolymphatic system **(endolymphatic hydrops).** This may result from insufficient fluid resorption in the endolymphatic sac or acquired blockage of the endolymphatic duct.

  4. Treatment. Acute attacks are treated with bed rest and vestibular sedative medications (see Table 4-3). In view of the uncertainty regarding the pathogenesis, together with the variable course (which may include prolonged remissions), it has been difficult to formulate or evaluate a rational pharmacologic program for the prevention of attacks of Ménière's syndrome. One recent study found that all forms of treatment, including placebos, resulted in approximately two-thirds of patients being temporarily relieved of their symptoms.

    A **low-sodium diet** and the use of **diuretics** (e.g., thiazides or acetazolamide) have been recommended in Ménière's syndrome, on the basis of the theory that these might correct fluid imbalance in the inner ear. The physiologic rationale for this therapy has never been demonstrated, and the popularity of diuretic–low-salt therapy has declined. Tranquilizers, neuroleptics, lithium, stellate ganglion blocks, and vasodilators (including nicotinic acid, isoxsuprine, papaverine, intravenous histamine) have been tried, but **none of these agents is superior to placebo.** The histamine derivative betahistine may have some modest benefit in preventing attacks of Ménière's syndrome.

  5. Surgery for intractable disease. A small number of patients with Ménière's syndrome will have recurrent uncontrollable and disabling attacks of vertigo. In these severe refractory cases, surgery may be necessary. **There is no "ideal" surgical treatment** for Ménière's syndrome. Cochlear endolymphatic sac shunt operations alleviate vertigo in 70% of patients, but there is a 45% incidence of increased hearing loss after this procedure. Intratympanic or systemic treatment with ototoxic drugs (e.g., gentamicin or streptomycin) may prevent acute vertigo but result in persistent disequilibrium and increased hearing loss. Destructive procedures (such as selective transtemporal vestibular nerve section, labyrinthectomy, or translabyrinthine vestibularectomy) are reserved for patients with persistent disabling vertigo and severe unilateral hearing loss.

  6. Differential diagnosis

    a. All patients with clinical signs and symptoms of Ménière's disease should be evaluated to exclude the possibility of a **cerebellopontine angle tumor** (e.g., acoustic schwannoma; see sec. **IV.C**). These tumors cause tinnitus, hearing loss, and disequilibrium but rarely cause acute vertigo.

    b. Infectious labyrinthitis, perilymph fistula, Cogan's syndrome, and hyperviscosity syndrome can produce attacks of vertigo, hearing loss, or both.

    c. Congenital syphilis. The onset of labyrinthine symptoms in congenital syphilis is often delayed to middle age and can mimic Ménière's syndrome. Treponemal organisms persisting in the temporal bone produce a chronic inflammatory process with endolymphatic hydrops and labyrinthine degeneration. The course is progressive, and both ears ultimately are involved. All patients suspected of having bilateral Ménière's syndrome should be evaluated for the possibility of **occult syphilis.** A fluorescent treponemal antibody absorption (FTA-ABS) test should be obtained since the routine screening tests (e.g., rapid plasma reagin or VDRL) may be negative in syphilitic labyrinthitis.

E. Labyrinthitis
  1. Bacterial labyrinthitis. Bacterial infection of the middle ear or mastoid, such as chronic otitis media, can produce toxins that inflame the cochlea, vestibular system, or both **(serous labyrinthitis).** The symptoms may be indolent at first but will gradually worsen if the infection is not treated. Direct bacterial infection of the labyrinth **(suppurative labyrinthitis)** can occur in patients who have bacterial meningitis or anatomic disruption of the membranes separating the middle and inner ears. Fulminant vertigo, nausea, hearing loss, headache, pain, and fever are present. Suppurative labyrinthitis is a potentially devastating condition. Prompt diagnosis and administration of appropriate antibiotics are imperative (see Chap. 8).

  2. Viral labyrinthitis. Audiovestibular symptoms can occur in association with common viral illnesses, including influenza, herpes virus, rubella, mumps, hepatitis, rubeola, and Epstein-Barr virus. Most patients improve spontaneously without permanent hearing or balance problems.

F. Physiologic vertigo syndromes. A mismatch among inputs from the vestibular, visual, and somatosensory systems that help maintain spatial orientation can result in vertigo. Vertigo can also be induced by physiologic stimulation of the normal stabilizing sensory systems.

  1. Motion sickness is caused by **unfamiliar body accelerations** or a **mismatch** between conflicting vestibular and visual stimuli to the brain. Persons in a closed ship cabin or the rear seat of a moving automobile perceive vestibular signals of acceleration that are contradicted by visual signals of a relatively stationary environment. The intensity of the ensuing nausea and vertigo is a function of the magnitude of the sensory mismatch. Motion sickness is reduced when ample peripheral vision of the true surroundings is provided. The medications listed in Table 4-3 are all effective in suppressing motion sickness when taken prophylactically.

  2. Vision-induced vertigo is caused by visual sensations of movement without concomitant vestibular and somatosensory inputs (e.g., as when one is watching movies of an automobile chase).

  3. Vertigo at heights is a common physiologic phenomenon that occurs when the distance between the subject and visible stationary objects in the environment becomes critically large. Many people have an immediate conditioned phobic reaction to heights that prevents adaptation to the physiologic visual-vestibular mismatch.

G. Transient brainstem ischemia
  1. Description
    a. Symptoms
      (1) Vertigo and **disequilibrium** are the most frequent symptoms in patients with vertebrobasilar disease and transient episodes of brainstem ischemia. However, these will seldom be the **only** symptoms of transient brainstem ischemia. It is usually erroneous to attribute recurrent episodes of vertigo to "vertebrobasilar insufficiency" unless some other manifestation of brainstem ischemia is present, such as **diplopia, dysarthria, facial or limb numbness, ataxia, hemiparesis, Horner's syndrome,** or **hemianopia.** As a general rule, repeated episodes of vertigo without other neurologic symptoms can be attributed to a peripheral vestibulopathy.
      (2) Unsteadiness and vague blurring of vision can accompany vestibular neuronitis as well as brainstem causes of vertigo and thus does not have localizing value. Acute hearing loss is not encountered in brainstem

vascular disease, with the rare exception of occlusion of the anterior inferior cerebellar artery (which may supply the inner ear via the internal auditory artery).

b. Differential diagnosis

(1) It is extremely **important** to distinguish patients with episodes of transient brainstem ischemia from patients with "benign" disorders, such as vestibular neuronitis, in order to initiate therapy to avert a serious **brainstem stroke** (see Chap. 10).

(2) Patients with transient brainstem ischemia will have an **absence of signs of residual damage between attacks.** However, careful neurologic examination during an attack of vertigo can reveal subtle signs (e.g., mild Horner's syndrome, skew deviation, internuclear ophthalmoplegia, vertical nystagmus, or "central" direction-changing nystagmus) that clearly localize the abnormality to the brainstem and not to the vestibular apparatus. **Positional nystagmus** is often elicited in patients with brainstem ischemia. The **Nylen Bárány maneuvers** may be helpful in distinguishing brainstem from vestibular disorders (see Table 4-4).

2. The **treatment** of transient brainstem ischemia is reviewed in Chap. 10. Other disorders affecting the brainstem, such as multiple sclerosis (Chap. 13) and tumors (Chap. 11), also commonly produce vertigo or disequilibrium.

H. Cerebellar infarction and hemorrhage

1. Clinical presentation. Patients with acute cerebellar infarction (or hemorrhage) in the territory of the posterior inferior cerebellar artery can present with severe vertigo and imbalance that can easily be mistaken for acute vestibular neuronitis. Dysarthria, Horner's syndrome, numbness, facial paresis, and other signs of lateral medullary dysfunction may not be present if the stroke is confined to the cerebellar hemisphere. Infarcts in the territory of the superior cerebellar artery cause disequilibrium of gait and limb ataxia without prominent vertigo.

2. Diagnosis. A high index of suspicion is necessary. Imbalance with a tendency to veer to the affected side occurs in both vestibular and cerebellar hemisphere dysfunction and is not helpful in differential diagnosis. Central nystagmus (e.g., direction-changing nystagmus with the rapid phase to the right on right gaze and to the left on left gaze) and hemiataxia of the limbs are subtle clinical clues of an acute cerebellar hemisphere infarct (or hemorrhage). A CT scan may *not* be adequate to demonstrate an infarct, particularly if done early after the onset of symptoms, but will visualize cerebellar hematomas. An MRI study is more likely to reveal the presence of a cerebellar infarct.

3. Course. Cerebellar infarcts and hematomas are often not massive and have a benign outcome: The patient gradually improves and is left with minimal sequelae. However, larger lesions are associated with cerebellar edema that can compress the brainstem and fourth ventricle, producing devastating consequences. These complications can be prevented (dehydration to prevent edema) or treated (surgical decompression), so it is important that patients with cerebellar infarctions or hemorrhages be promptly diagnosed and closely monitored throughout the acute phase of their illness.

I. Oscillopsia is the illusion that stationary objects are moving to and fro. The syndrome of oscillopsia, downbeat nystagmus, postural instability, and vertigo has been associated with disorders at the craniovertebral junction (e.g., cerebellar ectopia, Arnold-Chiari malformation) and cerebellar degenerations (e.g., olivopontocerebellar atrophy, multiple sclerosis). **Baclofen,** a putative gamma-aminobutyric acid agonist, can suppress the oscillopsia in these disorders and in other conditions causing "periodic alternating nystagmus." The usual baclofen dosage is 10–20 mg tid. The benzodiazepine clonazepam may also palliate some patients with brainstem-cerebellar disorders causing oscillopsia.

J. Vestibular epilepsy. Vertigo can occur as a predominant symptom in simple or complex partial seizures arising from cortical areas that receive vestibular projections (the superior temporal gyrus or parietal association areas). Tinnitus, nystagmus, and contralateral paresthesias may accompany the vertigo. The attacks are brief and can easily be mistaken for other causes of vertigo. Most patients will also experience "absences" or other more typical manifestations of temporal lobe epilepsy. Abnormalities on the EEG will help confirm the diagnosis. The seizures can be managed with anticonvulsant medication or resection of an underlying focal brain lesion.

K. Migraine (see also Chap. 2 sec. II.)

1. **Symptoms.** Vertigo can be a prominent symptom in attacks of **basilar artery migraine.** Concomitant visual symptoms, sensory symptoms, altered sensorium, and intense headache are also present during attacks.

2. **Diagnosis.** Recurrent vertigo in the absence of other symptoms may be a **migraine equivalent.** This is a diagnosis of exclusion but should be considered, especially if the patient has other manifestations of migraine.

3. **Treatment.** It is uncertain whether migraine-preventive medications (e.g., propranolol, amitriptyline) will eliminate attacks of vertigo in this group of patients.

L. Persistent vestibular dysfunction

1. **Description.** The **CNS** is able to recalibrate the relationship between vestibular, visual, and proprioceptive signals. Therefore, regardless of cause, acute vertigo usually resolves within several days due to CNS adaptation. However, some patients are unable to compensate for vestibular disturbances due to concomitant lesions in brain structures controlling vestibuloocular or vestibulospinal reflexes. Other patients are unable to adapt due to deficits in visual or proprioceptive sensory systems.

2. **Treatment.** Persistent vertigo, imbalance, and disequilibrium are potentially incapacitating problems. Pharmacologic treatment in such cases is largely empirical, and the results are disappointing. Patients with persistent symptoms are candidates for **"vestibular rehabilitation,"** an exercise approach to the remediation of disequilibrium and dizziness.

   a. The **goals** of these exercises are

   (1) To decrease dizziness.

   (2) To improve balance function in everyday situations.

   (3) To restore self-confidence.

   b. A typical **"vestibular exercise program"** consists of

   (1) **Vestibular habituation exercises.** Specific movements or positions that provoke the patient's vertigo and disequilibrium are repeated. These exercises are based on the rationale that the brain will habituate and attenuate the vertigo response after repeated exposure to the specific stimulus causing vertigo.

   (2) **Balance retraining exercises.** These exercises are designed to improve coordination of muscle responses and organization of sensory information for balance control.

IV. Diagnosis and treatment of disorders causing disequilibrium (see Tables 4-2 and 4-3)

A. Multiple sensory deficits

1. **Description.** Patients with diminished **proprioception** in the lower extremities can experience severe unsteadiness, imbalance, or a "drunken" feeling when attempting to walk. They will often use the term **dizziness** to describe their disequilibrium. Loss of proprioception commonly occurs in patients with peripheral neuropathy, vitamin B_{12} deficiency, tabes dorsalis, and myelopathies (such as cervical spondylosis). **Vision** also contributes significantly to spatial orientation and balance. These patients are particularly dizzy and unsteady in the dark, when there are fewer visual cues to compensate for the loss of proprioception.

   Patients with concomitant visual loss (e.g., cataracts, macular degeneration), extrapyramidal dysfunction, orthostatic hypotension, or vestibular disturbances may be particularly incapacitated by even mild proprioceptive deficits (the syndrome of "multiple sensory deficits").

2. **Treatment** involves correcting the underlying neurologic disorder when possible. Evaluation by a physical therapist and use of a cane or walker might prevent serious falls. A night-light is helpful to reduce the disequilibrium when the patient tries to walk to the bathroom in the middle of the night. These patients may benefit from a vestibular rehabilitation exercise program.

B. Cerebellar disorders (e.g., alcoholic cerebellar degeneration, tumors, infarcts, system degenerations) or **extrapyramidal diseases** (e.g., parkinsonism, progressiv supranuclear palsy) often cause unsteadiness and disequilibrium that the patien describes as dizziness.

C. Schwannomas and other cerebellopontine angle tumors
   1. Description
      a. Schwannomas (tumors of Schwann cells) commonly arise from the vestibula division of the cranial nerve in the internal auditory canal. As the tumor slowly expand into the cerebellopontine angle, there is usually an orderl progression of symptoms:
         (1) Hearing loss, tinnitus, and mild disequilibrium.
         (2) Headache.
         (3) Imbalance and incoordination.
         (4) Involvement of adjacent cranial nerves (facial numbness, paresthesia, o facial weakness).
         (5) Symptoms of increased intracranial pressure. Although unilateral hear ing loss with or without tinnitus is almost always the initial symptom patients often ignore this condition and seek medical attention only whe other symptoms such as headache, imbalance, or vague dizziness ensue
      b. Meningiomas, epidermoid tumors, and **other neoplasms** also may occur ir the cerebellopontine angle and produce similar symptoms.
   2. Diagnosis. Unresectable acoustic schwannomas cause major morbidity. The goal is to identify these schwannomas sufficiently early so that surgical remova is safe and leaves minimum deficit. Therefore, all patients with sensorineura hearing loss, particularly when combined with a vestibular abnormality, shoulc undergo evaluation to exclude a cerebellopontine angle tumor.
      a. Physical findings other than hearing loss are often not present. Decreasec corneal sensation, nystagmus, and facial hypesthesia are the most commonly elicited signs.
      b. The **audiologic battery** is useful in distinguishing cochlear disease from ret rocochlear lesions, such as acoustic schwannoma (see Table 4-1). Classic find ings in retrocochlear lesions include poor speech discrimination in relation tc pure tone threshold, no recruitment, tone decay, and impaired stapedial reflex
      c. An **MRI** with gadolinium is now the imaging procedure of choice for evaluating posterior fossa tumors and is capable of visualizing even small intracanalic ular tumors.
      d. High-resolution CT scanning (without *and* with intravenous contrast) with thin sections through the posterior fossa will detect all but relatively small intracanalicular tumors.
   3. Treatment. Most cerebellopontine angle tumors should be resected; in most instances, a surgical cure of acoustic schwannoma is possible (see Chap. 11) sparing facial nerve function. For small tumors (i.e., < 2 cm in diameter) auditory function can also be spared in some instances. Since these tumors are slow growing, some elderly patients may be followed with sequential neurologic examination and scanning rather than surgery.

D. Drug-induced disequilibrium. Intoxication with a variety of agents can produce disequilibrium, vertigo, and other labyrinthine symptoms (Fig. 4-3). Drug intoxi cations commonly produce a symmetric "gaze paretic nystagmus." With eye devia tion to the side, the eyes slowly drift back to the midline, and this is followed by a quick corrective jerk in the direction of gaze.
   1. Anticonvulsants. Most of the commonly used anticonvulsant drugs (e.g., phe nobarbital, phenytoin, ethosuximide, primidone, and carbamazepine) will pro duce **vestibuloocular signs** (e.g., nystagmus, vertigo) and **ataxia** as blood levels exceed the toxic range. The symptoms will disappear if the drugs are withheld, thereby allowing the blood levels to fall below the toxic range.
   2. Alcohol intoxication is regularly associated with unsteadiness of gait and dysarthria, suggestive of cerebellar dysfunction. Positional nystagmus and positional vertigo also commonly occur. The positional vertigo is due to variable rates of diffusion of alcohol into the cupula and endolymph, producing transient specific gravity changes that cause the cupula to act as a gravity sensor.

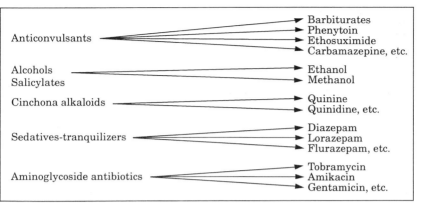

Fig. 4-3. Common causes of drug-induced disequilibrium.

   3. **Salicylates.** Tinnitus and vertigo are among the earliest signs of salicylate intoxication. Hearing loss may also occur, and its severity seems to be closely correlated with the blood salicylate level. When these symptoms appear in patients receiving chronic large doses of salicylates, it is an indication for discontinuing or reducing the dosage. The vestibular symptoms and hearing loss reverse within 2 or 3 days after withdrawal of the drug.
   4. **Aminoglycoside antibiotics are ototoxic drugs** (Table 4-5). Although all of these drugs produce both auditory and vestibular damage, vestibular symptoms are more frequently associated with streptomycin, gentamicin, or tobramycin, and auditory symptoms are more frequently associated with amikacin, kanamycin, or neomycin. These drugs produce hair cell damage in the inner ear. The ototoxicity of these agents is directly related to the blood drug levels and duration of therapy.
      a. The patients rarely complain of vertigo but rather complain of a **disequilibrium** or unsteadiness, particularly in the dark, where corrective visual cues cannot be utilized. **Oscillopsia** is another common symptom and tends to occur when the head moves (e.g., while walking), due to loss of vestibuloocular reflexes. Serial caloric studies can document a progressive bilateral loss of vestibular responsiveness.
      b. **Hearing loss** begins at high frequencies and at times may be delayed in onset.
      c. There is **no specific treatment** for the labyrinthine damage. Symptoms may begin to abate within a few days of stopping the antibiotic therapy; however, full recovery may take more than 1 year, and some patients, particularly the elderly, may suffer severe residual impairment of function.
      d. Several **precautions** can prevent serious aminoglycoside ototoxicity. The total daily dosage, duration of therapy, and blood drug levels should be closely monitored. These precautions are especially important in patients in whom there is renal insufficiency that interferes with the excretion of these drugs. All patients receiving aminoglycoside antibiotics should have frequent evaluation of their vestibular and auditory functions. The medication should be stopped when impairment first appears.
 V. **Hyperventilation syndrome and psychogenic dizziness**
   A. **Hyperventilation syndrome.** Some patients who complain of dizziness suffer from episodes of the hyperventilation syndrome. **Anxiety, panic attacks,** or related emotional disturbances trigger the episodes.
      1. **Description.** Hyperventilation results in hypocapnia, alkalosis, increased cerebrovascular resistance, and decreased cerebral blood flow. The patient complains of an ill-defined **light-headedness,** often in association with circumoral or digital **paresthesias, breathlessness, sweating, trembling, palpitations,** and **panic** (acute anxiety attack). Of great aid in diagnosis, as well as in therapy, is the

Table 4-5. Ototoxic drugs

Drug	Vestibular toxicity	Cochlear toxicity
Anticonvulsants		
Phenytoin	+ + +	
Barbiturates	+ + +	
Carbamazepine	+ + +	
Ethosuximide, etc.	+ + +	
Alcohols		
Ethanol	+ +	
Methanol	+ +	
Salicylates	+	+ + +
Cinchona alkaloids		
Quinine	+	+ + +
Quinidine	+	+ + +
Aminoglycosides		
Streptomycin	+ + +	+
Gentamicin	+ + +	+
Kanamycin	+	+ + +
Tobramycin	+ + +	+
Neomycin	+	+ + +
Other antibiotics		
Minocycline	+ + +	
Polymyxin-B	+ + +	
Colistin	+ + +	
Heavy metals		
Cisplatin	+	+ + +

Key: + = mild; + + = moderate; + + + = severe.

demonstration to the patient that the symptoms can be reproduced by voluntary hyperventilation for 3 minutes.

2. **Treatment. Prophylactic therapy** of the hyperventilation syndrome is based on the **reassurance** of the patient that these attacks do not represent a life threatening illness. Psychiatric consultation and behavioral therapy are appropriate in severe cases. Acute episodes of hyperventilation syndrome can be terminated by having the patient breathe into a bag (thereby allowing rebreathing of exhaled carbon dioxide and preventing the hypocapnia and alkalosis).

B. **Psychogenic dizziness**

1. **Description.** Some patients with **neuroses** or **psychoses** complain of dizziness that does not fit any recognizable condition (e.g., vertigo, syncope, or disequilibrium) and is not reproduced by any of the maneuvers in the dizziness simulation battery. Dizziness is a symptom in over 70% of patients with **anxiety neurosis** and in over 80% of patients with **hysterical neurosis.** The dizziness in these patients has often been present for years and may be continuous rather than episodic. Many of these patients equate dizziness with loss of energy, difficulty concentrating, and mental fuzziness.

2. It is important to reemphasize that acute vestibular disturbances are often accompanied by great anxiety and apprehension. Patients often report that they feel as if they might die during severe bouts of vertigo. Chronic vestibular disturbances can result in adverse changes in the patient's mood and outlook. Anxiety and depression are **not** the sine qua non of psychogenic dizziness but may accompany chronic vestibular disorders.

3. **Management**

   a. The management of patients with psychogenic dizziness is based on **reassurance and trust.** Patients often resent the implication that their syndrome may be psychological, so it is insufficient merely to tell the patient that there is nothing wrong physically—the patient will continue to worry about serious medical illness and will go "doctor shopping." The physician must describe the psychiatric syndrome to the patient in lay terms and be available to provide emotional support and follow-up.

    b. The **minor tranquilizers** of the **benzodiazepine** family (e.g., diazepam, lorazepam, oxazepam) may be useful in treating acute anxiety symptoms. However, drugs that are subject to misuse must be monitored closely in patients with anxiety or hysterical neuroses. When depressive symptoms are prominent, the tricyclic antidepressant agents are often helpful in relieving symptoms.

VI. Tinnitus

A. Definition. Tinnitus is an unwanted noise perceived by the patient that has no source in the external environment.

B. Description. Tinnitus associated with disorders of the middle ear, cochlea, or auditory nerve is generally described as ringing, roaring, "hollow sea shell," or buzzing. The character of the tinnitus alone does not determine the site of the disturbance. Identifiable causes of this type of tinnitus include noise-induced hearing loss, presbycusis, Ménière's syndrome, tympanosclerosis, and acoustic neuroma. These disorders are generally accompanied by hearing loss. All patients with tinnitus should be evaluated for the possibility of an acoustic neuroma. Over half of patients with ringing do not have hearing loss, and in these patients a cause of tinnitus is seldom identified.

C. Medications can produce tinnitus without hearing loss. Potential culprits include salicylates, quinidine, aminophylline, indomethacin, and caffeine. These drugs should be eliminated if possible in patients with tinnitus.

D. Pulsating tinnitus synchronous to the heartbeat usually is indicative of turbulent blood flow. These patients may be hearing their own bruit from a stenotic or tortuous carotid or vertebral artery. Vascular malformations and vascular tumors (e.g., glomus tympanicum tumor) can also cause pulsatile tinnitus. Treating the vascular abnormality can eliminate the pulsatile tinnitus.

E. Treatment. Tinnitus can be extremely annoying, and many patients become preoccupied by this symptom. It is often most noticeable at night, resulting in insomnia. Chronic anxiety and depression are common accompaniments of intractable tinnitus. Diagnosing and treating these concomitant emotional problems can help reduce the devastating effects of the tinnitus.

    1. Medications have been of little value in eliminating chronic tinnitus. Some patients are temporarily palliated by intravenous lidocaine, but this is not a practical long-term treatment.

    2. Masking devices. Most patients prefer to hear an external sound rather than their tinnitus. Some patients will benefit from leaving the radio playing at night or wearing a device that generates a "masking" sound. Unfortunately, these devices are no panacea for tinnitus.

VII. Disorders associated with presyncope.

Many patients use the term **dizziness** to describe a sense of **impending faint.** Other terms used by presyncopal patients to describe their symptoms include **light-headedness** and **giddiness,** although vertiginous patients commonly experience these symptoms as well. Symptoms associated with presyncope, such as nausea, pallor, diaphoresis, apprehension, and blurred vision, may also accompany vertigo; therefore, it is sometimes difficult to classify the patient's complaints of dizziness properly. In these patients, the dizziness simulation battery is especially useful (see sec. **I.E**). Although patients with acute vertigo will occasionally fall due to sudden loss of balance, disorders associated with vertigo rarely if ever cause transient loss of consciousness (syncope). Presyncopal dizziness is usually caused by cardiovascular reflex or hemodynamic disorders.

A. Cardiovascular reflex syncope is mediated via autonomic nervous system reflex mechanisms that lead to a vasodepressor response. The spells are characterized by a fall in total peripheral resistance leading to right heart underfilling and a drop in cardiac output. The spells occur in the standing or (less commonly) sitting position.

Premonitory symptoms such as nausea, pallor, light-headedness, and diaphoresis are very common in patients with reflex syncope.

1. **Vasovagal syncope** is generally triggered by fear, emotional stress, or pain. It is the most common cause of syncope in otherwise healthy young people.
2. **Situational syncope** (also known as **vagovagal or visceral reflex syncope**) includes
   a. Micturition and defecation syncope.
   b. Tussive (cough) syncope.
   c. Deglutition syncope.
   d. Postprandial hypotension, which may be an important cause of syncope in elderly patients with impaired baroreflex function that cannot compensate for splanchnic blood pooling after a meal.
3. **Carotid sinus hypersensitivity** can produce light-headedness and syncope by several mechanisms: cardioinhibitory type, vasodepressor type, or a "mixed" mechanism.
4. **Orthostatic hypotension** and syncope occur when the compensatory sympathetic reflex mechanisms that maintain blood pressure on standing are inadequate.
   a. **Primary autonomic insufficiency** occurs in the Shy-Drager syndrome and idiopathic orthostatic hypotension.
   b. **Secondary orthostatic hypotension** can occur in patients with:
      (1) **Autonomic neuropathies** (e.g., diabetes, alcoholism, amyloidosis).
      (2) **Medications** commonly cause orthostatic hypotension, including antihypertensive agents, nitrates, vasodilators, tranquilizers, antidepressants, phenothiazines, and other vasoactive drugs.
      (3) **Hypovolemia** from blood loss, vomiting, excess diuresis, and dehydration.
      (4) **Prolonged bed rest** can lead to cardiovascular deconditioning and hypotension on standing.
B. **Cardiac syncope** results from inadequate left heart output. Unlike cardiovascular reflex syncope, attacks of cardiac syncope are often of abrupt onset and may lack premonitory symptoms.
   1. **Mechanical (obstructive) cardiac syncope** is caused by left ventricular outflow tract obstruction (e.g., due to aortic stenosis, hypertrophic cardiomyopathy, pulmonary hypertension, cardiac tamponade, atrial myxoma, global myocardial ischemia).
   2. **Arrhythmic cardiac syncope** can be caused by ventricular tachycardia, atrioventricular block, sick sinus syndrome, bradycardia-tachycardia syndrome, long-QT syndrome, pacemaker malfunction, and so on.
   3. Cardiac syncope can be life-threatening, and evaluation of patients with recurrent unexplained syncope should focus on ruling out a serious cardiac disorder. The history, physical examination, and routine cardiac investigations will provide important clues in most patients. New cardiovascular diagnostic tests, such as electrophysiologic studies, tilt-table evaluation, and prolonged ambulatory monitoring with continuous loop ECG recorders, have provided diagnostic information in some cases of unexplained syncope.
C. **Cerebrovascular occlusive disease** does not cause syncope or presyncopal dizziness, and it is erroneous to refer to these symptoms as "transient ischemic attacks." The **rare** situation in which cerebrovascular disease causes syncope is in patients with **widespread** narrowing or occlusion of the cervical vessels that supply the brain, as might occur in
   1. **Advanced bilateral atherosclerosis with occlusion of multiple extracranial vessels.** These patients may experience primary orthostatic cerebral ischemia (orthostatic hypotension of the brain without systemic orthostatic hypotension).
   2. **Takayasu's disease.**
   3. **Subclavian steal syndrome.**

Selected Readings

Baloh, R. W., Honrubia, V., and Jacobson, K. Benign positional vertigo. *Neurology* 37:371, 1987.

Brandt, T. *Vertigo: Its Multisensory Syndromes*. London: Springer-Verlag, 1991.

Brandt, T., and Daroff, R. B. The multisensory physiological and pathological vertigo syndromes. *Ann. Neurol.* 7:195, 1980.

Drachman, D. A., and Hart, C. W. An approach to the dizzy patient. *Neurology* 2:323, 1972.

Kroenke, K., et al. Causes of persistent dizziness: A prospective study of 100 patients in ambulatory care. *Ann. Intern. Med.* 117:898, 1992.

Manolis, A. S., et al. Syncope: Current diagnostic evaluation and management. *Ann. Intern. Med.* 112:850, 1990.

Troost, B. T., and Patton, J. M. Exercise therapy for positional vertigo. *Neurology* 42:1441, 1992.

Zee, D. S. Perspectives on the pharmacotherapy of vertigo. *Arch. Otolaryngol.* 111:609, 1985.

Backache

Richard C. Hinton

I. **General approach to the patient with backache.** Backache is an extremely common symptom with many possible causes. Proper therapy, therefore, depends heavily on making the correct diagnosis. All patients complaining of backache should have the following **minimum evaluation:**
   A. **History,** with special reference to
      1. **Location** of the pain.
      2. **Radiation** of the pain.
      3. **Body position** that brings exacerbation or relief.
      4. **Trauma.**
      5. **Litigation.**
      6. **Drugs** used for pain and amounts required for relief.
      7. **Malignancy.**
   B. **Physical examination,** with special reference to
      1. Signs of **systemic infection.**
      2. Signs of **occult malignancy.**
      3. Local **tenderness,** or tenderness in sciatic notch.
      4. **Muscle spasm.**
      5. **Range of motion.**
      6. **Straight-leg raising.**
      7. **Rectal examination** (prostate sphincter tone).
   C. **Neurologic examination,** with special reference to
      1. **Affect** and mood.
      2. **Muscle weakness,** atrophy, or fasciculations.
      3. **Sensory loss** including the perineum.
      4. **Reflexes** (deep tendon, abdominal, anal, cremasteric).
   D. **Laboratory**
      1. **X ray** (posteroanterior, lateral, and oblique).
      2. **Complete blood count and erythrocyte sedimentation rate.**
      3. **Serum,** for
         a. Creatinine.
         b. Calcium.
         c. Phosphate.
         d. Alkaline phosphatase.
         e. Uric acid.
         f. Acid phosphatase (men only).
         g. Fasting blood sugar.
   E. **Further studies** (e.g., bone scan, 2-hour postprandial blood sugar, MRI, CT scan, and myelography) depend on the results of the above screening procedure. Usually this thorough basic evaluation will reveal the cause of the pain, and the problem can be categorized into one of the following diagnostic groups.
II. **Disk syndromes**
   A. **Pathophysiology.** The **intervertebral disk** serves the dual purpose of articulation, allowing flexibility of the spine, and cushioning, acting as a shock absorber to prevent damage to the bones.
      1. **Herniation,** or **rupture,** of an intervertebral disk refers to protrusion of the nucleus pulposus along with some part of the anulus into the spinal canal or

intervertebral foramen. Because the anterior longitudinal ligament is much stronger than the posterior longitudinal ligament, disk herniation almost always occurs in a posterior or posterolateral direction. The material usually bulges as a solid mass and retains continuity with the body of the disk, although fragments at times may protrude through the posterior longitudinal ligament, break off, and lie free in the spinal canal.

2. Some controversy exists concerning the **factors that lead to rupture** of the intervertebral disk. Many cases can be related to trauma, either acute severe injury or, more commonly, repeated minor injuries secondary to bending and lifting. Another contributing factor seems to be the degenerative changes in the disk that occur with aging: shrinking of the nucleus pulposus and thickening of the anulus fibrosus. Disk herniation occurs most commonly in the lumbar region, followed next in frequency by cervical disk rupture. Thoracic disk herniation is distinctly uncommon.

B. **Lumbar disk herniation**

1. **Clinical description.** Lumbar disk herniation is most common in adult white males, reaching a peak incidence in the fourth and fifth decades. It seems to occur more frequently in those whose occupation involves bending and lifting. Because the posterior longitudinal ligament in the lumbar region is stronger in its central portion, protruded disks tend to occur in a posterolateral direction, with compression of the nerve roots.

a. **Areas affected**

(1) The **last two lumbar interspaces** (L4–L5 and L5–S1) are most commonly affected, particularly L5–S1. L3–L4 is the next most common site. Rupture of higher lumbar disks is rare and almost always the result of massive trauma.

(2) Because of the anatomic relationships in the lumbar spine, a protruding disk usually compresses the nerve root emerging one level below it. The most common disk syndromes of **nerve root compression** are presented in Table 5-1. However, this anatomic arrangement is by no means invariable. Thus, although the nerve roots affected by a disk can be identified clinically, the exact level of the protruded disk cannot always be localized with great certainty.

(3) If there is a **free disk fragment,** it usually affects the root emerging above the herniated disk.

b. **Development of symptoms.** More than half of the patients will date their symptoms to some type of trauma, either a hard fall or a twisting or bending stress.

(1) The **initial complaint** is usually a dull, aching, often intermittent, low back pain of gradual onset, although at times the pain is of sudden onset and severe. This pain is felt to be secondary to stretching of the posterior longitudinal ligament, since the disk itself probably possesses no pain fibers. Characteristically the pain is **aggravated** by activity or exertion and by straining, coughing, or sneezing. It is usually **relieved** by lying on the unaffected side with the painful leg flexed. Often there is reflex spasm of the paravertebral muscles that causes pain and prevents the patient from standing fully erect.

(2) **Course of symptoms.** After a variable period of time, an aching pain begins in the buttocks and posterior or posterolateral aspect of the thigh and leg on the affected side, usually termed **sciatica.** This is often accompanied by numbness and a tingling that radiates into the part of the foot served by the sensory fibers of the affected root. These symptoms may be elicited by **Lesegue's test:** straight-leg raising with the patient lying prone. In the normal patient, the leg can be raised to almost 90 degrees without pain, while in the patient with sciatica, characteristic pain is produced by elevations of 30–40 degrees. Eventually, loss of sensation, muscle weakness, and loss of reflexes may ensue (see Table 5-1).

(3) In the uncommon situation where a **midline disk protrusion** occurs in the presence of a narrow spinal canal in the lumbar region, **cauda equina**

Table 5-1. Symptoms and signs in lateral rupture of lumbar disk

Disk	Root	Pain and paresthesias	Sensory loss	Motor loss	Reflex loss
L3–L4	L4	Anterior surface of thigh, inner surface of shin	Anteromedial surface of thigh, extending down along shin to inner side of foot	Quadriceps	Knee jerk
L4–L5	L5	Radiating down outer side of back of thigh and outer side of calf, and across dorsum of foot to great toe	Usually involves outer side of calf and the great toe	Extensor hallucis longus; less commonly, muscles of dorsiflexion and eversion of foot	None
L5–S1	S1	Radiating down back of thigh and outer side and back of calf, to foot and the lesser toes	Almost always involves outer side of calf, outer border of foot, and the lesser toes; less commonly, the back of the thigh	Gastrocnemius, and occasionally muscles of eversion of foot	Ankle jerk

compression may result, with paraparesis and loss of sphincter tone. A pseudoclaudication syndrome has been described, with pain in the legs on exertion, secondary to intermittent compression of the nerves of the cauda equina. The pathophysiology is possibly ischemia.

2. **Diagnostic tests**
   a. **Routine x rays** of the spine (including oblique projections) are not ordered as frequently as they were prior to the advent of CT scanning. They are at times useful in ruling out congenital anomalies or deformities, involvement of the spine with rheumatic diseases, and metastatic or primary tumors. In disk disease, the x rays may be normal or may show degenerative changes with narrowing of the intervertebral space and osteophyte formation.
   b. **Serum levels** of calcium, phosphate, alkaline and acid phosphatase, and glucose should be ascertained in every patient, since metabolic bone disease, metastatic tumors of the spine, and diabetic mononeuritis may all imitate intervertebral disk disease.
   c. **Lumbar puncture.** Although the cerebrospinal fluid may show mildly elevated protein in the presence of disk disease, lumbar puncture usually adds little to the diagnostic evaluation. If a complete spinal block is present, the protein may be very elevated with an abnormal Queckenstedt's maneuver.
   d. **Neurophysiologic studies. Electromyography (EMG)** may be normal in disk disease, or fibrillation potentials and positive sharp waves may be seen in muscles innervated by the affected root after a delay of a few weeks. At times EMG may be useful in differentiating root compression from peripheral neuropathy, since with root compression, conduction in the motor system is usually normal even in the presence of fasciculations and fibrillations, and sensory conduction is unimpaired. The Hoffmann reflex may be delayed or absent.
   e. **Myelography.** When the diagnosis of a disk syndrome is certain, and one is not concerned about the possibility of a cauda equina tumor or some other abnormality, myelography need not be performed unless surgery is contemplated. When surgery is being considered, myelography is carried out to determine the level of disk protrusion.
   f. A **CT scan** is useful in the diagnosis of disk disease and spinal stenosis. Sometimes myelography can be avoided when a high-resolution CT scan is available.
   g. An **MRI** is particularly useful in the diagnosis of compression of the spinal cord or cauda equina. It seems to be a little less accurate than a CT scan in the evaluation of nerve root compromise.
   h. Diskography has not been found particularly helpful in evaluating disk disease, since the results are often difficult to interpret. Furthermore, it has been suggested that the procedure itself may produce damage to the intervertebral disk.

3. **Treatment**
   a. **Conservative treatment.** The **majority of patients respond** to conservative therapy and do not require surgery.
      (1) In patients with **mild symptoms,** suggest
         (a) **Ways to avoid bending or straining;** instruct the patient in this as well as in proper posture.
         (b) **Resting in bed** when pain is present and avoidance of painful activities.
         (c) **Application of heat** to the low back area.
         (d) **Analgesics** as necessary.
         (e) **Exercises** designed to strengthen the erector spine and abdominal muscles.
         (f) A **lumbar corset,** to prevent excessive motion of the lumbar area.
      (2) In patients with **severe incapacitating pain:**
         (a) Strict **bed rest** on a firm bed may be necessary, in whatever position is most comfortable.
         (b) **Supporting boards** underneath the mattress are useful to provide a firm surface.

  (c) **Analgesics** are given during this period, as are antispasmodic agents such as diazepam, and anti-inflammatory agents such as aspirin and the nonsteroidal anti-inflammatory agents.

  (d) **If the symptoms remit,** activities are gradually increased after a few days or so, and the patient is then treated as in the case of mild symptoms.

  (e) **Pelvic traction** generally has **not** been found effective except to help enforce strict bed rest.

(3) In the past, strict **bed rest** was prescribed sometimes for 2–3 weeks. However, recent studies have concluded that earlier mobilization after a few days of bed rest is preferable.

b. **Surgery is more likely to be successful when there are objective signs of neurologic impairment.** Surgery produces good to excellent results in approximately two-thirds of patients; half of the remaining are improved. The **usual indications** for surgery are the following:

  (1) The most common indication for surgery is **failure to respond to conservative therapy.** The decision for surgery in this case must be made by the patient, with the guidance of the physician. Surgery is usually elected when the pain is severe, incapacitating, and unrelieved by conservative therapy, although at times the frequency of recurrences of less severe pain may lead some patients to choose surgery.

  (2) **Surgery without delay** is mandatory in the uncommon situation in which a **midline disk compresses the cauda equina,** with paraparesis and sensory loss in the legs along with loss of sphincter control.

  (3) When **nerve root compression is associated with motor loss,** especially quadriceps weakness or footdrop, surgery is usually indicated. Occasionally, mild weakness may remit with conservative therapy.

c. **Chemonucleolysis** is now available as a treatment for herniated lumbar disks and involves injection of the disk with chymopapain. This procedure is unlikely to benefit patients with sequestered disks, free disk fragments, or osteophytic nerve root compression, In addition to anaphylaxis, other side effects have been reported soon after injection with chymopapain, including paraplegia, cerebral hemorrhage, and transverse myelitis/myelopathy. The transverse myelopathy tends to begin acutely 2–3 weeks after chymopapain injection, and most cases have occurred when diskography was performed in conjunction with the procedure. Recent Food and Drug Administration recommendations include avoiding diskography as part of the chemonucleolysis procedure, verifying needle location, avoiding multiple-level injections, and using supplemented local anesthesia rather than general anesthesia.

C. **Cervical disk herniation**

1. **Clinical description.** Cervical disk rupture often follows a traumatic event after a variable period of time but frequently occurs without any preceding traumatic event.

  a. **Areas affected.** Cervical disk protrusion most commonly occurs at the C5–C6 or C6–C7 levels. In contrast to the lumbar region, the cervical posterior longitudinal ligament is weaker in its central portion, so the herniations may be midline posterior, compressing the cord, or posterolateral, with root compression. **Signs of cord compression** include spastic paraparesis and posterior column sensory loss in the legs, hyperactive leg reflexes, and bilateral Babinski's responses. Table 5-2 summarizes the **root syndromes** resulting from cervical disk rupture.

  b. **Development of symptoms.** Symptoms usually begin with recurrent attacks of **pain** in the posterior cervical area, often accompanied by **muscle spasm** in the paravertebral muscles. Later, the pain begins to radiate into the ipsilateral arm, with numbness and tingling in the distribution of the particular root involved. As with lumbar disk disease, the symptoms are usually aggravated by coughing, straining, or sneezing.

2. **Diagnostic tests.** The same guidelines for diagnostic evaluation presented for lumbar disk herniation (see sec. **II.B.2**) apply in general to cervical disk disease.

Table 5-2. Symptoms and signs in lateral rupture of cervical disk

Disk	Root	Pain and paresthesias	Sensory loss	Motor loss	Reflex loss
C4–C5	C5	Neck, shoulder, upper arm	Shoulder	Deltoid, biceps	Biceps
C5–C6	C6	Neck, shoulder, lateral aspect of arm, and radial aspect of forearm to thumb and forefinger	Thumb, forefinger, radial aspect of forearm, lateral aspect of arm	Biceps	Biceps, supinator
C6–C7	C7	Neck, lateral aspect of arm, and ring and index fingers	Forefinger, middle finger, radial aspect of forearm	Triceps, extensor carpi ulnaris	Triceps, supinator
C7–T1	C8	Ulnar aspect of forearm and hand	Ulnar half of ring finger, little finger	Intrinsic muscles of the hand, wrist extensors	None

3. Treatment

a. The measures for **conservative therapy** of cervical disk include cervical traction in addition to those outlined for the lumbar disk (see sec. **II.B.3.a**). A soft cervical collar may be helpful.

b. With regard to **surgery,** the previously mentioned indications for surgery for lumbar disk disease (see sec. **II.B.3.b**) apply to cervical disk disease as well, but one should bear in mind that **cervical cord compression** can occur and that it requires **early surgery**.

D. Thoracic disks

1. Clinical description. Thoracic disks are the rarest type of disk protrusion, accounting for less than 1% of all herniated disks.

a. Areas affected. The **lower four thoracic interspaces** are most frequently involved, with T11–T12 being most commonly affected. Because the extradural space is narrower in the thoracic region than in any other area of the spine (and because the majority of the disk protrusions are central), **cord compression** is more likely to occur than in the other disk syndromes.

b. Development of symptoms. At times, the onset of symptoms is acute or subacute and associated with trauma, but the **majority have a chronic course** unassociated with trauma.

(1) Initially, **back pain** is the most common symptom, occurring in the thoracic, lumbar, or sciatic region. Again, the pain is often aggravated by coughing, sneezing, or straining.

(2) Symptoms of **cord compression,** when they occur, arise from pressure on the cord or from compromise of the arterial supply to the cord.

(3) Paraplegia may occur suddenly.

(4) When the herniation is lateral, the **root compression** may mimic pleurodynia, angina, or visceral pain, depending on the level.

2. Diagnostic tests. Diagnostic evaluation proceeds according to the guidelines in the section on lumbar disks (see sec. **II.B.2**). Compared with the other disk syndromes, thoracic disk disease is more likely to be associated with **intervertebral disk calcification,** although the calcified interspace may not be the disk that has ruptured. If there are signs of spinal cord involvement, **myelography** should be performed promptly, and usually films must be taken with the patient lying supine.

3. Treatment

a. Many patients with root compression alone will respond go **conservative treatment** (see sec. **II.B.3**).

b. When cord dysfunction is present, **surgery** is necessary. This is technically the most difficult area for back surgery because of the narrow canal and the usually central herniation. Surgical results are probably best with the anterior transthoracic or transpleural approach.

III. Degenerative disease of the spine (spondylosis)

A. Pathophysiology. With advancing age, degenerative changes take place in the spine, consisting of dehydration and collapse of the nucleus pulposus and bulging in all directions of the anulus fibrosus. The anulus becomes calcified, and hypertrophic changes occur in the bones at the margins of the vertebral bodies, creating lips or spurs (osteophytes) (Figs. 5-1 and 5-2). With narrowing of the intervertebral space, the intervertebral joints may become subluxated and compromise the intervertebral foramina, which may also be encroached on by osteophytic processes.

B. Clinical description

1. Root compression indistinguishable from that produced by disk protrusion may occur, although the pain is usually less prominent with spondylosis.

2. Dysesthesias without pain may be present in the distribution of the roots affected, and corresponding muscle weakness and reflex changes may occur. These are more likely to be symptomatic in the cervical region, but they may occur in the lumbar area as well.

3. The **osteophyte formation** occurring in the more central portion of the vertebral body may **compress the spinal cord** in the cervical region, or the cauda equina may be compressed in the lumbar area in the presence of a narrowed canal

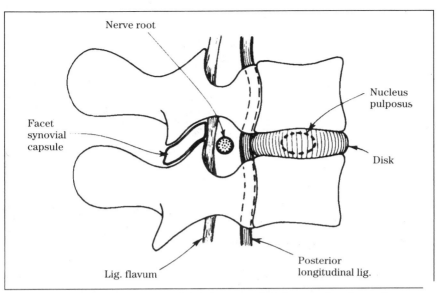

Fig. 5-1. The normal disk. The normal disk is composed of the central nucleus pulposus (a fibrogelatinous fluid), the cartilaginous plates covering the vertebral body surfaces, and the anulus fibrosis, which surrounds the nucleus pulposus and provides the bulk of the disk. The anterior and posterior longitudinal ligaments cover the respective surfaces of the disk.

(**lumbar stenosis**). In the cervical region, this produces spastic paraparesis, often with posterior column sensory loss, hyperactive reflexes in the legs, and bilateral Babinski's responses. Depending on the level, the arms may or may not be involved. An interesting situation often arises when the C5–C6 interspace is involved: The biceps reflex is diminished because of root compression, and the triceps reflex is hyperactive because of cord compression. When there is lumbar involvement, symptoms of cauda equina compression with paraparesis and sensory loss in the legs, along with loss of sphincter control, may result. A curious pseudoclaudication (or neurologic claudication) syndrome may also occur in which the patient notes back and leg pain on standing or walking; the pain is relieved by lying down.

C. **Diagnostic tests and treatment.** The diagnostic workup and conservative therapy should proceed in the same manner as for disk disease (see secs. **II.B.2**) and **II.B.3**). The **indications for surgery** also are the same as for disk disease: evidence of spinal cord compression, muscle weakness, or intractable pain. For root compression, a procedure is performed to enlarge the intervertebral foramina. When the spinal cord is compressed, a laminectomy is done to enlarge the spinal canal.

IV. **Spondylolysis and spondylolisthesis**
  A. **Pathophysiology. Spondylolisthesis** is forward displacement of one vertebral body onto the vertebral body below it. This most commonly occurs in conjunction with **spondylolysis,** a condition in which the posterior portion of the vertebral unit is split, causing a loss of continuity between the superior and inferior articular processes (Fig. 5-3). This is believed to result from fracture of the neural arch shortly after birth, although it rarely becomes symptomatic until later in life; the average age of patients seeking treatment is 35 years. The most common site of involvement is the last lumbar vertebra (L5), which subluxates onto the sacrum. Less commonly, spondylolisthesis may occur secondary to degenerative disease of the spine; this usually involves L5 or L4.

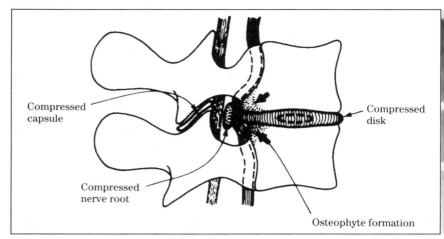

Fig. 5-2. Degenerative changes of the spine.

B. **Clinical description.** The most common symptom is **low back pain,** usually beginning early in life and gradually worsening, that is accentuated by extension movements. However, the pain may begin abruptly in association with an injury. **Leg pain** from compression of the nerve roots is less common. With severe deformity, cauda equina may be compressed.

C. **Treatment**
  1. **Conservative therapy** consists of restriction of activity and institution of flexion exercises. A corset may be beneficial to provide stability to the spine.
  2. **Surgery.** As the patient grows older, if conservative therapy has failed to halt progression of the condition, spinal fusion usually is indicated.

V. **Neurologic complications of diseases involving the spine**
  A. **Ankylosing spondylitis.** Early in the course of ankylosing spondylitis there is low back pain. In a small percentage of patients, this may radiate in a sciatic distribution, but neurologic findings are rare. Uncommonly, **compromise of the cauda equina** may occur, but this usually appears late in the course of the disease, at a time when the disease has become inactive. Ankylosing spondylitis progresses insidiously, with muscle wasting, pain, and sensory loss in the legs, together with loss of sphincter control. Treatment is symptomatic.
  B. **Rheumatoid arthritis** may result in serious neurologic complications from involvement of the cervical spine.
    1. **Pathophysiology.** The characteristic deformity is subluxation of one vertebra onto another. The most common situation is **atlantoaxial subluxation,** which may result in spinal cord compression. Another common site for subluxation is C3–C4. Pain without cord compression is more likely to occur with atlantoaxial subluxation, while painless cord compression is more common at C3–C4. These complications of rheumatoid arthritis generally occur only as a consequence of long-standing severe disease.
    2. **Treatment** involves immobilization of the affected joint. This can be accomplished temporarily with a **hard four-post collar,** but definitive therapy requires **spinal fusion** at the involved interspace.
  C. **Paget's disease** (osteitis deformans) often produces **back pain** but only rarely produces neurologic complications from involvement of the spine. However, many well-documented cases of **cord compression** have been reported. Compression may occur from narrowing of the spinal canal by hypertrophic bone, with subsequent direct compression, from interference with the arterial supply to the cord, or from extramedullary hematopoiesis. Cord compression may also result from vertebral

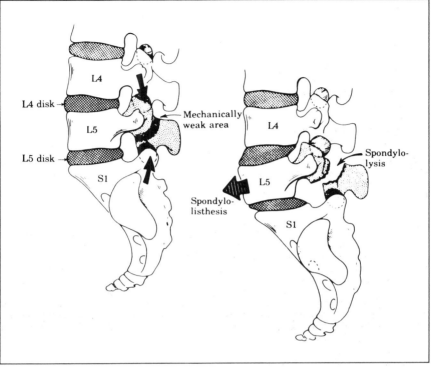

Fig. 5-3. Mechanism of spondylolysis. The pincer effect of the adjacent facets on the interposed isthmus is demonstrated with ultimate spondylolisthesis due to the restraining mechanism of the posterior articulation that is being detached.

collapse with dislocation of the vertebral bodies. There is no specific treatment for the back pain of Paget's disease, so **therapy** consists of palliation with back brace and analgesia.

D. **Metastatic disease frequently causes back pain** by involvement of vertebrae or spinal roots. It may produce **spinal cord compression** either because of collapse of extensively replaced vertebral bodies or by extramedullary (intradural or extradural) metastatic deposits.

1. **Diagnostic tests.** Plain x rays of the spine may show evidence of metastatic disease. However, even when plain x rays are normal, a bone scan is useful for diagnosis in patients with unexplained back pain. Lung, breast, and prostate cancer are the most frequent tumors producing back pain.

2. **Treatment** of the primary tumor or local radiation therapy to the involved vertebrae or both are useful palliative measures and often provide excellent **relief of pain. Spinal compression is an emergency** often requiring prompt myelography and surgical decompression, although some patients may be treated successfully with steroids and radiation therapy.

E. **Metabolic bone diseases** (e.g., osteoporosis, hyperparathyroidism, osteomalacia) frequently cause **back pain but rarely produce neurologic deficits by spinal cord or root compression. Treatment** is of the underlying condition if that is possible (i.e., discontinue steroids, give vitamin D and calcium, treat malabsorption or renal failure, remove parathyroid adenomas). Table 5-3 summarizes the differential diagnosis of various metabolic bone diseases that may present with back pain, based

Table 5-3. Differential diagnosis of various bone diseases that may cause back pain

Disease	Serum Ca^{2+}	Serum PO$_4$	Serum alkaline phosphatase
Hyperparathyroidism	↑	↓	N
Osteoporosis (primary or secondary to steroid excess, hyperthyroidism, or acromegaly)	N or ↓	N	N
Osteomalacia			
Vitamin D lack or resistance	↓	↑	↑
Chronic renal failure	↓	↑	N or ↑
Malabsorption	↓	↓	↑
Malignancy with osseous metastases	↑	N	↑

Key: ↑ = increased; ↓ = decreased; N = normal.

on serum calcium, phosphate, and alkaline phosphatase testing. If no specific treatment is possible (e.g., as in postmenopausal osteoporosis), palliative measures such as a back brace and analgesics are used.

VI. Spinal epidural abscess is a purulent infection of the epidural fat pad. In many cases this infection is preceded by **vertebral osteomyelitis.** The infection usually reaches the vertebra by hematogenous spread from a distal infection, although direct spread from local skin infection is known to occur. The disease is rare, but when it occurs it is usually associated with **severe back pain** and almost always with **local tenderness.** Spinal epidural abscess may cause **spinal compression.** Myelography is required for diagnosis, and treatment consists of surgical removal of the abscess and 4–6 weeks of intravenous antibiotic therapy.

VII. Psychiatric causes of back pain.

  A. Depression. In patients with chronic back pain in which the neurologic examination is normal and categorization into any of the previously discussed syndromes is not possible, depression is a common finding. Such patients should not be treated with analgesics or other modes of therapy meant for specific backache syndromes. Tricyclic antidepressants may be useful (see Chap. 9 for details).

  B. Back pain also may be seen in the context of various **characterologic diseases.** The prognosis in these cases is less favorable than in depression, and there is no effective therapy, although psychotherapy may meet with limited success. Analgesics (particularly opiates) should be avoided, since drug dependency is a very common complication in these patients. (Such patients often fail to have relief of their back pain while litigation is pending.)

Selected Readings

Cailliet, R. *Low Back Pain Syndrome* (3rd ed.). Philadelphia: Davis, 1981.

Cailliet, R. *Neck and Arm Pain* (2nd ed.). Philadelphia: Davis, 1981.

Chemonucleolysis. *FDA Drug Bull.* 14:14, 1984.

Frymoyer, J. W. Back pain and sciatica. *N. Engl. J. Med.* 318:291, 1988.

Matthews, W. B. The neurological complications of ankylosing spondylitis. *J. Neurol. Sci.* 6:561, 1968.

Smith, P. H., Benn, R. T., and Sharp, J. Natural history of rheumatoid cervical luxations. *Ann. Rheum. Dis.* 31:431, 1972.

Youmans, J. R. *Neurological Surgery,* Vol. 1. Philadelphia: Saunders, 1973.

Epilepsy

Raymond J. Fernandez and
Martin A. Samuels

Epilepsy may be defined as a **state of recurrent seizures.** Since seizures are due to aberrant electrical activity in virtually any part of the cerebral cortex (and perhaps even in the cerebellum and subcortical structures), one may expect that nearly every conceivable form of human experience could be caused by seizure discharges. However, although this is literally true, generally the term *epilepsy* (or **seizure disorder**) is used to characterize relatively stereotyped recurrent attacks of involuntary experience or behavior.

I. **Classification.** Many efforts have been made to classify the epilepsies by using various parameters: etiology, symptomatology, duration, precipitating factors, postictal phenomena, and aura. The most useful of these classifications with regard to therapy utilizes the **clinical symptomatology** of the seizures; this mode of classification also permits differentiation of true epilepsies from similar yet clinically distinct conditions.

A. **Classification of epilepsies**
   1. **Generalized**
      a. **Absence**
         (1) Typical (petit mal).
         (2) Atypical, including Lennox-Gastaut syndrome.
      b. **Tonic and/or clonic** (grand mal)
         (1) Intermittent convulsions.
         (2) Status epilepticus.
      c. **Myoclonic epilepsy**
         (1) Infantile spasms.
         (2) Benign myoclonus of infancy.
         (3) Juvenile myoclonic epilepsy.
         (4) Other, including subacute sclerosing panencephalitis and Lafora's disease.
      d. **Febrile seizures**
   2. **Partial** (focal)
      a. **Simple** (without impairment of consciousness)
         (1) Motor.
         (2) Sensory.
         (3) Autonomic.
      b. **Complex** (psychomotor or temporal lobe, with impairment of consciousness)
         (1) Automatism.
         (2) Psychic phenomena.
   3. **Neonatal.**
B. **Classification of paroxysmal conditions resembling epilepsy**
   1. Narcolepsy.
   2. Migraine.
   3. Paroxysmal abdominal pain.
   4. breath-holding spells.
   5. Hypercyanotic attacks.
   6. Shuddering attacks.
   7. Cardiovascular syncope.
   8. Hysteria.
   9. Malingering.

      10. Trigeminal neuralgia (tic douloureux).

      11. Paroxysmal vertigo.

  C. Within a single attack, it is most useful diagnostically and therapeutically to classify the seizure on the basis of its initial manifestations, if that is possible. Thus a partial motor seizure that becomes generalized (secondarily generalized) should be considered a partial rather than a generalized attack.

II. Evaluation of the patient. A seizure is only a symptom caused by excessive neuronal discharges. The precise cellular mechanism involved will not be discussed herein; it is sufficient to state that this symptom can be produced by protean abnormalities, both within and outside the nervous system. The major categories of these abnormalities are as follows:

  A. Genetic and birth factors

      1. Genetic influence (primary, idiopathic, cryptogenic, essential).

      2. Congenital abnormalities (including chromosomal abnormalities).

      3. Antenatal factors (infections, drugs, anoxia).

      4. Perinatal factors (birth trauma, asphyxia neonatorum, infections).

  B. Infectious disorders

      1. Meningitis.

      2. Epidural or subdural abscess.

      3. Brain abscess and granuloma.

      4. Encephalitis.

  C. Toxic factors

      1. Inorganic substances (e.g., carbon monoxide).

      2. Metallic substances (e.g., lead, mercury).

      3. Organic substances (e.g., alcohol).

      4. Drugs and drug withdrawal.

      5. Allergic disorders (injection or ingestion of foreign protein).

  D. Trauma or physical agents

      1. Acute craniocerebral injuries.

      2. Subdural or epidural hematoma and effusion.

      3. Posttraumatic meningocerebral cicatrix.

      4. Anoxia or hypoxia.

  E. Circulatory disturbances

      1. Subarachnoid hemorrhage.

      2. Sinus thrombosis.

      3. Encephalomalacia (thrombosis, embolus, hemorrhage).

      4. Hypertensive encephalopathy.

      5. Syncope.

      6. Cardiac arrhythmia. The prolonged QT syndrome associated with recurrent ventricular fibrillation, and sometimes associated with deafness, may on occasion be diagnosed on the ECG lead of the EEG. The QT interval, corrected for heart rate, should be measured, especially if the clinical diagnosis is syncope. The corrected QT interval (QT_c) is calculated by the following formula:

$$QT_c = \frac{QT \text{ in seconds}}{RR \text{ interval}}$$

      The QT_c should not exceed 0.45 in infants up to 6 months, 0.44 in children, and 0.425 in adolescents and adults.

  F. Metabolic or nutritional disturbances

      1. Electrolyte and water imbalance (hyponatremia, hypocalcemia, water intoxication, dehydration).

      2. Carbohydrate metabolism (hypoglycemia, glycogen storage disease).

      3. Amino acid metabolism (e.g., phenylketonuria).

      4. Fat metabolism (e.g., lipid storage diseases).

      5. Vitamin deficiency or dependency (e.g., pyridoxine dependency; biotinidase deficiency)

  G. Neoplasms

      1. Primary intracranial (astrocytoma, other gliomas, meningiomas).

      2. Metastatic (breast, lung, melanoma).

3. Lymphoma and leukemia.
4. Blood vessel tumors and vascular malformations.
H. Heredofamilial
1. Neurofibromatosis.
2. Tuberous sclerosis.
3. Sturge-Weber syndrome.
I. Febrile seizures
J. Degenerative diseases
K. Unknown causes

III. **Diagnostic approach.** The diagnosis of epilepsy rests mainly on the **history;** it must be considered in any patient who suffers from recurrent attacks of **stereotyped** involuntary behavior or experience. Particular diagnostic points relative to each of the types of seizures will be mentioned in the subsections in each category; however, the following general points apply broadly in the diagnosis of epilepsy.

   A. EEG. There is no diagnostic test that will reliably either diagnose or exclude epilepsy. The EEG is often normal, even in a patient with a known seizure disorder; and conversely, an abnormal EEG in the absence of symptoms does not automatically indicate treatment for seizures. It is relatively unusual for seizure activity to be recorded during an EEG. Therefore, the usefulness of the test is largely dependent on interictal abnormalities, particularly when focal or lateralized slow waves are observed—a finding that suggests a localized abnormality is responsible for the seizure. Various activation procedures may be utilized (e.g., hyperventilation, photic stimulation, and sleep) to exacerbate an underlying abnormality not recognizable on the ordinary tracing. Ambulatory and inpatient EEG monitoring is now available in many centers. This allows one to record much larger samples of EEGs, thus increasing the chance of observing an infrequent epileptic event. The EEG is especially important when one is evaluating **absence,** a seizure pattern often confused with complex partial seizures. In absence seizures, generalized spike and wave paroxysms are seen, whereas focal abnormalities may be seen with partial seizures.

   B. Etiology. Once the diagnosis of a seizure is made, a search for the etiology should ensue. The diagnostic course to be followed will vary depending on the type of seizure disorder identified and the age of the patient.

   1. **History.** To categorize a patient's seizure properly, it is necessary to obtain a careful history from both the patient and someone who has witnessed the seizure or seizures.

      a. **Focality of seizures.** Important historic points derive from whether the seizures are generalized from their onset or have some partial quality. **If they are partial,** it must be determined whether consciousness is altered. Examples of altered consciousness may include disorders of arousal mechanisms (e.g., drowsiness or momentary loss of consciousness), abnormalities in perception such as psychic phenomena (e.g., déjà vu, jamais vu, or paranoid or hostile feelings), or gustatory or olfactory hallucinations.

      b. The **family history** may reveal relatives with epilepsy or with diseases associated with seizures.

      c. The patient's **past medical history** may give a clue concerning remote infections, such as meningitis or encephalitis; or a history of stroke or head trauma may be elicited, either of which may be epileptogenic.

      d. **Pregnancy history.** The history of the pregnancy, labor, and delivery should be reviewed for evidence of complications known to be associated with seizures in later life. Most notable among these are
         (1) Prenatally determined due to developmental malformations, maternal drug abuse, or infections.
         (2) Complications of labor and delivery.
         (3) Complications of prematurity.

   2. **A general physical examination** may reveal a medical illness that may be associated with seizures. Special care should be taken in examining the **skin,** since neuroectodermal disorders (e.g., tuberous sclerosis, neurofibromatosis, and Sturge-Weber syndrome) can be diagnosed in this way.

3. **The neurologic examination** may show some lateralizing or localizing abnormality that would lead one to investigate more fully for an underlying cause of a patient's seizures.
4. Once a seizure has been categorized with regard to the predominant type of epilepsy from which the patient is suffering, further investigation and treatment may be considered.

IV. **General principles in management**
  A. Treat reversible metabolic conditions known to be associated with seizures, for example:
    1. Hyponatremia.
    2. Hypertension.
    3. Drug withdrawal (e.g., alcohol, barbiturates).
  B. Choose the proper drug for the seizure type, for example:
    1. Phenytoin, carbamazepine, phenobarbital, or valproate for generalized tonic-clonic seizures.
    2. Ethosuximide for typical absence seizures.
  C. Minimize the number of drugs.
  D. Simplify the dosage schedule.
  E. Check blood levels when necessary, for example:
    1. Approximately 2 weeks after adding a drug or changes in dosage.
    2. When drugs known to interact are used.
    3. Poor control of seizures.
    4. Symptoms or signs of drug toxicity.

V. **Generalized seizures**
  A. **Absence seizures**
    1. **Typical absence seizures (petit mal)**
      a. **Description.** Absence seizures are manifested by **brief attacks of loss of consciousness,** sometimes associated with 3/second minor activity, with 3/second generalized spikes and slow waves seen on the EEG. Absence seizures usually begin when the patient is between 4 and 8 years of age. Most seizures are simple absence attacks in which the patient does not lose body tone and does not fall. The attacks are usually 5–10 seconds in duration and rarely exceed 30 seconds. Minor motor activity occasionally is seen, facial twitching is usual, and, less often, automatisms such as lip smacking and repetitive swallowing are seen. Sometimes these automatisms are suggestive of complex partial (psychomotor, temporal lobe) epilepsy, but there is no aura and no postictal state, and the patient quickly returns to normal activity. The patient is rarely aware of these attacks, so the history must be obtained from an observer.
      b. **Diagnosis.** This form of epilepsy is unique in that **the clinical seizures and the EEG are of equal diagnostic importance.** The **EEG** shows a highly characteristic, generalized 3/second spike and slow-wave pattern. An **activation procedure,** particularly hyperventilation, is often required to bring out the abnormality. In the classic case, no further diagnostic evaluation is necessary.
      c. **Prognosis.** Most cases of classic absence seizures will **resolve spontaneously** by the time the person enters the third decade of life. However, some children also experience generalized tonic-clonic seizures before, together with, or subsequent to absence seizures. Although absence seizures will resolve by the third decade of life or earlier, generalized tonic-clonic seizures may persist. Four factors are associated with a good prognosis (i.e., patients who do not satisfy these criteria will be more likely to have generalized tonic-clonic seizures during childhood or in later life):
        (1) Onset between the ages of 4 and 8 years and normal intelligence.
        (2) No other seizure type present.
        (3) Easy control with a single drug.
        (4) Classic, 3/second generalized spike and slow-wave pattern on EEG, without other EEG abnormalities.
      d. **Treatment** (Tables 6-1 and 6-2)

Table 6-1. The treatment of typical absence (petit mal) seizures

Choice	Drug	Preparation	Dosage	Route
1	Ethosuximide (Zarontin)	250-mg capsules; 50-mg/ml syrup	20 mg/kg/d, divided into 2–3 doses, increasing to a maximum of 40 mg/kg/d	PO
2	Valproic acid (Depakene) Divalproex sodium (Depakote)[a]	250-mg capsules; 50-mg/ml syrup 125-, 250-, 500-mg tablets; 125-mg sprinkle capsules	15–60 mg/kg/d, divided into 2–4 doses	PO
3	Clonazepam (Klonopin)	0.5, 1.0, 2.0-mg tablets	0.01–0.03 mg/kg/d increasing to 0.1–0.2 mg/kg/d, divided into 3 doses	PO
4	Trimethadione (Tridione)	150-mg chewable tablets; 300-mg capsules; 40-mg/ml solution	20–40 mg/kg/d, divided into 3 doses (maximum 2.4 mg/d)	PO
5	Paramethadione (Paradione)	150- and 300-mg capsules; 300-mg/ml solution	20–40 mg/kg/d, divided into 3 doses (maximum 2.4 g/d)	PO
6	Methsuximide (Celontin)	150- and 300-mg capsules	5–20 mg/kg/d, divided into 3 doses (maximum 1.5 g/d)	PO
7	Phensuximide (Milontin)	500-mg capsules; 60-mg/ml suspension	5–20 mg/kg/d, divided into 3 doses (maximum 1.5 g/d)	PO
8	Acetazolamide (Diamox)[b]	125-mg tablets; 250-mg tablets; 500-mg sustained release capsules	10–25 mg/kg/d, divided into 3 doses (maximum 1 g/d)	PO
9	Ketogenic diet			

[a] Valproic acid should be used initially in patients with generalized tonic-clonic as well as absence seizures.
[b] This drug may be added to any of the above preparations but is of little use alone and should be discontinued if a ketogenic diet is used.

Table 6-2. Common toxicities and recommended monitoring for the major anticonvulsants

Drug	Plasma half-life	Major toxicity	Safety in pregnancy	Therapeutic range (serum)	Monitor
Adrenocorticotropic hormone (ACTH)		1. Glucose intolerance 2. Salt retention 3. Ulcer disease 4. Hypertension	Not safe		1. Stool guaiac every week 2. Electrolytes every week 3. Blood pressure 4. Infectious symptoms and signs; exposure to chickenpox requires treatment with VZIG (varicella-zoster immune globulin)
Acetazolamide (Diamox)		1. Hyperchloremic acidosis 2. Gastrointestinal upset 3. Nephrolithiasis	Not safe		1. Electrolytes every 3 mo 2. Serum calcium every 6 mo
Carbamazepine	9–15 hr (half-life falls if drug is used chronically)	1. Rash 2. Sedation 3. Dry mouth 4. Gastrointestinal upset 5. Jaundice 6. Aplastic anemia 7. Pancytopenia	Abnormalities reported	4–10 µg/ml	1. CBC every week for 2 mo, then every 3 mo 2. Liver function tests every 3 mo
Clonazepam (Klonopin)		Sedation	Unknown	0.013–0.72 µg/ml	1. Clinical response 2. Level of consciousness
Diazepam (Valium)	IV = 0.5–4.0 hr; PO = 24 hr	1. Sedation 2. Respiratory depression 3. Hypotension	Unknown		1. Clinical response 2. Level of consciousness
Ethosuximide (Zarontin)	24–36 hr	1. Gastrointestinal upset 2. Ataxia	Unknown	40–100 µg/ml	1. CBC every 6 mo 2. Liver function tests every 6 mo

Drug	Half-life	Teratogenicity	Therapeutic serum level	Adverse effects	Monitoring
(continued from previous page)				3. Sedation 4. Grand mal seizures 5. Vasculitis 6. Pancytopenia 7. Abnormal liver function tests	
Felbamate (Felbatol)	20–23 hr	Unknown	Not known	1. Anorexia 2. Vomiting 3. Insomnia 4. Headache	1. Clinical response
Lorazepam (Activan)	IV = 1–4 hr; PO = 12 hr	Unknown	30–100 ng/ml	1. Sedation 2. Respiratory depression	1. Clinical response 2. Level of consciousness
Mephobarbital (Mebaral)		Unknown	20–40 µg/ml	Same as phenobarbital	Same as phenobarbital
Methsuximide (Celontin)		Unknown	40–100 µg/ml	1. Gastrointestinal upset 2. Ataxia 3. Sedation 4. Pancytopenia 5. Abnormal liver function tests	1. CBC every 3 mo 2. Liver function tests every 6 mo
Midazolam (Versed)	1.2–12.3 hr	Unknown	Level if not correlated to the therapeutic effect	1. Sedation 2. Respiratory arrest 3. Hypotension	1. Clinical response 2. EEG 3. Respiratory function 4. Blood pressure
Paramethadione (Paradione)	12–24 hr	Probably dangerous (should be avoided if possible)	6–41 µg/ml	1. Photophobia 2. Sedation 3. Aplastic anemia 4. Nephrotic syndrome 5. Grand mal seizures 6. Dermatitis 7. Hepatitis	1. CBC every 3 mo 2. Urinalysis every 6 mo 3. Liver function tests every 6 mo

Table 6-2. (continued)

Drug	Plasma half-life	Major toxicity	Safety in pregnancy	Therapeutic range (serum)	Monitor

Phenobarbital (Luminal)	88–108 hr	1. Sedation
		2. Irritability (children)
		3. Learning difficulty
		4. Ataxia
		5. Rash
		6. Megaloblastic anemia
		7. Osteomalacia
			Probably unsafe	25–45 µg/ml	1. Level of consciousness
					2. Psychomotor development
					3. CBC every 6 mo
					4. Serum Ca^{2+} every 6 mo
					5. If anemic
					  a. Vitamin B_{12}
					  b. Folate

Phensuximide (Milontin)		1. Gastrointestinal upset 2. Ataxia 3. Sedation 4. Grand mal seizures 5. Pancytopenia 6. Abnormal liver function tests	Unknown	40–80 µg/ml	1. CBC every 3 mo 2. Liver function tests every 6 mo

Phenytoin (Dilantin)	12–36 hr	A. Local: GI upset
		B. Idiosyncratic
		  1. Dermatitis
		  2. Gingival hypertrophy
		  3. Hirsutism
		  4. Pseudolymphoma
		  5. Leukopenia, thrombocytopenia, agranulocytosis, aplastic anemia
		  6. Lupuslike syndrome
			Unsafe	5–20 µg/ml	1. CBC every 6 mo
					2. Calcium every 6 mo
					3. Ataxia
					4. Nystagmus
					5. Lymph nodes
					6. If anemic
					  a. Vitamin B_{12}
					  b. Folate

Drug (half-life)	Adverse effects	Use in pregnancy	Therapeutic serum level	Monitoring

	C. Dose-related
	  1. Cerebellar ataxia
	  2. Folate and vitamin B_{12} deficiency; megaloblastic anemia
	  3. Hypocalcemia and osteomalacia
	  4. Low bound thyroxine			

Primidone (Mysoline)
6–18 hr
	1. Sedation
	2. Megaloblastic anemia
	3. Ataxia
	4. Rash
		Probably unsafe	5–15 µg/ml
			Also serum phenobarbital level due to metabolism of primidone = 5–32 µg/ml
				1. Level of consciousness
				2. Nystagmus
				3. CBC every 6 mo
				4. If anemic
				  a. Vitamin B_{12}
				  b. Folate

Trimethadione (Tridione) 12–24 hr	1. Photophobia 2. Sedation 3. Aplastic anemia–neutropenia 4. Nephrotic syndrome 5. Grand mal seizures 6. Dermatitis 7. Hepatitis	Dangerous; should be avoided	20–40 µg/ml	1. CBC every 3 mo 2. Urinalysis every 6 mo 3. Liver function tests
Valproic acid (Depakene) 16–18 hr	1. Hepatic toxicity 2. Hemorrhagic tendency 3. Sedation 4. Nausea, vomiting 5. Pancreatitis 6. Serum amylase every 3 mo	Abnormalities reported (neural tube defects)	50–150 µg/ml	1. Liver function tests monthly for the first 6 mo and every 6 mo thereafter 2. CBC and platelet count every 3 mo thereafter

VZIG = varicella-zoster immune globulin.

(1) Ethosuximide (Zarontin). The treatment of choice for typical absence seizures is ethosuximide, 20–40 mg/kg/day, divided into two or three doses. The dosage usually begins with 20 mg/kg/day and is increased gradually at weekly intervals until the seizures are controlled or until the patient develops gastrointestinal upset, ataxia, or marked drowsiness. The patient can be followed clinically for toxicity, or the serum levels of ethosuximide can be measured (therapeutic range is 40–80 (μg/ml). Patients with typical absence seizures may also have generalized tonic-clonic seizures. If these occur, valproic acid should be used as the sole drug (Table 6-3). Rarely, a combination of ethosuximide and phenytoin or phenobarbital must be used.

(2) Valproic acid (Depakene and Depakote) should be used if ethosuximide is not effective. Valproic acid may also be used as the single drug in the management of patients with both typical absence and generalized tonic-clonic seizures. An initial dose of 15 mg/kg/day is recommended, with increases of 5–10 mg/kg/day at 1-week intervals until seizures are controlled or until there are clinical or biochemical signs of toxicity. The maximum recommended dose is 60 mg/kg/day divided into two to four doses. Therapeutic serum levels are 50–150 μg/ml.

    (a) Side effects. Although popular, valproic acid is not considered the drug of first choice because of its potentially serious side effects. Death due to liver failure has been reported in association with valproic acid treatment. Fatal hemorrhagic pancreatitis also has been reported. Elevation of the hepatic transaminase and serum ammonia levels may occur in patients on valproic acid, which may be dose-related. Bone marrow suppression resulting in clinically significant thrombocytopenia and neutropenia may occur. This usually responds to reduction in dosage, but discontinuation of the drug may be necessary. Less serious side effects are drowsiness and gastritis. Carnitine deficiency may occur secondary to long-term valproic acid treatment, and this complication should be prevented by supplementing carnitine (L-carnitine, Carnitor) when necessary. The dosage is 50–100 mg/kg/day, maximum 3 g/day. Carnitor is supplied as 300-mg tablets and as an oral solution containing 100 mg/ml.

    (b) Liver function tests, serum amylase levels, CBC, and platelet counts should be performed prior to treatment and at frequent intervals thereafter. A rise in the hepatic transaminase levels without associated symptoms or other biochemical abnormalities may be successfully managed by a reduction in dosage by at least 10 mg/kg/day. The drug should be discontinued if the patient develops signs of liver failure, pancreatitis, or biochemical abnormalities other than transient hepatic transaminase elevation. When valproic acid is given concurrently with phenobarbital, blood levels of the latter drug often increase. This often will require a reduction of phenobarbital dosage. Phenytoin blood levels may decrease with valproic acid usage.

(3) Clonazepam (Klonopin). There is evidence that clonazepam may be useful in the treatment of absence seizures. At present, however, it should be reserved for cases not controlled with ethosuximide or valproic acid. The drug has the advantage of having very few side effects, the most notable of which is sedation. Dosage of clonazepam is 0.1–0.03 mg/kg/day PO initially, divided into two or three doses; this is increased slowly to 0.1–0.2 mg/kg/day.

(4) Oxazolidinediones. In the very rare circumstance that control cannot be obtained with ethosuximide, valproic acid, or clonazepam, or if unacceptable toxicity or allergy is encountered, one of the oxazolidinediones may be utilized. Of the two available preparations, **paramethadione** (Paradione) is slightly less likely to produce side effects than is **trimethadione** (Tridione), but the former is often less effective. Despite the chemical similarity of the two drugs, failure of a patient to respond to one does not

Table 6-3. Treatment of atypical absence and the Lennox-Gastaut syndrome

Choice	Drug	Preparation	Dosage	Route
1	Valproic acid Depakene Depakote	250-mg capsules; 50-mg/ml syrup 125-, 250-, and 500-mg tablets; 125-mg sprinkle capsules	10–20 mg/kg/d, divided into 2–3 doses	PO
2	Felbamate (2-phenyl- 1,3-propanediol dicarbamate)	400- and 600-mg tablets; 120-mg/ml suspension	Initial dose 15 mg/kg/d; increase by 15 mg/kg/d at weekly intervals to maximum dose of 45 mg/kg/d; maximum dose 3600 mg/d. Higher doses may be used if necessary	PO
3	Clonazepam (Klonopin)	0.5-, 1.0-, and 2.0-mg tablets	0.01–0.03 mg/kg/d, increasing to 0.1–0.2 mg/kg/d	PO
4	Phenobarbital (Luminal)[a] or Phenytoin (Dilantin)[a]	15-, 30-, 60-, and 100-mg tablets; 4-mg/ml elixir 30- and 100-mg capsules; 50-mg chewable tablets; 6- and 25-mg/ml suspension	3–5 mg/kg/d, divided into 2–3 doses 5 mg/kg/d, divided into 1–3 doses	PO, IM PO
5	Ethosuximide (Zarontin)[b]	250-mg capsules; 50-mg/ml syrup	20 mg/kg/d, divided into 2–3 doses, increasing to 40 mg/kg/d	PO
6	Ketogenic diet			

[a] Used for associated tonic and/or tonic-clonic seizures.
[b] Rarely effective but relatively nontoxic.

preclude use of the other. The same principle holds for the tendency to produce side effects.

(a) **Side effects.** The most common side effects are **sedation** and **photophobia.**

(b) **Complications.** The most important possible complications are **nephrotic syndrome, neutropenia, aplastic anemia, exfoliative dermatitis,** and **hepatitis.** These complications seem to be idiosyncratic but usually are reversible on discontinuation of the drug. The patient should be screened quarterly with CBC, urinalysis, and liver function tests, since development of these toxicities is an absolute contraindication to the continued use of oxazolidinediones.

(c) Oxazolidinediones should be discontinued if a **dermatitis** develops.

(d) Oxazolidinediones are contraindicated in **pregnancy.**

(e) Oxazolidinediones may produce **tonic-clonic seizures,** but these often can be treated with concomitant use of phenytoin, phenobarbital, primidone, or carbamazepine without discontinuance of the oxazolidinedione.

(5) **Succinimides other than ethosuximide.** The next two drug choices for control of absence seizures, as listed in Table 6–1, are succinimide derivatives, closely related to ethosuximide, namely **methsuximide** (Celontin) and **phensuximide** (Milontin). Both are given in dosages of 5–20 mg/kg/day PO, divided into two or three doses, and both have toxic potential similar to that of ethosuximide, except that methsuximide does not seem to have the same tendency to produce tonic-clonic seizures as the rest of the succinimide drugs do.

The succinimides and oxazolidinediones may be used together in extreme circumstances, but it is recommended that they not be used concomitantly, since the tendency toward bone marrow toxicity may be partially additive.

(6) **Acetazolamide** (Diamox) is of limited value alone but is often of some use in combination with another anticonvulsant. Added to any of the above anticonvulsants, it occasionally improves seizure control. The dosage is 10–25 mg/kg/day PO, divided into three doses.

(7) A **ketogenic diet** helps to control absence seizures, but its use is reserved for cases that are difficult to control, since the diet is unpleasant and difficult for the patient to maintain. The acetazolamide should be discontinued prior to institution of the ketogenic diet.

2. **Atypical absence seizures, including the Lennox-Gastaut syndrome**

a. **Description.** Atypical absence seizures and the Lennox-Gastaut syndrome share many similarities and for this reason are discussed together. Patients in this category have absence plus a variety of seizure types including myoclonic, atonic, tonic, or tonic-clonic. There are idiopathic and symptomatic types, the latter being due to a wide variety of static or progressive diseases.

The Lennox-Gastaut syndrome usually begins during infancy or early childhood. The seizure types listed above occur in varying combinations, and there is evidence of developmental delay or regression depending on the underlying disease. The EEG shows a variety of abnormalities including interictal slow spike and wave complexes as well as spikes, polyspikes, and slowing and disorganization of the background.

b. **Diagnosis.** These forms of epilepsy are recognized by the characteristic history and EEG patterns listed above. They may be idiopathic but frequently reflect underlying degenerative or static brain disease.

c. **Prognosis.** Seizure control is extraordinarily difficult, and developmental outcome depends on the underlying process.

d. **Treatment** is extremely difficult, and control is rarely achieved (see Table 6–3).

(1) Valproic acid as sole therapy should be tried initially (see sec. **V.A.1.d.[2]**).

(2) Clonazepam may be tried next.

(3) Phenytoin or phenobarbital should be tried for tonic-clonic seizures (see secs. **V.B.5.a** and **V.B.5.b**).

(4) Ethosuximide is rarely effective but should be tried (see sec. **V.A.1.d.[1]**).

(5) Other modalities such as acetazolamide or ketogenic diet may be added to the above drug regimens.

(6) Felbamate (2-phenyl-1, 3-propanediol dicarbamate) can be effective in the treatment of the Lennox-Gastaut syndrome, especially by reducing the frequency of atonic episodes that often are particularly troublesome. It is recommended as add-on treatment, to be used along with drugs already being administered. It is necessary to reduce the dosage of other drugs to avoid toxic side effects due to drug interaction. See Table 6-3 for the dosage of felbamate.

3. Absence status epilepticus (nonconvulsive status epilepticus)

   a. Description. A patient in nonconvulsive status epilepticus may appear to be confused or stuporous, and the EEG shows continuous generalized spike and wave abnormalities.

   b. Diagnosis is based on the clinical picture and the EEG.

   c. Treatment consists of diazepam (0.3 mg/kg) by IV infusion over 10 minutes.

B. Intermittent generalized tonic-clonic (grand mal) seizures

   1. Description. Tonic-clonic (grand mal) convulsive epilepsy is defined as **recurrent episodes of sudden loss of consciousness, with associated major motor activity.** Tonic-clonic convulsions are characterized by sudden loss of consciousness in which the entire body usually becomes rigid in extension. The patient falls to the ground, sometimes with a cry, and may urinate and be temporarily apneic. After a period of tonic rigidity, clonic jerking of the face, trunk, and limbs ensues. The rate of clonic jerking gradually decreases, and the patient finally becomes limp and comatose. Consciousness gradually returns, often with a postictal state of confusion, headache, and drowsiness. Patients may display various combinations of these components; they may have purely tonic or purely clonic attacks, or any combination thereof.

   Although many patients describe a prodromal period of irritability that varies from a few minutes to several days before an attack, generalized tonic-clonic seizures do not have a true aura, as may be seen in focal seizures. Because of the **apoplectic nature** of the attacks, these patients—unlike patients with absence seizures—are subject to serious injury during an attack, due to accidents consequent to the sudden loss of consciousness.

   2. Diagnosis

   a. Age range and incidence

      (1) A **family history** of epilepsy is common, and the familial nature of this condition is generally recognized.

      (2) True tonic-clonic convulsive seizures usually begin **before the age of 30 years** but are rare before age 3–4 years. The vast majority of these patients will have **idiopathic epilepsy** and will respond readily to treatment with one or two drugs.

      (3) **Between the ages of 30 and 60 years,** the most common cause of tonic-clonic convulsions is still **idiopathic epilepsy,** although the risk of **intracranial tumor** is significantly higher than in the younger age groups.

      (4) **Over the age of 60 years,** the onset of tonic-clonic convulsions most likely represent **cerebrovascular disease** (usually postcerebral embolus), but tumor and idiopathic epilepsy remain important diagnoses as well. At no time in life does the onset of tonic-clonic convulsions primarily suggest brain tumor, although incidence of brain tumor peaks in middle life, and this diagnosis should certainly be excluded.

   b. It is very important to attempt to rule out partial seizures that have spread to become generalized (secondarily tonic-clonic seizures) as the cause of what is apparently a primarily tonic-clonic seizure. In older children and in adults, tonic-clonic seizures are very likely to be either idiopathic or metabolic, whereas partial seizures, with or without spread to tonic-clonic convulsions, represent focal brain disease and thus may have a graver prognosis. In infants (especially neonates) and young children, seizures are more likely to be partial, whether due to a diffuse or focal process.

It should be kept in mind that **the history is often insufficient** to definitely rule out partial seizure with spread, so many cases of what are apparently generalized tonic-clonic convulsions are in fact partial seizures with spread. Because these cases carry a more ominous prognosis with respect to focal brain disease, whenever the history is vague, one should assume that there is a possibility of partial seizures and act accordingly (i.e., carry out a more vigorous evaluation, as outlined in sec. **VI**).

3. **Prognosis.** In patients with classic generalized tonic-clonic seizures, the prognosis is good, because it is likely that the diagnosis will be idiopathic epilepsy, which can be controlled easily with drugs. Often, seizures that begin in the second or third decade become less frequent and even stop entirely, allowing total discontinuation of anticonvulsant medications. Patients with idiopathic tonic-clonic convulsions may experience exacerbation of their seizures with metabolic stresses, such as drug withdrawal, fever, hypoglycemia, and hyponatremia, all of which can produce tonic-clonic convulsions in nonepileptic people.

4. **Evaluation.** Most patients who suffer their first seizure should be hospitalized for the initial evaluation, since no predictions concerning etiology, future course, or facility of control can be made on one isolated examination. **Routine studies** on all patients who have suffered their first tonic-clonic convulsion should include the following:

   a. A careful **neurologic examination** should be aimed primarily at determining whether any focal or lateralizing aspects of the seizure state can be found either ictally or postictally.

   b. CBC.

   c. Serum electrolytes (sodium, potassium, chloride, bicarbonate).

   d. BUN.

   e. Serum calcium.

   f. Blood sugar.

   g. Liver function tests (SGOT, alkaline phosphatase, total bilirubin).

   h. Lumbar puncture for cerebrospinal fluid (CSF) if infection is suspected.

      (1) Cell count.

      (2) Glucose.

      (3) Protein.

      (4) Culture.

      (5) Syphilis serology.

   i. **Toxic screen** and **blood alcohol levels** are obtained if drug or alcohol ingestion is suspected.

   j. During a generalized tonic-clonic convulsion, the **EEG** shows generalized spikes. Postictally, it is generally slow, and interictally, the EEG may be totally normal. If an abnormality is seen, care is taken to exclude a focal or lateralizing abnormality, either ictally or postictally. However, if there is a nonfocal, nonlateralizing EEG, the prognosis is good.

   k. An **MRI** is the imaging method of choice and should eventually be performed. **CT scan** remains a useful test and is easier to perform, especially in an urgent situation such as trauma or suspected intracranial hemorrhage.

5. **Treatment** (Table 6-4). There are four major drugs for the treatment of generalized tonic-clonic seizures: phenytoin, phenobarbital, carbamazepine, and valproic acid. These four drugs are virtually equally effective. The decision as to which one to use in a particular patient depends on the relative side effects and patient's age.

   a. **Phenytoin**

      (1) **Administration**

         (a) **Therapeutic serum levels** of 5–20 μg/ml correlate well with the anticonvulsant properties of phenytoin. When given at 5 mg/kg/day (about 300 mg/day in an average adult), it takes 5–15 days to reach the therapeutic range. However, if a loading dose of 18 mg/kg (15–20 mg/kg; maximum 1 g) is given PO, the therapeutic range can be reached within a few hours. Since the biologic half-life of phenytoin is usually about 24 hours, the drug needs to be given only once per day.

Table 6-4. The treatment of generalized tonic-clonic convulsions and partial seizures

Choice	Drug	Preparation	Dosage	Route
1	Carbamazepine (Tegretol)[a] or	100-mg chewable tablets; 200-mg tablets; 100-mg/5-ml suspension	7–15 mg/kg/d, divided into 2–3 doses (adults usually require 200–800 mg/d)	PO
	Phenytoin (Dilantin)[b] or	30- and 100-mg capsules; 50-mg chewable tablets; 6-mg/ml suspension; 25-mg/ml suspension; 250-mg ampules	5 mg/kg/d; loading dose of 15 mg/kg may be given over 20 min	PO, IV
	Phenobarbital (Luminal)[c] or	15-, 30-, 60-, and 100-mg tablets; 4-mg/ml elixir	1–5 mg/kg/d, divided into 2–3 doses (adults usually require 60–120 mg/d)	PO, IM IV
	Valproic acid[d] Depakene Depakote	250-mg capsules; 50-mg/ml syrup 125-, 250-, 500-mg tablets; 125-mg sprinkle capsules	15–60 mg/kg/d, divided into 2–3 doses	PO
2	Combinations of drugs in Choice 1			
3	Primidone (Mysoline)	50- and 250-mg tablets; 50-mg/ml suspension	10–25 mg/kg/d, divided into 2–3 doses (adults usually require 300–1000 mg/d)	PO
4	Felbamate (Felbatol)	400- and 600-mg tablets; 120-mg/ml suspension	15–45 mg/kg/d, maximum 3600 mg/d	PO
5	Gabapentin (Neurontin)	100-, 300-, and 400-mg capsules	900–1800 mg/d, divided into 3 doses	PO

[a] Has not been approved by the Food and Drug Administration for use in children below the age of 6 years but is being used in younger children nevertheless.
[b] Not useful in young infants; generally avoided in children because of side effects.
[c] Should generally be avoided in school-aged children. May be replaced by mephobarbital (Mebaral) if persistent behavioral change develops. The dosage of mephobarbital is 2–10 mg/kg/d, divided into 2–3 doses; it is available in 30-, 50-, 100-, and 200-mg tablets.
[d] Especially useful in school-aged children if carbamazepine is not effective.

If the drug is given IV, the therapeutic range can be reached in minutes.

(b) **Dilantinization** should be considered much in the same way as digitalization. The rate at which a patient is dilantinized depends on the clinical situation. The therapeutic range can be reached in as little as 20 minutes or as long as 15 days. Obviously, the number of dose-related side effects will increase with the speed at which the patient is dilantinized, so the general rule of thumb is to proceed as slowly as is clinically safe. For example, if the patient has had only one seizure and will be in the hospital for several days for initial evaluation and observation, 5 mg/kg/day is administered PO (about 300 mg/day in an average adult), and therapeutic effects are expected in about 5 days. However, some patients have excessive phenytoin metabolism, in which case the therapeutic effects may not be demonstrated for as long as 2 weeks.

(c) **If the patient has had several seizures or cannot be hospitalized** for some reason, one might wish to administer 18 mg/kg in the first 24 hours, perhaps divided into three doses. The entire loading dose can be given at once if even more rapid dilantinization is desired. The latter method would result in therapeutic levels in 5–6 hours. Various approaches to dilantinization are outlined in Table 6-5.

(d) There is usually reasonably good correlation between serum phenytoin levels and the following **clinical signs:**

  (i) **Nystagmus** develops when the phenytoin level is about 10–20 $\mu g/ml$. It is very common to see bilateral horizontal nystagmus on lateral gaze when phenytoin levels are in the therapeutic range.

  (ii) **Ataxia** develops when the phenytoin level is about 30 $\mu g/ml$. The development of frank ataxia should warn the physician that the dosage should be decreased.

  (iii) **Lethargy** develops when the phenytoin level reaches about 40 $\mu g/ml$

(2) **Side effects.** The side effects of phenytoin are protean, but fortunately the most serious ones are infrequent and are usually reversible. The untoward effects can be divided into three categories: local, idiosyncratic, and dose related.

  (a) **Local side effects.** The only local side effect is gastric upset, which can usually be relieved if phenytoin is taken with meals or milk.

  (b) **Idiosyncratic side effects.** Several idiosyncratic effects are seen, many of which require discontinuation of the drug. For example, dermatitis may develop, with fever and eosinophilia. A lupuslike syndrome occasionally occurs, with positive antinuclear antibodies; and occasional blood dyscrasias occur, including leukopenia, agranulocytosis, thrombocytopenia, aplastic anemia, and pseudolymphoma. If any of these complications occur, phenytoin is discontinued in favor of another anticonvulsant. Gingival hypertrophy and hirsutism are common side effects of phenytoin, and although they are not in themselves contraindications to the use of the drug, they may be sufficiently bothersome cosmetically to indicate replacement of phenytoin by another anticonvulsant. For this reason alone, many neurologists use another anticonvulsant as the first choice in young patients.

  (c) **Dose-related side effects.** A number of dose-related side effects also exist, including cerebellar ataxia and nystagmus, as mentioned previously; a megaloblastic anemia due to interference with folic acid and vitamin B_{12} metabolism; low protein-bound thyroxine (T_4) due to competitive binding of phenytoin to the thyroid-binding globulin; immunosuppression clinically expressed as recurrent infections; and hypocalcemia with osteoporosis and elevated serum alkaline phosphatase. The latter effect is probably caused by phenytoin's effects on

Table 6-5. Various methods of dilantinization

Therapeutic range* reached (after initial dose)	Rate of administration	Route	Comment
20 min	15–20 mg/kg, maximum 1 gm, over 20 min	IV	Always with pulse, BP, and respiration monitored; given by syringe; not mixed in bottle.
4–6 hr	1000 mg stat in adults; then 300 mg/d (about 15 mg/kg stat in children; then 5 mg/kg/d)	PO	Local gastric upset is common; give with meals or milk.
24–30 hr	300 mg q8h for 3 doses in adults; then 300 mg/d (5 mg/kg/q8h for 3 doses in children; then 5 mg/kg)	PO	Mild ataxia is common initially.
5–15 d	300 mg/d in adults (5 mg/kg/d in children)	PO	No unusual side effects.

* The therapeutic range is 5–20 µg/ml of serum.

the liver, which accelerates vitamin D metabolism, producing a relative deficiency of vitamin D. It has been reported that long-term phenytoin use occasionally may be associated with cerebellar degeneration and polyneuropathy. Subtle interference with cognitive function may occur in children.

    (d) Treatment of side effects. Many of these side effects can be treated without stopping the phenytoin:

        (i) By lowering the dosage if it is above the therapeutic range.

        (ii) By administering folate, vitamin B_{12}, or vitamin D when indicated.

        (iii) By recognizing that an apparently low T_4 only represents an artifactual lowering of T_4 binding to thyroid-binding globulin.

(3) Drug interactions. Many commonly used drugs interfere with the metabolism of phenytoin, thus elevating its blood level. If frequent clinical examinations are done to monitor the blood level of phenytoin, the dosage can be lowered until the proper therapeutic range is reached for a particular patient. Serum levels of phenytoin may be helpful.

    (a) Drugs known to elevate the blood level of phenytoin or to increase the risk of toxic side effects:

        (i) Isoniazid (INH).

        (ii) Coumarin anticoagulants.

        (iii) Disulfiram (Antabuse).

        (iv) Chloramphenical (Chloromycetin).

        (v) Benzodiazepines (Librium, Valium, Serax, Clonopin).

        (vi) Methylphenidate (Ritalin).

        (vii) Phenothiazines.

        (viii) Estrogens.

        (ix) Ethosuximide (Zarontin).

        (x) Phenylbutazone (Butazolidin).

        (xi) Acute alcohol ingestion.

        (xii) Tolbutamide.

        (xiii) Halothane.

    (b) Drugs known to lower the blood level of phenytoin or to decrease its therapeutic effects:

        (i) Carbamazepine (Tegretol).

        (ii) Chronic alcohol abuse.

        (iii) Reserpine.

    (c) Drugs known to either lower or increase blood levels of phenytoin:

        (i) Phenobarbital.

        (ii) Valproic acid.

    (d) Drugs whose efficacy is impaired by phenytoin:

        (i) Corticosteroids.

        (ii) Coumarin anticoagulants.

        (iii) Oral contraceptives.

        (iv) Quinidine.

        (v) Vitamin D.

b. Phenobarbital is a barbiturate and has potent anticonvulsant properties.

    (1) Administration. The required dosage of phenobarbital is less predictable than that of phenytoin. Children require 3–5 mg/kg/day (the serum therapeutic range is 20–40 µg/ml), whereas adults usually require proportionally less, about 60–120 mg/day. The biologic half-life of phenobarbital is even longer than that of phenytoin (about 96 hours), and thus, theoretically, it can be given less frequently. However, the sedative effects of the drug usually preclude giving the entire daily dose at one time. Thus it is generally necessary to administer it in two or three divided doses.

    There is no limiting factor to increasing the dosage of phenobarbital, except sedation or behavioral and personality changes, and often much higher dosages than have been recommended are required to control seizures. The use of phenobarbital for continuous seizures is slightly different and is covered in sec. **V.C.**

(2) Side effects

(a) The major contraindication of phenobarbital is that it produces **sedation** when it is given in the anticonvulsant therapeutic range. Usually this effect will decrease as the patient becomes tolerant to the drug, but sometimes it does not. In patients in whom the sedative effects are tied closely to the anticonvulsant effects, phenobarbital sometimes cannot be used. Fortunately, this situation is rare. Furthermore, as the patient becomes tolerant to the sedative property of phenobarbital, the patient may also become tolerant to the anticonvulsant properties, in which case the dosage must be increased, producing drowsiness again. Usually, the drowsiness decreases after a few days or weeks, and the potent anticonvulsive effects remain. In school-aged children, the drug commonly causes hyperactivity and irritability and interferes with learning, so it is rarely used. Mephobarbital is rarely a useful substitute in this circumstance.

(b) Rarely, phenobarbital may produce a megaloblastic anemia, similar to that produced by phenytoin. This effect is responsive to folate or vitamin B_{12}, but sometimes this therapy results in exacerbation of seizures, requiring that another anticonvulsant be used.

(c) Relative vitamin D deficiency and osteomalacia may also be seen with phenobarbital use, but less frequently than with phenytoin.

c. Carbamazepine (Tegretol) is a dibenzazepine derivative that is related structurally to imipramine (Tofranil). The drug has gained widespread use as initial treatment because many of the behavioral, cognitive, and other side effects of phenobarbital and phenytoin can be avoided, especially in school-aged children.

(1) Administration. Dosage is 15–25 mg/kg/day, given PO in two or three doses. Barring abnormalities in the blood count or liver function tests, the dosage may be gradually increased from the lower to the higher doses until either unacceptable sedation or control of seizures occurs. A serum carbamazepine test is available, and the therapeutic range is 6–10 μg/ml. Carbamazepine may be used alone or in combination with either phenytoin or phenobarbital, or both, or with primidone. However, it is very rare that three drugs are required to control ordinary generalized tonic convulsions.

(2) Side effects include allergic skin rashes, sedation, dry mouth, gastrointestinal upset, cholestatic jaundice, aplastic anemia, and pancytopenia. As a result, patients should be followed closely, with quarterly CBCs and liver function tests, and the drug should be discontinued if there is evidence of significant bone marrow depression or liver dysfunction. Most of these side effects have been reversible, although irreversible and fatal blood dyscrasias have occurred very rarely.

d. Valproic acid. See **sec. V.A.1.d.(2).**

e. Primidone (Mysoline) is closely related chemically to phenobarbital, but it will occasionally help to control tonic-clonic convulsions when phenobarbital fails.

(1) Indications. Primidone may be used alone, but more often it is used in combination with phenytoin when phenobarbital fails. Phenobarbital and primidone are not used in combination because of their close chemical relation.

(2) Administration. The usual dosage for children under 6 years old is 10–25 mg/kg/day, divided into two or three doses. As with phenobarbital, adults require proportionally lower dosages, usually in the range of 300–750 mg/day. Children should be started on 10 mg/kg/day and the dosage gradually increased until either seizure control or unacceptable sedation occurs. Adults should be started at low dosages (50–125 mg/day), which can be gradually increased to the therapeutic range. Primidone can only be given PO.

(3) Side effects

(a) The major side effect is **sedation,** which may be severe and less likely to disappear with time, as it does with phenobarbital. This can sometimes be avoided by beginning with a low dosage and gradually increasing it to the therapeutic range (10–25 μg/ml).

(b) A syndrome of **vertigo** with **cerebellar ataxia** may develop in the first few days of therapy but generally resolves spontaneously.

(c) An **allergic rash** rarely develops, but when it does, primidone should be replaced with another anticonvulsant.

(d) A **megaloblastic anemia** may also develop occasionally, most often due to folate deficiency, but occasionally caused by vitamin B_{12} deficiency. This can be treated with folate, vitamin B_{12}, or both, without discontinuing the medication.

(e) Primidone has the same potential for **tolerance** and **withdrawal** as phenobarbital, and its ability to produce **life-threatening respiratory depression** in overdosage is the same as with other barbiturates.

(f) **Miscellaneous drugs.** Occasionally, drugs related to phenytoin or phenobarbital are useful when their parent compounds fail or are poorly tolerated. Mephobarbital (Mebaral), 2–10 mg/kg/day, and mephenytoin (Mesantoin), 5–10 mg/kg/day, are used most commonly for this purpose. The side effects are similar to those of their parent compounds.

6. Pregnancy. The question of how to manage epilepsy in the pregnant patient is difficult. However, there are some general principles to guide the physician.

a. The precise **effect on the fetus** of most anticonvulsants is not known. The use of anticonvulsants has been associated with a slightly increased incidence of serious congenital anomalies, but human studies are always limited by the fact that epilepsy itself may have similar effects. Because of the lack of evidence for safe use of most anticonvulsants, it is recommended that **as many anticonvulsants as possible be discontinued in pregnancy, particularly in the first trimester.**

b. Absence and partial seizures probably have no adverse effect on the mother or fetus, and thus anticonvulsants may be discontinued in some of these patients for the duration of the pregnancy. However, if absence or partial seizures are overwhelmingly disabling or dangerous to the patient, then the risk to the patient must be weighed against the unknown risk to the fetus.

c. It is generally agreed that frequent tonic-clonic convulsions during pregnancy are dangerous to the mother and fetus. Although the clinician should attempt to decrease anticonvulsants during pregnancy, this may not always be possible. If the seizures cannot be controlled, it is reasonable to use whatever anticonvulsant is required, since the risk to the fetus is probably greater with multiple tonic-clonic convulsions than it is with any of the anticonvulsants.

7. Toxemia of pregnancy refers to the syndrome of acute or subacute hypertension during gestation. **Preeclampsia** refers to the development of blood pressure above 140/90 mm Hg with proteinuria, persistent edema, or both. Hyperreflexia and headache are common features of preeclampsia but are not part of the definition. When seizures or coma is added to this syndrome, the condition is called **eclampsia.** It is generally agreed that the neurologic aspects of the illness are due to hypertensive encephalopathy. Toxemia occurs almost exclusively in the second half of gestation and is seen most commonly in poorly nourished primigravidas. The etiology is unknown. The condition is associated with a high maternal and fetal mortality; when it is diagnosed, pregnancy should be terminated if possible. Prior to the termination of pregnancy, the following treatment regimen is recommended:

a. Lower the blood pressure with nitroprusside, 3 μg/kg by continuous IV infusion. Propranolol, 1–5 mg IV, may be required to block the reflex tachycardia that is seen with nitroprusside use.

b. If seizures continue, check metabolic indices that may be associated with seizures, in particular the serum sodium.

c. If seizures persist despite correction of metabolic abnormalities and normalization of the blood pressure, treat with phenytoin, 15 mg/kg at 50 mg/min.

d. If phenytoin fails, perform a lumbar puncture, obtain a CT scan, and infuse diazepam (5–10 mg) by slow (over about 5 minutes) injection.

e. There is little evidence to support the use of magnesium in the treatment of toxemia.

8. Drug withdrawal seizures. Seizures may occur as part of the withdrawal syndrome from many drugs, the most common and important of which are **alcohol** and **barbiturates.** If they are caused only by withdrawal from these agents, they should be generalized tonic-clonic convulsions. However, if there appears to be a focal aspect to the seizure or a postictal (Todd's) paralysis in a patient suspected of withdrawing from drugs, the possibility of focal brain disease must be raised, and the diagnosis of simple drug withdrawal seizures cannot be made.

In general, drug withdrawal seizures are treated acutely, just as any other form of generalized tonic-clonic convulsions. There are, however, many commonly held misconceptions about these types of seizure, which the following points may help to clarify:

a. Phenytoin is useful in treating both **alcohol and barbiturate withdrawal seizures,** acutely and prophylactically. However, long-term anticonvulsant treatment with phenytoin or any other drug is often unsatisfactory, since patients rarely continue their medications faithfully when taking drugs or alcohol. Thus, most neurologists use phenytoin only when necessary to control severe convulsions, but not on a long-term basis. In the case of alcohol withdrawal seizures ("rum fits"), paraldehyde, which may be used for the control of other aspects of the withdrawal syndrome, is often helpful in preventing severe convulsions as well. Repletion of magnesium may also help to prevent alcohol withdrawal seizures.

b. Barbiturates in very large doses (sometimes more than 1 g of secobarbital [Seconal]) may be necessary to control **severe barbiturate withdrawal seizures.** In these cases, other anticonvulsants, including phenytoin, are often of little value. One can only suspect such a situation by obtaining a history from the patient's friends or relatives. Short-acting barbiturates, such as secobarbital, are more likely to produce a withdrawal syndrome than long-acting agents, such as phenobarbital. However, all **barbiturates can produce withdrawal seizures.** When administering barbiturates in doses higher than about 250 mg in acute situations, preparations should be made to perform endotracheal intubation if necessary.

c. When one is faced with a **known barbiturate addict who has discontinued use of the drugs abruptly,** it is usually wise to administer barbiturates prophylactically to prevent withdrawal seizure and then gradually decrease dosage of the drug over several days or weeks. The level of the patient's tolerance can be judged clinically by administering secobarbital, 200 mg PO, and observing for nystagmus and cerebellar ataxia 30 minutes later. If no toxicity is noted, secobarbital, 100 mg, can be administered every 30 minutes until nystagmus or cerebellar ataxia is noted. The total dose administered may be considered the patient's daily maintenance dose. This dose can then be tapered by 50–100 mg every other day to withdraw the drug completely and safely.

d. In most cases of **uncomplicated alcohol withdrawal seizures** (and many cases of barbiturate withdrawal seizures as well), the illness is self-limited and does not require anticonvulsant therapy.

C. Continuous tonic-clonic convulsions (convulsive grand mal status epilepticus)

1. Description. Generalized tonic-clonic status epilepticus is defined as either **continuous (30 minutes or longer) tonic-clonic convulsions or convulsions that are so frequent that each attack begins before the postictal period of the preceding one ends.** For example, the patient's motor movements may be continuous or stop intermittently. In the latter case, the patient may respond to stimuli or even follow simple commands, but before the patient regains total consciousness, another seizure may intervene.

2. The **diagnosis** of generalized tonic-clonic status epilepticus is not difficult. The patient exhibits tonic or clonic movements (or both) of all limbs. These movements are often associated with roving eye movements or clonic eye movements which may vary in direction from time to time. Without a history from an observer of the onset of the seizures, there is no way to be sure whether the seizures are classified as primarily generalized tonic-clonic seizures or whether they are the result of spread from a partial seizure. Since the latter holds a graver prognosis with respect to the underlying disease process that could have precipitated the attack (i.e., it implies focal brain disease), it is assumed that there is a focus until proved otherwise. In this way a serious focal brain lesion will not be overlooked, such as subdural hematoma, which may appear as continuous, generalized tonic-clonic epilepsy.

3. **Prognosis.** The outcome following an episode of status epilepticus depends on the underlying disease and the duration of the seizures plus associated metabolic abnormalities. In general, the outlook is more favorable in patients with idiopathic epilepsy or easily correctable metabolic abnormalities in contrast to patients with acute destructive brain insults such as hypoxia, encephalitis, or trauma. Systemic metabolic abnormalities such as hypoxia, acidosis, and hypoglycemia may result in a poor outcome. In addition, local biochemical tissue changes may occur after 20–30 minutes of status epilepticus, and within 60 minutes irreversible neuronal damage may be seen.

4. **Evaluation.** In every patient with continuous tonic-clonic convulsions, the following evaluation should be performed:

   a. A **careful history** (from friends or relatives) and **physical examination** should be aimed at

      (1) Signs of head trauma.

      (2) CNS infection.

      (3) Drug intoxication.

      (4) History of epilepsy and anticonvulsant use.

      (5) Any evidence of focal characteristics of the seizures themselves.

      (6) Recent surgery (e.g., thyroid or parathyroid surgery that might predispose a patient particularly to hypocalcemia).

   b. A history or physical signs of **insulin use** might lead one to consider hypoglycemia as a major possibility.

   c. An **ECG,** if technically possible (sometimes it can be done interictally), may show a long QT interval, which is evidence of possibly significant hypocalcemia or an underlying cardiac arrhythmia that precipitated the seizure episode and might recur.

   d. Before therapy is initiated, blood is drawn and sent to the laboratory for the following:

      (1) Serum glucose.

      (2) Serum calcium.

      (3) Serum sodium.

      (4) When specifically indicated, serum and urine may be sent for toxic screen, and serum is sent for anticonvulsant levels.

   e. Nearly all patients in tonic-clonic status epilepticus are febrile, so this alone is not an indication to do a **lumbar puncture.** Lumbar puncture is technically difficult in a convulsing person and may be deferred until after the seizures are controlled, unless strong indications are present (e.g., historic or physical evidence of possible bacterial meningitis).

5. **Treatment** (Figure 6-1)

   a. **When to treat. Seizures rarely require emergency intervention,** since the majority are brief and self-limited. A great deal of harm can be done by overdosing patients in an attempt to control non–life-threatening seizures with aggressive anticonvulsant therapy. Continuous, generalized tonic or clonic convulsions (or both) require deliberate, relatively rapid therapy on an

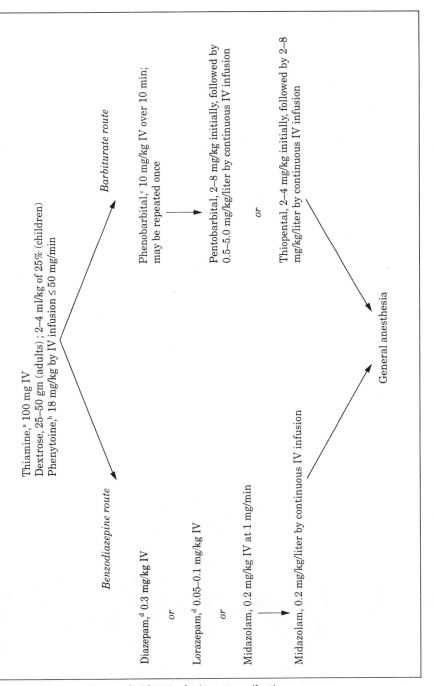

Fig. 6-1. Treatment of generalized tonic-clonic status epilepticus.
a Thiamine is given when alcoholism or malnutrition is suspected.
b Never dilute in glucose-containing fluids.
c Drug of first choice in neonates.
d In children, either diazepam or lorazepam usually initial drug, followed by phenytoin.

emergency basis. Even in this situation, **termination of the seizure within seconds or minutes is rarely required and should be sought only when the seizure activity has resulted in either severe hypoxia or acidosis, which in turn threatens the patient's life or has been prolonged (i.e., approaching 60 minutes).**

b. General measures

    (1) The patient is placed in a semiprone position, preferably with the head lower to prevent aspiration, until full consciousness is regained.

    (2) Care is taken to maintain an adequate airway. Usually this can be accomplished with an oral airway, but occasionally endotracheal intubation is required.

    (3) Oxygen may be administered by face mask.

    (4) The patient is placed in a safe environment with padded bed rails but is not restrained, since many intraictal injuries are caused by restraint in abnormal postures.

    (5) **After blood is drawn for initial chemical studies,** drug therapy is initiated (see Fig. 6-1).

c. Drug therapy

    (1) **Thiamine.** In adults, thiamine (100 mg IV) is always given before dextrose, to protect the patient against an exacerbation of Wernicke's encephalopathy, a relatively common disease among patients with status epilepticus.

    (2) **Dextrose.** All patients should receive dextrose (25–50 g by rapid IV infusion in adults, and 2–4 ml/kg of 25% dextrose by IV infusion in children).

    (3) **Sodium chloride**

        (a) In patients with seizures thought to be secondary to hyponatremia (serum sodium is usually lower than 120 mEq/liter), hypertonic (3%) sodium chloride should be given by slow IV drip. These patients are usually resistant to conventional anticonvulsant therapy.

        (b) In most cases, hyponatremia is not recognized until the serum sodium level is available; however, a history of compulsive water drinking, head trauma (causing the syndrome of inappropriate antidiuretic hormone), or hyponatremia in the past may raise a suspicion of this diagnosis. **Note that hypertonic saline infusions are dangerous and should be reserved for severely ill patients with strongly suspected or proved hyponatremia.** In these patients, an attempt should be made to correct only half the calculated sodium deficit with 3% saline, which should be sufficient to terminate the seizures. The rest of the deficit can be corrected by restricting free water intake and waiting for diuresis to occur. Excessively rapid correction of hyponatremia may result in cardiovascular overload or central pontine myelinolysis.

        (c) The formula for **calculating the required sodium infusion** is

mEq sodium required = (desired serum sodium − patient's serum sodium) × (0.6 × patient's weight in kg)

    (4) **Calcium.** In patients with hypocalcemia, 1 or 2 ampules of calcium gluconate, depending on the patient's size (90 mg of elemental calcium/ampule), should be given IV over a 5- to 10-minute period. In illness with an unknown etiology in which the suspicion of hypocalcemia is high (i.e., long QT interval on ECG or recent history of thyroid or parathyroid surgery), calcium should be given also, even before the serum calcium levels are available.

    (5) **Phenytoin** is a very effective anticonvulsant. It has the advantage of having very little effect on the patient's level of consciousness and EEG.

        (a) **Therapeutic levels.** Levels of phenytoin in the patient's serum correlate with its clinical effectiveness. Given IV (15 mg/kg, or about 1000 mg in adults, over 20 minutes), therapeutic levels of 10–20 µg/ml can be reached within a few minutes. Thus, initial anticonvulsant therapy for generalized tonic-clonic status epilepticus should be intravenous phenytoin, as described in sec. **V.B.5.a.**

(b) The injection is given preferably by a physician, and **blood pressure, respiratory rate,** and **ECG are monitored** during the injection, since occasional fatalities have been reported due to hypotension, heart block, and respiratory depression during excessively rapid phenytoin injections. **Phenytoin should be given undiluted,** since the drug may precipitate out in IV solutions. If phenytoin must be placed in solution, only saline should be used, and the solution should be administered with a controlled infusion pump.

(c) Intravenous phenytoin is **relatively contraindicated** in patients with known heart disease, particularly where conduction abnormalities are known to be part of the disease process. The injection itself requires up to 20 minutes, after which the patient should be observed for 20 or 30 minutes. Most seizures will improve significantly or stop during this time.

(6) **Benzodiazepines**

(a) **Diazepam** (Valium) is a benzodiazepine derivative that possesses some anticonvulsant activity. The drug has gained a great deal of popularity in the treatment of continuous generalized convulsions. It may, however, produce serious respiratory depression or hypotension, particularly in combination with barbiturates. Furthermore, since its anticonvulsant action is brief, it should never be given alone but always in combination with a long-acting anticonvulsant such as phenytoin. However, there are some situations in which this sequence is not effective or the patient is severely apneic or hypoxic, and as a result, enough time cannot be allowed for the conventional anticonvulsants to work. In this circumstance, diazepam may be very useful (0.25–0.40 mg/kg up to 20 mg by slow IV infusion) to control clinical seizure activity. Endotracheal intubation is very often required at this stage, and hypotension is a potential problem.

(b) Another benzodiazepine, **lorazepam** (Ativan), is also effective in this circumstance. Initially 0.05–0.10 mg/kg to a maximum dose of 4 mg is given over about 2 minutes. If seizures are not controlled, another 4 mg may be given in a similar fashion. Respiratory depression may occur, but overall the drug seems reasonably safe.

(c) **Midazolam** (Versed) is a short-acting benzodiazepine that may also be useful in the management of tonic-clonic status epilepticus. A slow IV infusion of 0.2 mg/kg may be given (i.e., about 1 mg/min), followed by a constant infusion of 0.2 mg/kg/hr. Monitoring by EEG is useful if the constant infusion is used.

(d) Either diazepam, lorazepam, or midazolam may be used, but **only one benzodiazepine should be administered to the same patient during a given attack of status epilepticus.**

(7) **Phenobarbital** is generally considered an effective drug for control of generalized tonic-clonic status epilepticus. It is the drug of choice in neonates.

(a) **Dosage.** Phenobarbital should be given IV if possible, 10 mg/kg in children and 90–120 mg in adults, either as the initial drug or as the second-line drug if phenytoin fails to control the seizures. This may be repeated every 10–15 minutes to a maximum dose of about 25 mg/kg in children and 1000 mg in adults.

(b) **Respiratory depression** is common with barbiturates, particularly when given IV; they should be given only when the facilities are available for emergency endotracheal intubation. In patients who received phenobarbital as the first-line drug, phenytoin may be used as the second (see sec. **V.C.5.c.[5]**).

(8) **General anesthesia** or pentobarbital-induced coma is the last resort for the control of tonic-clonic status epilepticus. In addition to controlling the muscular movements, these act as anticonvulsants and will often termi-

nate the most resistant forms of status epilepticus. Long-acting anticon vulsants should always be given before general anesthesia is adminis tered. Use of pentobarbital requires the availability of continuous EEG monitoring to document the production of an isoelectric EEG. For dosage regimen, see Chap. 1, sec. **VII.D.6.g.**

D. **Myoclonic epilepsy.** The term **myoclonus** is used to describe several different types of abnormal involuntary movements characterized by single or repetitive jerks of a body part. The phenomenon of myoclonus may be a symptom of a disease that involves numerous parts of the nervous system. However, some types of myoclonus are associated with paroxysmal discharges of the EEG, suggesting that it is epileptic in nature. Other types have no associated EEG abnormality, and these are not generally felt to be epileptic in nature. The latter variety includes many **biochemical disorders,** such as uremia and hepatic failure; nocturnal myoclonus, occurring as a person is about to fall asleep; myoclonus seen in some spinal cord lesions; and palatal myoclonus, which is thought to be caused by disease of the central tegmental tract of the brainstem. Action myoclonus, seen occasionally as a sequel to hypoxic brain damage or encephalitis, sometimes has associated EEG spikes and sometimes does not (see Chap.15).

1. **Infantile spasms**

   a. **Description.** Infantile spasms are defined as **massive flexor** (rarely extensor) **spasms of the extremities and trunk that begin in infancy,** usually between the ages of 4 and 9 months, and are associated with hypsarrhythmia. There are two varieties of infantile spasms: cryptogenic and symptomatic. In the cryptogenic variety, etiology is unknown, and the infant is normal neurolog- ically up until the onset of the spasms, with developmental regression typically occurring thereafter. Brain CT scanning and MRI are normal, at least at the onset. Possible etiologies in the symptomatic group include developmental brain abnormalities (particularly lissencephaly), congenital infections, neurocutaneous syndromes (e.g., tuberous sclerosis), complications of labor and delivery, and a variety of metabolic diseases. Infants in this category are usually abnormal developmentally and neurologically prior to onset of spasms. Both types of infantile spasms are characterized by general- ized flexor spasms of the neck, trunk, and extremities. The attacks occur in bouts several times a day, occurring sometimes as often as 50 times/day, often during periods of drowsiness.

   b. The **diagnosis** depends on the characteristic appearance of spells in an infant between the ages of 4 and 9 months, although occasionally the onset can be earlier or later (up to 2 years). The EEG shows an abnormality that is referred to as hypsarrhythmia (generalized asynchronous spikes and high-voltage slow, sharp activity), which is highly characteristic of this disorder. Diagnostic evaluation should include a search for a metabolic, infectious, or structural abnormality, which may be the cause of the spasms.

   c. The **prognosis** with infantile spasms is poor, particularly if there is an earlier onset, if there is delayed development prior to the onset of the seizures, or if there is evidence of a structural abnormality by CT scan or MRI. Many patients die in childhood owing to complications of the chronic underlying neurologic disease.

   d. **Treatment** (Table 6-6)

      (1) **Adrenocorticotropic hormone (ACTH)** may have some effect on the course of infantile spasms in that it may control the seizures and improve the EEG. However, there is no evidence that treatment with ACTH will alter the ultimate outcome. ACTH, 20–40 units IM, is given daily. If the initial response is good, a 2- to 3-week course of treatment is often all that is necessary. Up to 6–8 weeks of treatment or a higher dosage may be necessary if the initial response is less favorable. A repeat course of treatment is recommended if there is relapse after ACTH is stopped. It is important to monitor BP, stool for blood, electrolytes, and infectious symptoms and signs. Chickenpox exposure should be treated with ZIG (zoster immune globulin) as soon as possible.

Table 6-6. Treatment of infantile spasms

Choice	Drug	Preparation	Dosage	Route
1	Adrenocorticotropic hormone	40–80 units/ml	20–40 units/d for 2–3 wk if good initial response; 6–8 wk of treatment if initial response is less favorable	IM
2	Valproic acid	50 mg/ml	Initially 15 mg/kg/d, divided into 3 doses; increase by 5–10 mg/kg/d, weekly if necessary	PO
	Depakene Depakote	250-mg capsules; 50-mg/ml syrup 125-, 250-, and 500-mg tablets 125-mg sprinkle capsules		
3	Clonazepam	0.5-, 1.0-, and 2.0-mg tablets	0.01–0.03 mg/kg/d, divided into 3 doses, increasing by 0.25–0.50 mg every 3 days to maintenance dosage of 0.1–0.2 mg/kg/d	PO
4	Diazepam (Valium)	2-, 5-, and 10-mg tablets; 0.4-mg/ml syrup	1–2 mg q3h	PO
5	Ketogenic diet[a] or Acetazolamide[b]	25-mg tablets	10–25 mg/kg/d, divided into 3 doses	PO

[a] A ketogenic diet may be used with any of choices 1, 2, or 3, but it is of little use alone.
[b] Acetazolamide may be used with any of choices 1, 2, or 3, but it is of little use alone and should not be used in combination with the ketogenic diet.

(2) **Valproic acid** is sometimes effective in controlling myoclonus. The dosage is discussed in sec. **V.A.1.d.(2).** If used, it must be understood that the likelihood of serious liver toxicity is greater in infants than in older patients and especially if the infant is also developmentally delayed or is receiving additional antiepileptic drugs. In children below the age of 2 years, valproate should not be used in combination with another drug. The suspicion or documentation of an underlying metabolic disorder may be a contraindication to the use of valproate. This is especially true if the underlying disorder involves mitochondrial enzyme function. Carnitine should be supplemented in infants and young children who are in relatively high risk categories for serious liver toxicity. The carnitine dosage ranges from 50–100 mg/kg/day to a maximum of 3 g/day.

(3) **Clonazepam,** a benzodiazepine derivative that is related to diazepam, may be useful in the treatment of various types of myoclonus. It is started at 0.01–0.03 mg/kg/day PO and is gradually increased to 0.1–0.2 mg/kg/day, divided into three doses.

(4) **Diazepam** is occasionally effective in infantile spasms in dosages of about 1–2 mg PO q3h.

(5) **A ketogenic diet** can be used in combination with any of these drugs.

(6) **Acetazolamide** can also be used in combination with any of these therapies discussed, with the exception of the ketogenic diet.

2. **Benign myoclonus of infancy.** The seizure pattern is similar to that seen in infantile spasms, but there are no neurodevelopmental or EEG abnormalities. The cause is not known. Treatment is not necessary, and outcome is good.

3. **Juvenile myoclonic epilepsy.** The seizure pattern has a genetic basis and is carried in chromosome number 6. It usually begins between 12 and 18 years of age and typically consists of myoclonic jerks, which usually occur on awakening or shortly thereafter. The arms are involved to a greater degree than the legs. Consciousness may or may not be altered. Absence and generalized tonic-clonic seizures may also occur. Patients are otherwise normal neurologically. The EEG shows generalized repetitive spike and spike-wave discharges. Valproic acid is the drug of choice and is usually effective. Alcohol and sleep deprivation are potent triggers of seizures in this syndrome, and patients should be aware of this.

4. **Other causes of myoclonic epilepsy**

   a. **Description.** Myoclonic seizures may be seen in a wide variety of static, metabolic, and degenerative diseases, such as Lafora's disease, various lipidoses, and subacute sclerosing panencephalitis.

   b. **Diagnosis.** Diagnostic studies will be determined by the underlying cause or causes suspected.

   c. **Prognosis** will vary with the underlying illness.

   d. **Treatment**

   (1) **Valproic acid** may be effective in controlling the variety of seizure patterns seen in this syndrome with its associated slow spike-and-wave EEG abnormality.

   (2) **Mysoline** is the second-line drug and should be tried next if valproic acid is not effective.

   (3) **Clonazepam** and **diazepam** may be useful to control the myoclonus (see secs. **V.D.1.d.[3]** and **V.D.1.d.[4]**).

   (4) **Phenytoin** and **phenobarbital.**

E. **Febrile seizures**

1. **Description.** Uncomplicated febrile seizures are defined as brief generalized seizures in a child, usually between the ages of 6 months and 5 years, who is febrile prior to the seizure in the absence of CNS infection or other defined cause. Children who have had prior afebrile seizures are excluded from this category. If the definition of uncomplicated febrile seizures is strictly followed, it is possible to separate out a group of children who have a good prognosis:

   a. The child should be between 6 months and 5 years of age.

   b. There should be a clear history of fever prior to the onset of the seizure.

   c. The seizure should have no focal features.

d. The seizure should be short, usually less than 10 minutes in duration.

e. The child should be normal neurologically and developmentally, before and after the seizure.

f. There should be no family history of afebrile epilepsy.

g. Usually such seizures are over by the time the family can bring the child to the emergency room, and therapy is rarely required.

h. Lumbar puncture should be normal, free of any evidence of infection.

i. Routine laboratory studies, including electrolytes, glucose, calcium, phosphate, magnesium, and BUN are all normal.

j. When the possibility of lead poisoning exists, a lead level may also be determined.

2. Prognosis. If the above criteria are satisfied, the neurologic outcome is excellent, and the parents may be so advised. Overall, there is approximately a 30–40% recurrence rate of uncomplicated febrile seizures. The recurrence risk is higher if the initial seizure occurs prior to 1 year of age. If, however, the above criteria are not strictly satisfied, one is not dealing with an uncomplicated febrile seizure disorder and prognosis will vary, depending on the underlying condition. In such a patient, there may be recurrence of seizure activity with or without fever, and treatment with anticonvulsants may be necessary as described in sec. **V.C.** and Table 6-4. Risk factors that may indicate a greater likelihood of a patient's having afebrile seizures include neurologic or developmental abnormality, prolonged or partial seizure pattern, and a family history of afebrile epilepsy.

3. Treatment. By definition, little or no therapy is required to control a single uncomplicated febrile convulsion.

a. Control of fever

(1) Tepid baths.

(2) Acetaminophen, 5–10 mg/kg/dose q4h PO or PR.

(3) Nonsteroidal anti-inflammatory drugs are effective in reducing temperature in febrile children. Ibuprofen suspension (Pedia-Profen), 100 mg/5 ml can be used in infants 6 months and older. The dosage ranges from 5–10 mg/kg q6h, up to a maximum daily dose of 40 mg/kg.

(4) Aspirin may contribute to the pathogenesis of Reye's syndrome, and it should **not** be prescribed routinely, especially in children with chickenpox or those suspected of having influenza.

b. Seizure control is rarely necessary due to the self-limited nature of uncomplicated febrile convulsion.

c. Prophylactic therapy. In selected patients with recurrent febrile seizures, prophylactic therapy is necessary. Phenobarbital is rarely used because of its side effects and lack of efficacy in a significant number of patients. Recently, diazepam (Valium) was shown to be effective in preventing recurrences if given immediately at the onset of fever and continued until the patient was afebrile for 24 hours. Children who experience a seizure immediately at the onset of fever should be given diazepam in anticipation of fever, depending on prodromal symptoms and signs. The recommended dosage is 0.33 mg/kg PO q8h.

VI. Partial (focal) seizures

A. Description. The term **partial (focal) seizures** refers to seizures that arise from a particular focal region of the brain. A partial seizure may

1. Remain partial.

2. Spread to involve neighboring regions of cortex (jacksonian seizure).

3. Proceed to a generalized convulsion.

B. Diagnosis. In any seizure episode, it is the onset of the spell that determines whether or not it is a partial seizure. Since any area of the cerebral cortex may be involved with focal epileptic discharges, nearly every variety of human experience can be imitated by a seizure. Often, in fact, the nature of the behavior or the experience that precedes a generalized convulsion gives a clue to the focus from which the seizure emanated.

1. The disturbance of cortical function that precedes a generalized convulsion is referred to as the **aura.** By definition, an aura occurs only in partial epilepsy and is of strong differential value in diagnosing a patient who has had a generalized convulsion. Thus, occurrence of an aura confirms the diagnosis of a partial seizure with spread to a secondarily generalized convulsion.

2. A **postictal (Todd's) paralysis** also suggests a partial seizure. **This distinction is crucial, since partial seizures represent focal brain disease, whereas generalized seizures usually do not.**

3. In a patient with partial seizures, a careful search for the **underlying disease process** always should be made. A history of the exact nature of the partial seizures or the aura of secondarily generalized seizures may provide valuable information regarding the location of the abnormality. A focal or lateralizing EEG abnormality also may be helpful.

4. **Classification.** Partial seizures are usually divided into two major categories: simple and complex.

   a. **Simple partial seizures** consist of elementary sensations, simple movements, or speech disturbances. These disturbances may be motor, sensory, or autonomic. Examples of partial motor seizures are localized, repetitive movements of a body part, masticatory movements, speech arrest, adversive postures, or tonic postures. Sensory seizures may be somatic, visual, auditory, gustatory, vertiginous, or abdominal, and autonomic attacks may initiate nausea, vomiting, or diaphoresis. These seizures are thought to originate in the areas of the cortex that are known to subserve movement or sensation for the particular body parts involved. There is no impairment of consciousness.

   b. **Complex partial seizures** refer to apparently integrated purposeful activity, sometimes with amnesia and psychic phenomena, such as hallucinations, déjà vu (factitious familiarity with an unfamiliar environment), jamais vu (factitious unfamiliarity with a familiar environment), paranoid feelings, forced thinking, and affective disturbances. This group of disorders has been referred to as **psychomotor epilepsy,** which is thought to arise often from abnormalities in the limbic cortex (i.e., orbital frontal or temporal lobes). Most cases of **temporal lobe epilepsy** begin between the ages of 10 and 30 years. Cases that begin after the age of 30 years should raise the question of brain tumor, primary or secondary. In younger children, temporal lobe epilepsy may be difficult to distinguish from absence seizures. However, the presence of an aura and postictal confusion in the former often helps to make the distinction clinically. The EEG is often helpful, particularly if it shows the typical 3/second spikes and slow-wave pattern of typical absence seizures. A normal EEG interictally is of no help in making the distinction.

5. A partial seizure pattern unique to the pediatric patient is **rolandic** or **benign childhood epilepsy** with centrotemporal spikes. It usually begins between 5 and 10 years of age, although earlier or later onset is possible. Patients typically have nocturnal seizures predominantly involving facial and oropharyngeal muscles. Seizures may also occur while the patient is awake. The EEG shows characteristic central-midtemporal (rolandic) spikes, which typically are more frequent or are only present during sleep. The EEG background is normal. Patients are otherwise normal, and an anatomic abnormality is not identified if diagnostic criteria are met. Remission during adolescence, or sooner, can be expected. Not all children with benign focal epilepsy of childhood require treatment in spite of the impressive EEG abnormality that accompanies the syndrome. Children should be treated if seizures recur frequently, are prolonged, or occur randomly through the day rather than just typically at night.

C. **Evaluation**

1. A careful history and physical examination with special reference to evidence of **old strokes, congenital anomalies, remote infections, head trauma, cranial surgery,** and **neoplasm** (particularly cancer of the breast, lung, colon, kidney and melanoma).

2. **EEG.** (If the routine EEG is normal, activation procedures may be used, including sleep, hyperventilation, and photic stimuli, Occasionally special recording methods are used, such as nasopharyngeal or sphenoidal leads, in an attempt to record abnormalities in the temporal lobes—areas that are far from

the standard scalp electrodes.) Ambulatory or simultaneous EEG-video monitoring might be necessary.

3. An MRI is the imaging method of choice, and CT scan should be bypassed except in the emergency setting.
4. Lumbar puncture, with special reference to cell count, cytology, syphilis serology, and protein in selected patients.
5. Chest x ray.
6. CBC.
7. Erythrocyte sedimentation rate.
8. Stool guaiac.
9. Serum electrolytes.
10. Serum calcium and phosphate.
11. Liver function tests (SGOT, total bilirubin, and alkaline phosphatase).
12. Urinalysis.
13. BUN and serum creatinine.
14. Blood glucose.
15. Further studies, including arteriography, may be required if the screening studies discussed are abnormal, requiring further evaluation of a particular part of the nervous system.
16. In **children** with partial seizures, there is less likelihood of a serious underlying brain disease than in adults, and thus the evaluation is sometimes less extensive. If the evaluation is negative, treatment may be started, but careful, frequent follow-up examinations are necessary, since the primary disease process may become obvious only some time after the epilepsy begins.

D. **Prognosis.** The outlook depends on the underlying condition; even if the primary disease is benign (e.g., mesial temporal sclerosis) or no primary disease can be found, these seizures are generally much more difficult to treat than primary generalized convulsions. In the case of complex partial seizures, interictal behavioral abnormalities are a common accompaniment of the disease. Whether these psychiatric syndromes (e.g., schizophrenialike illness sometimes seen in patients with temporal lobe epilepsy) are due to the same primary disease that caused the epilepsy is unknown at the present time. However, it is generally agreed that **anticonvulsants have little or no effect on the interictal behavior disorders seen in these patients.** Many require antipsychotic drugs for the control of these disorders, and the prognosis for a normal life in these patients is poor. In partial seizures with simple symptoms, there is no concomitant psychiatric illness, but the seizures themselves may be very difficult to control without reaching drug toxicity.

E. **Treatment**
1. **Medical.** The drug treatment of partial seizures is the same as that for generalized tonic-clonic convulsions (see Table 6-4). Felbamate and gabapentin are recently approved drugs for the treatment of partial seizures. They are used mainly as adjunctive agents. Felbamate interaction requires a 20% to 30% reduction in the dose of the drug(s) being used. Gabapentin has no interaction with other antiepileptic drugs. Lamotrigine and vigabatrin are currently under investigation, but are not yet approved in the United States.

   An important principle of treatment is that **partial seizures, even when continuous (epilepsia partialis continua), are not an emergency and should not be treated as such.** It is also important to remember that control is difficult, and rapid control of focal phenomena is rarely, if ever, required. Thus one should proceed cautiously and methodically through the choices of drugs shown in Table 6-4, making sure not to produce unacceptable side effects in an effort to control small focal abnormalities.

2. **Surgical.** Occasionally, partial seizures are impossible to control medically, and surgical intervention is necessary. Some patients will require surgical removal of the offending focus. Other surgical treatments for medically resistant seizure patients include cortexectomy and partial corpus callosotomy. However, results in these extraordinarily severe cases are variable, so surgical treatment should be reserved for medical failures and should not be used as a first-line form of therapy. Exceptions to this rule are patients with partial seizures caused by a

surgically removable lesion, vascular malformation (e.g., arteriovenous malfo mation, cavernous hemangioma), or congenital anomaly. Such procedures r quire intraoperative electrocorticography and should be performed at specialize centers where such techniques are routinely employed.

Some neurosurgeons believe that the behavioral abnormalities sometim seen in temporal lobe epilepsy may be reversed by removal of the epileptogen focus. However, this is not a generally accepted notion, and at present, on medically uncontrollable seizures are an indication for surgery.

VII. Neonatal seizures

A. Description. Neonatal seizures refer to seizure activity during the first 30 days life. Unlike those in the older patient, seizures in the newborn are often subtle an more difficult to diagnose. Common manifestations of neonatal seizures include

1. Tonic eye deviation, rapid eye movements, or both.
2. Repetitive eyelid blinking.
3. Facial grimacing.
4. Fragmentary clonic movements of single extremities.
5. Tonic posturing of a single extremity.
6. Apnea, often associated with other seizure activity but sometimes the sol manifestation of the seizure.
7. Generalized tonic-clonic seizures, which occur but are uncommon.

B. The **diagnosis** rests on the clinician's ability to recognize the symptoms, which ar often only fragmentary movements that may be epileptic in nature. Treatment the seizure itself is rarely an emergency unless respirations are compromised. It more important to diagnose the patient's condition rapidly, so appropriate therap can be initiated promptly. Speed is important because several types of neonat seizures may result in irreversible cerebral damage. The common causes of neonat seizures are the following:

1. **Prenatally determined problems,** such as developmental brain malformation infections, or maternal abuse of drugs.
2. **Metabolic abnormalities**
   a. **Hypoglycemia,** which usually occurs within the first few hours of birth. I babies who are small for their gestational age, are premature, have diabeti mothers, or are septic, one should suspect possible hypoglycemia. Hypoglyce mia in the term infant can be defined as a blood glucose level belo approximately 35 dl within the first 72 hours and 45 dl thereafter. In th low-birth-weight infant, hypoglycemia is defined as a blood glucose leve below approximately 25 dl. Many pediatricians will start early feedings or a intravenous glucose infusion as prophylaxis against hypoglycemia. Als blood glucose should be monitored frequently in high-risk groups, sinc hypoglycemia can produce irreversible cerebral damage. It is obviously bette to prevent neonatal hypoglycemic seizures than to treat them once they occur
   b. **Hypocalcemia**
      (1) **Early-onset** hypocalcemia (within the first 3 days of life) is commonly see in babies with low birth weight, in premature infants, and in babies wh are small for their gestational age. There is often a history of pregnanc complicated by toxemia, perinatal distress, or mechanical birth trauma
      (2) **Late-onset** hypocalcemia (after the third day of life) is thought to be du to the high phosphate load the infant receives in the first few days of life The serum calcium level is usually below 7.5 mg/dl in both early- an late-onset hypocalcemia.
   c. **Hypomagnesemia** presents much the same picture as hypocalcemia and i found in the same high-risk groups, but is less common. Hypomagnesemi and hypocalcemia may coexist, and both must be treated.
   d. **Pyridoxine dependency** usually produces seizures within minutes or hour after birth, but there are recent reports of atypical cases with later onset.
   e. **Biotinidase deficiency** and treatment with biotin, 5–10 mg/day, should b considered in infants with unexplained seizures, especially if they ar refractory to standard drugs. It is not necessary to wait for the result of th serum biotinidase assay before starting biotin.

     f. Other metabolic abnormalities, including **aminoacidurias** and **drug withdrawal** (infants of addicted mothers).

  3. Both intrauterine and postnatally acquired **CNS infections** may produce seizures in the first month of life. The evaluation should include routine CSF examination and antibody titers for toxoplasmosis, rubella, cytomegalovirus, and herpesvirus.

  4. **Perinatal complications** resulting in severe asphyxia or mechanical trauma.

  5. **Genetic factors** can be important in the newborn, resulting in the syndrome of benign familial neonatal convulsions. Seizure onset is usually on day 2 or 3 of life, seizures tend to be brief and of mixed types, remission occurs in the majority of patients by 6 weeks of age, and neurodevelopmental outcome is usually good, although a number of patients have had later epilepsy and learning difficulties. This unique syndrome is linked to the long arm of chromosome 20.

C. Treatment (Table 6-7). Once blood is drawn and sent to the laboratory for analysis, therapy is begun at once. The sequence shown in Table 6-7 is self-explanatory. The use of short-acting drugs such as diazepam is no more effective than maximum doses of phenobarbital and phenytoin.

VIII. Discontinuation of medication in patients with seizures. There are no fixed rules concerning discontinuation of medication in patients with seizures. Most neurologists would consider stopping drugs only after a **long** (4–5 years) seizure-free interval, but a shorter interval is also acceptable if the patient is in a relatively low-risk category. In children, it is reasonable to attempt to discontinue treatment after 2 seizure-free years. When this is done, drugs should be **tapered slowly** over several months. During the period of tapering, the patient must be considered at risk for a seizure, and recommendations regarding daily activities are made accordingly.

A. Factors that favor a bad prognosis (i.e., make it more likely that seizures will recur)

  1. Development abnormalities, such as mental retardation.

  2. Abnormal neurologic examination.

  3. Long duration of epilepsy before control.

  4. Partial seizures.

  5. Combination of seizure types.

  6. Significant EEG abnormality.

B. Factors not associated with increased risk of recurrence

  1. Age of onset of epilepsy, although at least one recent study showed that seizures beginning after age 12 years were more likely to recur.

  2. Number of seizures before control.

Table 6-7. Treatment of neonatal seizures

Step	Drug[a]	Dosage	Route	Rate
1	Glucose	2–4 ml/kg of 25% dextrose	IV	Rapid (push)
2	Pyridoxine[b]	50 mg	IV	Rapid (push)
3	Calcium[c]	1–2 ml/kg of 10% calcium gluconate (maximum 10 ml)	IV	Over minutes[d]
4	Magnesium[c]	0.1–0.2 ml/kg of 50% $MgSO_4$	IV	Over minutes
5	Phenobarbital	10–30 mg/kg	IV	Over minutes
6	Phenytoin[d]	15–20 mg/kg	IV	Over 20 min
7	Biotin[e]	5–10 mg/day	PO	Daily

[a] A reasonable amount of time should elapse between steps to assess drug action.
[b] If possible, monitor the EEG during infusion of pyridoxine.
[c] If possible, obtain confirmation of low level before administering.
[d] Monitor ECG during infusion.
[e] Biotinidase should be measured in serum and a trial of biotin treatment can be carried out before results are available in a newborn with unexplained, refractory seizures.

      3. Age at discontinuation of medications.

      4. Family history of epilepsy.

IX. Daily activities in patients with seizures. Certain activities are of particular potential risk in patients with seizures because of potential harm to either the patient or others There are no rigid guidelines for the restriction of such activities as swimming, skiing, or driving an automobile.

    A. In general, people with epilepsy should not **swim** alone or **climb** to excessive heights, but these restrictions probably apply to everyone, especially children.

    B. Children should be allowed to ride **bicycles,** but not in traffic, and they should wear a protective helmet (as should everyone).

    C. Driving. In some localities, the law requires that a physician report any knowledge of seizures to officials responsible for issuing driver's licenses. In other places, this is not required and, in fact, may represent a breach of confidence between the physician and patient. It is strongly recommended that physicians become familiar with the local or state laws that apply to this issue. (Detailed information about the laws in each state regarding the legal rights of seizure patients may be obtained from the Epilepsy Foundation of America, 4351 Garden City Drive, Landover, MD 20785; (301) 459–3700.) From a purely medical point of view, most neurologists would consider patients **functionally normal** if they are seizure-free for 1 year and are reliably taking the prescribed anticonvulsant regimen. In patients in whom the seizures are not associated with loss of consciousness or change in cognitive function, driving may be considered safe as long as the patient is capable of operating a motor vehicle during a seizure.

X. Paroxysmal conditions resembling epilepsy. A number of paroxysmal disorders exist that may be related to epilepsy, either by virtue of their clinical similarity and possible confusions in diagnosis or by virtue of their possible, although unproved, true epileptic nature. It is important to diagnose these syndromes correctly, since some have specific therapies of their own, a few of which may actually conflict with anticonvulsant therapy.

    A. Narcolepsy

      1. Description

        a. Narcolepsy is defined as a group of disorders characterized by some or all of the following characteristics:

          (1) Sleep attacks (irresistible episodes of sleep).

          (2) Cataplexy (sudden attacks of loss of postural tone sparing consciousness, often stimulated by emotional experiences, e.g., laughter, passion, fear).

          (3) Sleep paralysis (total paralysis that lasts a few minutes, usually on awakening from sleep but sometimes just before falling asleep).

          (4) Hypnagogic hallucinations (vivid visual or auditory hallucinations or both just as the person is falling asleep).

          (5) The EEG may show the characteristic phenomenon of sleep-onset rapid eye movement (REM) sleep.

        The physiology of normal sleep is reviewed in Chap. 1, sec. **IX.**

        b. The essential abnormality in narcolepsy is thought to be defective activity of the reticular activating system (RAS). Some patients with narcolepsy will slip uncontrollably from the waking state directly into REM sleep (so-called sleep-onset REM), and it is believed that, as a result of this process, the rest of the syndrome evolves. For example, sleep paralysis and cataplexy are merely components of the paralysis that occurs during normal REM sleep (as already noted), and hypnagogic hallucinations are merely dreams, normally occurring in the REM sleep state.

        c. Patients with narcolepsy are most likely to fall asleep in situations that would normally produce drowsiness (i.e., postprandial and during boredom), presumably because of an underactive RAS, and are unable to maintain the waking state under stress. Patients who have more severe narcolepsy will, of course, fall asleep at inappropriate times, such as while driving a car.

        d. Studies of accident-prone drivers have revealed a much higher than expected number of narcoleptics. The relation between emotional experiences and cataplexy is unknown, but it is thought to be mediated through the RAS also.

2. The **diagnosis** depends on a characteristic history and the typical EEG pattern, although the latter will not occur in every episode of sleep. Thus, a normal sleep EEG does not rule out narcolepsy. Conversely, sleep-onset REM, found incidentally in asymptomatic patients, should not lead to treatment for narcolepsy. However, it should be considered in patients with hypersomnia, whether or not the other associated abnormalities are found. The EEG may be helpful if positive (i.e., if it shows sleep-onset REM); however, the diagnosis can be made legitimately with a normal EEG if the history is sufficiently characteristic.

It is possible to confuse narcolepsy with epilepsy, particularly if the sleep attacks come on very suddenly. However, a history of an irresistible tendency to sleep and the associated abnormalities should permit proper diagnosis by history alone.

3. **Prognosis.** The outlook for narcolepsy is generally good, and the patient usually responds dramatically to drug therapy.

4. **Treatment.** There is no single treatment for all the elements of narcolepsy. Individual patients must be treated for their predominant symptoms, sometimes combining drugs to attain adequate relief from the entire complex.

   a. **Sleep attacks, hypnagogic hallucinations, and sleep paralysis**

      (1) **Amphetamines** are known to suppress REM sleep. It is not known whether this characteristic of these agents is the reason for their effectiveness in narcolepsy. However, it is clear that amphetamines are often useful in controlling sleep attacks and are sometimes useful in controlling hypnagogic hallucinations and sleep paralysis.

         (a) Many problems are associated with **chronic use of amphetamines.** For example, many narcoleptics abuse these agents, constantly raising the dosage as their tolerance develops. Other patients find that under treatment they are less aware of an oncoming sleep attack, and this places them at even greater risk for accidents. Since amphetamines interfere with normal sleep, these patients often require increasingly higher doses during the day to protect against an even greater tendency for sleep attacks.

         (b) **Side effects** of amphetamine use include a syndrome of irritability, paranoid ideation, and psychosis. Furthermore, these agents are relatively contraindicated in patients with coronary artery disease and hyperthyroidism.

         (c) **Dosage.** Despite their drawbacks, when used carefully, amphetamines are still the best treatment of the major manifestations of narcolepsy. Whichever amphetamine preparation is used, therapy should begin with low dosages and be gradually increased until a satisfactory therapeutic effect is obtained. Some commonly used agents are as follows:

            (i) **Methylphenidate** (Ritalin), 20–200 mg/day PO, divided into two or three doses.

            (ii) **Methamphetamine hydrochloride** (Fetamin), 20–200 mg/day PO, divided into two or three doses.

            (iii) **Dextroamphetamine sulfate** (Dexedrine), 20–200 mg/day PO, divided into two or three doses.

      (2) **Monoamine oxidase (MAO) inhibitors** often have a striking therapeutic effect.

         (a) Serious **side effects,** such as orthostatic hypotension, hypertension, edema, and impotence are common, requiring discontinuance of the medication in a large number of patients.

         (b) **MAO inhibitors cannot be given in combination** with dibenzepine derivatives (e.g., tricyclic antidepressants, doxepin, carbamazepine), sympathomimetics (e.g., amphetamines), or food with high tyramine content (e.g., cheese, sour cream, Chianti wine, sherry, beer, pickled foods).

         (c) **Withdrawal** of MAO inhibitors may result in insomnia, hallucinations, and serious depression, with suicidal thoughts and severe anxiety. For this reason, they are recommended only when amphetamines canno be used and the symptoms of narcolepsy are unbearable. Even the **the drug should be administered only under strict supervision.**

  (d) **Dosage.** Some commonly available MAO inhibitors and their recom mended dosages are as follows:
  (i) **Phenelzine sulfate** (Nardil), 15–75 mg/day PO, divided into thre or four doses.
  (ii) **Tranylcypromine sulfate** (Parnate), 10–30 mg/day PO, divide into two doses.
  (iii) **Pargyline hydrochloride** (Eutonyl), 25–200 mg/day PO in a singl dose.
  (iv) **Isocarboxazid** (Marplan), 10–30 mg/day PO in a single dose.

  b. **Cataplexy.** Amphetamines and MAO inhibitors have little effect on cata plexy. However, it has been shown that the **tricyclic antidepressants** may b particularly effective in the relief of this symptom. Furthermore, they ar effective in much lower dosages than are required for the treatment o depression; this suggests a separate mechanism for their effect in thi syndrome. **Imipramine** (Tofranil), 50–100 mg/day PO, divided into one o three doses is commonly used in the management of cataplexy.

  c. **Sleep attacks and cataplexy.** Theoretically, the combination of a tricycli antidepressant and an amphetamine is dangerous, since the latter causes a release of catecholamines at the neuronal synapse; the former blocks re uptake of the catecholamine neurotransmitter. This combination could there fore produce hypertensive episodes, but actually one may generally us **imipramine** (25 mg tid) **together with methylphenidate** (5–10 mg tid) withou difficulty and with good control of both sleep attacks and cataplexy. **Tricycli antidepressants should not be used in combination with an MAO inhibitor**

B. **Migraine** (see also Chap. 2). Because of its paroxysmal attacks of neurologi symptoms, usually followed by headache, migraine has some relation to epilepsy However, the differential diagnosis between the two conditions usually is no difficult. In one situation, brainstem or basilar artery migraine, loss of consciousnes may occur due to vasomotor changes consequent to transient brainstem ischemia and this may imitate epilepsy. In some rare circumstances, the cerebral ischemia due to vasospasm may actually trigger bona fide convulsions, usually in a patien with known epilepsy. On the other hand, some patients with migraine have associated paroxysmal EEG abnormalities. Some of these patients experience relie of their headaches when treated with anticonvulsants, so a trial of phenytoin or phenobarbital is often warranted in these patients. (See Chap. 2 for the details o diagnosis and treatment of migraine.)

C. **Paroxysmal abdominal pain ("abdominal epilepsy").** A syndrome of paroxysmal abdominal pain occurs in children for which no gastrointestinal or intraabdominal cause can be found. Some of these patients will respond to conventional anticonvul sant therapy, a fact that has led some patients to believe that this pain is caused by an epileptic syndrome. Thus, in a child with recurrent apoplectic episodes of abdominal pain in which a thorough medical evaluation has revealed no cause, it is probably reasonable to perform an EEG and conduct a therapeutic trial of an anticonvulsant.

D. **Breath-holding spells**
  1. **Description.** Breath-holding or reflexive apneic spells usually begin during the first 2 years of life, but rarely before 6 months of age. A precipitating factor, such as fear, pain, anger, or frustration, leads to a brief bout of crying, during which the breath is held in expiration. Cyanosis then develops, which may be followed by loss of consciousness and a brief generalized convulsion. The exact mechanism for this type of spell and its physiologic consequences are not known, but the brief convulsion that is sometimes seen is presumably caused by cerebral hypoxia.
  2. **Treatment** consists of reassuring patients and giving them advice on how to protect the child during a spell. There is no doubt that behavioral influences may lead to an increase in the frequency of spells, and parents should be advised of this possibility.

3. **Differential diagnosis.** It is important to distinguish between breath-holding spells and true epilepsy because the prognosis and treatment differ. Anticonvulsants are not indicated in the treatment of breath-holding spells, and they are not effective in terminating the attacks. The spells almost always terminate by the age of 5 years, and they have no relation to the later development of epilepsy.

E. **Hypercyanotic attacks**

1. **Description.** In patients with **cyanotic congenital heart disease**, particularly tetralogy of Fallot, sudden episodes of increased cyanosis may occur and be followed by loss of consciousness and perhaps a convulsion. The mechanism for these attacks may be spasm of the already small infundibulum (right ventricular outflow tract). The pulmonary circulation, which is already compromised, is decreased further, and the blood becomes even poorer in oxygen than it is normally. Then cerebral anoxia increases suddenly, and loss of consciousness and, possibly, convulsions result.

2. The **treatment** is repair of the anomaly or at least surgical creation of an aortopulmonary shunt (Blalock-Taussig operation) until definitive repair is technically possible. No anticonvulsants are required. Treatment of the acute attack is administration of oxygen in as high a concentration as can be obtained.

F. **Shuddering attacks.** Sudden, brief shuddering or shivering movements may occur in infants and children, often with flexion of the trunk and extremities, but without alteration of consciousness. Patients and their EEGs are normal. A cause is not known, and treatment is not necessary.

G. **Cardiovascular syncope.** Syncope is loss of consciousness due to an acute decrease in cerebral blood flow. If it is prolonged, convulsions may occur, particularly in patients with known epilepsy. The causes of syncope are protean, but they must always be ruled out when the patient suffers from episodic loss of consciousness, with or without convulsions. It is important to make this distinction because the treatment of cardiovascular syncope varies significantly from the treatment of epilepsy. In fact, phenytoin, a commonly used anticonvulsant, is strongly contraindicated in syncope caused by heart block. Thus cardiovascular syncope must be carefully excluded before the patient is treated for epilepsy.

1. The **major causes** of syncope are the following:
    a. Heart block.
    b. Arrhythmias (usually ventricular tachycardia or ventricular fibrillation).
    c. Carotid sinus hypersensitivity.
    d. Vasovagal attacks.
    e. Aortic stenosis.
    f. Asymmetric septal hypertrophy.

2. **Diagnosis**
    a. The diagnosis is not difficult to make **if the attack is observed,** since in cardiovascular syncope there is **hypotension,** whereas epilepsy alone does not produce hypotension. The heart rate may be very slow (as in heart block, carotid sinus hypersensitivity, or vasovagal syncope) or very rapid and weak or absent altogether (as in tachyarrhythmias).
    b. **If an attack is not observed,** the differential diagnosis between cardiovascular syncope and epilepsy can be very difficult. Also, whenever there is doubt concerning the mode of onset of the attacks, particularly in elderly patients, cardiovascular syncope should be considered, and several days of Holter ECG monitoring should be performed. This, of course, will not entirely rule out very infrequent arrhythmias or episodes of heart block, but it is the best procedure available.

3. **Treatment.** Carotid sinus massage may be performed under controlled circumstances, and a detailed cardiologic evaluation is often useful to exclude significant aortic valvular disease or asymmetric septal hypertrophy. No anticonvulsant therapy is required and is, in fact, contraindicated in heart block.

H. **Conversion (hysteria)** (see Chap. 9) may present a difficult problem in two ways when it occurs in a patient with apparent seizures.

1. **Hyperventilation** may result in a loss of consciousness and tetany, simulating

epilepsy. This condition can be remedied by using a rebreathing bag for acute therapy. It is not really an epileptic phenomenon.

2. **Hysterical seizures** may be very difficult to distinguish from true epilepsy. Furthermore, many patients with hysterical seizures also have authentic epileptic seizures. The normal EEG is of some help, but, as stated previously, many patients with bona fide epilepsy display repeatedly normal EEGs, thus making this an inadequate criterion. Prolonged ambulatory EEG monitoring, when available, may be helpful, and if an episode is recorded, the distinction between epileptic and nonepileptic events can be made. An experienced clinician can sometimes distinguish a poor imitation of a true convulsion, but when the patient is able to imitate a convulsion accurately, there is no practical method of distinguishing hysterical attacks from real ones.

One helpful criterion is whether the patient is incontinent or not. It is said that all persons are incontinent during a tonic-clonic convulsion unless their bladders are empty. Thus patients who have multiple attacks will certainly be incontinent during some of them, whereas many patients with hysterical seizures are never incontinent. However, this criterion is of no help in patients who are incontinent or in patients with conversion attacks that mimic absence or partial seizures, which do not show incontinence as a part of the bona fide seizure pattern.

I. **Malingering.** Seizures imitated by malingerers pose a problem similar to that of hysterical seizures. Imitations of generalized convulsions are very rarely associated with incontinence, even less so than in hysterical seizures. The only way for physicians to distinguish other forms of imitations is to use their experience with respect to the appearance of real epilepsy. However, even the most experienced observer can be misled, and occasionally malingerers are treated with anticonvulsants. Again, recording an event with prolonged EEG monitoring will be diagnostic.

J. **Tic douloureux** (see Chap. 2). Trigeminal neuralgia and some other neuralgialike syndromes have certain characteristics in common with epilepsy. They occur intermittently, usually with an apoplectic onset, and may respond to anticonvulsants, particularly phenytoin and carbamazepine. It is rare, however, that they actually pose a difficult differential diagnosis from true epilepsy.

K. **Paroxysmal vertigo** (see Chap. 4). Several syndromes of paroxysmal vertigo exist that may be confused occasionally with epilepsy, namely **benign positional vertigo** (Bárány's vertigo) and **Ménière's syndrome.** Usually these two syndromes can be distinguished from epilepsy on the basis of history and physical examination. The former may have a clear history of positional exacerbation of vertigo, and the patient will experience vertigo and nystagmus if the head is positioned properly during the neurologic examination. The latter shows episodes of vertigo that are always associated with concomitant hearing loss in the affected ear. Although the hearing loss will fluctuate with the attacks of vertigo, over time decreased hearing will be noted, and this can be documented by neurologic examination and audiometry. Vertigo may be a manifestation of complex partial seizures but is usually associated with some clouding of consciousness or change in mental state during the vertiginous episodes.

Selected Readings

Browne, T. R., and Feldman, R. L. *Epilepsy: Diagnosis and Management.* Boston: Little, Brown, 1983.

Callaghan, N., Garrett, A., and Goggin, T. Withdrawal of anticonvulsant drugs in patients free of seizures for two years *N. Engl. J. Med.* 318:942, 1988.

Camfield, C., et al. Outcome of childhood epilepsy: A population-based study with a simply predictive scoring system for those treated with medication. *J. Pediatr.* 122:681, 1993.

Committee on Drugs of the American Academy of Pediatrics. Behavioral and cognitive effects of anticonvulsant therapy. *Pediatrics* 76:644, 1985.

Donaldson, J. O. *Neurology of Pregnancy.* Philadelphia: Saunders, 1978. Pp. 211–250.

The Felbamate Study Group in Lennox-Gastaut Syndrome. Efficacy of felbamate in childhood epileptic encephalopathy (Lennox-Gastaut syndrome). *N. Engl. J. Med.* 328:29, 1993.

Jones, K. L., et al. Pattern of malformations in the children of women treated with carbamazepine during pregnancy. *N. Engl. J. Med.* 320:1661, 1989.

Kumar, A., and Bleck, T. P. Intravenous midazolam for the treatment of refractory status epilepticus. *Crit. Care Med.* 20:483, 1992.

Porter, R. J., and Morselli, P. L. (eds.) *The Epilepsies.* Boston: Butterworth, 1985.

Ronen, G. M., et al. Seizure characteristics in chromosome 20 benign familial neonatal convulsions. *Neurology* 43:1355, 1993.

Rosman, N. P., et al. A controlled trial of diazepam administered during febrile illnesses to prevent recurrences of febrile seizures. *N. Engl. J. Med.* 329:79, 1993.

Salbert, B. A., Pellock, J. M., and Wolf, Barry. Characterization of seizures associated with biotinidase deficiency. *Neurology* 43:1351, 1993.

Scott, A. K. Management of epilepsy. *Br. Med. J.* 288:986, 1984.

Shinnar, S., et al. Discontinuing antiepileptic medication in children with epilepsy after two years without seizures. *N. Engl. J. Med.* 313:976, 1985.

Solomon, G. E., Kutt, H., and Plum, F. *Clinical Management of Seizures* (2nd ed.). Philadelphia: Saunders, 1983.

Thurston, J. H., et al. Prognosis in childhood epilepsy. *N. Engl. J. Med.* 306:831, 1982.

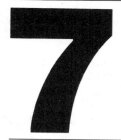

Brain Death and Persistent Vegetative State

Thomas M. Walshe III

I. Brain death

A. Definition

1. **Medical definition.** The criterion for the diagnosis of death traditionally has been cessation of the circulation and asystole. In certain cases, however, the cardio respiratory function can be maintained artificially while the brain is irreversibly destroyed.

   a. The concept of **death defined by brain viability,** termed **brain death,** has developed in the past 25 years, following advances in resuscitation technology.

      (1) Brain death often results from **acute anoxia,** as in cardiorespiratory arrest or prolonged hypotension, that devastates the brain but spares the less sensitive organs so that they can be revived.

      (2) **Brain tumor, trauma,** and **stroke** may also cause complete destruction of the brain but allow artificial maintenance of the other organs.

   b. The **pathology of brain death** (the so-called respiratory brain) is widespread necrosis and edema without inflammatory reaction. Transtentorial (temporal lobe) and cerebellar tonsillar herniations occur. Brain swelling causes increased intracranial pressure and an absence of cerebral blood flow.

   c. The **clinical recognition of brain death** has become important because the brain-dead patient may provide high-quality organs for transplantation. Moreover, the high cost of supportive and resuscitative care makes it desirable to recognize the brain-dead patient as early as possible.

2. **Legal definition.** The legal definition of death is taken from **Black's Law Dictionary,** which states that death is ". . . **defined by physicians** as a total stoppage of the circulation of the blood and a cessation of the animal and vital functions consequent thereupon, such as respiration, pulsation, etc."

   a. The American Bar Association, the American Medical Association, the National Conference of Commissioners on Uniform State Laws, and the President's Commission for the Study of Ethical Problems in Medicine have proposed a model statute to better standardize the definition of death. The proposed statute is entitled the "Uniform Determination of Death Act" and states the following:

   > An individual who has sustained either (1) irreversible cessation of circulation and respiratory functions or (2) irreversible cessation of all functions of the entire brain, including the brainstem, is dead. A determination of death must be made in accordance with acceptable medical standards.

3. **Other sanctions.** The concept of brain death has been accepted by the Roman Catholic Church and by attendees at the First World Meeting on Transplantation of Organs. At the twenty-second World Medical Assembly, in the Declaration of Sydney, the physician was deemed responsible for the definition of death, and cerebral death was named as an acceptable criterion. In 1972, the American Neurological Association accepted brain death as a definition of death.

B. Criteria

1. **Exclusions**

   a. **Before the criteria can be applied,** the diagnostic and therapeutic measures needed to correct the underlying illness must have been undertaken.

b. If there is suspicion of **intoxication with CNS depressants,** the diagnosis of brain death cannot be made.

    (1) Blood levels of drugs do not always correlate with mortality in drug overdose. The criteria for brain death can be applied only when drug levels have been allowed to drop to therapeutic or lower levels for an adequate time. Longer periods of observation are necessary in patients intoxicated at the onset of coma.

    (2) The signs suggesting brain death do not persist for more than 36 hours in most cases of uncomplicated drug intoxication. Careful neurologic observation reveals gradually increasing reflex activity in such cases, which indicates improvement. Usually, the earliest reflex to return is the pupillary light response. If the patient continues to improve, oculocephalic, corneal, and other reflexes return. The EEG may be isoelectric in some cases of drug overdose but usually shows fast activity superimposed on generalized slowing.

    (3) Endogenous toxins from renal, hepatic, or other organ failure also preclude making the diagnosis of brain death.

    (4) Paralytic agents when used in severely ill patients may produce such profound weakness that the cranial reflexes are absent. Brain wave and cerebral blood flow are preserved.

c. **Hypothermia** of less than 90° F (32° C) also precludes the application of the criteria for brain death. Hypothermia occurs in patients with brain death, but the temperature is usually higher than 90° F (32° C), and the hypothermia is not found initially.

d. Patients with **cardiogenic shock** cannot be judged by the criteria. Blood pressure must be above 90 mm Hg systolic to use the criteria.

e. The concept of brain death is specific. It does not apply to **patients existing in a persistent vegetative state** or to other severe degrees of brain damage. Decisions concerning these patients need to be based on other criteria.

2. **Standard of practice.** The specific criteria for brain death are usually established by individual hospitals and reflect the local laws. Local practice is based by the general criteria presented in Table 7-1. A history and examination that establish the diagnosis of an untreatable structural brain lesion are necessary for the diagnosis of brain death. In general, the criteria attempt to define signs that indicate that there is no nervous system function above the spinal cord.

3. **Duration.** The diagnosis of brain death usually is not even considered for several hours after the onset of artificial support. The Harvard ad hoc committee recommended that the signs be consistent for 24 hours, but recent analysis of brain death cases shows that over half the patients with proved brain death suffer cardiac arrest before the 24-hour waiting period is over. Therefore, if the signs are clear and there is no suspicion of drug intoxication, the diagnosis can be made if the syndrome persists for at least 6 hours in adult. When the history and examination are unequivocal, a single examination is sufficient. Making the diagnosis before cardiac decompensation and arrest occur provides the highest quality of organs for transplantation (see sec. **I.B.7**).

4. **Reflex activity**

a. The pupils are often dilated but may be in midposition in brain death. The most **helpful reflex signs** in diagnosing brain death are fixed pupils and absent corneal, oculocephalic, and vestibular reflexes. Gag, cough, and respiratory reflexes are also absent.

b. **Spinal cord reflex** activity persists in as many as two-thirds of patients with angiographically proved brain death. The presence of these reflexes indicates a functional spinal cord but does not exclude brain death. Although they are usually absent, the deep tendon reflexes may persist in brain death. Spinal cord reflexes must be separated from decerebrate and decorticate postures, which would exclude the diagnosis of brain death.

c. Induced **movements** and **muscle tone** do not always preclude the diagnosis of brain death unless there is movement of the face. The full decerebration posture is inconsistent with brain death, but partial movements resembling

Table 7-1. Criteria for brain death

Criteria	Comments
Established cerebral lesion	Clear history of anoxia, trauma, or other event; CT scan helps to identify a lesion
Absence of endogenous or exogenous toxins	Complete medical workup
Body temperature greater than 90° F (32° C)	Hypothermia may produce an isoelectric EEG, which is reversible with rewarming
Adequate observation time	Shorter in cases in which a brain lesion has been identified; children and drug cases require longer periods for certainty
Unresponsiveness	No behavior response to noxious stimuli; no reflex response, such as increased heart or respiratory rate, to noxious or other stimuli
Apnea	If necessary to prove apnea exists, ventilate the patient with pure O_2 or O_2 and CO_2 for 10 min; withdraw ventilator and insert nasal catheter with O_2 at 6–10 liters; 10 min of apnea produces hypercapnia > 60 mm Hg, which is sufficient stimulus; blood gases can be used to confirm the level of hypercapnia
Absent cranial reflexes	Fixed pupils and immobile eyeballs on ice water irrigation of auditory canals; absent corneal reflex and pharyngeal reflexes; no spontaneous blinking, swallowing, or vomiting
Isoelectric EEG	Absent EEG activity occasionally occurs in patients who do not have brain death (e.g., patient with drug overdose); if EEG activity is present, diagnosis of brain death cannot be made

decerebration do not indicate brain survival. Spontaneous movement may also occur in brain death, but the movements are never voluntary or complex. Simple random jerks of the limbs are the most commonly observed movements in brain death.

   d. The **snout reflex, jaw jerk, abdominal reflexes,** and **plantar responses** also may persist and are not indicative of brain survival.

5. **EEG**
   a. The EEG is a very helpful test in the diagnosis of brain death, although it is not mandatory. In the absence of drug intoxication, patients who have an isoelectric EEG for 12–24 hours do not survive.
   b. Because of the **high gains needed,** it is necessary to use leads to monitor external movement and the ECG. An electrode on the right hand serves to measure external movement; since there is no muscle activity, there will be no muscle artifact. The study is run at standard gains, and again at twice standard gains, for at least 30 minutes to ensure the absence of brain waves. There should be no EEG response to pain or other stimuli.
   c. **When any brain wave is present, the diagnosis of brain death cannot be made.**

6. **Absent cerebral blood flow.** A persistent absence of cerebral blood flow determined by radionuclide angiography is diagnostic of brain death. However, a **conventional angiogram is seldom necessary** when clinical observation and EEG are available. Funduscopy that shows sludging of blood in the retinal veins ("boxcars") is clinical evidence of absent cerebral blood flow.

7. **Physician responsibility.** The **psychosocial implications of death** are always difficult for both the physician and the patient's family. The difficulty is compounded in patients in whom there are superficial signs of survival.

    a. Once the diagnosis has been determined, the physician should explain **the meaning of the syndrome carefully to the patient's family.** To prevent confusion and misunderstanding, the physician should be sure that the family realizes that the patient is dead before stopping organ maintenance or suggesting organ donation.

    b. The **clinical record** must reflect the decision-making process and should document the signs carefully. Two physicians, neither of whom is a member of the transplantation team, should agree on the diagnosis in the record.

C. Summary

    1. The diagnosis of brain death is made by a physician on the basis of the observation of a number of **clinical signs** that indicate absence of brain function.

    2. The **EEG** corroborates the diagnosis and is done when possible.

    3. Documentation of absent cerebral blood flow is confirmatory but usually not necessary.

    4. Death is declared and documented in the record **before** organ maintenance is stopped.

    5. Careful explanation to the family is of paramount importance.

II. Persistent vegetative state

A. Description. Patients who do not meet the criteria for brain death but who are severely brain damaged cannot be managed as those with brain death, even if they remain permanently unconscious. Some patients appear permanently asleep (comatose) without even the outward appearance of consciousness. Others appear to be awake and have a sleep-wake cycle; they are, however, unable to experience the environment or to respond to stimuli in any way. Patients in the latter group are said to be in a vegetative state, and when it lasts for more than a month it is called a persistent vegetative state (PVS). Because the diagnosis is not as intuitive as in patients who are permanently comatose, a set of criteria has been established for PVS. The management for PVS and permanent loss of consciousness is the same.

B. Diagnosis

    1. The **criteria** for defining PVS are the following:

        a. History of extensive destruction of brain from any cause.

        b. Abnormal CT scan or MRI showing loss of brain substance.

        c. Absence of sedative, toxic, or systemic complications that alter the level of awareness.

        d. Wakeful state with periods of sleep.

        e. Absent awareness of environment and self.

        f. Absent ability to communicate.

        g. Only reflex or random motor activity to stimulus.

        h. Spontaneous pulse, respiration, and blood pressure.

        i. Duration of at least 1 month.

    2. The PVS may follow trauma, cardiac arrest, or drug overdose or may present as an end stage of chronic degenerative disease.

    3. A careful **neurologic examination** performed by an experienced physician is necessary to establish the absence of any awareness of environment or ability to react with more than reflex responses.

    4. A **CT scan** is used in identifying destructive brain lesions and in establishing a neurologic diagnosis. When a CT scan is not sufficient, angiography or other radiographic tests should be used.

    5. The patient must be observed for a sufficient time to establish the permanence of the syndrome. At least 1 month (and longer in children) is needed to show that there is no improvement. Serial neurologic examinations should document failure to improve even minimally.

    6. The patient's state should be determined only when there are no concomitant medical or toxic conditions. The diagnosis of PVS cannot be made when the patient either has an acute illness or is on medication that reduces mentation.

C. Prognosis

    1. The **neuropathology** usually involves destruction of the neocortex, hippocampus, and basal ganglia. There is relative sparing of the brainstem.

    2. In cases of **nontraumatic coma,** it is not possible to predict which patients will

enter the PVS. There are, however, several unfavorable signs, which, when observed early, are suggestive of poor outcome.
   a. Absent motor responses at admission.
   b. Absent normal responses at 1 day.
   c. Poor motor responses at 3 days despite awakening at day 1.
   d. Persistent roving conjugate eye movements at 1 week.
   e. Persistent coma at 1 week.
   f. The vegetative state at 1 week.
   3. Patients with **head trauma** have a slightly better chance of recovery than patients with anoxic-ischemic injury when the unfavorable signs exist.
   4. Recovery from the PVS seldom occurs. Most patients die of medical complications and those who live for long periods do not regain the functions of a social human being.
D. Management
   1. Feeding by artificial means is not necessary, since the patient has no awareness of nutrition. The decision should be made considering the wishes of the family.
   2. Proper care of bowel and bladder is needed to reduce nursing demands. A urinary catheter may be needed as a convenience.
   3. It is not mandatory to treat infection, renal failure, cardiac failure, or other medical problems in a permanently vegetative patient. The patient should not be put on a respirator.
   4. Decisions on the degree of care should be based on the availability of medical resources, the wishes of the patient when known, and the wishes of the family. When there is a small possibility that the diagnosis is not PVS, vigorous treatment should be pursued until the diagnosis is clear. If the family insists on vigorous treatment, the physician should comply as long as resources are available.
   5. When the physician or nursing staff cannot comply with the wishes of the family, it is best to transfer the patient to the care of those who feel comfortable with the family's wishes. When there is no way to resolve conflict between the family and the medical staff, the court may appoint a guardian.
   6. It is best to identify a single family member with whom to make plans. That person can involve appropriate family members. At times a meeting between the family and the medical team is helpful in establishing an acceptable plan.

Selected Readings

Ad Hoc Committee of The American Encephalographic Society. Cerebral death and the electroencephalogram: Report of the ad hoc committee of EEG criteria for determination of cerebral death. *J.A.M.A.* 209:1505, 1969.

ANA Committee on Ethical Affairs. Persistent vegetative state: Report of the American Neurological Association Committee on Ethical Affairs. *Neurology* 33:386, 1993.

Bates, D., et al. A prospective study of nontraumatic coma: Methods and results in 310 patients. *Ann. Neurol.* 2:211, 1977.

Benzel, E. C., et al. Apnea testing for the determination of brain death: A modified protocol. Technical note. *J. Neurosurg.* 76:1029, 1992.

Black, P. M. Brain death. *N. Engl. J. Med.* 299:388, 1978.

Cranford, R. E., and Smith, H. L. Some critical distinctions between brain death and the persistent vegetative state. *Ethics Sci. Med.* 6:199, 1979.

Dougherty, J. H., et al. Hypoxic-ischemic brain injury and the vegetative state: Clinical and neuropathologic correlation. *Neurology* 31:991, 1981.

Goldie, W. D., et al. Brainstem auditory and short latency somatosensory evoked responses in brain death. *Neurology* 31:248, 1981.

Korein, J. (ed.). Brain death: Interrelated medical and social issues. *Ann. N.Y. Acad. Sci.* 315:1, 1978.

Korein, J., and Maccario, M. On the diagnosis of cerebral death: A prospective study on 55 patients to define irreversible coma. *Clin. Electroencephalogr.* 2:178, 1971.

Levy, D. E., et al. Factors influencing the recovery from non-traumatic coma. *Ann. Intern. Med.* 94:293, 1981.

Mohandas, A., and Chou, S. N. Brain death: A clinical and pathological study. *J. Neurosurg.* 35:211, 1971.

Pius XII. The prolongation of life. *The Pope Speaks.* 4:393, 1958.

Report of the committee on irreversible coma and brain death. *Trans. Am. Neurol. Assoc.* 102:192, 1977.

Report of the President's Commission for the Study of Ethical Problems in Medicine and Biomedical and Behavioral Research. *Deciding to Forego Life-Sustaining Treatment.* Washington, D.C.: U.S. Government Printing Office, March 1983.

Starr, A. Auditory brainstem responses in brain death. *Brain* 99:543, 1976.

Van Till, H. A. H. Diagnosis of death in comatose patients under resuscitation treatment: A critical review of the Harvard report. *Am. J. Law Med.* 2:1, 1976.

Ventura, M. G., and Masser, P. G. Defining death: Developments in recent law. *Crit. Care. Clin.* 1:397, 1985.

Walker, A. E., Didmond, E. L., and Moseley, J. The neuropathological findings in irreversible coma. *J. Neuropathol. Exp. Neurol.* 34:295, 1975.

Wilson, K., et al. The diagnosis of brain death with Tc–99 HMPOA. *Clin. Nucl. Med.* 18:428, 1993.

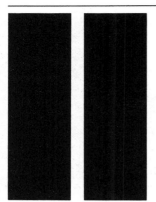

Neurologic Diseases

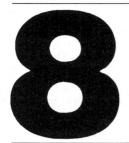

Infectious Diseases

Stephen M. Sagar and
Dawn McGuire

I. Bacterial meningitis
A. Diagnosis
1. Indications for lumbar puncture (LP)

a. Examination of the cerebrospinal fluid (CSF) is the only means of making a definite diagnosis of meningitis and identifying the infecting organism. Untreated bacterial meningitis is virtually 100% fatal within hours to days. Because of the urgency of starting specific therapy, it is imperative to examine a sample of CSF as soon as possible.

b. Identification of an organism in a parameningeal or systemic source of infection is not adequate to guide therapy. In over 25% of cases, blood cultures fail to yield an organism.

c. All material for bacteriologic examination should generally be obtained prior to beginning antibiotic therapy. However, positive bacteriologic culture can frequently be obtained up to 4 hours after the first dose of antibiotics, and bacterial antigens can be detected in CSF up to several days after initiation of therapy. When radiologic studies need to be performed prior to LP, antibiotic therapy should not be delayed. When brain imaging is not mandatory, however, most clinicians would perform an expeditious LP and obtain all other bacteriologic cultures before administering the first dose of antibiotics.

d. Risks of LP. Diffusely elevated intracranial, pressure occurs in nearly all cases of bacterial meningitis and is not in itself a contraindication to LP. In the presence of a mass lesion, however, withdrawal of CSF from the lumbar space and the continuing leak of CSF through the dural defect may cause a pressure difference between the supra- and infratentorial compartments. This can lead to downward herniation of brain. **Although the risk is real, delay in diagnosing bacterial meningitis is fatal far more often than is an imprudent LP.** Therefore, the risks and benefits of LP must be carefully weighed in each case.

(1) In the presence of a known intracranial mass lesion, such as tumor, abscess, or hemorrhage, LP can be especially hazardous.

(2) Papilledema or retinal hemorrhages rarely occur in uncomplicated bacterial meningitis. A CT evaluation should precede LP.

(3) A clear history of a progressive focal neurologic deficit preceding the onset of meningitis suggests the presence of an abscess, tumor, subdural fluid collection, or other mass lesion. A CT scan should precede LP.

(4) Certain complications of bacterial meningitis (cortical vein thrombosis with venous infarction of the brain, arterial infarction, subdural empyema, subdural effusion, disseminated intravascular coagulation [DIC] with a bleeding diathesis) may increase the risks of LP but usually occur later in the course rather than at presentation.

(5) Skin or soft tissue infection in the area through which the needle must pass is a contraindication to LP.

(6) Signs of possible herniation such as altered pupillary responses, new focal neurologic deficits, rapidly declining mental status, or Cushing's reflex (hypertension and bradycardia) must be evaluated radiographically prior to LP. Evidence of shift of midline structures, obliteration of CSF pathways, or frank herniation is an absolute contraindication to LP.

(7) Seizures, isolated cranial nerve palsies, focal neurologic signs, ataxia, and depressed mental status all can occur early in the course of bacterial meningitis in the absence of a mass lesion. These symptoms alone do not increase the risk of LP but should be evaluated radiographically prior to LP.

e. It is a good practice to have a secure IV in place when the LP is performed. Hyperosmolar agents can then be infused if necessary, and antibiotics can be begun immediately on obtaining the CSF sample.

f. Alternatives to LP

(1) The LP may be deferred while emergency radiologic studies are performed to confirm or exclude the presence of a mass lesion. As discussed in **1.c,** an initial dose of antibiotics should be administered immediately.

(2) The CSF may be obtained by a **ventricular tap** through an open fontanelle in an infant or by means of a burr hole in children and adults. This procedure should be performed only by an experienced neurosurgeon, and it carries its own high risks. Furthermore, ventricular fluid is not entirely equivalent to subarachnoid fluid. In some cases of meningitis, the ventricular fluid may be sterile and may result in a falsely negative CSF culture.

(3) **In rare instances** (limited almost entirely to pediatric practice), when the diagnosis of bacterial meningitis seems indisputable on clinical grounds, when the infecting organism may be predicted with a high degree of confidence, and when the patient is at significant risk of herniation, antibiotics may be started without obtaining a sample of CSF. In these instances, blood cultures are taken and LP is performed 8–24 hours after both antibiotics and antiedema therapy are initiated. By following this procedure, the risk of LP is lessened, and the CSF formula may still be purulent, allowing the diagnosis to be confirmed. If the appropriate antibiotic is chosen, however, there is little chance of culturing an organism from the CSF.

2. Technique for LP

a. Preparing the patient

(1) A blood glucose should be drawn within 15 minutes of beginning the procedure.

(2) To minimize the patient's anxiety, the procedure is explained to the patient, and all steps are described during the procedure.

(3) **Positioning the patient**

(a) Whenever possible, the LP is performed with the patient lying on his or her side with knees and hips flexed. The patient may be left relatively relaxed while being prepped and draped, and only when the physician is prepared to introduce the needle are the patient's hips and back maximally flexed. Care must be taken to avoid airway obstruction when flexing the neck of an infant; risk of respiratory compromise is especially high in infants with cyanotic heart disease.

(b) The L3–L4 interspace is palpated at the level of the superior iliac crests, and any scoliosis or abnormalities of the spine are noted.

(c) If the puncture cannot be performed with the patient lying on his or her side, it may be done with the patient in a sitting position, leaning forward onto a table. It is essential that the patient's spine be perfectly vertical. The CSF pressure cannot be measured accurately in this position; however, once puncture of the dura is achieved, the patient can be carefully repositioned in the lateral decubitus position and the opening pressure obtained.

(4) **Preparing the skin**

(a) Wash the patient's back with iodine-soaked sponges; begin at the site of the proposed puncture and wash in concentric circles. Wash with iodine 2 or 3 times, and then wash with alcohol-soaked sponges 3 times, taking care to wash off all the iodine.

(b) To avoid introducing iodine into the subarachnoid space on the LP needle, change gloves before proceeding.

(c) Cover the patient with a sterile drape.

b. **Introducing the needle**

(1) Have all the equipment for the puncture ready before introducing the needle (i.e., 20-gauge LP needle, stopcock attached to a manometer and appropriately positioned, and three or four sterile tubes with stoppers).

(2) Anesthetize the skin with a small wheal of lidocaine or procaine at the exact site of the proposed puncture. The skin wheal is painful and should be raised slowly with an intradermal injection of 0.1–0.2 ml of anesthetic. A further 0.2–0.5 ml may be injected into deeper layers of the dermis, but there is no need to inject anesthetic deep into the muscle because this is usually more painful than the single passage of a 20-gauge needle.

(3) Introduce a 20-gauge LP needle, with the stylus in place, through the skin in the center of the skin wheal. Direct the bevel of the needle with its flat surface parallel to the long axis of the patient's spine; thus, the needle will spread, rather than cut, the dural fibers that run longitudinally. Direct the needle tip 10–15 degrees cephalad (more or less toward the umbilicus), and introduce the needle slowly but steadily until the needle is felt to pierce a tough membrane or is thought to be near the dura. At this point, the needle is introduced in steps of 2–3 mm, and the stylus is removed between each step to check for CSF return. Once CSF return is obtained, the needle is introduced 1–2 mm farther, and the bevel is turned perpendicular to the long axis of the spine. Care must be taken not to introduce the needle too far because puncture of the venous plexus anterior to the spinal canal is the most common cause of a "traumatic tap."

(4) If CSF return cannot be obtained at the L3–L4 interspace, the L2–L3 or L4–L5 spaces may be tried. After repeated LPs, a patient may develop a persistent CSF leak, keeping CSF pressure so low that it will not flow through a 20-gauge needle unless the patient's head is elevated.

(5) Each time the stylus is withdrawn, be ready to attach the stopcock and manometer to the needle as quickly as possible to minimize unnecessary CSF loss and obtain an accurate opening pressure.

c. **Collecting the CSF**

(1) Measure the CSF pressure by allowing fluid to flow into the manometer. Evidence that the needle is properly positioned in the subarachnoid space includes good respiratory variation of the fluid level in the manometer. The patient should be as relaxed as possible; the legs and hips can be extended slightly from the maximally flexed position when the pressure is measured.

(2) Collect the fluid into at least three sterile tubes. One scheme is as follows:

(a) Tube No. 1: Collect 2 ml for protein and glucose. This tube is centrifuged, and the sediment is used for microscopic examination.

(b) Tube No. 2: Collect 1–2 ml for bacteriologic culture.

(c) Tube No. 3: Collect 1 ml for cell count and 1 ml for serology.

(3) If the **opening pressure** is high, there is little advantage in collecting less fluid in an attempt to minimize the risk of herniation. Much of the danger from the LP is from leakage of CSF through the dural defect created by the needle.

(4) In virtually all cases of bacterial meningitis, the CSF pressure is found to be elevated. Thus, the patient should be observed closely (no less often than every 15 minutes for the next 4 hours) and hyperosmolar agents administered if the patient shows evidence of neurologic deterioration.

(5) If the patient's condition deteriorates during the performance of the LP or if the patient is considered to be at a high risk of herniation, the stylet is replaced into the needle and the needle is left in place. Mannitol, 1.0–1.5 g/kg, is infused over 20–30 minutes, and high-dose steroid therapy is begun with dexamethasone (Decadron), 10 mg, given by rapid IV infusion. After the mannitol has been infused, the needle is withdrawn.

d. Withdrawal of the needle. Cases have been reported in which nerve roots were trapped by an LP needle when the stylet was replaced; the root was avulsed as the needle was withdrawn. When the needle is withdrawn, the stylet should not be in place.

e. Examination of the CSF

(1) CSF formula (Table 8-1). The CSF formula in bacterial meningitis will be purulent (elevated cell count, predominantly polymorphonuclear leukocytes), with low glucose (<40 mg/dl) and elevated protein (>50 mg/dl) concentrations. However, in some cases the CSF profile can be misleading:

(a) In a "partially treated" bacterial meningitis.

(b) Early in overwhelming infection, especially with *Streptococcus pneumoniae*, where there can be a poor polymorphonuclear response.

(c) When the patient is markedly leukopenic or immunosuppressed.

(d) When meningitis is caused by bacteria that induce a lymphocytic rather than neutrophilic CSF profile (e.g., *Listeria monocytogenes*, *Treponema pallidum*, *Borrelia burgdorferi*, *Leptospira interrogans*).

(2) Microscopic examination. The following examinations are performed, as indicated, on the sediment of fresh, centrifuged CSF:

(a) Gram's stain.

(b) Acid-fast bacilli (AFB) stain. The greater the volume of CSF examined, the higher the yield of this procedure. Therefore, the CSF sediment may be concentrated by allowing four or five drops of CSF to dry sequentially on one area of a slide.

(c) India ink preparation is not as good a screening test for *Cryptococcus* species as is Gram's stain, in which the organisms appear as large gram-positive cocci. When Gram's stain suggests fungus, India ink can be used to identify the cryptococcal capsule. Identification of **cryptococcal antigen** titers in CSF by latex agglutination is the most sensitive means of detecting cryptococcal meningitis.

(d) Wet smear for fungi and amebae.

(e) Examination of polymorphonuclear cells with **polarized light** to look for keratin fragments. These fragments indicate chemical meningitis, secondary to the spillage of the contents of a dermoid cyst or craniopharyngioma.

(3) Bacteriologic examination

(a) Routine cultures for bacteria. CSF is smeared on a blood agar plate or a chocolate agar plate or slant or is inoculated into a nutrient broth. It is essential to inoculate all cultures as soon as possible after the LP.

(b) If indicated, fluid may be cultured for mycobacteria, fungi, and amebae.

(4) Special studies

(a) Meningitis due to *Neisseria meningitidis, Haemophilus influenzae,* and *S. pneumoniae* may be rapidly diagnosed, even in the absence of a positive Gram's stain, by the documentation of the presence of specific bacterial antigens in the CSF. The **latex particle agglutination** and **coagglutination tests** have replaced counterimmunoelectrophoresis for rapid detection in CSF.

(b) Serologic test for syphilis. Peripheral blood serology should be used as a screening test for syphilis and the CSF serology examined only when the peripheral serology is positive **or** there is clinical suspicion of CNS syphilis.

(c) Viral isolation studies or viral antibody titers as indicated based on clinical suspicion.

(d) Immunoassays for fungal antigens. **Latex particle agglutination** for cryptococcal antigen is more sensitive than Gram's stain or India ink preparation for the diagnosis of cryptococcal meningitis. **Complement**

Table 8-1. The cerebrospinal fluid formula

Purulent profile	Lymphocytic–low-glucose profile	Lymphocytic–normal-glucose profile
Elevated WBC, predominantly polymorphonuclear leukocytes, low sugar, and high protein	Elevated WBC, predominantly lymphocytes, low sugar, and high protein	Elevated WBC, predominantly lymphocytes, normal sugar, and high protein

Infectious
  Bacterial meningitis
  Viral meningitis in the early phase
  Embolic cerebral infarction with endocarditis
  Parameningeal infections (e.g., subdural empyema, brain abscess, cortical vein thrombophlebitis)
	Tuberculous meningitis
	Fungal meningitis
	Bacterial meningitis that is either in the resolving or partially treated phase or with certain organisms (e.g., spirochetes, *Leptospira, Listeria monocytogenes*)
		Viral meningitis or encephalitis
		Bacterial meningitis in the resolving or partially treated phase
		Parameningeal infections (e.g., intracranial abscess, sinusitis, mastoiditis, cortical vein thrombophlebitis)

Tuberculous meningitis in the early phase Acute hemorrhagic leukoencephalitis	Viral meningitis	Fungal and tuberculous meningitis in the early phase Parasitic infestation (e.g., toxoplasmosis, trichinosis)

Noninfectious
  Chemical meningitis (e.g., contrast media, detergents, keratin released from tumors, foreign agents)
  Behçets disease
  Mollaret's recurrent meningitis
	Carcinomatous meningitis
	Sarcoidosis of the meninges
		Postinfectious encephalomyelitis
		Active demyelinating diseases

Source: Adapted from N. E. Hyslop, Jr. and M. N. Swartz, Bacterial meningitis. *Postgrad. Med.* 58:120, 1975.

fixation tests can be obtained from the State Department of Heal
Laboratory when coccidioidomycosis or histoplasmosis is suspecte

3. Additional studies

a. Once the presumptive diagnosis of bacterial meningitis has been made, t
patient is reassessed for factors that may have increased the risk of meni
gitis. These factors include

  (1) Recent head trauma with **skull fracture,** usually basilar, giving organism
  access to the intracranial cavity.

  (2) The presence of a **"CSF leak,"** usually due to head trauma and involvi
  a defect in the cribriform plate.

  (3) Recent **intracranial surgery.**

  (4) **Meningomyelocele.**

  (5) **Immune deficiency.** Patients with defects in cell-mediated immunit
  including transplant recipients, are especially susceptible to intracellul
  parasites such as *Listeria*. Patients with poor humoral immunity or wl
  have been splenectomized are at risk for infection with encapsulat
  organisms. Neutropenic patients are at increased risk for infection wi
  Pseudomonas aeruginosa and the Enterobacteriaceae.

  (6) The presence of a **parameningeal focus** of infection: sinusitis, otit
  (usually chronic), mastoiditis, osteomyelitis of the skull, occult bra
  abscess, and infected pilonidal sinuses.

  (7) A source of systemic sepsis, especially **endocarditis.**

b. Routine tests in all patients with presumptive bacterial meningitis:

  (1) Hematologic
    (a) CBC with differential.
    (b) Examination of a peripheral blood smear.

  (2) Metabolic
    (a) BUN and creatinine.
    (b) Blood glucose.
    (c) Electrolytes.
    (d) Urinalysis.
    (e) If nephrotoxic drugs are to be used, a baseline **creatinine clearan**
    (Cl_{cr}) is obtained.

  (3) Radiologic
    (a) Chest x ray.
    (b) An MRI or CT scan (with bone windows) of the head to seek a possib
    parameningeal focus of infection.

  (4) Blood, urine, and throat cultures.

c. Special studies for special circumstances:

  (1) When there is evidence of a **CSF leak,** and in all cases of **recurre**
  meningitis without an obvious cause, a radioactively labeled tracer or
  dye solution is injected into the subarachnoid space, and pledgets a
  placed in the nasal cavity or ear canal. The pledgets are then examine
  over time to document CSF rhinorrhea or otorrhea. Glucose oxidase te
  strips are not a reliable means of detecting CSF leaks.

  (2) In **neonatal meningitis,** the mother is examined for signs of infectio
  Amnionitis, endometritis, maternal urinary tract infections, and septic
  mia are known to predispose to neonatal meningitis. A knowledge of tl
  identity and antibiotic sensitivity of maternal perinatal infections ma
  help to guide therapy for the neonate.

B. General medical care of a patient with bacterial meningitis

1. Systemic complications

a. Shock

  (1) Septic shock, if present, should be treated with volume replacement an
  pressors, as indicated.

  (2) Shock associated with hemorrhagic infarction of the adrena
  (Waterhouse-Friderichsen syndrome) is an uncommon complication
  meningococcal meningitis. It is associated with severe purpura ar
  fulminant meningococcemia. In a patient with bacterial meningitis an

shock, emergency treatment with replacement doses of corticosteroids is warranted until the patient has stabilized and the medical situation is better evaluated.

   (3) Disseminated intravascular coagulation (DIC) may accompany septic shock. In a recent prospective study, DIC complicated bacterial meningitis in over 8% of patients, occurring predominantly in the first week of illness.

   (4) Adult respiratory distress syndrome (ARDS), or "shock lung," is another consequence of microcirculatory failure, causing severe hypoxemia and refractory pulmonary edema. ARDS was seen in 3.5% of patients in a prospective study of complications of bacterial meningitis, with 100% mortality.

  b. Volume status. Because of the likely presence of brain swelling and increased CSF pressure in CNS infection, care is taken not to overhydrate the patient. If the patient is not hypotensive, approximately 1200–1500 ml of normal saline is adequate daily fluid intake in adults, and about 1000 ml/m² body surface area is adequate in children. The volume of fluid in which the antibiotics are administered and any oral intake are included in this total. These restrictions may be gradually relaxed as the patient's infection responds to therapy, especially if the CSF pressure is decreasing. Solutions that contain more than 50% "free water" (e.g., 5% D/W) should not be administered, except in small volumes when they are used to dissolve the antibiotics.

  c. Fever. Salicylates, acetaminophen, and baths in tepid water may all be used to lower body temperature. Patients usually become afebrile within 2–5 days of initiation of appropriate antibiotic therapy. If fever persists or recurs, reassessment, including repeat LP, is indicated. Inadequate drug therapy and complications such as cortical venous thrombophlebitis, subdural empyema, or extracerebral metastatic infection must be considered, as well as drug fever. A syndrome of fever, arthritis, and pericarditis is seen in about 10% of patients with meningococcal meningitis, usually beginning 3–6 days after initiation of therapy.

  d. Isolation. Patients with meningococcal infections or meningitis of unknown etiology are placed under respiratory precautions for the first 24 hours of antibiotic therapy or until meningococcal disease has been ruled out. Precautions may be necessary in patients with bacterial infections that have broad drug resistance to prevent the organisms from infecting other susceptible patients.

 2. Treatment of predisposing factors

  a. Parameningeal infections are treated concurrently with meningitis, with surgical drainage if necessary.

  b. Foci of systemic sepsis may require more prolonged antibiotic therapy than the meningitis (e.g., infective endocarditis, osteomyelitis, and wound infection).

  c. Minor CSF leaks need not be repaired until after the CNS infection is under control.

C. Systemic antibiotic therapy of bacterial meningitis

 1. General principles

  a. Patients are **hospitalized** for the entire course of treatment, and the entire course of antibiotics is administered parenterally.

  b. The minimum **duration of antibiotic therapy** necessary is unknown, but in meningitis with the common organisms (*S. pneumoniae, H. influenzae,* and *N. meningitidis*), the practice is to treat at full dose of parenteral antibiotics for at least 10 days and at least 7 days after the patient becomes afebrile. If any surgery is performed near the end of therapy, the antibiotics are continued at least 72 hours after surgery. In infections with less-sensitive organisms (e.g., enteric gram-negative organisms) or after trauma or surgery, when pockets of organisms can infect poorly perfused tissues, it is reasonable to prolong the duration of antibiotic therapy to 3 weeks or longer.

  c. In complicated cases, **when the organism is relatively difficult to treat** (e.g., enteric gram-negative rods, *Listeria, Staphylococcus aureus*), an LP should be performed about 72 hours after initiation of antibiotic therapy. The CSF cell count, differential cell count, protein, and glucose are determined, and the CSF is examined microscopically and cultured appropriately to document that it has been sterilized. An LP at the conclusion of therapy has not proved useful in predicting those patients who will relapse.

- **d.** **In meningeal infections with organisms that are relatively sensitive to antibiotics with good CSF penetration** (e.g., streptococcal species, *N. meningitidis,* and *H. influenzae*), the CSF should be sterile within 24 hours of beginning therapy, and the differential cell profile should be predominantly mononuclear. (The CSF protein level may continue to be high and the CSF glucose may remain low for 2 weeks or longer despite curative therapy.) Other organisms, especially gram-negative rods, may continue to be cultured from the CSF for as long as 72 hours after the initiation of therapy. Persistence of the infecting organism in the CSF beyond the expected interval, however, may imply a need to change antibiotics or to add intrathecal antibiotics. It may also indicate the presence of an occult parameningeal focus of infection seeding the CSF.
- **e.** **Drug toxicity.** In the treatment of bacterial meningitis, the highest doses of drugs that can be tolerated are generally used, and often the patients have underlying hepatic, renal, or hematologic disease. Therefore, the patient must be observed carefully for the development of drug toxicity.
- **f.** Antibiotics that penetrate poorly into the CSF are avoided in the treatment of bacterial meningitis, including the **tetracyclines** and the **first- and second-generation cephalosporins.**

2. **Pharmacology of antibiotics used in the chemotherapy of bacterial meningitis**
   a. **Chloramphenicol**
      (1) **Pharmacokinetics.** Half-life = 1.5–3.5 hours. The CSF concentration is 30–80% of plasma concentration. The drug is inactivated primarily in the liver by glucuronidation, and the inactive metabolites are excreted in the urine. Therefore, the dosage does not have to be decreased in renal failure but should be decreased in severe hepatic insufficiency.
      (2) **Dosage**
          (a) Chloramphenicol is **not recommended** for use **in neonates.** It is not bactericidal to enteric bacilli, and risk of side effects is high in infants under 1 month of age.
          (b) **Infants over 1 month old:** 50 mg/kg/day IV, divided into two doses at 12-hour intervals.
          (c) **Children:** 100 mg/kg/day IV, divided into four doses at 6-hour intervals.
          (d) **Adults:** 4–6 g/day IV, divided into four doses at 6-hour intervals.
      (3) **Toxicity**
          (a) **Hypersensitivity reactions** include rash, fever, angioedema, stomatitis, and idiosyncratic bone marrow suppression with pancytopenia. Aplastic anemia occurs in fewer than 1 in 40,000, but it is irreversible. It occurs usually after prolonged exposure or on a second exposure.
          (b) Dose-related and reversible **bone marrow suppression** occurs with plasma drug levels of 25 μg/ml or higher. Recovery usually occurs about 12 days after the drug is stopped.
          (c) **Gray baby syndrome** and **cardiovascular collapse** occur in premature infants and neonates with inadequate hepatic glucuronyltransferase activity.
      (4) **Precautions**
          (a) **Bone marrow function** must be checked frequently. The CBC, differential, platelet count (or peripheral smear), serum iron, total iron-binding capacity (TIBC), and reticulocyte count should be checked 3 times weekly. The first sign of bone marrow suppression is increased serum iron and increased saturation of TIBC.
          (b) Extreme care must be used if the drug is given to **children less than 1 month old.**

(c) If used **in combination with penicillin,** the first dose of penicillin is given at least 30 minutes before the first dose of chloramphenicol, and succeeding doses of the two drugs should not be given within 30 minutes of each other.

(d) Chloramphenicol penetrates the CSF and reaches levels sufficient to be bactericidal against *H. influenzae, S. pneumoniae,* and *N. meningitidis.* However, bactericidal levels against most enteric gram-negative rods are not achieved after intravenous administration, and chloramphenicol is not adequate treatment for these organisms.

b. The penicillins

(1) Penicillin G

(a) Pharmacokinetics. Penicillin G is excreted primarily by the kidney and partially in bile. The half-life is approximately 30 minutes in adults but is 3 hours in neonates less than 1 week old. The half-life increases in renal failure. In meningitis, CSF levels are variable, ranging between 5% and 30% of concentrations in blood, and are generally therapeutic.

(b) Dosage

(i) Neonates: 50,000–100,000 units/kg/day IV, divided into two doses.

(ii) Infants: 250,000 units/kg/day IV, divided into four to six doses.

(iii) Children: 12×10^6 units/day, divided into six doses.

(iv) Adults: 24×10^6 units/day IV, divided into six doses.

(v) In renal failure ($Cl_{cr} < 10$ ml/min):
Children: same doses as above.
Adults: 2×10^6 units q4h IV.

(c) Toxicity

(i) Hypersensitivity reactions include rash, fever, eosinophilia, angioedema, anaphylaxis, serum sickness, and encephalopathy.

(ii) Seizures can occur with high doses of intrathecal use.

(iii) Penicillin G is available as a sodium or potassium salt, and it may create a significant **salt load** in infants or in patients with heart or renal failure.

(iv) Precautions. Potassium salt has 1.7 mEq of potassium per 10^6 units.

(2) Ampicillin

(a) Pharmacokinetics. Half-life = 1.5 hours. Ampicillin is excreted primarily by the kidneys; therefore, the dosage must be reduced in renal failure. Penetration into CSF is similar to that of penicillin G.

(b) Dosage

(i) Neonates: 50–100 mg/kg/day IV, divided into two doses.

(ii) Infants 2 weeks to 2 months old: 100–200 mg/kg/day IV, divided into three doses.

(iii) Infants over 2 months old: 300–400 mg/kg/day IV divided into four doses.

(iv) Adults: 12 g/day IV, divided into four to six doses.

(v) In renal failure (adults): 2–3 g given at the following intervals:

Cl_{cr} (ml/min)	Dosage interval
80	q6h
50–80	q6h
10–50	q9h
< 10	q12h

(c) Hypersensitivity reactions are the same as with penicillin G. An ampicillin rash does not necessarily represent hypersensitivity and, in itself, does not preclude continuation of the drug, its future use, or the use of other penicillins.

(3) The broad-spectrum penicillins, **carbenicillin, ticarcillin, piperacillin, mezlocillin,** and **azlocillin,** are antibiotics similar in pharmacokinetics and antibacterial action to ampicillin, except they have greater activity against *P. aeruginosa, Proteus* strains, and *Enterobacter.*

(a) Dosage
  (i) Carbenicillin:
    Neonates during the first week of life and **infants** weighing less than 2000 g: 400/mg/kg/day IV, divided into four doses.
    Infants after the first week of life if weight is greater than 2000 g: 400–600 mg/kg/day IV, divided into 6–12 doses.
    Adults: 24–36 g/day IV, divided into 12 doses.
  (ii) Ticarcillin:
    Neonates: 200–450 mg/kg/day IV, divided into four to six doses (the package insert and *Physicians' Desk Reference* have detailed instructions for computing the dosage in neonates).
    Infants: 300 mg/kg/day IV, divided into six doses.
    Children and adults: 200–300 mg/kg/day IV, divided into 6–12 doses.
  (iii) Piperacillin, mezlocillin, and azlocillin:
    Children: 75 mg/kg IV q4h, up to 24 g/day.
    Adults: 240–360 mg/kg/day IV, divided into six doses.
  (iv) In renal failure

Cl_{cr} (ml/min)	Dosage interval
> 100	q4h
50–80	q4h
10–50	q6–8h
< 10	q8–12h

(b) Toxicity is similar to that of penicillin G; abnormal platelet aggregation with bleeding diathesis has been reported with carbenicillin and ticarcillin.

(c) Precautions. Carbenicillin and ticarcillin contain 5.2 mEq/g of sodium. Since ticarcillin is administered at a lower dosage than carbenicillin, it is to be preferred when a large sodium load must be avoided. Piperacillin (1.85 mEq/g), mezlocillin (1.85 mEq/g), and azlocillin (2.17 mEq/g) are even lower in sodium, but there is less experience with their use in gram-negative meningitis than with either carbenicillin or ticarcillin. **None of the broad-spectrum penicillins is to be used alone in the treatment of gram-negative meningitis,** especially *Pseudomonas,* since antibiotic resistance commonly develops during monotherapy. An aminoglycoside is usually added.

(4) Oxacillin
  (a) Pharmacokinetics. Half-life = 0.5–1.0 hour. Oxacillin is excreted by the kidneys and liver. Penetration into CSF is similar to that of penicillin G.
  (b) Dosage
    (i) Neonates, 1 week old: 50–100 mg/kg/day IV, divided into two to three doses.
    (ii) Neonates, 2–4 weeks old: 100–200 mg/kg/day IV, divided into two to three doses.
    (iii) Infants and children: 200 mg/kg/day IV, divided into four to six doses.
    (iv) Adults: 12 g/day IV, divided into four to six doses.
    (v) In renal failure: Dosage adjustment is usually unnecessary, but some clinicians limit dosage to 1 g IV q4–6h if the Cl_{cr} is less than 10 ml/min.
  (c) Toxicity is the same as for penicillin G; interstitial nephritis has also been reported.
(5) Nafcillin
  (a) Pharmacokinetics. Half-life = 30 minutes. Ninety percent is excreted in bile. Penetration into CSF is similar to that of penicillin G.
  (b) Dosage. Same as for oxacillin.
  (c) Toxicity. Same as for oxacillin.

c. Aminoglycosides
(1) Pharmacokinetics
(a) Penetration into CSF with systemic administration is very low in the presence of a normal blood-brain barrier and variable but low with inflamed meninges. Levels in CSF are higher in neonates. Aminoglycosides are excreted unchanged in the urine primarily by glomerular filtration.

(b) **Half-life**
- (i) **Streptomycin:** 2–3 hours.
- (ii) **Gentamicin:** 2 hours.
- (iii) **Tobramycin:** 1.5–3.0 hours.
- (iv) **Kanamycin:** 3–4 hours.
- (v) **Amikacin:** 2 hours.
- (vi) **Netilmicin:** 2 hours.

(c) Serum drug levels achieved after a given dose may vary widely among individuals.

(2) Dosage
(a) **Systemic gentamicin, tobramycin, and netilmicin**
- (i) **Premature and term infants less than 1 week old:** 5 mg/kg/day IV, divided into two doses.
- (ii) **Neonates older than 1 week:** 7.5 mg/kg/day IV, divided into three doses.
- (iii) **Infants and adults:** 5 mg/kg/day IV, divided into three doses.
- (iv) **In renal failure:** 1.0–1.3 mg/kg qxh, where x = serum creatinine value × 8.

(b) **Systemic kanamycin and amikacin**
- (i) **All ages:** 15 mg/kg/day, divided into two doses.
- (ii) **In renal failure:** 7 mg/kg qxh, where x = serum creatinine value × 9.

(c) **Intrathecal gentamicin and tobramycin**
- (i) **Neonates:** 1 mg q24h.
- (ii) **Adults:** 4–8 mg q24h.

(3) Toxicity
(a) **Vestibular disturbance** is dose-related and occurs more readily in the presence of inflamed meninges. The labyrinthine disorder typically occurs in four stages:
- (i) A prodrome of 1–2 days of headache.
- (ii) An acute stage of nausea, vomiting, and vertigo, lasting 1–2 weeks.
- (iii) A chronic labyrinthitis, with gait ataxia as the main symptom, lasting about 2 months.
- (iv) Gradual compensation, by means of visual and proprioceptive cues, so that balance can be maintained except when the eyes are closed. Recovery may take 12–18 months and may be incomplete.

(b) **Hearing dysfunction** occurs less readily than vestibular dysfunction and is also dose-related. Older patients are more susceptible. Tinnitus is often the first symptom, and audiometry shows a high-tone hearing loss as the first sign, gradually progressing to involve the lower tones. Tinnitus persists as long as 2 weeks after the drug is stopped.

(c) The aminoglycosides are weak **neuromuscular blockers,** an effect that has no importance in patients with normal pulmonary function. However, it can be important in patients with myasthenia gravis, chronic obstructive pulmonary disease, or acute respiratory failure and in the immediate postoperative period when other neuromuscular blockers may still be active.

(d) **Nephrotoxicity.** Acute tubular necrosis with impaired glomerular filtration may occur and is associated with prolonged therapy and high trough aminoglycoside concentrations. Dehydration, shock, oliguria, and concurrent administration of other nephrotoxic drugs may potentiate the renal toxicity.

(e) **Hypersensitivity reactions.** Rash, eosinophilia, blood dyscrasia, exfoliative dermatitis, stomatitis, fever, lymphadenopathy, and anaphylaxis are **unusual** reactions of therapy.

(f) **Intrathecal use** is frequently associated with paresthesias of the legs and, occasionally, transverse myelitis or spinal arachnoiditis. Injection of excessive amounts of aminoglycoside into the ventricles has produced seizures, encephalopathy, and death.

(4) Precautions

(a) Follow renal function and urinalysis at least twice weekly.

(b) Observe the patient carefully for any sign of vestibular or auditory dysfunction.

(c) **Serum drug levels** vary widely among individuals on a given dose of aminoglycoside. Thus, serum drug levels should be measured just before and 0.5–1.0 hour after a dose is given, once a steady-state concentration is achieved, and at least weekly thereafter if the renal function is normal. Levels should be obtained more frequently if the renal function is abnormal. If direct injection of the drug into the CSF is indicated, the CSF level should be checked before the second dose and before every other dose thereafter.

(i) Therapeutic **peak** drug levels of gentamicin and tobramycin are 6–8 μg/ml (20–25 μg/ml for kanamycin and amikacin).

(ii) **Trough** levels should be less than 1 μg/ml for gentamicin and tobramycin (< 6 μg/ml for kanamycin and amikacin) to prevent excessive accumulation of drug.

(d) If maximum doses are to be used or a prolonged course is anticipated, a **baseline audiogram** should be obtained before initiation of therapy and at any sign of hearing loss.

(e) If an aminoglycoside must be used in patients with respiratory disease or neuromuscular disease affecting respiration, respiratory function is checked before beginning therapy, after the first dose, and then as indicated. In myasthenia, depending on severity, respiratory function may need to be checked as often as every 4 hours. **Neuromuscular blockade** can be counteracted with intravenous calcium or an anticholinesterase agent (neostigmine or pyridostigmine).

(5) Synergistic action with penicillins. Gram-negative rods such as *Pseudomonas* or *Proteus* species may be sensitive both to a broad-spectrum penicillin or third-generation cephalosporin and to an aminoglycoside. The aminoglycosides work synergistically with these beta-lactam antibiotics, and **combination therapy is warranted in treating meningitis caused by gram-negative rods.**

d. Erythromycin

(1) Pharmacokinetics. Half-life = 1.5–2.0 hours. Erythromycin is excreted in the bile. There is no need to decrease the dosage in renal failure. Penetration into CSF is similar to that of penicillin G.

(2) Dosage

(a) **Neonates:** 20 mg/kg, divided into two doses.

(b) **Children:** 40–50 mg/kg/day IV, divided into four doses.

(c) **Adults:** 4–8 g/day IV, divided into four doses.

(3) Toxicity

(a) **Hypersensitivity reactions** include rash, fever, eosinophilia, and cholestatic jaundice (with the estolate form).

(b) Intravenous use frequently causes **phlebitis.**

(c) High-tone **hearing loss** has been reported.

(4) Precautions. If used IV, infuse over 0.5–1.0 hour in 250 ml of solution.

e. Vanomycin

(1) Pharmacokinetics. Half-life = 6 hours. Levels in CSF with inflamed meninges are similar to those with penicillin. Vancomycin is excreted by the kidneys, so the dosage must be adjusted in renal insufficiency.

(2) Dosage
  (a) Premature infants and neonates: 6–15 mg/kg/day IV, divided into four doses.
  (b) Children: 44 mg/kg/day IV, divided into two or three doses.
  (c) Adults: 2 g/day IV, divided into two doses.

(3) Toxicity
  (a) Hypersensitivity reactions include rash, fever, and anaphylaxis.
  (b) High-tone **hearing loss,** which is unusual with plasma concentrations less than 30 μg/ml.
  (c) Nephrotoxicity.

(4) Precautions
  (a) Concurrent administration with other oto- or nephrotoxic drugs should be avoided.
  (b) Follow renal function at least twice weekly.
  (c) Serum drug levels should be obtained just before and 1 hour after a dose is given, 24 hours after initiation of therapy, and at least weekly (more frequently if renal function is deteriorating).
    (i) Peak range is 15–35 μg/ml at steady state.
    (ii) Trough levels should be less than 10 μg/ml.
  (d) When maximum doses are to be used, obtain a **baseline audiogram,** and repeat it at any sign of hearing loss.

f. Cephalosporins
  (1) The third-generation cephalosporins, **ceftriaxone, cefotaxime,** and **ceftizoxime,** achieve concentrations in the CSF 10–30 times the mean bactericidal concentration for many pathogens. They are widely used in bacterial meningitis.
  (2) In general, these agents are effective for meningitis caused by *N. meningitidis, S. pneumoniae,* and *H. influenzae* (including beta-lactamase–producing strains) as well as against many enteric gram-negative rods, including most strains of *Escherichia coli* and *Klebsiella.* These agents are therefore useful for the **initial therapy of acute meningitis** in nonimmunosuppressed hosts, both children and adults. These agents are not active against *Listeria, S. aureus,* or anaerobic bacteria, so they must be used in conjunction with other agents for the initial therapy of neonatal meningitis, in postneurosurgical patients and immunosuppressed hosts, and in cases where *Pseudomonas* is a likely pathogen.
  (3) Ceftazidime, unlike the other third-generation cephalosporins listed, has activity against *Pseudomonas.* Its use **should be reserved for cases where *Pseudomonas* is suspected.**
  (4) Toxicity. Cephalosporins are generally well tolerated, but **hypersensitivity reactions** (typically rash or fever) occur. Penicillin-allergic patients may or may not have allergy to cephalosporins. Bone marrow suppression occurs rarely. Diarrhea is relatively common with third-generation cephalosporins. Nephrotoxicity has been reported with concomitant administration of cephalosporins and aminoglycosides or furosemide.
  (5) Ceftriaxone
    (a) Pharmacokinetics. Half-life = 6–9 hours. Excretion is 60% renal and 40% hepatic.
    (b) Dosage
      (i) Children: 80–100 mg/kg/day IV divided into four doses.
      (ii) Adults: 4–6 g/day IV divided into two or three dosages.
      (iii) The dosage requires adjustment in the presence of **combined renal and hepatic insufficiency.**
    (c) The clinical experience in treating bacterial meningitis with **ceftriaxone** is greater than that with other cephalosporins. Many clinicians regard it as the **agent of choice** for the initial treatment of meningitis

of unknown etiology and in the treatment of organisms known to be sensitive, especially enteric gram-negative rods.

(6) Cefotaxime

(a) **Pharmacokinetics.** Half-life = 1 hour. Excretion is renal.

(b) **Dosage**

(i) **Children:** 200 mg/kg/day IV divided into six doses.

(ii) **Adults:** 12 g/day IV divided into six doses. The dosage must be adjusted in renal failure.

(c) Cefotaxime is almost as active as penicillin against pneumococci. Like ceftriaxone, it can be used alone in the initial treatment of bacterial meningitis in immunocompetent adults.

(7) Ceftizoxime

(a) **Pharmacokinetics.** Half-life = 1.4–1.8 hours. Excretion is renal.

(b) **Dosage**

(i) **Children:** 600 mg/kg/day IV divided into three doses.

(ii) **Adults:** 9–12 g/day IV divided into three doses. The dosage must be adjusted in renal failure.

(8) Ceftazidime

(a) **Pharmacokinetics.** Half-life = 0.9–1.7 hours. Excretion is renal.

(b) **Dosage**

(i) **Children:** 90–150 mg/kg/day IV divided into three doses.

(ii) **Adults:** 6–12 g/day IV divided into three doses. The dosage must be adjusted in renal failure.

(c) Although the spectrum of action and pharmacokinetics of ceftazidime are similar to those of the other third-generation cephalosporins used to treat meningitis, it has enhanced activity against *Pseudomonas*. Because of the potential for development of drug resistance during therapy, most experts favor using ceftazidime in combination with an aminoglycoside for *Pseudomonas* meningitis. Cures with monotherapy have been reported.

g. Aztreonam has a monocyclic beta-lactam nucleus that confers stability against beta-lactamase–producing **gram-negative aerobes,** including *Pseudomonas*. It has been used successfully as monotherapy in gram-negative meningitis in an open-label trial and **can be used in penicillin-allergic patients.**

(1) Pharmacokinetics. Half-life = 1.7–2.0 hours. Excretion is renal, and dosage must be adjusted in renal failure.

(2) Dosage

(a) **Infants:** 90–120 mg/kg/day IV divided into three or four doses.

(b) **Children greater than 2 years old:** 150–200 mg/kg/day IV divided into three or four doses.

(c) **Adults:** 3–8 g/day IV divided into three or four doses.

(3) Toxicity. Aztreonam is generally well tolerated. Eosinophilia is common; rash, diarrhea, and abnormal liver function tests occur occasionally. Thrombocytopenia and seizures have been reported rarely.

3. Initial choice of antibiotics

a. Identification of the infecting organism must be made, and the drug sensitivities determined. Until this information is available, the initial choice of antibiotics is guided by the following factors:

(1) Gram's stain. If a high-quality Gram's stain shows an identifiable organism in abundance, the patient is treated for that organism. In addition, coverage should be given for other likely infecting organisms given the age of the patient.

(2) Age of the patient. In the absence of complicating conditions (e.g., immunologic disease, recent intracranial surgery or head trauma), the epidemiology of infection changes with the age of the patient.

(a) **Neonatal meningitis** generally originates from two sources:

(i) Infections acquired during delivery, which usually appear within the first week of life; the pathogenic organisms are those found in the female genital tract, such as enteric gram-negative bacilli, group B streptococci, and *L. monocytogenes.*

   (ii) After about 1 week of age, meningitis is more often a result of systemic sepsis from respiratory, skin, or umbilical infections, and the predominant organisms are *S. aureus,* group B streptococci, and organisms present in hospital nurseries, such as *Pseudomonas* and *Proteus* species. Opportunistic pathogens such as *Flavobacterium septicum* or *Salmonella* species must also be considered.

   (iii) The temporal division is not sharp, however, because neonates may develop delayed infections from organisms presumably acquired during delivery, and hospital-acquired organisms may cause infection within the first days of life. Consequently, the first 2 months of life may be considered as a unit.

(b) Children and adolescents.

   (i) **After the age of 2 months,** the child loses the protection of maternal antibodies and becomes susceptible to the common organisms that cause childhood meningitis, primarily *H. influenzae* and *N. meningitidis.* There are rare cases of gram-negative or staphylococcal infection, which are usually associated with surgery, trauma, or systemic sepsis. The incidence of ***H. influenzae* meningitis peaks at the age of 1 year,** then drops off steadily as most children develop antibodies to the group B capsular antigen, either naturally or through vaccination.

   (ii) **After the age of 4 years,** *H. influenzae* meningitis is much less common, leaving **meningococcus** as the most frequent agent for the remainder of the first two decades of life.

(c) Adults. After the age of 20 years, most adults have developed immunity to meningococcus, and **pneumococcus** becomes the leading cause of bacterial meningitis. With its many type-specific capsular antigens and lack of cross-immunity among types, no permanent immunologic protection can develop against the pneumoccocus. Virtually all other bacterial meningitis in adults occurs in the setting of some predisposing condition, such as trauma, surgery, or immunosuppression. Elderly and debilitated patients, including alcoholics, are at increased risk for infection with gram-negative rods, particularly *E. coli.* In addition, cases of *H. influenzae* meningitis are being recognized more frequently among older adults, and at least 20% of the strains are beta-lactam resistant.

(3) Predisposing factors

(a) Head trauma. Closed head injury, with skull fractures or defects in the cribriform plate, can give bacteria access to the subarachnoid space. Usually the meningitis occurs within 2 weeks of injury, and **pneumococcus** is the infecting organism. With open head injuries and delayed onset of meningitis, a wide variety of organisms, including gram-negative bacilli and staphylococci, may invade the CNS. Meningitis associated with CSF rhinorrhea is due to pneumococcus in a high percentage of patients, even long after trauma.

(b) Parameningeal infections. Sinusitis, chronic otitis, and mastoiditis may lead to the development of meningitis, which is due to **pneumococcus** in most cases, less commonly to *H. influenzae,* and occasionally to *S. aureus.* It should be emphasized that **the presence of an organism in a parameningeal focus of infection does not guarantee that organism to be the etiology of the meningitis,** and the initial antibiotic is not chosen on that basis alone. Any organism that infects the ears or sinuses should be covered by the initial therapy; but unless there is confirmation by a strongly diagnostic CSF Gram's stain, other likely organisms must be covered as well.

(c) Postneurosurgical meningitis. The organism is introduced at surgery or shortly thereafter, before healing of the incision. Most often it is a skin organism or one of the wide variety of organisms acquired in the hospital environment. Consequently, broad-spectrum coverage is necessary until an organism can be identified. *Staphylococcus epidermidis* is an especially common pathogen infecting intraventricular shunts.

(d) **Anatomic defects.** Meningomyeloceles, midline dermal sinus tract including pilonidal sinuses, and tumors of the head and neck that invade the skull and meninges may give organisms access to the subarachnoid space. Thus, these conditions are sought in all patients with meningitis caused by unusual organisms. In the presence of these defects, initial antibiotic coverage must include staphylococci, streptococci, and enteric gram-negative organisms in addition to the common organisms for the particular age group.

(e) **Evidence of systemic sepsis.** Purpuric or petechial skin lesions may point to a diagnosis of meningococcemia, and bacilli often can be seen in or cultured from such lesions. However, staphylococcal septicemia, acute bacterial endocarditis, and, rarely, septicemia with enteric gram-negative organisms, may produce similar skin lesions.

Pneumonia may accompany meningitis and is often the primary infection, with meningitis occurring as a consequence of septicemia. Just as with sinus and ear infections, however, initial therapy should not be chosen purely on the basis of the respiratory pathogen.

(f) **Underlying systemic illness**
  (i) **Splenectomy and sickle cell anemia** predisposes to pneumococcal sepsis and meningitis.
  (ii) **Navahos and individuals with the HLA-B12 haplotype** may be at increased risk of *H. influenzae* B infection.
  (iii) **Systemic malignancy,** especially hematologic malignancy, induces vulnerability to a much wider range of organisms than that affecting the normal host, especially if the WBC count is depressed. Patients with malignancy and a normal peripheral WBC count are most often infected with *Cryptococcus,* but *Listeria* should also be considered, along with the more usual pathogens such as pneumococcus. When the WBC count falls below 2700, gram-negative rod meningitis becomes more likely.
  (iv) **Transplant recipients** and other patients on **immunosuppressive therapy,** as well as patients with **renal failure,** are susceptible to infection with fungus, enteric gram-negative rods, and hospital-acquired pathogens such as *Pseudomonas, Acinetobacter,* and *Serratia* species. Dialysis patients are particularly likely to become infected with skin organisms, such as staphylococci and streptococci.
  (v) Patients with **AIDS** are susceptible to infections with *Toxoplasma,* fungi (especially *Cryptococcus*), herpesviruses, and mycobacteria. Patients with AIDS may have simultaneous CNS infections with more than one pathogen (see sec. **XVII**).

(g) **Epidemiology.** In nonhospitalized patients, knowledge of community epidemics helps determine the appropriate therapy. In hospitalized patients with malignancy, immunosuppression, or anatomic defects that predispose to the development of meningitis with unusual organisms, initial antibiotic therapy should cover the organisms known to be present in the patient's hospital environment. Thus one should take into account antibiotic sensitivities of hospital flora in choosing a therapeutic regimen. Broad-spectrum antibiotic coverage should be used if there is any doubt about the infecting organism, particularly in patients with inadequate host defenses or with hospital-acquired infections.

b. **Recommendations for initial antibiotic therapy** (Table 8-2)
  (1) **Neonatal meningitis** (in infants younger than 2 months old)

Table 8-2. Initial therapy of bacterial meningitis

Clinical situation	Drug of choice	Alternative
Neonates	Ampicillin and gentamicin **or** Ampicillin and ceftriaxone	Vancomycin and gentamicin
Infants and children	Ampicillin and chloram-phenicol **or** Ceftriaxone	Erythromycin and chloramphenicol
Adults	Ampicillin and ceftriaxone	Erythromycin and chloramphenicol
Neurosurgical infection	Oxacillin and gentamicin	Vancomycin and gentamicin
Basilar skull fracture or CSF leak	Ampicillin **or** Penicillin	Erythromycin and chloramphenicol
Immunosuppression or malignancy	Ticarcillin and gentamicin	Erythromycin (or vanco-mycin) and gentamicin

    (a) Ampicillin, 50–100 mg/kg/day IV, divided into two doses, **and one of the following:**
        (i) Gentamicin, 5.0 mg/kg/day IV or IM, divided into two doses in premature infants and in term infants in the first week of life; or 7.5 mg/kg/day IV or IM, divided into three doses in neonates after the first week of life; **or**
        (ii) Amikacin, 15 mg/kg/day, divided into two doses if gentamicin-resistant organisms are common in the hospital nursery.
    (b) Alternative. Ampicillin, 50–100 mg/kg/day IV divided into two doses, **and ceftriaxone,** 100 mg/kg/day divided into two doses.
    (c) For penicillin-allergic patients. Vancomycin, 6–15 mg/kg/day divided into four doses, **and one of the following:**
        (i) Gentamicin or amikacin in the same dosage as in **(a)(i)** or **(a)(ii), or**
        (ii) Tobramycin, 3.0–4.5 mg/kg/day IV divided into three doses.
  (2) Infants and children (over 2 months old)
    (a) Ampicillin, 300–400 mg/kg/day IV, in four or six divided doses, **and one of the following:**
        (i) Chloramphenicol, 50–100 mg/kg/day IV, in four divided doses, **or**
        (ii) A **third-generation cephalosporin** (e.g., ceftriaxone, 100 mg/kg/day IV).
    (b) Alternative. Chloramphenicol, 50–100 mg/kg/day IV, divided into four doses, **and erythromycin,** 25–50 mg/kg/day, divided into four doses.
  (3) Adults (community-acquired meningitis)
    (a) Ampicillin, 12 g/day IV, divided into four or six doses. If ampicillin-resistant strains of *H. influenzae* are common in a particular area, it is reasonable to add **ceftriaxone,** 4–6 g/day IV divided into two doses.
    (b) Alternative. Chloramphenicol, 4 g/day IV, divided into four doses, **and erythromycin,** 4 g/day IV, divided into four doses.
  (4) Patients with basilar skull fractures or CSF leaks. Treatment is the same as in **(3)** if acquired outside the hospital and the same as in **(5)** if hospital-acquired.
  (5) Postneurosurgical infections
    (a) Oxacillin, 200 mg/kg/day IV in infants and children (other than neonates; see sec. **I.C.2.b.[4]**) and 10–12 g/day IV in adults, divided

into four doses (or **nafcillin,** same dosages as for oxacillin), **and one of the following:**

  (i) **Gentamicin,** 5.0 mg/kg/day IM or IV, divided into two doses, in premature infants; 7.5 mg/kg/day IM or IV, divided into three doses, in neonates; 5 mg/kg/day IV, divided into three doses, in children and adults with normal renal function; **plus intralumbar gentamicin,** 10 mg/day in adults and 1–2 mg/day in infants; **or**

  (ii) **Tobramycin** at the same dosages as for gentamicin, **or**

  (iii) **Amikacin,** 15 mg/kg/day IV divided into two doses, plus 30 mg/day intrathecally in adults.

  (b) **Alternatives:**

  (i) **Erythromycin,** 20 mg/kg/day IV, divided into two doses, in neonates; 40–50 mg/kg/day IV, divided into four doses, in children; 4–8 g/day IV, divided into four doses, in adults; **and gentamicin** 5 mg/kg/day IV divided into two doses; **or**

  (ii) **Vancomycin,** 2 g/day IV divided into two doses, **and gentamicin** (5 mg/kg/day IV divided into two doses), **tobramycin** (same dosage as gentamicin), **or amikacin** (15 mg/kg/day IV divided into two doses).

  (6) **Underlying immunosuppression or malignancy**

  (a) **Ticarcillin,** 240–360 mg/kg/day IV divided into six doses, **and gentamicin (or tobramycin or amikacin** [see **(5)(b)(ii)** for dosage]).

  (b) **Alternative: Erythromycin (or vancomycin) and gentamicin** (see **(5)(b)(i)** and **(ii)** for dosage).

c. **Antibiotic therapy of bacterial meningitis of known etiology**

  (1) As soon as the identification of the infecting organism has been made and its antibiotic sensitivity is known, the broad-spectrum coverage is changed to the optimum antibiotic available for the pathogen (Table 8-3). This antibiotic is continued for the remainder of the course.

  (2) The third-generation cephalosporins are a major improvement in the therapy of **gram-negative meningitis.** However, resistance is common among strains of *Enterobacter, Pseudomonas,* and *Serratia.*

  (a) The suggested initial therapy of meningitis caused by an **unidentified gram-negative rod** is as follows:

  (i) **Systemic aminoglycoside: gentamicin, tobramycin, or netilmicin,** 5–6 mg/kg/day IV; **or amikacin,** 15–20 mg/kg/day IV, when gentamicin-resistant *Pseudomonas* strains are a possibility; **and**

  (ii) **Intralumbar or intraventricular aminoglycoside: gentamicin or tobramycin,** 5–10 mg/day IV, **or amikacin,** 20–25 mg/day IV, **and**

  (iii) **Systemic cephalosporin: ceftriaxone,** 4–6 g/day IV divided into two doses, or an equivalent cephalosporin.

  (b) **Once antibacterial sensitivities are known,** the antibiotics can be adjusted. For *Enterobacter* and *Pseudomonas* infections, the combination of a broad-spectrum penicillin (carbenicillin, ticarcillin, piperacillin, mezlocillin, or azlocillin) or ceftazidime, 6–12 g/day IV, divided into three doses, plus an aminoglycoside administered both IV, and intrathecally is the therapy of choice (see **2.c.(2)(c)** for dosage).

  (c) **Trimethoprim-sulfamethoxazole** has been used in treating gram-negative meningitis with some success, but experience with its use is limited. It may have a role in the treatment of unusual pathogens and in treating patients allergic to the standard antibiotics. The dosage in adults is 15–20 mg/kg/day IV divided into four doses.

  (d) **Aztreonam,** 3–8 g/day IV divided into three or four doses, has also been used successfully in treating gram-negative meningitis.

  (3) *H. influenzae* presents a special problem in antibiotic choice. An increasing percentage of isolates in the United States are **resistant** to ampicillin by virtue of their ability to produce an enzyme, beta-lactamase, which renders the ampicillin molecule inactive. As a consequence, hospitals in which ampicillin-resistant *H. influenzae* has been recovered from spinal fluid use chloramphenicol or a third-generation cephalosporin as the

Table 8-3. Antibiotic therapy of bacterial meningitis of known etiology

Organism	Drug of choice	Alternative[a]	Optional intrathecal drug
Gram-positive organisms			
Streptococcus pneumoniae (pneumococcus)	Penicillin G	Third-generation cephalosporin Chloramphenicol Erythromycin	
Streptococcus, group A and B	Penicillin G	Erythromycin	
Streptococcus, group D (enterococcus)	Penicillin and gentamicin	Vancomycin and gentamicin	Gentamicin
Staphylococcus	Oxacillin or nafcillin	Vancomycin	Bacitracin
Listeria monocytogenes	Ampicillin	Penicillin G Trimethoprim-sulfamethoxazole Chloramphenicol	
Gram-negative organisms			
Meningococcus	Penicillin G	Third-generation cephalosporin Chloramphenicol	
Haemophilus influenzae	Ampicillin[b] or third-generation cephalosporin	Chloramphenicol	
Enteric gram-negative rods (*Escherichia coli, Proteus* species, *Klebsiella* species)	Third-generation cephalosporin or ticarcillin plus gentamicin[c]	Gentamicin IV and IT	Gentamicin
Pseudomonas aeruginosa	Ticarcillin (or ceftazidime) plus gentamicin	Gentamicin IV and IT	Gentamicin

Key: IT = intrathecally.
[a] For patients allergic to penicillin.
[b] Ampicillin is recommended for *H. influenzae* only when the organism is known to be sensitive to the drug.
[c] Antibiotics should be chosen with attention to sensitivity testing; other semisynthetic penicillins or aminoglycosides may need to be substituted.

first-line drug for *H. influenzae* meningitis. A direct assay of beta lactamase activity of the isolate is a more reliable indication of ampicillin sensitivity than is the standard disk inhibition method. There have been only rare reports of *H. influenzae* isolates that are resistant to chloramphenicol.

D. Intrathecal antibiotic therapy of bacterial meningitis

1. **Rationale.** Because of the relatively low CSF drug concentrations obtained with some antibiotics, there have been many attempts to treat CNS infections with direct subarachnoid injections. This procedure is used to expose the organisms in the meninges and CSF to higher concentrations of antibiotics than can be achieved with systemic administration alone.

2. There are several **problems** with the intrathecal approach.

   a. Many drugs are **toxic to the CNS** when they come in contact with the surface of the brain or spinal cord in high concentrations. For example, penicillin and its derivatives cause seizures and encephalopathy. Also, many drugs, when injected into the lumbar subarachnoid space, have been reported to cause paresthesias, radiculopathies, or transverse myelitis, and there have been reports of arachnoiditis following repeated intrathecal administration of drugs.

   b. **Drugs do not diffuse freely throughout the CSF.** When administered into the lumbar space, they reach negligible concentration in the ventricles and relatively low concentrations in the basilar cisterns.

   c. Patients with CNS infections may have **blocks in CSF flow** at various levels limiting drug access to some parts of the subarachnoid space.

   d. **The concentration of antibiotic in the CSF varies widely** from patient to patient following a given intrathecal dose and can be affected by the dynamics of CSF flow as well as the presence of hydrocephalus.

3. **Aminoglycoside antibiotics** can be injected safely into the subarachnoid space. They may, however, produce paresthesias in the extremities and eighth cranial nerve damage, especially in high concentrations. Nevertheless, in reasonable doses, these drugs can be used safely for a brief course of intrathecal therapy. **Techniques of administration** are as follows:

   a. **Intralumbar.** An LP is performed in the usual manner, and 5–10 ml of CSF is removed for analysis, including **drug-level measurement,** cell count, protein, sugar, and culture. The drug to be administered is dissolved either in 5 or 10 ml of sterile saline **without bacteriostatic preservative** or in CSF and is injected through the LP needle slowly.

   b. **Intracisternal.** Drugs may be injected into the basilar cistern by those skilled in the technique of cisternal puncture. The advantage over lumbar injection is that higher levels of antibiotic may be achieved at the base of the brain and over the convexity. This technique is essentially the same as intralumbar injection, but the drug is injected over 1 minute to minimize the time the needle remains in the cistern, where it can potentially damage the medulla. Cisternal puncture is **not recommended for repeated administration** of drugs and should be undertaken only by those with considerable experience with the technique.

   c. **Intraventricular.** An indwelling catheter that connects one lateral ventricle to a small silicone rubber reservoir **(Ommaya reservoir)** may be implanted surgically. The self-sealing reservoir can be repeatedly punctured percutaneously, thereby giving ready access to the intraventricular space, either for the sampling of CSF or the injection of drugs. Very high drug levels may be achieved in the ventricles, and adequate levels are reached in the cisternal and lumbar CSF. With aminoglycosides, a 5-mg dose injected intraventricularly may yield therapeutic drug levels (4–6 µg/ml) throughout the CSF for as long as 24 hours after injection. The disadvantages of this method of administration are that the patient is subjected to a neurosurgical procedure with its possible complications, and the devices can become plugged, disconnected, or infected during use. Drug administration using the reservoirs requires meticulous **aseptic technique.**

4. Precautions to be taken with intrathecal antibiotic administration
   a. Measure the **CSF drug level** with each dose to ensure that antibiotic is not accumulating excessively in the CSF.
   b. Follow the **CSF protein** and **cell count** for signs of a CSF block (greatly elevated protein) or chemical meningitis (increasing CSF white cell count, often with polymorphonuclear leukocytes predominating, and increasing protein).
   c. **Culture** the CSF with each injection. An increasing cell count may indicate iatrogenic CNS infection as well as chemical meningitis.
   d. Be aware of the possibility of blockages of CSF flow, denying the antibiotic access to regions of the subarachnoid space that may harbor "loculated infections." A radioactively labeled colloid may be injected into the ventricle to determine the **patency of CSF pathways** by radiologic methods. In patients with obstructive hydrocephalus, combined intraventricular administration of antibiotic through a drainage catheter and intralumbar administration may be required.
5. Indications for intrathecal therapy. Intrathecal therapy is reserved for those patients in whom systemic therapy alone is not likely to be curative. In these patients, the organism requires higher drug levels than are attainable in CSF by intravenous administration. Definite indications for the use of intrathecal antibiotic administration have not been defined, but it should be limited to certain rare situations.
   a. Gram-negative meningitis
      (1) If the bacteria are sensitive to ampicillin or a third-generation cephalosporin, these drugs achieve bactericidal concentrations in the CSF with intravenous administration. Experience has shown them to be adequate as single agents against most susceptible pathogens. Strains of *Pseudomonas, Serratia, Acinetobacter (Mima, Herellea)*, and some *Proteus* species are usually resistant to these antibiotics. Most clinicians would use an aminoglycoside administered systemically and intrathecally as part of the initial therapy when these organisms are suspected.
      (2) If the organism is resistant to ampicillin and the cephalosporins, or if the infection fails to respond adequately to a full course of therapy, an aminoglycoside may be used both systemically and intrathecally, in combination with an appropriate broad-spectrum penicillin.
      (3) The indications for intraventricular administration of an aminoglycoside via an Ommaya reservoir are not established. In the absence of good evidence for the superiority of the ventricular route, it is reasonable to begin with intralumbar therapy and resort to intraventricular therapy only for
         (a) Highly resistant organisms (as determined by the minimal bacteriocidal concentration of the antibiotic used).
         (b) Infections that fail to respond to intralumbar therapy
         (c) Patients with known block to CSF flow that prevents drugs administered into the lumbar subarachnoid space from reaching the basilar cisterns.
   b. Staphylococcal meningitis. Bacitracin in doses of 5000–10,000 units may be injected into the subarachnoid space in the treatment of meningitis due to penicillinase-producing *S. aureus*. However, this therapy is indicated only in moribund patients and those failing to respond to systemic administration of oxacillin or nafcillin in high doses. The technique of administration is the same as that for the aminoglycosides.
   c. Enterococcal meningitis (Streptococcus faecalis) is a rare disease, at times occurring in neonates or as a complication of surgery or bacterial endocarditis. Although sensitive to ampicillin in vitro, this organism requires combined therapy with penicillin and an aminoglycoside to cure serious infections. Consequently, the combination of penicillin G and gentamicin is administered systemically. Intrathecal gentamicin may be added if response to intravenous therapy is inadequate.

E. Corticosteroid therapy of bacterial meningitis

 1. **Infants and children.** Dexamethasone, 0.15 mg/kg body weight q6h for the first 4 days of antibiotic therapy, has been shown to reduce the risk of hearing loss and other neurologic sequelae in infants and children with bacterial meningitis. Therefore, many experts recommend its routine use in childhood meningitis in nonimmunosuppressed hosts. **Administration early** in treatment is essential.

 2. **Adults.** Some experts recommend the routine use of anti-inflammatory doses of corticosteroids (prednisone, 40–80 mg/day or equivalent) in nonimmunosuppressed adults with bacterial meningitis. There are no systematic studies verifying the efficacy of this practice.

 3. High-dose corticosteroids are used for the therapy of **cerebral edema** associated with severe meningitis (see sec. **I.H.1**).

 4. Maintenance doses of corticosteroids are administered if there is a suspicion of **adrenal necrosis** (Waterhouse-Friderichsen syndrome) (see sec. **I.B.1.a.[2]**).

F. Prophylactic treatment of contacts

 1. **Choice of contacts for treatment.** Patients with meningococcal disease are infectious and can spread the organism to others by the respiratory route until they have been on antibiotics for 24 hours. About 3 per 1000 family members of index cases will develop meningococcal disease. Others will become asymptomatic carriers and can expose other susceptible people to the organism. Therefore, it is recommended that the following groups be treated with antibiotics when an index case is diagnosed:

    a. Family and household members.

    b. Others in contact for prolonged periods with an index case. This does not include acquaintances or school classmates.

    c. Hospital staff members on whom the patient has breathed directly. There is no need to treat any hospital personnel who have merely been in the room with the patient.

 2. **Treatment.** The current recommendations for prophylactic therapy are as follows:

    a. If the organism is known to be sensitive to sulfonamides, the preferred antibiotic is **sulfadiazine,** 1 g PO q12h for 2 days in adults, 500 mg PO q12h in children ages 1–12 years, and 500 mg/day PO in infants.

    b. When the drug sensitivity of the organism is unknown or when it is known to be sulfadiazine-resistant, the preferred drug is **rifampin,** 600 mg PO q12h for four doses in adults, 10 mg/kg q12h for four doses in infants and children over 1 month of age, and 5 mg/kg q12h for four doses in infants under 1 month of age. The alternative in adults is **minocycline,** 200 mg PO, then 100 mg PO q12h for five doses (not to be used in children).

    c. Secondary cases of meningococcal disease usually occur within 4 days of the index case. Therefore, one should not await results of antibiotic sensitivity testing before treating those at risk but should **treat all close contacts of the index case immediately on diagnosis.** However, both rifampin and minocycline have significant side effects (GI upset and dizziness), so only those at real risk should be treated prophylactically. Neither drug should be used during pregnancy.

    d. **Close contacts** (e.g., those with oral contact with the patient, hospital personnel whose mucosa has been exposed to infected secretions) should be treated with **procaine penicillin G,** 600,000 units IM q8h for six doses, then penicillin V, 500 mg PO q8h for 8 days.

 3. A quadrivalent meningococcal **vaccine** (groups A, C, Y, W135) is immunogenic in adults and in children over 2 years of age. Its use should be considered in close household contacts of index cases as an adjunct to chemoprophylaxis and in asplenic children or those with complement deficiencies. It should be used only when the meningococcal type is known early during the index infection, as the vaccines require 5 days to confer protection. Serogroup B, for which there is not yet a vaccine, causes most of the sporadic meningoccocal disease in the United States. In epidemics of meningococcal disease, the Centers for Disease Control (CDC) should be consulted concerning the use of the vaccine.

 4. **Children younger than 6 years of age** who are household or day-care contacts of

patients with *H. influenzae* meningitis should receive rifampin, 20 mg/kg PO qd for 4 days.

G. Shunt infections. Infections of shunts that are implanted for the treatment of hydrocephalus make up a special category of postneurosurgical infections. These infections are usually acquired at surgery. Consequently, the spectrum of organisms is the same as that of other neurosurgical infections. Staphylococci (especially *S. epidermidis*), streptococci, and anaerobes are the organisms in the vast majority of infections; gram-negative enteric bacteria are unusual but significant pathogens. Meningococcus and pneumococcus are rare causes of shunt infections. The initial antibiotic coverage is the same as that for the other postneurosurgical infections already discussed.

   1. Diagnosis. CSF obtained by LP grows the infecting organism in only about three-fourths of shunt infections. Thus, the blood, surgical wound (if it is fresh), urine, and fluid obtained from a direct puncture of the shunt-valve reservoir, in addition to the lumbar CSF, are cultured. Peritonitis may occur with ventriculoperitoneal shunt infections, and the ascitic fluid may yield the organism.

   2. The **treatment** of a shunt infection is as follows:

     a. Surgical removal of the shunt.

     b. Appropriate systemic antibiotic coverage (see sec. **I.C.3.b.[5]**).

     c. Once the shunt is removed, the infection usually responds to systemic antibiotics, and there is no need for intrathecal therapy. When constant ventricular drainage is required after shunt removal, however, antibiotics can be instilled through the drainage cannula with little added morbidity.

H. Complications of bacterial meningitis

   1. Increased intracranial pressure (ICP) is common in bacterial meningitis.

     a. Etiology. Increased ICP usually occurs because of impaired CSF absorption due to accumulation of fibrin and inflammatory cells around the arachnoid villi and resolves with treatment of the infection. In addition, increased ICP can occur through two other mechanisms: hydrocephalus and brain edema. The latter is typically a diffuse process caused by bacterial and leukocyte products that increase capillary permeability (vasogenic edema) and compromise the integrity of cell membranes (cytotoxic edema). Brain edema may also be focal, secondary to arteritis or cortical venous thrombophlebitis with ischemia and brain infarction.

     b. Treatment. The pressure generally returns rapidly to normal as the infection responds to therapy. If the patient is afebrile, awake, and alert, without focal signs, it can safely be assumed that the increased CSF pressure has resolved. The therapy for increased ICP in association with meningitis is conservative. There is no need to treat intracranial hypertension per se unless there are signs of severe generalized brain edema or localized mass effect with risk of herniation. Bradycardia in association with elevated blood pressure, the **Cushing's reflex,** may signal increased ICP; however, hypotension and shock more commonly accompany increased ICP.

       (1) If the patient is doing well clinically, avoid repeated LPs.

       (2) Fluid balance. Avoid overhydrating the patient or administering large amounts of free water. In adults with adequate perfusion, 1500 ml of normal saline per day is sufficient, including the volume of fluid in which the antibiotics are administered. In children, one-third to one-half maintenance with half-normal saline in 5% D/W is recommended. When patients can regulate their own fluid intake, they should be limited to less than 2000 ml of total daily intake (PO plus IV) until the CSF pressure is no longer elevated. **In patients receiving mannitol, normal saline (309 mOsm/liter) should be used for all IV fluids, including, where possible, diluents for medications.**

       (3) Steroids are administered in high doses initially and then rapidly tapered once the infection is under control. One protocol consists of dexamethasone (Decadron), 10 mg IV for the first dose, then 4–6 mg IV q6h until the infection is under control. The dose is then tapered to zero over 5–10 days, assuming the total course is less than 3 weeks. If high doses are given for longer than 2 weeks, more gradual tapering is necessary, since the risk of adrenal insufficiency increases. The usual precautions necessary with high-dose steroid administration (i.e., the monitoring of blood glucose and stool guaiacs and concern for masked infection) are followed. Steroid begin to exert an effect only after 12–16 hours.

(4) **Hyperosmolar agents.** When using hyperosmolar agents, the physician must guarantee a patient urinary system; in comatose patients, a Foley catheter is required. Both mannitol and glycerol are associated with hyperosmolar, hyperglycemic, nonketotic coma in diabetics. Blood glucose and serum electrolytes should be followed frequently in diabetics and a least every other day in nondiabetics.

(a) **Mannitol,** 1.0–1.5 g/kg, may be given for acute increased ICP where there is danger of transtentorial herniation. Doses of 0.25–0.5 g/kg may be repeated twice at 4-hour intervals, to cover the period before steroids take effect. In children, 0.25–1.00 g/kg may be given over 10–30 minutes. Smaller doses may be as effective as larger ones and may be given more often, if necessary. Some data show that after mannitol is given, a "rebound" increase in ICP occurs. In meningitis this effect can be minimized by using steroids and by treating the infection. The **serum osmolality** should be checked immediately after administration of each dose and should not be allowed to rise above 320 mOsm/liter. **The goal of therapy is controlled hyperosmolality not hypovolemia.**

(b) **Furosemide** (0.5 mg/kg) can be used as an adjunct to mannitol to decrease ICP. It facilitates removal of sodium and water from brain and reduces CSF formation.

2. **Seizures** are a frequent manifestation of meningitis, especially in infants and children, and generally do not affect prognosis. Epilepsy is uncommon (3–7%) after recovery. However, seizures may also signal more serious complications of meningitis, including

   a. Bacterial encephalitis.
   b. Cortical vein thrombosis with venous infarction.
   c. Subdural effusion or empyema.
   d. Infectious vasculitis.
   e. Brain abscess (rare as a complication, except in neonates).
   f. Metabolic abnormalities. Hyponatremia from the syndrome of inappropriate antidiuretic hormone (SIADH) secretion is a particularly common complication of meningitis.

3. **Hydrocephalus**

   a. **Communicating hydrocephalus** may complicate bacterial meningitis due to obstruction of CSF flow by thickened and fibrotic meninges. Usually the site of obstruction is at the base of the brain. This syndrome may occur early or late in the course of the infection and should be suspected if the patient's mental status fails to return to normal as the infection clears or deteriorates after initial improvement. This condition is not a medical emergency and may resolve spontaneously without shunting. The same considerations apply in deciding whether, and when, a shunt should be implanted as with other cases of communicating hydrocephalus (see Chap. 3).

   b. **Noncommunicating hydrocephalus** rarely occurs as a complication of meningitis and is due to partial or complete obstruction of CSF flow at the aqueduct of Sylvius or at the fourth ventricular outlet.

   (1) **Total obstruction** of ventricular outflow is rare. It usually causes coma, which can mistakenly be assumed to be due to the infection itself. However, total obstruction of ventricular outflow is an emergency and will rapidly lead to death unless it is corrected. The presence of **coma, bilateral Babinski's signs, and paralysis of upward gaze** should suggest the diagnosis, which can be confirmed by CT scan or MRI. Papilledema is not necessarily present. Since this syndrome generally occurs early, when the CSF is still infected, the acute treatment is constant ventricular

drainage rather than shunting. After the CSF is sterile, a ventriculoperitoneal or ventriculoatrial shunt may be placed.

    (2) Partial obstruction at the aqueduct or fourth ventricular outflow is not an emergency, but it requires careful observation for signs of total obstruction.

4. Subdural effusion. Infants less than 1 year of age are subject to the accumulation of sterile collections of fluid in the subdural space as a complication of bacterial meningitis (most often *H. influenzae*).

    a. Description. The signs are nonspecific: vomiting, irritability, persistent fullness of the fontelle, or increasing head circumference.

    b. The **diagnosis** is made by transillumination of the skull or CT scanning, and it is confirmed by tapping the subdural space percutaneously through the patent fontanelle.

    c. Treatment is aimed at maintaining normal ICP. Repeated percutaneous aspiration of the fluid is usually adequate, and the fluid ceases to reaccumulate after the infection is treated. Subdural taps are not indicated if there are no signs or symptoms of increased ICP and no focal neurologic deficits. The membrane that surrounds the effusion may have to be excised surgically in rare cases if the fluid continues to reaccumulate after repeated taps.

5. Subdural empyema is a rare complication of meningitis.

    a. Description. Subdural empyema is suggested by the development of papilledema, persistently increased ICP, persistent fever, focal signs, or seizures.

    b. The **diagnosis** can be made by CT scan or MRI. The EEG and technetium brain scan are of little value in the diagnosis of this condition, and LP is dangerous.

    c. Treatment is immediate and aggressive surgical drainage. Appropriate stains and cultures are performed at surgery, and appropriate antibiotic therapy is continued for at least 1 week postoperatively.

6. Persistent fever during the treatment of bacterial meningitis suggests one of several conditions: an occult focus of infection requiring surgical drainage or prolonged antibiotic therapy (e.g., osteomyelitis, an occult abscess either in the brain or elsewhere, or subdural effusion), drug fever, or inadequate antibiotic therapy.

7. Persistent neurologic deficit

    a. A **focal neurologic deficit** may indicate destruction of brain tissue by encephalitis or infarction, or the presence of a mass lesion, such as a subdural effusion or empyema. Brain abscess complicating meningitis is rare after the neonatal period.

    b. Cranial nerve palsies may occur but usually resolve. **Hearing deficits** are the most frequently persistent cranial nerve abnormalities. Children should be evaluated with brainstem auditory evoked responses or audiometry.

    c. Venous thrombosis occurs as a result of cortical vein thrombophlebitis. The only known treatment is antibiotics to prevent progression of the process. Anticoagulation is of no known benefit.

    d. Vasculitis is relatively common, especially in children, and usually resolves with appropriate antibiotic therapy. However, with involvement of the large arteries at the base of the brain, stroke and permanent neurologic deficit can occur.

8. Medical complications

    a. Bacterial meningitis may lead to **SIADH** with hyponatremia and increased risk of seizures.

    b. Systemic sepsis may lead to DIC shock, ARDS, and metastatic abscess formation (see sec. **I.B**).

    c. Antibiotics used in high doses, as is necessary for meningitis, subject the patient to their associated risks (see sec. **I.C**).

    d. The risks associated with steroids and hyperosmolar agents have been discussed (see sec. **I.H.1.b[4]**).

II. Tuberculous infection of the CNS

  A. Diagnosis

    1. Tuberculous meningitis. "Any subacute febrile meningitis with a low spinal fluid sugar content is tuberculous meningitis until proven otherwise" (Adams R., *N. Engl. J. Med.* 290:1130, 1974). The diagnosis of tuberculous meningitis must often be made before culture results become available because *Mycobacterium tuberculosis* requires at least 4 weeks to grow in vitro. The diagnosis suggested by the clinical symptoms (fever, headache, lethargy, vomiting, and cranial nerve palsies), is supported by evidence of active pulmonary disease (present in only about one-third of cases, usually miliary) or by a positive PPD (present in about 50% of cases), and is confirmed by observing acid-fast organisms on a Ziehl-Neelsen–stained CSF sample. Nuchal rigidity is not often seen early in the disease. The CSF usually shows a lymphocytic pleocytosis with a low glucose; however, polymorphonuclear predominance may be seen early in the disease. The protein is nearly always elevated, frequently leading to the formation of a clot, or **pellicle,** on standing. The diagnostic yield of the CSF may be augmented in various ways:

   a. The probability of growing the organism is directly related to the quantity of CSF cultured. Consequently, **10–15 ml of CSF** should be removed for culture with each diagnostic LP.

   b. Concentration of the organisms will aid in microscopic identification by the AFB smear.

   (1) The pellicle can be smeared and is an excellent source of the organism

   (2) The CSF can be centrifuged and the sediment smeared if no pellicle forms

   c. Chemical and immunologic tests, including ELISA and latex particle agglutination, have been either technically difficult or unreliable, or both. Polymerase chain reaction to amplify tubercle bacillus DNA is under investigation as a detection method.

   d. Repeated CSF examinations may show a characteristic pattern of falling sugar, rising protein, and rising or stable cell count. **An initially normal CSF does not rule out tuberculous meningitis.**

   2. Other CNS complications. Tuberculosis may also infect the brain parenchyma producing diffuse **encephalitis** or a focal **tuberculoma,** with or without meningeal involvement. In the absence of meningitis or tuberculosis in other organs, the diagnosis may be extremely difficult and often is made only after tissue biopsy. *M. tuberculosis* also may invade blood vessels and cause a CNS **vasculitis** with associated brain infarction.

B. Treatment

   1. Antibiotics

   a. First-line drugs

   (1) Isoniazid (INH) is effective, is relatively nontoxic, and penetrates the meninges well. However, **organisms resistant to isoniazid, as well as rifampin, are increasingly common.** The dosage in adults is 5 mg/kg/day in a single oral dose. In children, the dosage is 10–20 mg/kg/day. The total daily dose should not exceed 300 mg. All patients over 6 years old should receive **pyridoxine,** 50 mg/day, to prevent pyridoxine-deficiency syndromes, which include neuropathy, encephalopathy, seizures, and anemia (see Chap. 14).

   (2) Rifampin, 600 mg/day PO in adults and 10–20 mg/kg/day PO in children, not to exceed 600 mg/day.

   (3) Pyrazinamide, 15–30 mg/kg/day PO in both children and adults, divided into three or four doses. The maximum daily dose is 2 g.

   (4) Ethambutol, 15–25 mg/kg/day PO in both adults and children. The maximum daily dose is 2.5 g.

   b. Second-line drugs for use in cases of resistant organisms or patient sensitivity to first-line drugs:

   (1) Streptomycin, 15 mg/kg/day (maximum 1 g/day) in adults and 20–40 mg/kg/day in children as a single daily IM injection. Because of eighth nerve and renal toxicity, the maximum dose should not be administered for more than 12 weeks.

   (2) Ciprofloxacin, 750 mg PO bid. Cycloserine penetrates into the CSF well, and CSF drugs levels approximate serum levels.

(3) Ethionamide, 0.5–1.0 g daily PO divided into two to four doses. Penetration into CSF is excellent, but GI, liver, and CNS toxicity is common.

c. Antibiotic regimen

(1) For the first 2 months and until antibiotic sensitivity is known, **four drugs** are recommended:

(a) Isoniazid, 300 mg/day, **and**

(b) Rifampin, 600 mg/day, **and**

(c) Pyrazinamide, 15–30 mg/kg/day, **and**

(d) Streptomycin, 15 mg/kg/day IM, **or**

(e) Ethambutol, 15–20 mg/kg/day.

(2) The regimen is adjusted after antibiotic sensitivities are known. Many clinicians reduce the regimen to two drugs (generally isoniazid and rifampin) after 2–3 months of therapy.

(3) The minimum necessary duration of therapy is unknown, but patients with tuberculous meningitis are typically treated for 6 months to 1 year. **In general, tuberculosis is treated 50% longer in patients with concurrent HIV infection.**

(4) The CDC recommends that therapy be monitored until patient compliance can be demonstrated. **Noncompliant patients** may have antibiotics administered under medical supervision on a **twice weekly schedule:**

(a) Isoniazid, 15 mg/kg (maximum 900 mg), twice per week, **and/or**

(b) Rifampin, 600 mg, twice per week, **and/or**

(c) Pyrazinamide, 50–70 mg/kg, twice per week, **and/or**

(d) Ethambutol, 50 mg/kg, twice per week.

2. Steroids. Some have advocated the use of systemic, or even intrathecal, steroids in tuberculous meningitis. The aim is to inhibit the inflammatory response and thereby prevent some of the complications of infection, which result as much from the inflammation and granuloma formation as from direct destruction by the bacteria.

a. Theoretical indications for the use of steroids in addition to antituberculous chemotherapy are as follows:

(1) To reduce elevated ICP due to brain swelling.

(2) To reduce inflammatory exudate in the subarachnoid space and associated risk of obstructive hydrocephalus or spinal block.

(3) To decrease vascular inflammation (arteritis) of the vessels at the base of the brain and associated risk of infarction.

b. Patients with a normal mental status and no neurologic deficit probably would **not** benefit from steroid therapy.

c. Clinical indications for steroid use are

(1) Deterioration in level of consciousness.

(2) Progressive focal neurologic signs. Findings should be elevated radiographically when possible.

d. The **dosage** of steroids for increased ICP is the same as for increased pressure of other types: dexamethasone, 10 mg IV as a first dose, then 4–6 mg IV q6h (adults and children). Mannitol may also be used in acute situations. Prednisone, 60 or 80 mg/day, or its equivalent, is usually chosen as an anti-inflammatory agent. The high dose is generally maintained for 2–3 weeks and is then slowly tapered over about 1 month.

3. Contacts of the patient should be treated prophylactically according to the recommendations of the American Thoracic Society (see **Selected Readings**).

4. Tuberculomas are treated medically with regimens identical to those used for tuberculous meningitis. **Indications for surgical excision** include size greater than 2 cm in diameter, elevated ICP due to edema around the lesion that is refractory to medical therapy, intractable epilepsy, lack of response to appropriate antibiotics, and situations where the diagnosis is in question. Biopsy of tuberculomas has been reported to cause tuberculous meningitis and should be carried out with caution.

5. Follow-up and complications

a. Repeat LPs are performed at 1 month, 6 months, and 2 years after beginning

therapy if the patient is clinically stable. The appearance of a new neurolog
sign or symptom should prompt an LP or other diagnostic tests as indicate
   b. The major late neurologic complication of tuberculous meningitis is **hydr
   cephalus.** Treatment depends on the site and degree of the CSF block (s
   Chap. 3).
   c. Relapses. The main reason for relapse is noncompliance with treatmer
   Inadequate therapy has caused an alarmingly high incidence of **organism
   resistant to multiple drugs.** At the first indication of a relapse, the patient
   hospitalized, the antibiotic sensitivity of the organism is rechecked, a
   pending those results, appropriate changes in the drug regimen are mad
   These changes may include the administration of the drugs under supervisio
   as well as substitution or addition of alternative drugs.
6. Toxicity of antituberculous chemotherapy
   a. Isoniazid
      (1) Hepatic. About 10% of patients on isoniazid develop elevated SGOT leve
         Usually, the SGOT returns to normal even if isoniazid is continued. Tr
         hepatitis occurs in only 1% of cases. It can occur months after beginnir
         therapy and can produce jaundice, permanent liver damage, and eve
         death. The risk of developing hepatitis increases with age, is not dos
         dependent, and may occur principally in rapid acetylators of isoniazi
      (2) Neurologic. Pyridoxine-deficiency syndromes, including neuropathy, an
         mia, encephalopathy, and seizures may occur if pyridoxine supplement
         tion is not provided. This does not occur in children under the age of
         years. Optic atrophy occurs rarely.
      (3) Psychiatric. Euphoria, mania, and frank psychosis may occur and gene
         ally do not represent pyridoxine deficiency.
      (4) Hypersensitivity reactions are rare.
      (5) Precautions
         (a) Provide pyridoxine supplementation at a dose at least one-tenth th
            isoniazid dose for patients over 6 years of age.
         (b) Evaluate monthly for symptoms of hepatitis. Perform liver functio
            tests at baseline and when symptoms suggest hepatotoxicity.
         (c) Isoniazid may precipitate phenytoin toxicity by interfering with tha
            drug's metabolism.
   b. Streptomycin
      (1) Neurologic. Eighth cranial nerve damage (vestibular and hearing distu
         bances) limits the maximum dose of streptomycin that can be used. Dose
         of 1 g/day or less are reliably tolerated for 2–3 months.
      (2) Renal. As with all aminoglycosides, dose-related renal impairment ma
         occur, but in the absence of preexisting renal disease, doses of streptomy
         cin up to 1 g/day are tolerated.
      (3) Hypersensitivity reactions are unusual.
      (4) Precautions
         (a) Renal function is checked prior to use, and the dosage is adjuste
            accordingly.
         (b) Evaluate monthly for symptoms and signs of labyrinthine dysfunc
            tion. **If administered to pregnant women, streptomycin may caus
            congenital deafness in the fetus.**
   c. Ethambutol
      (1) Neurologic. Visual changes with optic nerve dysfunction can occur a
         doses higher than 15 mg/kg/day. However, this problem usually reverse
         if the drug is withdrawn promptly. The most sensitive indicators are test
         of color vision and visual acuity.
      (2) Precautions. Evaluate monthly for visual symptoms.
   d. Rifampin
      (1) Gastrointestinal upset is common with rifampin administration.
      (2) Hypersensitivity reactions, thrombocytopenia, hepatocellular injury, and
         skin eruptions are rare.
      (3) Drug interactions. Rifampin increases the rate of hepatic metabolism o

many drugs, including warfarin, anticonvulsants, and estrogen-containing contraceptives.

    (4) Precautions. Patients should be warned that rifampin turns the urine, tears, and sweat orange. Soft contact lenses can be permanently discolored.

  e. Pyrazinamide

    (1) Hepatic. Hepatocellular toxicity occurs in about 15% of patients at a dose of 3 g/day. Fatal hepatic necrosis occurs rarely.

    (2) Gastrointestinal upset is common.

    (3) The drug may precipitate attacks of **gout** and may exacerbate **diabetes mellitus.**

    (4) Hypersensitivity reactions are relatively common.

    (5) Precautions. Evaluate monthly for symptoms of hepatitis. Perform liver function tests at baseline and when symptoms suggest hepatotoxicity.

  f. Ciprofloxacin

    (1) Neurologic. Central nervous system toxicity is rare, but seizures, psychosis, and tremors have been reported.

    (2) Gastrointestinal upset occurs occasionally.

    (3) Hypersensitivity reactions are relatively common.

    (4) Precautions. Ciprofloxacin, like all the quinolones, is contraindicated in children and should not be given to pregnant women.

  g. Ethionamide

    (1) Hepatic. Hepatocellular toxicity occurs in about 5% of patients taking the drug; diabetics appear to be at higher risk.

    (2) Neurologic. Reversible CNS toxicity, with depression, drowsiness, tremor, and olfactory disturbances, may occur. Seizures are rare.

    (3) Gastrointestinal upset is common.

    (4) Severe postural hypotension can occur.

    (5) Precautions. Evaluate monthly for symptoms of hepatitis. Liver function tests should be performed at baseline and when symptoms suggest hepatotoxicity.

III. Brain abscess

  A. Diagnosis

    1. Clinical presentation. Brain abscess generally manifests itself as the subacute progression of focal neurologic signs, headache, and altered mental status. Seizures occur in 25–50% of patients. Systemic signs of infection, such as fever and peripheral leukocytosis, are present only in about half of patients. Erythrocyte sedimentation rate usually is elevated.

    2. There may be evidence for a contiguous or systemic source of infection.

    3. Differential diagnosis may include brain tumor, chronic subdural hematoma, chronic meningitis, or viral encephalitis. Signs of meningeal irritation are usually absent or mild. However, if the abscess ruptures into the ventricular system, the ensuing ventriculitis and meningitis produce marked meningeal signs.

    4. The definitive diagnosis is often made only at surgery, although a characteristic **CT scan** or **MRI** in the appropriate clinical setting may strongly suggest the diagnosis.

  B. Localizing the lesion

    1. A **CT scan and MRI** are highly reliable in localizing abscesses. Furthermore, in the appropriate clinical setting, the typical "ring-enhancing" lesion (i.e., a thin, usually regular, contrast-enhancing ring around a low-density center) is relatively specific for brain abscess. Cystic tumors or infarcts with rims of neovascularization can give a similar appearance, but the CT absorption values of their centers are generally higher than those of abscess. The CT scan and MRI can also distinguish between an unencapsulated area of brain infection (cerebritis) and an encapsulated abscess.

    2. Arteriography is relatively poor in localizing brain abscess.

    3. An **LP** may be hazardous when a brain abscess is present, and the CSF rarely discloses the organism responsible for infection. Examination of the CSF can help rule out bacterial meningitis, but in most patients the history and examination will distinguish abscess from meningitis.

4. **Skull x rays or CT scan.** All patients with suspected brain abscess should have complete skull x-rays or CT scan with bone windows early in their course to search for parameningeal infection. Adequate views of the mastoids and sinuses are essential, since brain abscess due to sinusitis usually occurs adjacent to the infected sinus. Frontal or ethmoidal sinus infections are associated with abscesses in the frontal lobe, while either frontal or temporal abscesses complicate maxillary and sphenoid sinusitis. Abscess associated with mastoiditis or otitis commonly occurs in the temporal tip or cerebellar hemisphere.

C. **Pathophysiology.** Brain abscess formation involves two stages.

1. Initially, a diffuse and poorly marginated area of infection is associated with edema and destruction of brain tissue. During this **cerebritis** stage, the CT scan shows a nonspecific low-density area that enhances diffusely with IV contrast material. **At this stage, the infection is curable with antibiotic therapy alone and is not amenable to surgical therapy.**

2. Over a period of 4–9 days, the center of the infection turns into semiliquid pus and necrotic brain tissue. Once this stage is reached, the infection may not be curable by medical therapy alone. Gradually, **encapsulation** by gliotic tissue occurs and a free abscess forms. A CT scan with contrast demonstrates the characteristic ring lesion.

D. **Treatment**

1. **Surgery.** The traditional treatment of brain abscess is drainage of the abscess cavity, either by needle aspiration or by total excision.

   a. Presently, the best surgical treatment for abscess is controversial, and there are advocates of aspiration and defenders of total surgical excision. With the advent of CT-guided stereotactic biopsy and intraoperative ultrasound, an abscess in virtually any area of the brain can be aspirated relatively safely. For deep lesions, stereotactic aspiration is the procedure of choice. However, a superficial lesion in a readily accessible area (e.g., the frontal tip) should be considered for complete excision, since this eliminates the risk of recurrence.

   b. For patients at risk from increased ICP, immediate surgery is necessary to reduce mass effect, either by aspiration or complete excision.

2. **Medical therapy**

   a. **Antibiotics.** Preoperatively, the patient is started on appropriate antibiotics (see sec. **III.D.4.d**). The pus from the abscess is gram-stained and cultured for aerobic and anaerobic bacteria and for fungi. The results of these studies guide postoperative antibiotic choice. Antibiotics are continued for at least 4 weeks postoperatively, and the entire course is given parenterally and in "meningeal doses."

   b. **Antiedema therapy.** Patients in immediate danger of herniation are treated with mannitol, 1.0–1.5 g/kg IV over 20–30 minutes. Patients with severe brain edema may be treated with high-dose steroids. Generally, dexamethasone, 16–24 mg/day, is given in four to six divided doses preoperatively and for several days postoperatively. If the patient is stable, the dexamethasone dose is tapered over 1–2 weeks. There is no evidence that steroids lead to spread of the local infection of brain. However, steroids may reduce contrast enhancement on CT scan and lead to the false impression of a reduction in abscess size. There is experimental evidence that steroids interfere with the formation of an abscess wall and diminish antibiotic penetration into the abscess, so routine use is not recommended.

   c. **Anticonvulsants,** such as phenytoin (Dilantin), are used in patients with abscesses involving the cerebral cortex.

3. **Antibiotic therapy alone** is used in selected patients:

   a. In patients with **cerebritis** only.

   b. In patients with **multiple abscesses or surgically inaccessible lesions.**

   c. In patients who are poor surgical candidates and who are not in immediate danger from increased ICP. A CT scan should be performed and the therapy assessed weekly. If no shrinkage is noted by 4 weeks, surgical treatment should be considered. **Abscesses larger than 3 cm are generally refractory to medical therapy alone.**

4. **Initial selection of antibiotics**
   a. The most common sources of brain abscess are the following:
      (1) **Direct spread of infection from a contiguous source**
         (a) Otitis.
         (b) Paranasal sinus infection.
         (c) Meningitis (rare).
         (d) Orbital cellulitis.
      (2) **Hematogenous spread**
         (a) Congenital heart disease with a right-to-left shunt or systemic arteriovenous fistula.
         (b) Pulmonary infection.
         (c) Bacteremia from other extracranial infections or from dental or other procedures.
      (3) **Traumatic**
         (a) Penetrating head trauma.
         (b) Intracranial surgery.
   b. Any possible source of infection is cultured, and a Gram's stain is done. As with meningitis, one cannot assume that the abscess is infected with the same organism that is obtained from the presumed source of infection. Moreover, many brain abscesses contain **multiple organisms,** particularly **anaerobes.** As a result, **the organism** or organisms recovered from a brain abscess **cannot be predicted from the clinical situation** with the degree of confidence that is possible with meningitis.
   c. It is not known whether the ability of an antibiotic to penetrate into the CSF is as important in the therapy of brain abscess as it is in the therapy of meningitis. One might expect, however, that in the cerebritis stage there are organisms in areas of the brain with a relatively intact blood-brain barrier; therefore, drugs that penetrate the blood-brain barrier are preferred.
   d. **Recommended empiric therapy**
      (1) **Sinusitis and congenital heart disease.** Penicillin G, 16–24 million units/day IV divided into six doses, **or** ampicillin, 12 g/day IV divided into six doses; **and** metronidazole, 30 mg/kg/day divided into four doses.
      (2) **Otitis media, mastoiditis, and lung abscess.** Penicillin or ampicillin, as in sec. **III.D.4.d(1)** and ceftriaxone, 4–6 g/day IV divided into two doses, **and** metronidazole.
      (3) **Posttraumatic and postsurgical.** Oxacillin (or nafcillin), 10–12 g/day IV, divided into six doses, **and** ceftriaxone.
      (4) **Unknown source.** Same as in sec. **III.D.4.d.(2).** If there is evidence of *Pseudomonas* infection, an anti-*Pseudomonas* penicillin (e.g., carbenicillin or ticarcillin) and ceftazidime can be used.

IV. **Subdural empyema**
   A. **Diagnosis.** In adults, subdural empyemas occur most commonly in association with ear or sinus infection. They occur less commonly after head trauma or intracranial surgery and, rarely, in association with meningitis or bacteremia. Fever and peripheral leukocytosis may **not** be present initially. Clinical deterioration can be extremely rapid, with progression from mild hemiparesis to coma and death within hours. **Surgical treatment should not be delayed because a patient appears "clinically stable."** In children, subdural empyema occurs most frequently as a complication of meningitis.
   1. **MRI** is the preferred method of detecting subdural fluid collections.
   2. **CT scan** may miss small collections of fluid adjacent to the skull, but it is otherwise reliable.
   3. In infants, the diagnosis can be made by **transillumination** of the skull and **subdural tap.**
   4. **LP** is potentially hazardous and is **contraindicated** when a subdural empyema is suspected.

B. Treatment

1. **Surgery. Immediate** surgical drainage is indicated, followed by a course of high-dose antibiotics determined by the results of the Gram's stains and culture performed at surgery.

2. **Antibiotics.** The patient receives one preoperative dose of antibiotic. The appropriate regimen is chosen according to the clinical situation and guided by the same principles as in treatment of brain abscess (see sec. **III.D.4.d**).

3. The customary **duration** of postoperative antibiotics is 3 weeks. Presence of focus of infection such as osteomyelitis dictates a longer course.

4. **Increased ICP** may be treated, as in brain abscess, using mannitol initially and if more than a few hours of therapy are necessary, steroids.

V. Spinal epidural abscess

A. Diagnosis

1. **Clinical presentation.** The presence of a spinal epidural abscess is suggested by the onset of severe back pain and local tenderness, followed within a few days by radiculopathy and later by myelopathy. In acute cases, the patient is febrile and has an elevated WBC count and erythrocyte sedimentation rate. In chronic cases, however, the patient may lack systemic signs of sepsis. It is crucial to make the diagnosis in the early stages, before spinal cord compression occurs.

2. **Bacteriology.** The most common infecting organisms are *S. aureus*, enteric gram-negative rods, and aerobic streptococci. Anaerobic organisms are infrequent causes of spinal epidural abscess.

3. **Diagnostic tests**

   a. **MRI**, if available on an emergency basis, is excellent in localizing epidural abscess.

   b. **Myelography** can also localize the abscess and, if coupled with CT scanning, is extremely sensitive for areas of osteomyelitis. Moreover, myelography provides an opportunity to obtain a CSF sample.

   c. **A CSF sample** can be helpful in providing evidence for a coexistent bacterial meningitis. Moreover, the infecting organism may be cultured from CSF in many cases. If a CSF sample is to be obtained, **care should be taken** to avoid the involved area so as **not to pass the spinal needle through the abscess** and induce meningitis. If necessary, CSF can be obtained by lateral cervical or cisternal puncture.

   d. **Cultures.** As in other CSF infections, blood, urine, and any clinically apparent focus of infection are cultured prior to institution of antimicrobial therapy. The most common associated infection is vertebral osteomyelitis.

B. Treatment

1. **Surgery.** The infection is drained as soon after diagnosis as possible. **Either acute or chronic epidural abscesses can lead to paralysis within hours.** Acute abscesses contain semiliquid pus that can be drained easily. Chronic abscesses are composed of granulation tissue, which can be removed surgically. In either case, appropriate cultures and stains for aerobic and anaerobic bacteria as well as fungi should be performed at the time of surgery.

2. **Antibiotics.** A single dose of antibiotic may be given preoperatively. The postoperative antibiotic therapy is determined by the results of the stains and cultures done at the time of surgery. Initially, **oxacillin,** 2 g IV (40 mg/kg in pediatric patients), or **vancomycin** (in penicillin-allergic patients), 1 g IV (20 mg/kg in children), should be given. If a gram-negative infection is suspected, **gentamicin,** 1 mg/kg IV or IM, or **ceftriaxone,** 2 g IV, is given as well. The antibiotics are continued for 3–4 weeks unless there is evidence of vertebral osteomyelitis, in which case a 6- to 8-week course is indicated.

3. **Steroids.** Although there are no good data supporting the use of steroids in spinal epidural abscess, high-dose steroids may be used in an attempt to minimize spinal cord edema. Dexamethasone, 10 mg IV, can be given preoperatively, followed by 4–6 mg IV, IM, or PO q6h postoperatively. This dose is continued for 7–10 days, followed by a 10- to 14-day steroid taper.

VI. Neurosyphilis

A. Diagnosis. The incidence of syphilis increased dramatically in the 1980s and continues to rise. The chief goal of detection and treatment of early syphilis is to prevent disability from tertiary disease, including CNS complications. Neurologic symptoms rarely appear earlier than the secondary stage. However, treponemes reach the CNS early in infection, and CSF is consistent with an aseptic meningitis in up to one-third of asymptomatic patients. It is crucial to identify and treat patients in the primary and early secondary stages, therefore major damage can occur.

1. In **primary syphilitic chancres,** in **secondary skin lesions,** and, very rarely, in CSF or fluid from the anterior chamber of the eye, treponemes can be identified by **dark-field examination.** This provides hard evidence of active infection.

2. *Treponema pallidum* cannot be cultured routinely, and if the dark-field examination does not yield a diagnosis, one must rely on serologic tests. When the clinical presentation suggests neurosyphilis, both a nontreponemal serologic test for syphilis (STS) and a serum fluorescent treponemal antibody absorption test (FTA-ABS) should be performed.

   a. **Serologic tests for syphilis** (STS, **nontreponemal** tests). The Venereal Disease Research Laboratory (VDRL), Hinton, rapid plasma reagin, Kolmer's, and Kahn tests all depend on detecting, in the patient's serum or CSF, antibodies to lipoidal substances in the treponemal cell wall or resulting from the treponeme-host interaction.

      (1) These tests are inexpensive and can be used in mass screening programs.

      (2) These tests are less sensitive than the treponemal tests in detecting early evidence of infection, but after they become positive, they are the earliest of the serologic tests to revert to negative after treatment. Thus the effectiveness of therapy or the possibility of reinfection can be evaluated, based on the antibody titers obtained.

      (3) In late neurosyphilis, the serum STS may be negative in as many as one-third of cases. **A negative serum STS does not rule out neurosyphilis.** The CSF STS may be positive despite a negative peripheral blood serology, but **even a negative CSF STS does not absolutely rule out the diagnosis of neurosyphilis in an appropriate clinical setting.** In fact, an initially negative CSF STS may become positive during treatment.

      (4) Biologic false-positive STS tests are common and are associated with old age, pregnancy, and rheumatic and inflammatory disease (e.g., systemic lupus erythematosus and bacterial endocarditis). A positive STS should be confirmed by a more specific treponemal test.

   b. **Treponemal tests**

      (1) The **FTA-ABS** depends on the presence of antibodies that are specific for *T. pallidum.*

         (a) It is the most sensitive serologic test routinely available, being the first one to turn positive after infection and the last to revert to negative after therapy. The FTA-ABS may remain positive indefinitely, even with adequate therapy, so it cannot be used to judge the adequacy of therapy or possible reinfection.

         (b) The FTA-ABS is much more expensive than the STS. It should be performed only when specifically indicated (e.g., in the evaluation of possible tertiary syphilis) and not as a routine screening procedure.

         (c) A positive FTA-ABS rules out a biologic false-positive STS.

         (d) Of patients with late neurosyphilis, 5–10% have a negative FTA-ABS, so even this test may not completely rule out neurosyphilis.

         (e) The clinical significance of a positive CSF FTA-ABS is not known. Therefore, a **CSF FTA-ABS is not useful for diagnostic purposes.**

B. **Asymptomatic neurosyphilis** is defined as an abnormal spinal fluid in the absence of neurologic disease but in the presence of serologic evidence of syphilis. It can occur as early as the primary stage, but progression to symptomatic neurosyphilis is preventable with adequate therapy.

   1. **Diagnosis**

      a. An LP is performed in all patients with inadequately treated syphilis beyond 1 year's duration, even in the absence of neurologic signs and symptoms. Moreover, all patients previously treated for primary or secondary syphilis should undergo LP if they are possible treatment failures, as suggested by persistently high or rising STS titer.

b. The fluid is analyzed for cells, protein, and STS. The diagnosis of neurosyphilis is confirmed by a positive CSF STS, but **the cell count is the best indicator of disease activity.** The significance of a positive CSF STS in the setting of normal CSF profile is unclear.

c. In HIV-infected patients with a positive serum STS, an LP should be performed, even if treatment for primary or secondary syphilis has been documented. Conventional therapy may not be adequate to treat early syphilis in such patients, and the index of suspicion for neurosyphilis must be high. However, nonspecific CSF abnormalities are common at all stages of HIV disease and complicate interpretation.

2. Treatment

a. Penicillin is the drug of choice and is effective in preventing progression to symptomatic disease in immunocompetent patients. There are several possible regimens, but **only high-dose aqueous penicillin G achieves treponemicidal drug levels in CSF:**

(1) **Aqueous penicillin G,** 4 million units IV q4h for 14 days, **or**

(2) **Procaine penicillin G,** 2.4 million units/day IM, **plus probenecid,** 500 mg PO qid for 14 days, **or**

(3) **Benzathine penicillin G,** 2.4 million units IM weekly for three doses.

b. Alternative therapy for penicillin-allergic patients has not been well studied. The following are the usual recommendations:

(1) **Tetracycline,** 500 mg PO qid for 30 days, **or**

(2) **Erythromycin,** 500 mg PO qid for 30 days.

3. Follow-up examination

a. The patient is seen and the CSF examined approximately every 3–6 months for the first year, and the serum STS is checked. In 12–24 months, the STS should revert to negative or achieve a low stable titer. A normal CSF profile 1 year after treatment indicates cure.

b. Indications for retreatment

(1) Failure of the CSF **cell count** to revert to normal within 6 months; protein level should be falling but may not be normal at 6 months.

(2) Some clinicians consider a rising **CSF STS** titer or one that has not decreased by more than one dilution by the end of the first year as an indication for retreatment.

C. Symptomatic neurosyphilis

1. Diagnosis

a. When *T. pallidum* invades the CNS, several **types** of disease may result:

(1) **Meningeal and vascular**

(a) Cerebromeningeal: diffuse or focal (gumma).

(b) Cerebrovascular.

(c) Spinal meningeal and vascular.

(2) **Parenchymatous**

(a) Tabes dorsalis.

(b) General paresis.

(c) Optic atrophy.

b. The diagnosis must often be based on clinical grounds because in late neurosyphilis both the peripheral and CSF STS, less commonly the FTA-ABS, may be negative. The **CSF must be abnormal,** with increased WBCs and elevated protein, to make the diagnosis of meningovascular syphilis or general paresis. Rarely, *T. pallidum* can be visualized in the CSF by dark-field examination. The CSF is occasionally normal in tabes dorsalis, particularly in long-standing disease.

2. Antibiotic therapy

a. Adequate therapy for late neurosyphilis is unknown, and clinical progression can occur despite massive doses of antibiotics. It is possible that some of the manifestations of late neurosyphilis are caused by autoimmune mechanisms rather than by direct infection.

b. **The preferred treatment for neurosyphilis is high-dose parenteral penicillin.**
   (1) **Aqueous penicillin G,** 12–24 million units/day IV, divided into six doses for 14 days, **or**
   (2) **Procaine penicillin G,** 2.4 million units IM daily, **plus probenecid,** 500 mg PO qid for 14 days.
   (3) Either program should be followed by weekly injections of **benzathine penicillin G,** 2.4 million units IM, for 3 weeks.
c. **In patients allergic to penicillin,** alternatives are not well studied, and optimal doses and duration of therapy are not known. Rational programs include
   (1) **Tetracycline,** 500 mg PO qid for 30 days, **or**
   (2) **Erythromycin,** 500 mg PO qid for 30 days, **or**
   (3) **Chloramphenicol,** 1 g IV q6h for 6 weeks, with bone marrow function followed carefully and the dosage adjusted accordingly (see sec. **I.C.2.a**), **or**
   (4) **Ceftriaxone,** 2 g IV or IM daily, for 14 days.
3. **Steroids** have no proven effect in the treatment of late neurosyphilis. Prednisone, 40 mg daily, or its equivalent may decrease the CSF cell count, but there is no evidence that it affects the outcome of therapy or the long-term disability. Steroids are clearly indicated for syphilitic uveitis and syphilitic involvement of the inner ear with a hearing deficit and labyrinthine dysfunction. In these diseases, it is customary to administer prednisone, 80 mg every other day.
4. **Follow-up**
   a. The CSF should be examined weekly during treatment to document a falling WBC count. Most clinicians continue treatment beyond the usual duration if the CSF cell count is not falling. After treatment, the patient is seen every 3–6 months for the first year. At each visit, the serum STS is checked, and an LP is performed at least every 6 months. If the patient is stable after 1 year, with a normal CSF cell count and a falling or fixed low value of the CSF protein, yearly return visits are sufficient, with a final LP 2 years after treatment.
   b. As in asymptomatic neurosyphilis, if the therapy is effective, the CSF cell count is normal within 6 months after treatment. The CSF protein may be elevated for a longer time and may never return to normal, but it should plateau at a fixed low level.
   c. The STS may be positive for the life of the patient in both the serum and the CSF. In either case, the **CSF STS titer is of limited help in following the patient, the CSF cell count and clinical course being the essential data on which therapy is based.**
5. **Complications of neurosyphilis**
   a. **Communicating hydrocephalus** due to blockage of CSF flow at the base of the brain may follow neurosyphilis. Hydrocephalus should always enter into the differential diagnosis when "general paresis" progresses despite antibiotic therapy. The treatment is ventricular shunting.
   b. **Lightning pains** complicating tabes dorsalis have a poor prognosis. Phenytoin and carbamazepine may be tried, but they are often of no benefit.
   c. **Charcot's joints.**
   d. **Perforating ulcers.**
   e. **Parenchymal or meningeal gummas.**
   f. Spinal pachymeningitis.
D. **Congenital neurosyphilis**
   1. The **diagnosis** of congenital syphilis is often difficult to make, since the neonate's serum STS and FTA-ABS and even the CSF STS may be positive because of passively transferred maternal antibody in the absence of infection in the child. Long-bone x rays to detect metaphysitis and other bony lesions may aid in diagnosis.
      a. The **newborn's IgM FTA-ABS** can be tested, and the total IgM in the cord blood can be measured to aid in the diagnosis. However, if the mother acquired syphilis late in pregnancy, serology may be negative in both mother and infant.

   b. An **LP** is performed in all infants at risk of congenital syphilis. Cells in the CSF without another cause must be considered diagnostic of congenital neurosyphilis in the appropriate setting. However, up to about 1 month of age, CSF in the healthy newborn may contain a mildly elevated WBC count (30–40 cells) and protein (up to 150 mg/dl).

   c. **Treatment.** Some experienced clinicians recommend that congenital secondary syphilis be treated with a regimen effective for neurosyphilis. **Aqueous penicillin G,** 250,000 units/kg/day IV for at least 10 days, will achieve treponemicidal drug levels in CSF.

E. Jarisch-Herxheimer reaction

   1. The Jarisch-Herxheimer reaction is a febrile response that is believed to be caused by a release of large amounts of treponemal products into the circulation within the first 24 hours of therapy. It is characterized by fever, chills, myalgia, headache, tachycardia, tachypnea, elevated WBC count, and decreased blood pressure. During the reaction, the rash of secondary syphilis, if present, may worsen. It is a frequent occurrence on initiation of antisyphilitic therapy, usually beginning about 2 hours after the first dose of antibiotics, peaking at about 7 hours, and resolving in 24 hours.

   2. The standard therapy is hydration and antipyretics. It is important that the Jarisch-Herxheimer reaction not be confused with an allergic reaction to penicillin. Some physicians administer a dose of steroids with the initiation of therapy for secondary or tertiary syphilis in an attempt to prevent this reaction.

VII. Other spirochetal infections

A. Lyme disease is caused by *B. burgdorferi,* a spirochete that is transmitted by ixodid ticks, including the deer tick. Disease is endemic along the Atlantic coast of the United States and in some parts of the West and Midwest. The disease is also common in Western Europe. The prevalence of infected ticks appears to be increasing; this, along with increased recognition of the signs and symptoms, has made Lyme disease the most commonly reported tick-borne disease in the United States.

   1. **Description**

      a. **Stage 1.** The illness begins with a flulike syndrome, in some cases associated with an expanding ringlike skin rash with central clearing (**erythema chronicum migrans**). The tick itself is pinhead size, so the tick bite may not be apparent on clinical examination.

      b. **Stage 2.** After several weeks or months, a fluctuating **meningoradiculitis** may occur, with headache, stiff neck, and cranial nerve or spinal root involvement. In the United States facial nerve palsy, often bilateral, is the most common focal sign, but in Europe a polyradiculopathy involving spinal roots is more common. Cardiac involvement may also occur at this stage.

      c. **Stage 3** is usually associated with arthritis, involving predominantly large joints. However, CNS complications can occur months to years after initial infection, including seizures, encephalopathy, dementia, ataxia, and a demyelinating syndrome that may mimic multiple sclerosis.

   2. **Diagnosis**

      a. With neurologic involvement in stages 2 and 3, **CSF** examination usually reveals a lymphocytic pleocytosis with elevated protein.

      b. **Serum** IgG antibody titers to *B. burgdorferi* are generally high with active nervous system disease. The CSF serology is usually positive in stage 2 disease, but, like syphilis, it may be negative in tertiary Lyme disease.

      c. Because of cross-reacting antigens, patients with Lyme disease may have a false-positive syphilis serology. Conversely, false-positive Lyme serologies may be found in syphilis, leptospirosis, and relapsing fever.

   3. **Treatment**

      a. **Early disease and in patients with isolated seventh cranial nerve palsy and normal CSF**

         (1) **Tetracycline,** 500 mg PO qid, **doxycycline,** 100 mg PO bid, **or minocycline,** 100 mg PO bid, for 21–30 days.

         (2) **Amoxicillin,** 500 mg PO tid (20 mg/kg/day divided into three doses in

children), **plus probenecid,** 500 mg PO tid, is used for pregnant or lactating women, children under 8 years old, and patients allergic to tetracyclines, for 21–30 days.

(3) **Erythromycin,** 250 mg PO qid (30 mg/kg/day PO divided into four doses for children), is an alternative for penicillin-allergic patients, for 21–30 days.

b. **Patients with abnormal CSF, polyradiculopathy, or parenchymal CNS disease** are treated with high-dose parenteral penicillin.

(1) **Penicillin G,** 20–24 million units/day IV in six divided doses for 2–3 weeks, is standard.

(2) The alternative is **Ceftriaxone,** 2 g IV daily (75–100 mg/kg/day in children) for 14 days, **or cefotaxime,** 2 g IV q8h for 14 days.

(3) **Chloramphenicol,** 250 mg IV q6h for 14 days, has been used successfully in penicillin-allergic patients.

c. Patients may experience a **Jarisch-Herxheimer reaction** at the initiation of therapy. This can be treated as in syphilis (see sec. **VI.E**).

B. **Brucellosis** is caused by several *Brucella* species, which are small, gram-negative coccobacilli. Disease occurs in meat packers and those exposed to unpasteurized milk or cheese.

1. **Description**

a. **Early disease** is usually self-limited and resembles a flulike illness, but it may be associated with an acute lymphocytic meningitis.

b. **Late disease** may produce a chronic meningoencephalitis. Radiculopathies, myelitis, or encephalomyelitis may dominate the clinical picture.

2. **Diagnosis**

a. The CSF demonstrates a lymphocytic pleocytosis with elevated protein. The glucose may be low or normal. The CSF pressure may also be elevated.

b. *Brucella* can be cultured from blood or CSF in a significant proportion of patients.

c. The diagnosis is generally made by serology. Peripheral agglutination titers in active infections are usually greater than 1 : 160. Positive CSF agglutination titers are confirmatory of neurologic involvement.

3. **Treatment**

a. **Rifampin** is administered in combination with either a **third-generation cephalosporin, trimethoprim-sulfamethoxazole, or doxycycline.** Prolonged therapy, for 6 weeks up to 1 year, is required. The duration depends on the clinical response and repeat CSF examinations.

b. For acutely ill patients, parenteral therapy in doses used for the treatment of acute meningitis may be required. For chronic therapy, oral trimethoprim-sulfamethoxazole or doxycycline is obviously preferred over a parenteral cephalosporin.

c. The most widely used chronic regimen consists of rifampin, 600 mg PO daily, and trimethoprim-sulfamethoxazole, 160 mg PO qid.

C. **Leptospirosis** is caused by *L. interrogans.* The majority of cases involve a self-limited flulike syndrome, often with conjunctival suffusion and muscle tenderness, that occurs during the initial "leptospiraemic phase" of disease. A minority of infections produce more severe illness (**Weil's disease**), usually affecting the liver or kidney. Neurologic involvement is an uncommon complication of the "immune phase" of disease and can be seen about 2 weeks into the illness. Acute aseptic meningitis, myelitis, encephalitis, and cranial nerve palsies may occur, with spontaneous recovery in weeks to months. Exceptionally, CNS involvement is fatal. Leptospirosis generally occurs from contact with the urine of infected animals, and human disease is most common in farm workers, veterinarians, and pet owners. The disease is relatively common in the tropics, but in the United States it occurs with significant frequency only in southern states and along the west coast.

1. **Diagnosis.** *Leptospira* can be cultured from the CSF during the first 10 days of illness. However, the diagnosis is generally based on the clinical situation and detection of a fourfold rise in **serum agglutination titers** between acute and convalescent serum. A single titer of greater than 1 : 200 supports the diagnosis.

2. Treatment. Antibiotic therapy is administered if the diagnosis is made within the first 5 days of illness. **Antibiotics are not likely to benefit patients who present with immune-phase neurologic involvement.**

   a. Penicillin G, 1 million units IV q6h for 7–10 days, is commonly used.
   b. The **alternative** drug for penicillin-allergic patients has not been defined, but doxycycline, erythromycin, or chloramphenicol is a reasonable alternative

VIII. Fungal infections of the CNS

A. Description. The usual clinical picture is that of chronic meningitis; however, intra-parenchymal fungal infections may occur with symptoms that resemble bacterial brain abscess. Fungal infection of the CNS may occur in immunocompetent hosts, but risk is highest in hosts with compromised immune function due to cancer, lymphoma immunosuppressive therapy, or AIDS. Specific antifungal therapy can be curative even in immunocompromised hosts. The vast majority of cases of fungal meningitis in this country are caused by *Cryptococcus neoformans, Coccidioides immitis,* and *Candida albicans. Aspergillus* species, *Histoplasma capsulatum,* and *Blastomyces* rarely involve the CNS. Phycomycetes (mucormycosis) produce a characteristic rhi-nocerebral syndrome with or without associated meningeal inflammation. *Nocardia* and *Actinomyces,* although not true fungi, can infect the CNS and behave clinically like fungal pathogens. Each of these organisms has its distinctive features, but the basic approach to their therapy is similar (Table 8-4).

B. Amphotericin B

1. Clinical usefulness. Amphotericin B is an effective agent, both in vitro and in vivo, against virtually all known fungi, although resistance to the drug has been reported.

   a. Almost universal **toxicity** from the drug accompanies its use, ranging from fever and rigors to renal failure. **Side effects** of amphotericin B are as follows:

   (1) Dose-related effects
      (a) Short-term systemic effects
         (i) Fever, chills.
         (ii) Nausea, vomiting.
         (iii) Anorexia, malaise, headache.
         (iv) Hypotension.
      (b) Renal toxicity
         (i) Impaired glomerular function; decreased glomerular filtration rate and Cl_{cr}. This may progress to oliguric renal failure.
         (ii) Impaired tubular function; distal renal tubular acidosis; hypokale-mia, which may be severe.
      (c) Anemia secondary to bone marrow suppression.
      (d) Local toxicity
         (i) Intravenous administration: phlebitis.
         (ii) Intrathecal injection: parasthesias, nerve palsies, back pain, para-plegia, chemical meningitis, arachnoiditis, and CSF blocks.
         (iii) Intracisternal injection: hydrocephalus.
         (iv) Intraventricular injection: ventriculitis, encephalopathy, seizures, and death.

   (2) Idiosyncratic effects
      (a) Shock.
      (b) Thrombocytopenia.
      (c) Acute liver failure.
      (d) Seizures.
      (e) Cardiac arrest, ventricular fibrillation.

   b. Clinically, the most important toxic effects are **renal.** About one-half of patients receiving a total of 4 g and 85% of those receiving 5 g of amphotericin B are left with permanent renal insufficiency of clinical significance. Usually, the dosage of amphotericin administered to a given patient is limited by renal toxicity, which often occurs at a dosage of 0.5–0.7 mg/kg/day. Hypokalemia is common and requires close monitoring and potassium replacement as neces-sary. It is recommended that amphotericin B be used according to a strict protocol (see sec. **VIII.K** for guidelines for the use of amphotericin B).

Table 8-4. Antifungal therapy

Organism	Primary therapy	Optional adjunctive therapy	Comments
Cryptococcus	Amphotericin, 0.5 mg/kg/day IV 5-Fluorocytosine (5-FC), 150 mg/kg/day PO	Subarachnoid amphotericin B	Each isolate should be tested for 5-FC sensitivity Not sensitive to 5-FC
Coccidioides	Amphotericin B, 1.5 mg/kg/day IV Amphotericin B, 0.5 mg IT, 2 doses/wk	Intraventricular amphotericin B	
Candida	Amphotericin B, 1.5 mg/kg/day IV	5-FC, 150 mg/kg/day PO Subarachnoid amphotericin B	Each isolate should be tested for 5-FC sensitivity
Aspergillus	Amphotericin B, 1.5 mg/kg/day IV 5-FC may be tried	5-FC, 150 mg/kg/day PO Subarachnoid amphotericin B	Each isolate should be tested for 5-FC sensitivity
Phycomycetes	Amphotericin B, 1.5 mg/kg/day IV	Subarachnoid amphotericin B	Not sensitive to 5-FC
Histoplasma	Amphotericin B, 1.5 mg/kg/day IV	Subarachnoid amphotericin B	Not sensitive to 5-FC
*Blastomyces****	Amphotericin B, 1.5 mg/kg/day IV	Subarachnoid amphotericin B	Not sensitive to 5-FC

* Hydroxystilbamidine, although useful in pulmonary blastomycosis, is not recommended as a first-line drug for CNS blastomycosis.

   c. **Prolonged courses of therapy** at potentially toxic doses are necessary to treat
      fungal meningitis. However, relapse can occur even when the drug is
      continued until the patient is clinically well and the CSF is normal.
   d. **The drug levels** in the CSF associated with intravenous use are extremely
      low, and this probably accounts for the relapse rate. Injection of the drug
      directly into the subarachnoid space has been used, analogous to the use of
      intrathecal or intraventricular aminoglycosides in gram-negative meningitis
      and the problems are similar (see sec. **I.D**).
      (1) Intralumbar injections do not deliver high concentrations of drug to the
          basilar cisterns, the main site of most fungal infections, and virtually no
          drug enters the ventricles. Furthermore, subarachnoid blocks to CSF flow
          are frequent in fungal meningitis, complicating the problem of distribu-
          tion of drug through the subarachnoid space.
      (2) Amphotericin B produces **irritative side effects** when injected into the
          subarachnoid space. Intrathecal injection frequently gives temporary
          paresthesias, but progressive arachnoiditis, subarachnoid blocks, and
          transverse myelitis have occurred as well. A single intraventricular
          injection of 1 mg has produced encephalopathy and death within hours.
          Risks of repeated intraventricular injection include all the potential
          complications of Ommaya reservoirs.
   e. Even when fungal infection is cured, the inflammatory reaction induced by
      the fungus may lead to spinal block, hydrocephalus, and cranial nerve palsies.
      The meninges over the convexities can become severely thickened and cause
      bilateral mass effect with risk of herniation.
2. **Systemic therapy.** Despite its toxicity, amphotericin B remains the first-line
   drug in essentially all fungal infections of the CNS. Its detailed use is described
   in the guidelines for the use of amphotericin B (see sec. **VIII.K**). A low dose is
   given initially and increased incrementally to the maximum tolerated daily dose,
   or to a maximum of 0.7–1.5 mg/kg/day. The usual adult dosage is 50 mg/day.
   During chronic administration, renal function is followed closely, and the dosage
   is decreased if the serum creatinine begins to rise above 3.5 mg/dl. In the absence
   of hard data on the necessary dosage of amphotericin, various modifications of
   this approach have been suggested in an attempt to minimize the toxicity and
   discomfort associated with the daily administration of amphotericin B at high
   doses. These include
   a. **Administration of twice the daily dose on an alternate-day basis.** The
      advantage of this program is that fewer total injections are given, so phlebitis
      is less of a problem, and on the days during which patients do not receive the
      drug, they are free of fever, anorexia, and other debilitating effects of the
      drug. Nephrotoxicity is not reduced.
   b. **Determination of the minimal inhibitory concentration (MIC)** of drug in the
      patient's serum against the fungus isolated, and adjustment of the daily dose
      of amphotericin B to achieve a serum drug level that is twice the MIC. This
      generally results, for *Cryptococcus* species, in a dosage of 0.5–1.0 mg/kg/day.
      There are no data, however, that show serum levels of amphotericin correlate
      with clinical effectiveness.
3. **Intrathecal therapy**
   a. **Indications.** Subarachnoid administration should be considered in the follow-
      ing settings:
      (1) In patients who have failed to respond to systemic therapy or who relapse
          after a full course of systemic therapy.
      (2) In patients who are moribund at the initiation of therapy.
      (3) In severely immunosuppressed patients.
      (4) In patients with **coccidioidal** meningitis.
   b. **Routes of subarachnoid injection**
      (1) Intraventricular. If subarachnoid therapy is used, intraventricular injec-
          tion of amphotericin B by means of an Ommaya reservoir and indwelling
          intraventricular cannula constitutes the most reliable route of therapy.
          This is the preferred method at most institutions.

(2) **Intracisternal** injections of amphotericin B are used routinely at some centers, but this approach is not recommended unless the injections are done by a person very experienced in the technique.

(3) **Intralumbar.** The drug, suspended in a solution heavier than CSF, such as 10% D/W, can be injected into the lumbar space and the patient then placed in the Trendelenburg position for a period of time so that the drug can flow by gravity to the basilar cisterns. However, there is no wide experience with this technique.

c. The patency of CSF pathways from the site of injection to the base of the brain must be demonstrated before initiation of subarachnoid therapy and repeatedly throughout the course of therapy if there is any indication of a block to CSF flow.

C. **Fluorocytosine (5-FC)** is active against *Cryptococcus, Candida, Aspergillus, Torulopsis,* and chlorblastomycosis; however, not all strains of these fungi are sensitive to the drug, and resistance may develop during therapy. Therefore, **5-FC sensitivity must be documented in each case** in which the drug is used. Fluorocytosine has not been demonstrated to be effective when used alone against life-threatening infections. The following uses can be recommended (see dosage guidelines in sec. **VIII.L**):

1. In **cryptococcal disease,** 5-FC and amphotericin B are synergistic in their action, and combination therapy suppresses the appearance of 5-FC–resistant organisms. Consequently, it is reasonable to initiate therapy with the combination of amphotericin B and 5-FC and to use amphotericin B at less than the maximum dose (0.5 mg/kg/day). If the patient is moribund at the initiation of therapy, fails to respond to this regimen, or relapses after the therapy has been completed, amphotericin B can be increased to its maximum tolerated dose, in combination with 5-FC, and the addition of subarachnoid therapy can be considered. **The hematologic toxicity of 5-FC has limited its usefulness in HIV-infected patients.**

2. There is insufficient experience with fungal disease other than cryptococcosis to know whether the combination of 5-FC plus amphotericin B, at a dosage of 0.5 mg/kg/day, is as effective as amphotericin B at a maximum dosage in treating organisms that are sensitive to 5-FC. In severe infections with sensitive organisms and in moribund patients, 5-FC should be added to full-dose amphotericin B, the latter given both systemically and by a subarachnoid route.

3. After the patient has received a course of amphotericin B or amphotericin B plus 5-FC, 5-FC may be given alone to prolong the course of therapy.

4. Fluorocytosine is secreted by the kidneys. When given in combination with amphotericin B, renal dysfunction induced by amphotericin may result in progressively increasing serum levels of 5-FC. It is important, therefore, to monitor **serum levels** of 5-FC and to maintain serum concentrations in the 60–80 μg/ml range.

D. **Ketoconazole** has activity against coccidioidomycosis, histoplasmosis, and *Candida* infection. It is administered orally and penetrates poorly into the CSF, so that therapeutic levels against fungi are not reached at the usual oral dosage of 400–800 mg/day. Higher dosages have produced therapeutic responses in a few patients with **coccidioidal meningitis.** The major toxicity is nausea and hepatocellular dysfunction, which rarely can progress to fatal hepatic necrosis.

E. **Fluconazole**

1. Fluconazole has been used as both initial treatment and maintenance therapy in **cryptococcal meningitis.**

   a. Currently, it is recommended at a dosage of 200–400 mg/day PO as **maintenance or suppressive therapy** in cryptococcal disease in **AIDS** patients.

   b. In patients with **mild disease,** it can be used as initial therapy for cryptococcal meningitis at a dosage of 400 mg/day for 10–12 weeks.

2. In an uncontrolled study of **coccidioidal meningitis,** fluconazole (400 mg/day) was associated with a 70% response rate in previously untreated patients.

3. **Side effects.** Fluconazole is generally well tolerated but is occasionally associated with GI upset and, rarely, with hepatitis or allergic reactions.

F. **Duration of therapy.** The duration of therapy necessary to cure fungal infections of the CNS is unknown. In many patients the infection is probably never cured, in the sense that every organism is not eliminated and viable organisms remain. There are cases of cryptococcal meningitis in which the India ink stain remains positive for months after therapy is stopped, but the patient remains clinically well.

1. If the patient responds clinically to the initial therapy, that regimen should be continued
   a. For at least 6 weeks. Four weeks of therapy may suffice in a carefully selected subset of patients who meet all of the following criteria: meningitis without neurologic signs; no underlying systemic disease or immunosuppressive therapy; pretreatment CSF cell count greater than 20/μl; serum cryptococcal antigen titer less than 1 : 32; and after 4 weeks of therapy, a negative CSF India ink preparation and CSF cryptococcal antigen titer less than 1 : 8.
   b. For 1 month after the last positive CSF culture.
   c. Until there is no evidence of active CNS infection:
      (1) A stable or improving neurologic examination, **or**
      (2) A normal or only mildly elevated, stable CSF cell count.
   d. Until there is no evidence of active systemic infection.
   e. Until drug toxicity precludes further therapy.
2. **The need for prolonging therapy**
   a. Persistently positive CSF cultures or positive India ink preparations in cryptococcal disease require prolonging therapy. A persistently elevated CSF protein is not in itself an indication for prolonging therapy. A lifelong course of antifungal therapy is generally administered to AIDS patients with cryptococcal meningitis (see sec. **XVII**).
   b. In cryptococcal disease, failure of the serum or CSF antigen titer to fall by more than two dilutions during therapy carries a poor prognosis and should lead to prolonged treatment.
   c. Coccidioidal antigens may also be measured in the CSF, but their relation to prognosis has not been as clearly evaluated as it has for cryptococcal antigens.
   d. Oral 5-FC may be given alone after the course of combination therapy or after amphotericin B alone has been completed. Since there are presumably few viable organisms present, 5-FC resistance is less likely to develop.
   e. Some experts recommend the administration of subarachnoid amphotericin B weekly for life in coccidioidomycosis.
   f. The subarachnoid injection of amphotericin B may be continued, either alone or in combination with oral 5-FC, even after systemic amphotericin B has been stopped because of renal toxicity.
G. **Use of steroids**
   1. **Elevated CSF pressure.** In fungal meningitis, as in other infections of the CNS, high-dose steroids are used for the treatment of elevated CSF pressure due to brain swelling or focal infection of brain parenchyma. Hydrocephalus should be ruled out by CT scan or MRI in all such cases.
   2. Hydrocortisone may be injected along with intrathecal amphotericin B in an attempt to minimize local irritative effects (see sec. **VIII.K**).
H. Fungal meningitis is associated with an impressive granulomatous response at the base of the brain and at the lining of the ventricles. This can obstruct CSF flow and cause **hydrocephalus.** If hydrocephalus occurs late, after the CSF is sterile, a ventriculoatrial or ventriculoperitoneal shunt can be placed. If the CSF is still infected, constant ventricular drainage must be used or, if the CSF block is outside the ventricular system and the hydrocephalus is not life-threatening, definitive treatment may be deferred until the CSF can be sterilized.
I. **Intraparenchymal fungal infections of the CNS.** Fungi can invade the parenchyma of the brain and cause abscess or granuloma formation. This process may occur with or without an associated meningitis. *Aspergillus* is the organism that most typically causes focal intraparenchymal disease, but any fungus that infects the CNS may cause intraparenchymal infection, including *Cryptococcus, Candida,* and *Mucor.* The prognosis for intraparenchymal disease is worse than that for meningeal involvement alone. The diagnostic approach and treatment are similar to those for bacterial brain abscess, with surgical excision of accessible lesions. If the etiologic

agent is known or strongly suspected preoperatively, antifungal therapy in the maximum tolerated dosages should be started 48 hours before surgery. Multiple or inaccessible lesions may have to be treated medically, in which case the dosage of amphotericin B is pushed to its maximum, and 5-FC is added if the organism is sensitive. Intraparenchymal lesions caused by *C. neoformans* often can be treated medically and followed with serial CT scans, in a manner similar to the treatment of focal bacterial cerebritis (see sec. **III.D.3**).

J. Actinomycetes and *Nocardia* species are acid-fast organisms with properties that are intermediate between those of bacteria and fungi. When they infect the CNS, it is usually by causing brain abscess, with symptoms of an expanding mass lesion. Spinal cord abscess and meningitis may also occur. Rarely, an intracranial epidural abscess can complicate cranial osteomyelitis. Unlike the fungi, these organisms respond to antibacterial drugs. Single abscesses may require surgical excision. The drugs of choice are as follows:

1. Actinomycetes

a. Penicillin G, 24 million units/day in adults and 200,000 units/kg/day in children in 12 divided doses for at least 8 weeks. The optimum duration of therapy is not known, but some would prolong treatment for 5 months.

b. In penicillin-allergic patients, **erythromycin,** 4 g/day IV in adults, and 50 mg/kg/day IV in children in four divided doses.

2. *Nocardia* species

a. Trimethoprim-sulfamethoxazole, 15–20 mg/kg/day IV (trimethoprim dose, administered as a solution containing trimethoprim and sulfamethoxazole in a ratio of 1 : 5), divided into four doses. The drugs should be dissolved in at least 75 ml of 5% D/W immediately before administration and infused slowly over 1.0–1.5 hours. With renal impairment (Cl_{cr} 15–30 ml/min), halve the dose. The drug should not be used if Cl_{cr} is less than 15 ml/min.

b. Cycloserine, 15 mg/kg/day PO in four divided doses, in combination with sulfamethoxazole for severe disease, moribund patients, multiple intracranial abscess, or failure to respond to sulfamethoxazole alone.

K. Guidelines for the use of amphotericin B

1. Intravenous administration

a. Initial doses. When beginning treatment with amphotericin B, it is prudent to start with a small dose and build up to full therapeutic doses over 5–10 days. The first dose is generally 1 mg. Each succeeding dose is doubled until 16 mg/day is reached, and thereafter the dose is increased in increments of 10 mg until the full therapeutic dose, usually 50 mg/day, is reached. If therapy is interrupted for more than 10 days, the procedure is repeated. In life-threatening fungal infections, the full therapeutic dose must be achieved more rapidly. In that case, a 1-mg test dose is administered. If that dose is tolerated, a dose of 0.2 mg/kg is administered, and succeeding daily doses are increased in 0.2 mg/kg increments.

b. The infusion mixture is administered through a central catheter over 4–6 hours. The rate of infusion may be varied according to the severity of the side effects encountered. Generally, the immediate side effects tend to diminish with repeated doses.

c. Amphotericin B can produce acute hyperkalemia during and immediately following the infusion, so that patients receiving high doses, especially those with renal insufficiency, may require hourly monitoring of serum potassium levels. Chronically, the distal tubular toxicity of amphotericin B can produce both sodium and potassium wasting. Some clinicians replete patients with up to 300 mEq/day of sodium. Serum potassium should be monitored and dietary potassium supplemented as required.

d. Monitoring of drug toxicity. Renal and bone marrow function are closely observed during therapy. The following tests are performed before initiating therapy and at least twice a week while systemic amphotericin B is being administered:

(1) CBC.

(2) Peripheral blood smear, platelet count, or both.

      (3) Reticulocyte count.
      (4) BUN or creatinine.
      (5) Serum electrolytes.
      (6) Bilirubin.
      (7) SGOT.
      (8) Alkaline phosphatase.
      (9) Urinalysis.

    e. The maximum dosage is 1.5 mg/kg/day IV. Typically, adults receive 50 mg/dose. Tolerance of more than 1.0 mg/kg/day is uncommon. Dosage reduction is recommended when plasma creatinine rises over 3.5 mg/dl. Adequate hydration must be maintained to minimize azotemia.

  2. Intrathecal administration

    a. Premedicate the patient with an antiemetic, and perform an LP in the usual manner. With each dose, CSF is removed and the cell count, protein, sugar, and culture are checked to monitor the progress of the therapy. Fungal antigen titers, if available, are checked weekly.

    b. The first dose should be 0.025 mg dissolved in 5 ml of CSF. Hydrocortisone, 5–15 mg, may be added to the injection to reduce side effects. A dose is given every other day and is increased slowly by 0.025-mg increments with each dose until the maximum dose of 0.5 mg is achieved. At that point, the frequency of administration is decreased to twice a week.

L. Guidelines for the use of 5-FC. Fluorocytosine is well absorbed when taken PO, and CSF concentration reaches 80–100% that of serum.

  1. The **dosage** is 75–150 mg/kg/day divided into four doses.

  2. In **renal failure,** the frequency of doses (25–40 mg/kg) must be reduced as follows:

Cl_{cr} (ml/min)	Dosage interval
100	q6h
40–25	q12h
25–12	q24h
12	q48h

  3. The **sensitivity** of the organism being treated must be checked at the initiation of therapy and at least monthly thereafter.

  4. Serum levels should be monitored regularly, especially in the presence of decreased renal function. The therapeutic concentration is 50–100 µg/ml.

  5. Toxicity

    a. Gastrointestinal upset, with anorexia, nausea, vomiting, and diarrhea, is the most frequent untoward effect.

    b. Hepatic. Elevation of SGOT and alkaline phosphatase may occur, possibly in association with hepatic necrosis. Liver function should, therefore, be checked weekly during therapy.

    c. Hematologic. Anemia, leukopenia, or thrombocytopenia may occur. These reactions are dose-dependent and occur primarily in azotemic patients. Because of the renal toxicity of amphotericin B, the combination of 5-FC and amphotericin B is especially likely to lead to bone marrow dysfunction. Fluorocytosine may be especially myelosuppressive in AIDS patients. Blood counts are checked at least twice weekly in all patients during therapy with 5-FC.

IX. Viral meningitis

  A. Description. Viruses often infect the subarachnoid space and leptomeninges, with little or no parenchymal involvement of the CNS. The clinical syndrome is that of an acute febrile illness, with headache, meningismus, and often vomiting. The neurologic signs are sparse. There may be lethargy, irritability, mild drowsiness, isolated transient cranial nerve dysfunction, or minor reflex changes. Seizures, aside from febrile convulsions, or any severe and persistent neurologic deficits imply an encephalitic component to the illness. There may be associated findings of systemic viral infection, and these may help to identify the etiologic agent.

    The total duration of the illness is 10–14 days, and the course is benign, without significant sequelae in over 90% of cases. About 10% of patients require prolonged convalescence, and rarely there are permanent residual deficits, usually spasticity or intellectual impairment. Death from aseptic meningitis is exceedingly rare. A careful history may reveal evidence of concurrent viral illness in family members or other contacts of the patient.

B. **Etiology.** The most common single agent is **mumps,** especially where mumps vaccine use is limited, but the enteroviruses, primarily **coxsackievirus** and **echovirus,** constitute the most common viral group that infects the meninges. **Lymphocytic choriomeningitis** (LCM), **herpesviruses,** and **arthropod-borne viruses** are less frequently identified. **Human immunodeficiency virus (HIV)** can cause both acute and chronic aseptic meningitis but far more commonly causes asymptomatic CSF abnormalities. A similar clinical picture can be produced by certain nonviral agents. Leptospirosis is an unusual cause of the syndrome in the United States, and mycoplasmosis is a rare cause. All other agents account for less than 1% of cases of aseptic meningitis in the United States.

C. **Diagnosis.** The most important clinical problem in aseptic meningitis is to verify that the CSF is indeed aseptic (i.e., no bacterial, mycobacterial, or fungal agent is causing the infection). Leptospires and mycoplasmas, although bacteria, are included in the causes of aseptic meningitis, since they do not grow on the usual culture media, and they cause a benign neurologic disease that is indistinguishable from viral illness. The **CSF profile** is lymphocytic, with normal glucose, but very early in the course the CSF may have a polymorphonuclear predominance. A repeat LP 8–24 hours after the first will show a shift to lymphocytic predominance in these cases. Identification of the specific infecting organism is useful in confirming the diagnosis and for epidemiologic purposes, but it has no therapeutic importance.

D. Treatment consists of supportive measures. There is no known specific therapy.

E. **Complications**
   1. **Hydrocephalus.** There are reported cases of hydrocephalus following mumps meningitis. Mumps, and possibly other viruses, can cause an ependymitis throughout the ventricular system. The resultant scarring can lead to aqueductal stenosis as a late complication, and ventriculoatrial or ventriculoperitoneal shunting is required.
   2. **Residual neurologic deficits** occur rarely.

X. **Viral encephalitis**
A. **Description.** Viral encephalitis is usually an acute febrile illness. It is often associated with headache, meningismus, and behavioral change or depressed mental status. Examination of the CSF usually reveals a lymphocytic pleocytosis and elevated protein, but indices may be normal early on. Infection of cortical neurons may cause seizures or focal deficits. Coma may occur. The disease is more prolonged than aseptic meningitis, lasting 2 weeks to several months. There is significant mortality during the acute illness (about 10% for all cases of clinically recognized viral encephalitis), and there is a high incidence of permanent and disabling sequelae.

B. **Etiology.** The most frequent etiologic agents identified in this disease are **mumps, herpes simplex virus 1 (HSV-1),** and **arboviruses.** Enteroviruses are unusual causes of encephalitis, as are varicella and Epstein-Barr viruses and mycoplasma. Rabies encephalitis is rare in the United States. The prognosis depends on the etiologic agent.
   1. **Herpes simplex** is the most common cause of sporadic, focal encephalitis in the United States. Mortality is 10–40%, with a corresponding high incidence of serious residual deficits. Most infections are due to **HSV-1** and characteristically produce destructive lesions of the **inferior frontal and anterior temporal** lobes. Hence dementia, personality disorders, memory loss, and aphasia are frequent sequelae of infection. Culture of the CSF usually does not yield virus. A CT scan or MRI showing inflammation and edema in the characteristic areas or an EEG with periodic sharp wave activity temporally on a background of focal or diffuse slowing should prompt empiric treatment with intravenous acyclovir. Brain biopsy remains the gold standard of diagnosis. **Successful therapy depends on a high index of suspicion leading to early diagnosis.**
   2. The **arboviruses** have a variable prognosis.

    a. Eastern equine encephalitis is the most severe, with a 70–90% incidence of death or disabling sequelae.

    b. The morality from **western equine encephalitis** and **St. Louis encephalitis** is 2–20%. The disease is usually benign, although it may be severe in younger children and the elderly.

    c. California encephalitis (including the La Crosse virus) and **Venezuelan equine encephalitis** generally cause benign infections; death and disability are unusual.

  3. Encephalitis caused by mumps or LCM virus is benign except in rare instances.

  4. Neonatal viral encephalitis may occur and has a poor prognosis. Neonatal encephalitis due to **herpes simplex virus 2 (HSV-2)** is usually a fulminant, generalized, and rapidly fatal disease. Unlike in adult HSV-1 encephalitis, the yield of CSF viral culture in neonatal HSV-2 encephalitis is high.

C. Treatment

  1. Edema. In viral encephalitis, the CSF pressure may be very high, and focal areas of infection with edema, vascular engorgement, or hemorrhage may act as a mass lesion. Herniation can occur. Osmotic agents may be used in acute situations, and high-dose steroids may be used over the longer run (see sec. **I.H**). There is experimental evidence that steroids can potentiate the spread of herpes in nervous tissue, so steroids should not be used in viral encephalitis without definite indications. In addition, since much of the edema is cytotoxic, steroids may be of limited benefit.

  2. Seizures resulting from viral encephalitis may be extremely difficult to control, but their treatment is identical to that of seizures of other etiologies (see Chap. 6).

  3. Specific antiviral therapy

    a. Herpes simplex encephalitis. Acyclovir, 10.0–12.5 mg/kg IV q8h, is administered immediately on making the diagnosis of herpes simplex encephalitis. The patient should be adequately hydrated, and each dose should be slowly infused over 60 minutes to prevent the drug from precipitating in the renal tubules. The optimum duration of therapy is unknown, but 10–14 days is common.

      (1) Pharmacokinetics. Acyclovir is excreted by the kidney and has a half-life of about 3 hours with normal renal function. The dosage must be reduced in renal insufficiency. Concentrations in CSF reach about 50% of plasma levels.

      (2) Toxicity. Acyclovir is generally well-tolerated, but local irritation, nausea, and headache can occur with IV infusion. About 1% of patients receiving intravenous acyclovir develop encephalopathy, which can be difficult to distinguish from the underlying encephalitis. Abnormal bone marrow and hepatic function have been reported in immunocompromised patients.

      (3) Because the diagnosis of herpes simplex encephalitis is often unclear on clinical grounds, the precise indications for the use of acyclovir are undefined. The lack of toxicity of acyclovir has led to its use in many clinical circumstances where the diagnosis of herpes simplex encephalitis is entertained, but where definite proof from viral culture or brain biopsy is lacking.

      (4) Acyclovir is less toxic and more effective than vidarabine (ara-A) for the therapy of herpes encephalitis.

    b. Cytomegalovirus (CMV) infections. Cytomegalovirus can cause ventriculitis, encephalitis, myelitis, polyradiculopathy, and retinitis in immunocompromised hosts. It is a common pathogen in transplant recipients and AIDS patients.

      (1) Ganciclovir (DHPG) has broad-spectrum antiviral activity against herpesviruses but has achieved widest clinical use in CMV infections. It has demonstrated efficacy in CMV retinitis and is used, although without documented effect, in CMV encephalitis and myelitis. Improvement of CMV polyradiculitis has been demonstrated in a few cases.

        (a) Dosage. Ganciclovir, 5.0 mg/kg IV q12h, is infused over 1 hour. The dosage must be adjusted in renal insufficiency. The total duration of therapy is generally 14–30 days, depending on the clinical response. In AIDS patients, maintenance therapy at a dosage of 5 mg/kg daily or 6 mg/kg/day, 5 days/week, may have to be administered for life to prevent relapse.

- (b) **Pharmacokinetics.** Ganciclovir is excreted by the kidney and has a plasma half-life of 3–4 hours. CSF levels reach 38% those in the plasma.
- (c) **Toxicity.** The toxicity is dose-related and is directed primarily at rapidly dividing cells. Inhibition of spermatogenesis, bone marrow suppression, and GI reactions are common. Encephalopathy is uncommon.

(2) **Foscarnet** has a spectrum of antiviral activity similar to that of ganciclovir. It is effective in CMV retinitis and can be used as a second-line agent in patients with gancyclovir-resistant CMV causing nervous system disease.

- (a) **Dosage** is 60 mg/kg IV q8h for 14 days, infused over 1 hour by **infusion pump only.** In AIDS patients, maintenance therapy, 90–120 mg/kg/day IV, is recommended, administered as a 2-hour pump infusion.
- (b) **Pharmacokinetics.** Foscarnet is excreted by the kidney and has a plasma half-life of 3.3 hours. Levels in CSF reach 40% of those in plasma.
- (c) **Toxicity.** Renal toxicity is dose-limiting in up to 23% of patients. Derangements of calcium, potassium, phosphate, and magnesium levels can occur. The dosage must be adjusted in renal failure. **Acute overdose can cause seizures or cardiac arrhythmias and is potentially fatal.**

XI. **Rabies** is transmitted to humans by animal bites and causes severe brainstem encephalitis with high mortality. The usual incubation period in humans is 30–60 days for bites on the extremities, but incubation periods as long as 6 months have been reported. Bites on the face and neck can have an incubation period as short as 2 weeks. The clinical disease usually begins with personality change and a period of excitement. Then focal neurologic signs, especially those referable to the brainstem, develop. The characteristic hydrophobia is caused by dysphagia and hyperirritability of the respiratory tract and pharynx. Death results from respiratory failure or cardiac arrhythmia; the latter is associated with myocarditis in some cases. In rare cases, the clinical syndrome may begin with ascending paralysis of the Guillain-Barré type. The disease is nearly 100% fatal during the acute stage, but with intensive respiratory support and nursing care, complete recovery has been reported. **Rabies vaccine and antiserum should be administered to anyone with an animal bite sustained in an unprovoked attack.** Foxes, bats, and skunks are the major animal reservoirs in the United States.

XII. **Poliomyelitis.** A special form of viral infection of the CNS is caused by enteroviruses that target the anterior horn cells of the spinal cord. The clinical picture is one of an acute febrile illness with lower motor neuron paralysis. Fortunately, immunization has made infection with poliovirus rare. Cases continue to be reported sporadically, either secondary to poliovirus in nonimmunized individuals or, rarely, secondary to other enteroviruses. The treatment is purely supportive.

XIII. **"Slow viruses" and progressive multifocal leukoencephalopathy**

- A. **Jakob-Creutzfeldt disease** and **kuru** are transmissible diseases, but the agent, a small "proteinaceous infectious particle" **(prion)** has not been completely characterized. Kuru, once endemic in part of Papua New Guinea, was spread mainly by ingestion of infected human brain tissue and is now rare. Jakob-Creutzfeldt disease has a worldwide distribution and is a subacutely progressive **dementing illness,** usually beginning in middle age and progressing relentlessly to coma and death. **Ataxia** and **myoclonus** are striking features clinically. The CSF is normal, but the EEG is distinctive and characterized by periodic sharp wave complexes. There is no known specific therapy (see Chap. 3).
- B. **Subacute sclerosing panencephalitis** is a syndrome that occurs in childhood, is almost always the result of measles infection, but is rarely caused by rubella. The

first symptoms are personality change and intellectual deterioration, followed b the development of myoclonic seizures, ataxia, and visual impairment. There ai reports of spontaneous remissions, but only after permanent damage has occurred the brain. Usually, the disease progresses to death in a matter of months or a fe years. The **CSF** may contain a few lymphocytes, but, most important, it contains **highly elevated gamma globulin** with elevated titers of **anti-measles antibodie** Oral isoprinosine and intraventricular interferon-α have been used in a sma series, with neurologic improvement in a few patients.

  C. **Progressive multifocal leukoencephalopathy (PML)** is caused by the papovavir JC or, rarely, SV-40. The disease usually begins with focal neurologic signs ar symptoms and progresses within a few months to global impairment and death. Th virus causes demyelination of white matter in the brain (leukoencephalopathy with a marked absence of inflammatory response or edema. Although JC virus ubiquitous, and anti-JC antibodies are found in the majority of individuals, activ disease is seen only in patients with disorders of cellular immunity. Most cases ai seen among **AIDS** patients, but transplant recipients and patients with lymphom are also at risk. There is no proven effective therapy, and PML rarely stabilize spontaneously. Intrathecal cytosine arabinoside has been associated with improve ment in a few patients.

XIV. **Toxoplasmosis**

  A. **Description.** *Toxoplasma gondii* is an intracellular parasite that infects humar and animals. Infection is usually asymptomatic, but it can cause several varieties disease. It is the **most common opportunistic CNS pathogen in AIDS** (see sec. XVI

    1. **Congenital toxoplasmosis** classically causes a syndrome of choreoretiniti retardation, and intracranial calcifications, often associated with microcephal; hepatosplenomegaly, jaundice, and rash. Any of the components of the syndrom may be missing in a given patient.

    2. **Acquired toxoplasmosis** usually occurs in a host with defective cellular immu nity and may produce encephalitis, meningitis, or, most commonly, an intrace rebral mass lesion. Spinal cord abscess and myositis have been reportec Definitive diagnosis requires identification of the organisms in a tissue biops;

  B. **Diagnosis.** Serologic tests for toxoplasmosis are generally not helpful in th diagnosis of acute infections, since at least 40% of the population has IgG antibodie directed against *Toxoplasma*. In immunocompetent individuals, a fourfold rise i titers is indicative of active infection. In AIDS, where CNS toxoplasmosis i common, such a rise is rarely seen. However, the measurement of a baselin anti-*Toxoplasma* IgG titer at the time of diagnosis of AIDS may aid the diagnosis active toxoplasmosis in the appropriate clinical setting. It should be emphasize that anti-*Toxoplasma* titers can be nondetectable in up to 20% of AIDS patients wit cerebral toxoplasmosis; therefore **negative titers do not rule out toxoplasmosis a** the etiology of brain lesions in AIDS. When brain biopsy is necessary to establis the diagnosis, MRI is more sensitive than CT scanning in disclosing surgicall accessible lesions. *Toxoplasma* brain abscesses are characteristically multiple an ring-enhancing with contrast; however, single, nonenhancing, and diffusely enhanc ing lesions are also seen. **A trial of 10 days to 2 weeks of anti-*Toxoplasma* therap is reasonable in an AIDS patient with brain lesions consistent with toxoplasmosi** If lesions do not regress radiographically, brain biopsy should be considered.

  C. **Treatment.** Prompt treatment of the **acquired** disease often results in a cure. Th **congenital** disease is treated only in an attempt to prevent progression of th disease; the CNS damage that is present at birth is irreversible. There is a high spontaneous remission rate of acquired toxoplasmosis in immunocompetent indi viduals, but active CNS disease is an indication for treatment. AIDS patients shoul have lifelong maintenance therapy to prevent relapse. The recommended therapy i as follows:

    1. **Sulfadiazine,** 100 mg/kg/day (maximum 8 g/day), in combination with **py rimethamine,** 1 mg/kg/day, up to 100 mg/day. A 100- to 200-mg loading dose c pyrimethamine should be given. Trimethoprim, a folate antagonist similar t pyrimethamine, cannot be used in place of pyrimethamine because it has n activity against toxoplasmosis.

2. **Folinic acid** (Leucovorin), 10 mg/day, may be given to counteract the hematologic toxicity of pyrimethamine.
3. **Toxicity** from sulfadiazine and pyrimethamine is common. Problems leading to discontinuation of therapy include hypersensitivity reactions and bone marrow suppression. Patients with AIDS who are taking azidothymidine (AZT) may require a reduction in AZT dosage to prevent synergistic bone marrow toxicity.
4. **The optimum duration** of therapy is unknown. Radiographic reevaluation is performed after 10 days to 2 weeks of therapy to document regression of lesions. Patients with AIDS are usually treated for life. **Maintenance therapy** with pyrimethamine, 25–50 mg/day, folinic acid, 5 mg/day, and sulfadiazine, 1–2 gm/day, is standard; pyrimethamine, folinic acid, and clindamycin, 600 mg/day can also be used. The role of prophylaxis in AIDS patients with positive *Toxoplasma* serology has not been defined.
5. **Alternative regimens.** Pyrimethamine alone or in combination with clindamycin, 1200–2400 mg/day in four divided doses, is used in sulfa-allergic patients.

XV. **Amebic meningoencephalitis.** *Naegleria,* a genus of free-living amebas commonly present in warm freshwater, can cause an acute meningoencephalitis with purulent CSF and hemorrhagic brain lesions. They can be identified as mobile, large organisms on a wet preparation of fresh CSF. There is no known generally effective therapy. All forms of antibiotic therapy, including metronidazole (Flagyl), sulfamethoxazole and trimethoprim, amphotericin, and assorted antibacterial agents, have been tried.

XVI. **Herpes zoster (shingles)** is caused by reactivation of latent varicella-zoster virus chronically resident in dorsal root and cranial nerve ganglia. Fifty percent of cases involve thoracic dermatomes, with pain and paresthesias preceding the vesicular eruption. When the seventh cranial nerve is involved, there is a lower motor neuron facial palsy, and the vesicles appear in the external auditory canal or the tympanic membrane (Ramsay Hunt syndrome).

A. Patients with symptomatic herpes zoster, especially young patients, have an **increased incidence of immunodeficiency states,** particularly HIV infection and lymphoma. Such conditions should be sought by physical examination and appropriate blood testing.
B. **Steroids** should be avoided in the acute period and, if possible, should be decreased or discontinued if their use preceded the infection.
C. **Treatment of pain** may be difficult both acutely and chronically (post-herpetic neuralgia). Carbamazepine, imipramine, or local application of capsaicin cream may be of value in a minority of patients. The treatment of chronic pain is discussed in Chap. 9.
D. **Acyclovir,** 5 mg/kg IV q8h for 7 days, hastens the healing of cutaneous lesions and decreases the duration of acute pain. However, the incidence and severity of post-herpetic neuralgia are unaffected by antiviral therapy. Immunocompromised patients should be treated with acyclovir in an effort to prevent dissemination of the infection.
E. **Nonimmune contacts** of patients with cutaneous lesions of herpes zoster are at risk for primary infection with the virus (chickenpox).

XVII. **Acquired immunodeficiency syndrome (AIDS)** is a multisystem infection by the human immunodeficiency virus type 1 (HIV-1). Neurologic disease affects one-half to two-thirds of patients and can occur at any stage of the infection, but is more common in the setting of late-stage AIDS. A variety of mechanisms have been implicated in **primary** neurologic complications of HIV disease, including direct infection by the HIV virus, autoimmune disease, and neurotoxic effects of both viral products and the immune response to the virus. **Secondary** complications are due to opportunistic infections and neoplasms, as well as neurotoxic side effects of therapy.

A. **Primary HIV infection of the nervous system.** HIV is a neurotrophic as well as lymphotrophic member of the lentivirus subfamily of retroviruses, all of which target the nervous system of the host. HIV has been isolated from the CSF and brain of AIDS patients with various neurologic syndromes, and the synthesis of HIV-specific immunoglobins within the blood-brain barrier has been demonstrated. HIV has also been isolated from the CSF of asymptomatic seropositive patients, including those with normal CSF. HIV enters the nervous system early, causing **latent**

infection in brain macrophages; the virus is found only rarely in neurons or other parenchymal cells.

1. **Acute infection.** Although the initial CNS infection is usually asymptomatic neurologic disease may be the first manifestation of HIV and may occur at the time of seroconversion when immunologic indices are normal.

   a. An acute, reversible **encephalopathy** may occur. Confusion, memory loss, and disorder of mood are seen.

   b. **Acute aseptic meningitis,** with headache, stiff neck, photophobia, and arthralgias, may occasionally be accompanied by a maculopapular rash.

   c. Isolated **cranial neuropathies,** particularly Bell's palsy, and **acute ascending or transverse myelitis** have also been reported.

2. **Chronic infection**

   a. **HIV-associated cognitive-motor complex, or AIDS dementia complex,** occurs in at least 30% of AIDS patients, almost exclusively in the setting of severe immunosuppression. There is a progressive "subcortical" dementia, sometimes associated with loss of balance or leg weakness. Early on, the symptoms may be mistaken for depression, since difficulties with **concentration and memory, apathy,** and **psychomotor retardation** are common presentations. A **treatable affective disorder must be carefully ruled out.** Mania, organic psychosis, and, rarely, catatonia may occur. Seizures can occur, attributable only to HIV infection, but this must be a diagnosis of exclusion after appropriate clinical and radiologic evaluation. Grasp reflexes and other frontal release signs, tremor, cogwheel rigidity, long tract signs (e.g., extensor plantar responses), clumsy fine motor movements, and myoclonus are common. A CT scan usually reveals diffuse cortical atrophy and enlarged ventricles, and MRI may show multifocal or diffuse increase in white matter signal on T2-weighted images. On pathologic examination, white-matter pallor is the most common finding. Multinucleated giant cells—syncytia or infected macrophages—are pathognomonic for HIV encephalitis.

   b. Recurrent or chronic **meningeal irritation** may be associated with cranial neuropathies, particularly of the fifth, seventh, and eighth cranial nerves.

   c. **HIV-associated myelopathy** (vacuolar myelopathy) clinically resembles the combined systems degeneration of vitamin B_{12} deficiency. There is a **painless spastic paraparesis** and dorsal column sensory loss (loss of proprioception and vibration sense), sometimes associated with incontinence, that progresses over weeks to months. Coexistent HIV-associated dementia is common. **Vitamin B_{12}** deficiency, neurosyphilis, human T-cell lymphotropic virus type 1 myelopathy, and spinal cord tumor should be ruled out.

   d. **Peripheral neuropathies** (Table 8-5) are common, multifactorial in etiology and poorly understood. Some probably represent immune-mediated injury others (particularly progressive lumbosacral polyradiculopathy) can represent secondary infection. Toxic neuropathies are common with antiretroviral agents such as didanosine and zalcitabine and with chemotherapeutic agents used to treat Kaposi's sarcoma.

   e. **Lumbrosacral polyradiculopathy,** while occasionally a self-limited complication of HIV disease, often represents a treatable, potentially lethal complication of opportunistic infection with **CMV.**

      (1) **Description.** Patients present with a subacute onset of leg weakness with or without back and radicular pain. Bowel and bladder involvement often follows early on. Deep tendon reflexes in the lower extremities are depressed or absent, and there may be perianal anesthesia.

      (2) **Diagnosis.** Electromyography and nerve conduction studies can aid in diagnosis. Unlike many other AIDS-associated diseases, CSF examination can be relatively specific: a high WBC count (>500 WBCs/µl) with polymorphonuclear predominance is often, but not always, seen. Protein is usually elevated, and glucose can be normal or low. CSF should be sent for CMV culture, but **therapy should be begun empirically prior to culture results,** since improvement is usually seen only when therapy is initiated early. CMV culture is positive only in about one-half to two-thirds of cases

Table 8-5. Peripheral neuropathies associated with HIV infection

Neuropathy	Motor weakness	Sensory complaints	Urinary retention	EMG/NCV* picture	Treatment
Distal symmetric	+	+++	–	Small-fiber axonopathy	?AZT
Sensory ataxic neuropathy	–	+++	–	Large-fiber ganglioneuronitis	Unknown
Guillain-Barré	+++	+	–	Demyelinating; + axonal if severe	Plasmapheresis
Chronic inflammatory demyelinating polyneuropathy	+++	+	–	Demyelinating + axonal	Plasmapheresis ?Gamma globulin
Mononeuritis multiplex	++	++	–	Multifocal axonopathy	Plasmapheresis
Progressive polyradiculoneuropathy (cauda equina syndrome)	+++	++ (especially sacrogenital)	+	Axonal +/– demyelinating	?Ganciclovir

* EMG = electromyogram; NCV = nerve conduction velocity.

(3) The **differential diagnosis** includes lymphomatous meningitis and neuro-syphilis; therefore CSF evaluation should include a high volume (10–20 ml) sample for cytology and a CSF VDRL. In addition, **a mass in the cauda equina or conus medullaris must be ruled out radiographically.** A careful evaluation for CMV retinitis or other organ involvement should be undertaken; however, CMV polyradiculopathy can be seen in the absence of other CMV disease, as well as presenting during therapy or CMV disease in other organs.

(4) **Treatment** is with ganciclovir or foscarnet; in some patients, combined chemotherapy may be warranted (see sec. **X.C.3.b**). Resistant organisms have been reported.

3. **The CSF in HIV infection**
   a. Seropositive patients, even in the absence of neurologic disease, often have a mild to moderate CSF mononuclear pleocytosis, elevated protein, and mildly decreased glucose concentration (but >35 mg/dl).
   b. There is no association between the degree of pleocytosis and the ability to culture HIV from the CSF or between positive CSF HIV culture and neurologic complications.
   c. Despite the common, nonspecific CSF abnormalities seen in HIV infection, **patients who have neurologic signs and symptoms, CD4 (helper T cell) counts below 200, and the triad of CSF pleocytosis, elevated protein, and low CSF glucose are likely to have a treatable opportunistic infection.**
   d. The presence of viral p24 antigen in CSF may correlate with progressive dementia.

4. **Anti-HIV chemotherapy**
   a. **Azidothymidine (zidovudine)** specifically inhibits retroviral reverse transcriptase and has activity against HIV-1.
      (1) The **indications** for AZT are undefined but include patients who have the diagnosis of AIDS or AIDS-related complex (ARC). Whether all HIV-infected patients should receive the drug is controversial, as is the optimum time for initiation of therapy. The drug is of clear benefit in the **AIDS encephalopathy in children.** Clinical trials have demonstrated some benefit in cognitive function in **adults,** but follow-up has been limited to 16 weeks.
      (2) The **dosage** is 200 mg 6 times/day PO or 1.5 mg/kg q4–8 h IV. The dosage may require adjustment if bone marrow depression occurs. Lower doses may be equally effective for long-term use with less bone marrow suppression.
      (3) **Pharmacokinetics.** The drug is metabolized in the liver, and the glucuronidated metabolite is excreted by the kidneys. The serum half-life is about 1 hour, and penetration into the CSF is excellent.
      (4) **Toxicity.** Bone marrow suppression is common. It is generally dose-related and reversible. The myelotoxicity is potentiated by vitamin B_{12} or folate deficiency or by concurrent therapy with other cytotoxic drugs. Headache and mild behavioral abnormalities may also occur. Myopathy is an uncommon but serious complication and often improves on discontinuation or lower-dose therapy.
      (5) **Drug interactions.** Probenecid, cimetidine, lorazepam, and indomethacin interfere with the clearance of AZT and may potentiate its toxicity.
   b. **Didanosine (ddI) and zalcitabine (ddC)** also inhibit retroviral reverse transcriptase and have activity against HIV-1.
      (1) **Indications.** Neither ddI nor ddC is as effective as AZT in delaying disease progression and prolonging survival in AIDS patients with no prior treatment. However, in patients previously treated with AZT (for 2 months or longer), ddI is associated with slower disease progression when compared with AZT. Didanosine is often used as **monotherapy** in the treatment of patients **after prior treatment with AZT.** The effectiveness of combined chemotherapy of ddI or ddC with AZT is under investigation. Didanosine is comparable to AZT in improving neurologic func-

tion in children. Neurologic end points have not been well studied in adults.

(2) Dosage

   (a) Didanosine: patients over 75 kg, 300 mg bid; 50–75 kg, 200 mg bid; 35–49 kg, 125 mg bid.

   (b) Zalcitabine: 0.75 mg tid.

(3) Toxicity. Both drugs can cause pancreatitis (which may be fulminant with ddI); painful peripheral neuropathy, especially with higher dosages and after prolonged therapy, is fairly common with both drugs and usually resolves 2–6 weeks after discontinuation.

B. Opportunistic infections of the CNS. Patients with AIDS are at increased risk of CNS infection with toxoplasmosis, cryptococcosis, tuberculosis, progressive multi-focal leukoencephalopathy, CMV, and herpes zoster. Whether HIV increases the risk of neurosyphilis remains controversial. Patients with AIDS do not have a greatly increased risk of acute bacterial meningitis or bacterial brain abscess.

   1. The treatment for these infections in HIV-infected individuals is the same as for other patients, except that **prolonged courses of therapy** may be required. After the acute course of therapy for cryptococcal meningitis, tuberculous meningitis, or CNS toxoplasmosis is complete, most clinicians continue therapy with appropriate antibiotics at a reduced dosage (generally on a once or twice per week schedule).

   2. *T. gondii* is the most common opportunistic pathogen affecting the CNS in AIDS. It may present as a focal mass lesion or a meningoencephalitis. Seizures are common. The CSF is not helpful in diagnosis, and LP may be contraindicated (see sec. **I.A.1.d**). Definitive diagnosis requires biopsy of accessible lesions. However, therapy is often administered empirically, based on CT scan or MRI findings (see sec. **XIV**).

   3. Cryptococcal meningitis is the second most frequent opportunistic infection of the CNS in AIDS. It typically presents as a subacute meningitis. Cell count, protein, and glucose in the CSF can be normal in up to 20% of cases, but CSF cryptococcal antigen is detected in 90–95%. **India ink** preparation is an **inadequate screen** for cryptococcal meningitis. The therapy is discussed in sec. **VIII.**

   4. Central nervous system infection with *C. albicans* and *C. immitis,* as well as more common fungi, occurs with increased frequency in AIDS.

   5. It is common practice to treat all immunocompromised patients, including those with AIDS, with a 10-day course of acyclovir for cutaneous **varicella-zoster** eruptions (shingles).

   6. There is no available effective therapy for progressive multifocal leukoenceph-alopathy. Experimental therapies include intrathecal or intravenous cytosine arabinoside and interferon alfa.

   7. Herpesviruses. The treatments of infections with herpes simplex virus (see sec. **IX**), CMV (see sec. **IX**), and varicella-zoster virus (see sec. **XVI**) have been discussed. Although the optimum duration of therapy for these infections has not been established in AIDS, it is customary to administer more prolonged courses of antiviral therapy than are used in immunocompetent hosts.

C. Focal brain lesions. Patients who are HIV-positive frequently present with the subacute onset of diffuse or focal neurologic signs or with seizures. When CT scan discloses one or more low-intensity, ring-enhancing lesions in the brain, the differential diagnosis is broad and includes toxoplasmosis, lymphoma, tuberculoma, fungal abscess, stroke, and bacterial abscess or metastatic cancer given the appropriate clinical setting. Kaposi's sarcoma and bacillary angiomatosis rarely involve the brain. More than one pathologic process may be involved, and radio-graphic presentations of these diseases (e.g., contrast patterns and edema) can vary. Nonenhancing white-matter lesions with no associated edema or mass effect are suggestive of either PML or HIV encephalitis. However, **pathologic diagnoses cannot be made radiographically.** Because it is not realistic to perform brain biopsies of all such lesions, an empiric approach must be developed.

   1. An MRI is more sensitive than CT scanning in detecting brain lesions in AIDS.

2. One reasonable approach is based on the distinction between single and multiple lesions.

a. **Multiple contrast-enhancing lesions,** or lesions with mixed enhancement patterns, are treated empirically with anti-*Toxoplasma* therapy (see sec. **XIV**). Patients who deteriorate during therapy or who fail to respond both clinically and radiographically are considered for brain biopsy.

b. Accessible **solitary lesions** are biopsied unless highly suggestive of toxoplasmosis (e.g., a cortical or deep-gray ring-enhancing lesion). Up to one-quarter of toxoplasmic abscesses present as single lesions on CT.

3. Some clinicians recommend treating all AIDS patients with focal brain lesions, regardless of number or pattern of enhancement, with therapy for toxoplasmosis, providing *Toxoplasma* serology is positive. Patients with negative serology and those who fail to respond to therapy are biopsied. However, negative serology does not exclude the diagnosis of toxoplasmosis; up to 20% of patients with pathologically proven toxoplasmic abscesses have nondetectable serum anti-*Toxoplasma* antibodies.

4. The bone marrow suppressive effects of therapy for toxoplasmosis may require a reduction of AZT dose.

D. **Neoplasms.** Patients with HIV infection are at increased risk for **primary CNS lymphoma, lymphomatous meningitis,** and, rarely, involvement of the brain with Kaposi's sarcoma. The management of CNS lymphoma is discussed in Chap. 11.

XVIII. **Cysticercosis** is the most common parasitic CNS disease. Infestation of the CNS with larvae of the pork tapeworm *Taenia solium* is acquired by ingesting food contaminated by tapeworm eggs.

A. **Description.** The infection may be asymptomatic or may cause one of several neurologic syndromes: **epilepsy, hydrocephalus, stroke, chronic basilar meningitis, dementia, encephalitis,** and acute **chemical meningitis.** Spinal cord or retinal involvement is rare. Focal progressive neurologic deficits associated with intraparenchymal cysts may occur. The parasite is endemic to Mexico, Central and South America, Eastern Europe, China, and Southeast Asia. Patients with cerebral cysticercosis do not necessarily have signs of intestinal infection with tapeworm; that is, their stools may not contain ova or parasites, and peripheral blood eosinophilia is uncommon.

B. The **diagnosis** is suggested by the epidemiology and by a CT scan showing either punctate calcifications or fluid-filled parenchymal cysts. Contrast enhancement occurs in active lesions—that is, when larvae die and evoke inflammation and edema. Intraventricular cysts, which can cause life-threatening **hydrocephalus,** usually are not seen on CT; MRI is more sensitive in this setting. The diagnosis may be strengthened by a positive immunoblot for anticysticercus antibodies in serum or CSF and confirmed by brain biopsy, if necessary. **Patients and family members should have stool examinations for evidence of tapeworm and treatment where appropriate, since reinfection can occur.**

C. **Treatment**

1. **Praziquantel,** 50 mg/kg/day PO in three divided doses for 14 days, will kill surviving larvae in patients with active infestation. Praziquantel may cause headache, dizziness, and GI upset. Hypersensitivity reactions are rare.

2. **Albendazole,** 15 mg/kg/day in three divided doses for 21 days has compared favorably in treatment of parenchymal and subarachnoid neurocysticerosis. It is possible that shorter courses of albendazole are equally effective.

3. Patients with active neurocysticercosis who respond to chemotherapy develop an acute inflammatory reaction to the dying organisms. This reaction may produce headache, seizures, increased ICP, or focal neurologic deficits. Most are self-limited and can be managed with analgesia and anticonvulsants as necessary. More severe reactions will respond to **corticosteroids** (e.g., dexamethasone, 8 mg IV or PO q8h), but there is evidence that corticosteroids decrease the plasma level of praziquantel and may increase albendazole levels. Steroids are not used routinely but should be used in the setting of increased ICP, intraventricular cysts, or high intraparenchymal cyst burden. Steroids may also be of use in the acute, encephalitic form of neurocysticercosis and in chemical meningitis.

4. There is no indication for chemotherapy of **inactive neurocysticercosis,** as the larvae are dead. Edema or enhancement of the cyst on CT scan or MRI is taken as evidence of active disease.
5. There are only limited indications for **surgical excision** of cysts: when the diagnosis in in doubt, rapidly enlarging fourth ventricle cysts, or incipient herniation. Even with obstructive hydrocephalus due to intraventricular cysts, ventricular shunting without excision of the cysts is usually effective.

Selected Readings

BACTERIAL MENINGITIS

Durand, M. L., et al. Acute bacterial meningitis in adults. *N. Engl. J. Med.* 328:21, 1993.

Fong, I. W., and Tomkins, K. B. Review of *Pseudomonas aeruginosa* meningitis with special emphasis on treatment with ceftazidime. *Rev. Infect. Dis.* 7:604, 1985.

Lentnek, A. L., and Williams, R. R. Aztreonam in the treatment of gram-negative bacterial meningitis. *Rev. Infect. Dis.* 1:S586, 1991.

Pfister, H. W., Feiden, W. and Einhaupl, K. M. Spectrum of complications during bacterial meningitis in adults: Results of a prospective clinical trial. *Arch. Neurol.* 50:575, 1993.

Schaad, U. B., et al. Dexamethasone therapy for bacterial meningitis in children. *Lancet* 342:457, 1993.

Schwartz, M. N., and Dodge, P. R. Bacterial meningitis: A review of selected aspects. *N. Engl. J. Med.* 272:725, 1965.

Tunkel, A. R., Wispelwey, B., and Scheld, W. M. Bacterial meningitis: Recent advances in pathophysiology and treatment. *Ann. Intern. Med.* 112:610, 1990.

TUBERCULOUS MENINGITIS

American Thoracic Society and the Centers for Disease Control. Treatment of tuberculosis and tuberculosis infection in adults and children. *Am. Rev. Respir. Dis.* 134:355, 1986; 136:482, 1987.

BRAIN ABSCESS

Kaplan, K. Brain abscess. *Med. Clin. North Am.* 69:345, 1985.

Mampalam, T. J., and Rosenblum, M. L. Trends in the management of bacterial brain abscesses: A review of 102 cases over 17 years. *Neurosurgery* 23:451, 1988.

SPINAL EPIDURAL ABSCESS

Danner, R. L., and Hartman, B. J. Update of spinal epidural abscess: 35 cases and review of the literature. *Rev. Infect. Dis.* 9:265, 1987.

NEUROSYPHILIS AND OTHER SPIROCHETAL DISEASES

Al Deeb, S., et al. Neurobrucellosis: Clinical characteristics, diagnosis, and outcome. *Neurology* 39:498, 1989.

Dans, P. E., et al. Inappropriate use of the cerebrospinal fluid Venereal Disease Research Laboratory (VDRL) test to exclude neurosyphilis. *Ann. Intern. Med.* 104:86, 1986.

Dorfman, D. H., and Glaser, J. H. Congenital syphilis presenting in infants after the newborn period. *N. Engl. J. Med.* 323:1299, 1990.

Gourevitch, M. N., et al. Effects of HIV infection on the serologic manifestations and response to treatment of syphilis in intravenous drug users. *Ann. Intern. Med.* 118:350, 1993.

Hook, E. W., and Marra, C. M. Acquired syphilis in adults. *N. Engl. J. Med.* 326:1060, 1992.

Luft, B. J., et al. A perspective on the treatment of Lyme borreliosis. *Rev. Infect. Dis.* 11:S1518, 1989.

Steere, A. C. Lyme disease. *N. Engl. J. Med.* 321:586, 1989.

FUNGAL INFECTIONS

Dismukes, W. E., et al. Treatment of cryptococcal meningitis with combination amphotericin B and flucytosine for four as compared with six weeks. *N. Engl. J. Med.* 317:334, 1987.

Drugs for treatment of deep fungal infections. *Med. Lett. Drugs Ther.* 30:30, 1988.

Galgian, J. N., et al. Fluconazole therapy for coccidioidal meningitis. *Ann. Intern. Med.* 119:28, 1993.

Perfect, J. R. Cryptococcosis. *Infect. Dis. Clin. North Am.* 3:77, 1989.

Schwartz, M. N. Chronic meningitis: Many causes to consider. *N. Engl. J. Med.* 317:957, 1987.

VIRAL INFECTIONS

Collaborative DHPG Treatment Study Group. Treatment of serious cytomegalovirus infections with 9-(1,3-dihydroxy-2-propoxymethyl) guanine in patients with AIDS and other immunodeficiencies. *N. Engl. J. Med.* 314:801, 1986.

Corey, L., and Spear, P. G. Infections with herpes simplex viruses. *N. Engl. J. Med.* 314:686, 1986.

Whitley, R. J. Viral encephalitis. *N. Engl. J. Med.* 323:242, 1990.

Yalaz, K., et al. Intraventricular interferon and oral isoprinosine in the therapy of subacute sclerosing panencephalitis. *Neurology* 42:488, 1992.

ACQUIRED IMMUNODEFICIENCY SYNDROME (AIDS)

Dismukes, W. E. Cryptococcal meningitis in patients with AIDS. *J. Infect. Dis.* 157:624, 1988.

Hollander, H., McGuire, D., and Burack, J. H. Diagnostic lumbar puncture in HIV-infected patients: Analysis of 138 cases. *Am. J. Med.* 96:223, 1994.

McGuire, D., and So, Y. T. Neurologic Dysfunction in HIV: Intracranial Disorders. In P. T. Cohen, M. Sande, and P. Volberding (eds.), *AIDS Knowledge Base.* Boston: Little, Brown, 1994.

Porter, S. B., and Sande, M. Toxoplasmosis of the central nervous system in the acquired immunodeficiency syndrome. *N. Engl. J. Med.* 327:1643, 1992.

Price, R. W., et al. The brain in AIDS: Central nervous system HIV-I infection and AIDS dementia complex. *Science* 239:586, 1988.

Yarchoan, R., et al. Clinical pharmacology of 3'-azido-2', 3'-dideoxythymidine (zidovudine) and related dideoxynucleosides. *N. Engl. J. Med.* 321:726, 1989.

CYSTICERCOSIS

Alarcon, F., et al. Neurocysticercosis: Short course of treatment with albendazole. *Arch. Neurol.* 46:1231, 1989.

Del Brutto, O. H., and Sotelo, J. Neurocysticercosis: An update. *Rev. Infect. Dis.* 10:1075, 1988.

Takayanagui, O. M., and Jardim, E. Therapy for neurocysticercosis: Comparison between albendazole and praziquantel. *Arch. Neurol.* 49:290, 1992.

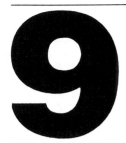

Neuropsychiatric Disorders

George B. Murray

I. Depression. The most common serious psychiatric disorder found in general medical practice is depression. It is primarily a disorder of affect, but it can influence the cognitive sphere as well. The causes of depression are unknown, although there are theories ranging on a spectrum from purely psychosocial stress events to a purely biochemical transmitter dysfunction.

A. Classification. Many attempts have been made to classify depression, but not everyone agrees to such classifications. The two most prevalent classifications are reactive versus endogenous depression and primary versus secondary depression.

    1. Reactive depression is thought to result primarily from psychosocial stress, as for example a grief reaction, whereas **endogenous depression** is thought to be more a result of specific biologic dysfunction.

    2. Primary depression is that usually seen by a psychiatrist or general practitioner in which there is no other medical or surgical illness involved. The primary depression may take on the somatic cloak of fatigue, GI symptoms, or other more generalized medical illness. **Secondary depression** follows some other medical or surgical illness, but this does not necessarily imply that the medical or surgical illness caused the depression.

B. Diagnosis

    1. Major depression. Since 1980 with the publication of the *Diagnostic and Statistical Manual,* 3rd edition (DSM-III), there has been more or less solid agreement on the criteria for making the diagnosis of major depression. Those criteria are outlined in Table 9-1.

        a. A handy mnemonic for these criteria is: SIG E CAPS. This is to signify a prescription for depression of "energy capsules." The initials stand for a disorder of one of the criterion symptoms.

        S—*sleep* disorder
        I—lack of *interest*
        G—*guilty* feelings
        E—loss of *energy*
        C—lack of *concentration* or thinking disorder
        A—loss of *appetite* or weight loss
        P—*psychomotor* retardation or agitation
        S—*suicidal* reflection or thoughts of death

        Thus, if the physician finds that the patient has been in a depressed mood, has a loss of interest or has been anhedonic for at least 2 weeks, and has a minimum of five of these symptoms, then a major depression is probably the diagnosis. Notice that the diagnosis is a clinical decision and not made by various paper and pencil tests.

        b. Laboratory studies are sometimes helpful but are not used often in general clinical practice.

            (1) The **dexamethasone suppression test (DST)** was touted as a method for diagnosing endogenous depression. It has been largely abandoned by clinicians interested in depression. It is now used most often in academic studies on depression. The result of the DST is considered abnormal if

Table 9-1. Major depression criteria

At least five of the following symptoms have been present during the same 2-week period and represent a change from previous functioning; at least one of the symptoms is either (1) depressed mood or (2) loss of interest or pleasure:

(1) Depressed mood most of the day, nearly every day, as indicated either by subjective account or observation by others

(2) Markedly diminished interest or pleasure in all, or almost all, activities most of the day, nearly every day

(3) Significant weight loss or weight gain when not dieting, or decrease or increase in appetite nearly every day

(4) Insomnia or hypersomnia nearly every day

(5) Psychomotor agitation or retardation nearly every day

(6) Fatigue or loss of energy nearly every day

(7) Feelings of worthlessness or excessive or inappropriate guilt nearly every day

(8) Diminished ability to think or concentrate, or indecisiveness, nearly every day

(9) Recurrent thoughts of death, recurrent suicidal ideation without a specific plan, or a suicide attempt or a specific plan for committing suicide

Source: Adapted from *Diagnostic and Statistical Manual of Mental Disorders* (4th ed.) (DSM-IV). Washington, D.C.: American Psychiatric Association, 1994.

cortisol levels are higher than 5 μg/dl in blood samples drawn 8, 12, and 16 hours after a single midnight dose of 1 mg of dexamethasone.

(2) The **thyroid-releasing hormone (TRH) test** has also been used in testing patients thought to be clinically depressed. About one-half of depressed patients fail to show a rise above 7 μU/ml of thyroid-stimulating hormone after administration of TRH.

(3) **Blood levels of antidepressants** are not drawn regularly as, for example, are blood levels in the use of anticonvulsants. However, there are levels that correspond approximately to therapeutic doses. They are generally used when one does not see a therapeutic benefit with a specific antidepressant. In this setting, a blood level is apt to show a subtherapeutic, antidepressant level possibly because of noncompliance, poor absorption, poor bioavailability, or rapid metabolism. Table 9-2 gives the approximate

Table 9-2. Approximate antidepressant plasma levels

Antidepressant	Therapeutic level (ng/ml)
Amitriptyline	AMI + NOR > 90–200
Amoxapine	AMO + 8-OH > 100–300
Bupropion	> 50 and < 100
Desipramine	40–160
Doxepin	DOX + DMD > 100
Imipramine	IMI + DMI > 180–225
Maprotiline	200–300
Nortriptyline	> 50 and < 150
Protriptyline	160–240

Key: AMI = amitriptyline; NOR = nortriptyline; AMO = amoxapine; 8-OH = hydroxyamoxapine; DOX = doxepin; DMD = desmethyldoxepin; IMI = imipramine; DMI = desipramine.

therapeutic levels of known antidepressants. Therapeutic blood levels for the newer antidepressants, as fluoxetine, bupropion, paroxetine and sertraline, are not agreed upon as yet.

   c. Approximately 90% of patients with major depressive disorders show some form of **sleep alteration.** Endogenous and nonendogenous forms of major depressive disorder show characteristic sleep EEG patterns. Patients with endogenous depression can be distinguished from those with nonendogenous depression on the basis of short rapid eye movement (REM) sleep latencies, that is, sleep to REM latencies of less than 62 minutes.

2. So-called **masked depression** is often difficult to diagnose. Some patients present with several somatic manifestations, but usually one is the cardinal complaint, such as fatigue, weakness, anorexia, insomnia, headache, dizziness, constipation, abdominal pain, or chronic pain. Usually these patients must be evaluated for their specific somatic complaint before depression can be absolutely diagnosed. However, the ultimate proof of masked depression consists of extinction of the somatic complaint with antidepressant treatment. Often, clinically ill patients will have a major depression that increases the pain or complaint of the somatic illness. On treating the depression in this setting, one often notes improvement in the patient's suffering due to the somatic illness.

3. Minor depression is listed in DSM-IV, but only as a depressive disorder not otherwise specified. It still remains strongly rooted in the research diagnostic criteria of Feighner. The criteria for diagnosis are similar to those of major depression except for the requirement of depressed mood or anhedonia for the same 2-week period and only two of the symptoms represented in SIG E CAPS (see sec. **I.B.1.a**).

4. Dysthymia (formerly known as depressive neurosis) consists of a chronic disturbance of mood involving depressed mood for most of the day, more days than not, for at least 2 years. In addition, during these periods of depressed mood there must be at least two of the following associated symptoms:

   a. Poor appetite or overeating

   b. Insomnia or hypersomnia

   c. Low energy or fatigue

   d. Low self-esteem

   e. Poor concentration or difficulty making decisions

   f. Feelings of hopelessness

   People with dysthymia may have a superimposed major depression (double depression). It is also quite common that people with dysthymia have a personality disorder, the most common of which are borderline, histrionic, narcissistic, avoidant, and dependent personality disorders. Dysthymia in these people with personality disorders is sometimes called characterologic depression. *The ICD–10 Classification of Mental and Behavioral Disorders* describes it as including depressive neurosis, depressive personality disorder, neurotic depression and persistent anxiety depression.

5. Bipolar disorder (manic-depressive illness). The essential features of bipolar disorder is one or more manic episodes. A manic episode is a distinct period during which the predominant mood is either elevated, expansive, or irritable with various associated symptoms, such as flight of ideas, pressure of speech, and grandiosity. For such a disorder to be called bipolar, there must be at least one episode of major depression. There are many subcategories of bipolar disorder, and the phenomenon of "rapid cycling" is not rare. Because of the complexity, a psychiatrist should be involved in the management of such patients. Mania can also be seen independently of depression and therefore is not part of bipolar disorder. Secondary mania is not infrequently seen following certain medications, head injury, or complex partial seizure.

6. Pseudodementia of depression is the syndrome in which dementia is mimicked or caricatured by a major depression. Pseudodementia is not a diagnosis; it is a descriptive term. A physician who sees a fair number of Alzheimer patients will undoubtedly encounter some with an apparent dementia who, in fact, will have the pseudodementia of depression. It is also possible that people with Alzheimer's disease may have a minor or major depression comorbidly. The only absolute way one can determine whether some patients have dementia or pseudodementia is to treat the patient with suspected pseudodementia for depression, and as the depression clears, the patient's cognitive findings return to baseline. See Chap. 3 for more clues for distinguishing dementia from the pseudodementia of depression.

C. **Treatment.** There are three major treatment modalities for major depression: psychotherapy, medication, and electroconvulsive therapy (ECT). Treatment of major depression is generally satisfactory, but refractory depressions are not uncommon in many patients. Dysthymia is difficult to treat effectively with any modality.

1. **Psychotherapy.** More emphasis was placed on psychotherapeutic treatment of depression in earlier years. No good studies are available that show the efficacy of psychotherapy in the resolution of any types of depression. The most common types of therapy used are the insight oriented, cognitive, and various subtypes of these two. Cognitive therapy seems to be very helpful in minor depression.

2. **Medication.** Many medically oriented psychiatrists feel that medication is the sine qua non of treatment, along with brief supportive psychotherapy. Most presently available drugs are polycyclic antidepressants. Table 9-3 gives a summary of various side effects, dosages, and uptake blocking of the polycyclics.

3. **Dosage of polycyclic antidepressants.** To minimize side effects with these medications, it is generally better to begin treatment at low dosages, usually 25–50 mg at bedtime (protriptyline is an exception [see Table 9-3]). About 2 days later the dosage can be increased to about 100 mg, and then about 3 days later to about 150 mg. If the patient shows side effects (e.g., orthostatic hypotension), one should maintain the dosage at the same level for several more days before increasing. If the side effects are too bothersome, change to another polycyclic. A single bedtime dose is usually helpful in compliance; however, some antidepressants like fluoxetine or protriptyline may be too energizing to give all in the evening. In elderly patients, even lower starting doses (e.g., 25 mg/day) and slower rates of dosage acceleration may be required.

4. **Side effects.** The most common side effects seen with these medications are a variety of anticholinergic effects (e.g., dry mouth, urinary retention, aggravation of glaucoma, constipation). Sedation may be a problem or a desired therapeutic effect depending on the patient's needs. Different medications are high or low in sedative potency (see Table 9-3). Antidepressant medications do have the potential, save fluoxetine, for producing cardiac arrhythmias. They can lengthen the QT interval, thereby increasing the vulnerable period for serious ventricular arrhythmia. As a matter of course, these medications are very rarely prescribed prior to 4 weeks after myocardial infarction. Any question with regard to their use in patients with cardiovascular disease should be discussed with a cardiologist.

5. **Monoamine oxidase inhibitors** (MAOIs) are being used more than previously. In some patients, they are used as a first-line medication, especially if someone in the patient's family has had success with an MAOI. A diet to eliminate tyramine must be followed while on these medications.

6. **Lithium.** Although lithium's primary use is in bipolar disorder, it is also used in unipolar depression as an adjunct in stabilizing the person's mood. It is now also being used in low dose added to antidepressant for refractory depression.

7. **Alprazolam** (Xanax) is included here because of the probably antidepressive qualities of this benzodiazepine. It has been used especially in patients soon after myocardial infarction.

8. **Suicide** is always a possibility in severe depression. If suicide is strongly suspected, it is prudent to get psychiatric consultation. Overdosage of polycyclic antidepressants is a common cause of suicide attempts.

9. **Mania.** The usual treatment for mania is to start a neuroleptic along with lithium. Secondary mania, if secondary to partial seizure, often cools down to normalcy on carbamazepine. Valproate and clonazepam have also been effective in secondary mania.

Table 9-3. Polycyclic antidepressants

Antidepressant	Effect on biogenic amine uptake		Sedative potency	Anticholinergic potency	Orthostatic hypotension	Cardiac arrhythmia potential	Target dose (mg/day)	Dosage range (mg/day)
	5-Hydroxytryptamine	Norepinephrine						
Tricyclics								
Doxepin	++	+	High	Moderate	Moderate	Yes	200	75–400
Amitriptyline	++++	++	High	Highest	High	Yes	150	75–300
Imipramine	++++	++	Moderate	Moderate	High	Yes	200	74–400
Trimipramine	+	+	High	Moderate	High	Yes	150	75–300
Protriptyline	+++	++++	Low	High	? Moderate	Yes	30	15–60
Nortriptyline	+++	++	Moderate	Moderate	Lowest	Yes	100	40–150
Desipramine	+++	++++	Low	Low	High	Yes	150	75–300
Other								
Amoxapine	++	+++	Moderate	Low	? Low	Yes	200	75–300
Maprotiline	+	++	High	Low	? Low	Yes	150	75–300
Trazodone	+++	0	High	Lowest	Moderate	Yes	150	50–600
Fluoxetine	++++	0	Low	Low	Low	Low	20	40–80
Alprazolam	0	0	Moderate	Low	Low	Low	4	0.5–10.0
Monoamine oxidase inhibitors			Low		High	Low		

Source: Data from N. H. Cassem, Pain. In E. Rubenstein and D. D. Federman (eds.), *Scientific American Medicine: Current Topics in Medicine.* New York: Scientific American, 1983; and E. Richelson, Pharmacology of antidepressants. *Psychopathology* 20(Suppl. 1):1, 1987.

II. Hysteria

A. Description. There are many meanings of the word *hysteria*.

1. There are at least six major ways that the word is used:
   a. Hysterical conversion reaction.
   b. Hysterical personality.
   c. Hysteria as a form of repetitive somatizing behavior (Briquet's syndrome)
   d. As a contagious group process.
   e. To connote a process in psychoanalytic theory.
   f. As a layman's term for exaggerated behavior or exaggerated symptoms.
2. In neurology, the term *hysteria* is usually used to describe conversion reactions and/or dissociative reactions. All physicians after adequate workup have en countered various conversions or dissociations such as paralyses, anesthesias movement and gait disorders, urinary retention, pain syndromes, seizures visual loss, amnesia, fugue states, and unresponsive states.

B. Histrionic personality disorder used to be known in psychiatry as hysterical personality disorder, but because of the rather pejorative quality of the historical concept of the "wandering uterus," the term was changed from *hysterical* to *histrionic* in 1980. A personality style is made up of traits that are enduring patterns of perceiving relating to, and thinking about the environment and oneself. When these traits are inflexible and maladaptive and cause either significant impairment in social or occupational functioning or subjective distress, they constitute a personality disorder.

1. **Diagnosis.** According to DSM-IV, the histrionic personality disorder is seen as a pattern of excessive emotionality and attention-seeking beginning by early adulthood. For the diagnosis to apply, patients must have at least five of the following eight characteristics:
   a. Uncomfortable in situations in which they are not the center of attention.
   b. Interaction with others is often characterized by inappropriate sexually seductive or provocative behavior.
   c. Display rapidly shifting and shallow expression of emotions.
   d. Consistently use physical appearance to draw attention to themselves.
   e. Style of speech is excessively impressionistic and lacking in detail.
   f. Self-dramatization, theatricality, and exaggerated expression of emotion.
   g. Suggestibility, that is, easily influenced by others or circumstances.
   h. Consider relationships to be more intimate than they actually are.
2. **Management features.** People with the histrionic personality disorder are commonly seen in medical practice. Histrionic patients are seen by generalists, internists, neurologists, and all other medical and surgical specialists. It should be borne in mind that *most* people with conversion disorder do not have a histrionic personality disorder.

C. Somatization disorder, also known as **Briquet's syndrome,** describes a syndrome of recurrent and multiple somatic complaints of several years' duration for which medical attention has been sought but that are apparently not due to any physical disorder. This diagnosis is primarily made in women. The onset occurs before age 35. It is never monosymptomatic and often includes a history of excessive surgical operations. It is the best studied syndrome in the whole field of hysteria. It is estimated to occur in 1–2% of the female population. If this diagnosis is suspected, psychiatric referral is strongly suggested.

D. Conversion reaction

1. **Description**
   a. The term *conversion reaction* was coined in 1893 by Freud to refer to a condition with qualities of excitation attached to certain unbearable ideas, which are transmuted into some bodily form of expression. Limb anesthesias, pseudoseizures, and tunnel vision are all fairly common examples of this. Conversion phenomena differ from malingering, since in conversion the patient does *not* have **conscious control** over the symptom. Most adult patients with conversion reactions are women, and the average age is about 40 years old.
   b. **LaBelle indifference** is **sometimes** present. This is not to be confused with stoicism.

    c. Many entities thought to be conversion reactions have turned out later to be, in fact, organic conditions. In a review of six studies, the rate varied from 13–30%.

2. Diagnosis. There are four important factors in diagnosing conversion disorder.

    a. Physical functioning is lost or altered, suggesting a physical disorder.

    b. Psychological factors are judged to be etiologically related to the symptom because of a temporal relationship between the symptom and a psychosocial stressor that is apparently related to a psychological conflict.

    c. The person is not conscious of intentionally producing the symptom.

    d. The symptom is not a culturally sanctioned response pattern and cannot, after appropriate investigation, be explained by a known physical disorder.

3. Pseudoseizure, once called hysterical seizure, is referred to by some as psychogenic seizure. The relationship between hysteria and epilepsy is notoriously confusing. A true pseudoseizure, as distinguished from malingering, is an apparent seizure with a subjective change in consciousness without ictal discharge. Three cautions are necessary:

    a. If it is a true conversion symptom, then the symptomatology must not be under the patient's control and a secondary gain must be discoverable.

    b. The surface EEG is not very helpful in detecting ictal discharge in deeper limbic structures; therefore, a surface EEG with no spiking evident does not, in fact, categorically rule out true seizure.

    c. Pseudoseizures are most common in patients with true epilepsy. The most difficult to distinguish cases are those patients who have pseudoseizures and complex partial seizures. Implanted electrodes in limbic structures have shown that what were once called pseudoseizures often are true seizures. The importance of making the distinction is obvious in the treatment. Holter monitor EEG has proved a useful, albeit not infallible, tool in understanding pseudoseizures.

4. Treatment. There is no standard treatment for conversion disorder.

    a. In some few patients, direct confrontation may be helpful, but this is discouraged unless the physician is quite sure of a very healthy, positive doctor-patient relationship. The use of hypnosis has been used sometimes with great efficacy, but again, a positive outcome is not assumed.

    b. A sodium amytal interview has often been helpful and in some cases clearly makes the diagnosis.

    c. Probably the most used and most helpful treatment is to suggest to patients that they will gradually recover and that there is nothing seriously wrong, and to allow patients "to save face" by not confronting them with a psychoanalytic explanation for the conversion reaction.

E. Dissociative disorders. The essential feature of "dissociation" is a sudden, temporary alteration in the integrative functions of consciousness, identity, or motor behavior. Often the layman will speak of a dissociation of consciousness as being "spaced." Important personal events cannot be recalled. A sudden temporary alteration in identity or integrative functions may result in the forgetting of one's usual identity and a totally or partially new identity will be assumed. This brings with it a feeling of unreality.

    An alteration in motor behavior is exemplified by a psychogenic fugue. One can be so overwhelmed by unconscious material that consciousness may be impaired in a psychogenic stupor or psychogenic unresponsiveness. All of these are characterized by attempts to escape from excessive tension and anxiety by separating off some parts of personality function from the rest.

1. Psychogenic amnesia. Usually this disorder is observed in adolescents and young adults and rarely in the elderly. It is often found in young people in the military.

    a. Amnesia begins suddenly and usually follows a severe psychosocial stress. It can be seen in posttraumatic stress disorder.

    b. Psychogenic amnesia is almost always anterograde.

    c. Malingering is one of the diagnoses that should be excluded, although it can be difficult to do so.

    d. Hypnosis, a sodium amytal interview, or both, may be helpful.

  2. Psychogenic fugue. The essential feature here is a sudden, unexpected travel away from home or customary work locale with assumption of a new identity and an inability to recall one's previous identity. Elements of disorientation and perplexity may exist, and in recovery there is often no recollection of the events.

    a. There have been some dramatic psychogenic fugues reported in the media. In most cases, however, the fugue is less elaborate and consists of little more than brief, apparently purposeful travel. Any new identity is usually partial.

    b. Little is known of elements such as age of onset, complications, prevalence, sex ratio, or family pattern in this entity.

    c. Just as in psychogenic amnesia, a differential diagnosis must include multiple personality, cursive epilepsy of complex partial seizure, and malingering.

    d. There is no standard treatment for this entity. Clear diagnosis and reassurance usually give the best results.

  3. Depersonalization disorder is sometimes referred to as self-estrangement. The major diagnostic point is the occurrence of one or more episodes of feeling outside of one's personality, an experience that causes social or occupational impairment.

    a. It is estimated that 30–70% of young adults may have depersonalization without significant impairment.

    b. Many people have mild depersonalization. This is not infrequent with the use of marijuana or during acute stresses (e.g., earthquake).

    c. Often the experience of one's self-identity is altered by some perception or experience (e.g., finding out that one is homosexual at a party), and the reality of one's identity is lost or skewed.

    d. These patients are not psychotic, since they have intact reality testing, but the feelings of unreality are ego-dystonic.

    e. Derealization is frequently present, where one feels the perception of one's surroundings are not as real as they usually appear.

    f. Onset after the age of 40 is rare.

    g. The course is generally chronic and marked by remissions and exacerbations.

III. Pain. All physicians come in contact with acute and chronic pain in their practice. Pain control has become a much more sophisticated area in medical practice in the last 20 years.

  A. In general, pain is categorized and managed into two areas: acute and chronic pain.

    1. It is always of primary importance to try to find the **cause** of any pain, so that it can be addressed before other treatments are started.

    2. Specific treatment of specific types of pain is preferable if it can be determined (e.g., carbamazepine for trigeminal neuralgia).

    3. For **generalized pain,** it is a rule of thumb that treatment starts with mild nonnarcotics and then moves up the scale to more potent narcotics depending on the pain and the patient's comfort. Table 9-4 lists the major analgesics used in common practice along with their duration of action and the efficacy of their mode of delivery.

    4. Placebos are sometimes used as a diagnostic tool, but this use is actually not very helpful, since over 33% of people will have a positive placebo response. The response in an individual can vary in the same person at different times. The postulated mechanism of action of the placebo effect is that the placebo activates a descending pain modulation system, which in part involves release of endogenous opiates. Placebo effects also appear to be influenced by the doctor-patient relationship, the significance of the placebo treatment to the patient, and setting of the treatment.

    5. There are many **ancillary techniques** used in the management of pain, especially in trying to alleviate chronic pain. In these ancillary techniques, the disciplines of anesthesia, neurosurgery, and psychiatry play a major role. Such techniques as the use of epidural morphine, nerve blocks, behavioral conditioning, neurosurgical lytic lesions, and cingulotomy are usually available at larger medical centers.

Table 9-4. Oral and parenteral narcotic analgesics for severe pain

Analgesic	Route	Equianalgesic dose (mg)	Duration (hr)	Plasma half-life (hr)	Comments
Narcotic agonists					
Morphine	IM	10	4–6	2.0–3.5	Standard for comparison; also available in slow-release tablets
	PO	60	4–7		
Codeine	IM	130	4–6	3	Biotransformed to morphine; useful as initial narcotic analgesic
	PO	200	4–6		
Oxycodone	IM	15	3–5	—	Short acting; available alone or as 5-mg dose in combination with aspirin and acetaminophen
	PO	30	4–5		
Heroin	IM	5	4–5	0.5	Illegal in U.S.; high solubility for parenteral administration
	PO	60	4–6		
Levorphanol (Levo-Dromoran)	IM	2	4–7	12–16	Good oral potency; requires careful titration in initial dosing because of drug accumulation
	PO	4	4–5		
Hydromorphone (Dilaudid)	IM	1.5	4–6	2–3	Available in high-potency injectable form (10 mg/ml) for cachectic patients and as rectal suppositories; more soluble than morphine
	PO	7.5	4–6		
Oxymorphone (Numorphan)	IM	1	4–5		Available in parenteral and rectal-suppository forms only
	PR	10	4–5		
Meperidine (Demerol)	IM	75		3–4 (normeperidine 12–16)	Contraindicated in patients with renal disease; accumulation of active toxic metabolite normeperidine produces CNS excitation
	PO	300			

Table 9-4. (continued)

Analgesic	Route	Equianalgesic dose (mg)	Duration (hr)	Plasma half-life (hr)	Comments
Methadone (Dolophine)	IM	10		15–30	Good oral potency; requires careful titration of the initial dose to avoid drug accumulation
	PO	20			
Mixed agonist-antagonist drugs					
Pentazocine (Talwin)	IM	60	4–6	2–3	Limited use for cancer pain; psychotomimetic effects with dose escalation; available only in combination with naloxone, aspirin, or acetaminophen; may precipitate withdrawal in physically dependent patients
	PO	180	4–7		
Nalbuphine (Nubain)	IM	10	4–6	5	Not available orally; less severe psychotomimetic effects than pentazocine; may precipitate withdrawal in physically dependent patients
	PO	—			
Butorphanol (Stadol)	IM	2	4–6	2.5–3.5	Not available orally; produces psychotomimetic effects; may precipitate withdrawal in physically dependent patients
	PO	—			
Partial agonists					
Buprenorphine (Temgesic)	IM	0.4	4–6	?	No psychotomimetic effects; may precipitate withdrawal in tolerant patients
	SL	0.8	5–6		

Source: Adapted from K. M. Foley, The treatment of cancer pain. *N. Engl. J. Med.* 313:84, 1985.

B. Acute pain. Most physicians can effectively treat acute pain in their practice.
   1. The tolerance of pain differs in individuals according to the attention drawn to it, the person's personality, and the possible psychiatric state of the patient.
   2. In the treatment of acute pain, especially in the hospitalized patient, there is little propensity for the patient to become addicted to a narcotic, whereas narcotic addiction is not infrequent in chronic pain.
C. Chronic pain is usually defined as pain that persists for about 6 months or more. It may be due to nonmalignant or malignant conditions and is usually distinguished from the continuous pain of the terminally ill.
   1. In chronic pain, it appears that the **limbic system** has a larger role than in acute pain. Suffering as distinct from nociception and pain enters the chronic picture. It is thought that the paleospinothalamic tract, having multiple connections in the limbic system, plays an important role in chronic pain and that the fast-tracking neospinothalamic tract has a lesser role.
   2. In any **assessment** of pain, whether acute or chronic, there are three factors that should always be considered:
      a. The astute use of anatomic dermatome reference points.
      b. Identification of pain of the deafferentation type.
      c. The assessment of the suffering and pain behavior components in the patient.
   3. Deafferentation pain is chronic pain that follows direct injury to the peripheral or central nervous system.
      a. Forms
         (1) Reflex sympathetic dystrophy.
         (2) Phantom limb.
         (3) Causalgia.
         (4) Postherpetic neuralgia.
         (5) Thalamic pain.
      b. Descriptions
         (1) Causalgia is a burning or searing sensation.
         (2) Dysesthesia feels like pins and needles, numbness, or tingling.
         (3) Formication feels like insects crawling on the skin.
         (4) Hyperpathia is the painful response to a light touch of a shirt or a breeze. This pain responds poorly to known therapies and in general narcotics are not the answer. Usually a referral to a pain center is needed.
   4. Psychiatric factors in chronic pain. One of the major difficulties in the treatment and management of chronic pain is that there is usually much more to the patient's presentation than just pain alone, even though that is the only thing the patient will talk about. Psychiatric factors can influence the "volume" or "gain" on the pain of any lesion. This can be seen on any Sunday when professional football players are injured after a particularly savage hit and then they return two or three plays later. If they had been hit that way standing on a street corner, their subsequent behavior might include a day or two in bed. This psychological decrease in volume on pain is well-known in combat veterans also. The following factors usually increase the volume of pain:
      a. Depression. Since in chronic pain the suffering component is more evident than in acute pain, where the nociceptive component is more stark, we presume that the limbic system has a regulatory influence on the intensity of felt pain. If the patient has a major depression, any gloominess, dysphoria, or irritability from that depression will amplify any painful sensation that is felt. Some pain specialists feel that almost all chronic pain is the result of severe depression.
      Diagnosing depression in the chronic pain patient is the first step. Polycyclic antidepressants have an analgesic quality that is relatively mild over and above their antidepressant quality.
      b. Anxiety. Many people with chronic pain may be anxious or even fearful, which influences the chronic pain they suffer. Although benzodiazepines are helpful in the anxious patient, for chronic-pain patients small doses of nonsedating, high-potency neuroleptics tend to decrease anxiety greatly and often are instrumental in reducing narcotic analgesics. When the clinician

sees fearfulness, the use of haloperidol, 0.5 mg bid, may be quite helpful in chronic pain control.

    c. Psychogenic pain. When no physical findings adequately account for the pain and there appear to be psychological factors that could be causal, the patient is said to suffer from psychogenic pain. There should be a temporal relationship between the onset of pain and a secondary gain. As an example, a naval aviator who previously had a terrifying carrier landing may find that he has an excruciating headache in the briefing room prior to his next scheduled flight. Another psychological factor could be that the patient get support from those around them that they would not get without the pain.

    d. Personality disorder. Chronic pain can be the arena where manipulation occurs through the distorted personality. The antisocial personality disorder, the dependent personality disorder, and the borderline personality disorder are probably the most bothersome of personality disorders with regard to pain behavior. The focus of the doctor-patient interaction will always be the pain or narcotic analgesics and not the distortion of personality that the patient has. It may be important to get psychiatric confirmation of personality disorder in these cases.

IV. Neuropsychiatric features of medical and neurologic illness

  A. Psychosis is occasionally found in patients who have dementing illness, basal ganglia disease, or stroke. The two major expressions of psychosis are delusion and hallucination.

    1. A **delusion** is a firm, fixed belief without any objective evidence for that belief. A patient may have a near-delusion, that is, an overvalued idea. This does not strictly mean that the patient has psychosis, but there is some reason why he is investing this idea with much greater affect.

    2. Hallucinations can be visual, auditory, olfactory, or somatosensory. Olfactory and dermatologic sensory hallucinations are not unusual; the most common are auditory and visual. Auditory hallucinations are more often seen with delusions whereas visual hallucinations are often seen alone.

    3. Treatment. After a metabolic disorder, seizure disorder, fever, or any other entity that might produce delusion or hallucination is ruled out, treatment can be initiated. The usual treatment is with neuroleptics. We tend to prefer high-potency, low-dosage haloperidol. Small doses, 0.5–2.0 mg, are to be tried first since most of these patients will have impaired brain to begin with. Visual hallucinations are usually well taken care of, auditory hallucinations not quite as well as visual, and delusions may not be able to be eradicated totally but usually show some improvement on neuroleptics.

  B. Obstreperous behavior can be seen either with or without psychosis.

    1. Cause. One must search for a possible known cause of obstreperous behavior, such as a medical side effect, a partial seizure, or the patient's acting on a delusional system. Usually there is no known cause of this behavior.

    2. Treatment. The most common treatment of obstreperous behavior is, again, with neuroleptics, using the lowest dosage possible. There has been some success with innovative treatments, that is, carbamazepine and trazodone at low dosages.

  C. Stroke. About 400,000 people per year suffer thromboembolic stroke. Neuropsychiatric features are common in stroke.

    1. Depression is common with stroke. One study found that 27% of stroke patients had major depression and 20% had minor depression within 2 weeks of the stroke. Six months later that 47% rose to 60% depressed, all untreated. Those stroke patients who are treated for their depression do much better in rehabilitation. It has been shown that 60% of stroke patients with depression have their stroke in the left anterior hemisphere. Treatment by antidepressants of post-stroke depression has been successful with both nortriptyline and trazadone. Recently, some success has been seen in post-stroke depression with the faster-acting psychostimulants.

    2. Subcortical dementia is a mildly controversial entity that can be seen in stroke patients. Not infrequently these patients are thought to have major depression when, in fact, they have only apathy. This apathy has been successfully treated with psychostimulants, such as methylphenidate or dextroamphetamine in low dosage.

3. Post-stroke a patient may develop **partial seizures** wherein the only symptomatology may be delusion, hallucination, or both.

D. **Basal ganglia disease** is looked on today in a more holistic manner, that is, concern is not merely with the motor problems but also with neuropsychiatric features of the disease.

1. **Parkinson's disease** patients may well have delusions, hallucinations, or depression. It is important to judge clinically whether these may be secondary to the medication that the patient is using. Depression has been seen in as many as 41% of parkinsonian patients, and most of these patients have a history of cognitive impairment while they are in major depression. More than 50% of patients will reveal depressive symptomatology during the evolution of the disease. Nortriptyline is effective in treating this depression; ECT is also quite effective in Parkinson's disease and has improved the quality of motor movement as well.

2. **Huntington's disease** also shows an inordinate amount of depression, with a suicide rate much higher than other basal ganglia diseases.

E. **Multiple sclerosis** causes fatigue with its patchy demyelination. Depression in multiple sclerosis patients has been estimated to be between 14 and 27%. Patients benefit from tricyclic antidepressant use. Amantadine has been helpful in reducing fatigue. Lability of mood has been estimated to be about 18% in multiple sclerosis patients and generally responds to low-dose neuroleptics.

F. **Alzheimer's disease** can be accompanied by depression, delusions, hallucinations, and obstreperousness. In a study of 120 outpatients with probable Alzheimer's disease, 13% had major depression, 30% had minor depression, 7% had hallucinations, and 4% had delusions. One-third of the patients had no other neuropsychiatric diagnosis than Alzheimer's disease.

Selected Readings

Bouckoms, A. J., et al. Chronic nonmalignant pain treated with long-term oral narcotic analgesics. *Ann. Clin. Psychiatry* 4:185, 1992.

Cummings, J. L. Subcortical dementia: Neuropsychology, neuropsychiatry and pathophysiology. *Br. J. Psychiatry* 149:682, 1986.

Cummings, J. L. Organic psychosis. *Psychosomatics* 29:16, 1988.

Devinsky, O., et al. Dissociative states and epilepsy. *Neurology* (NY) 39:835, 1989.

Diagnostic and Statistical Manual of Mental Disorders (4th ed.) (DSM-IV). Washington: American Psychiatric Association, 1993.

Foley, K. M. The treatment of cancer pain. *N. Engl. J. Med.* 313:84, 1985.

Ford, C. *The Somatizing Disorders: Illness as a Way of Life.* New York: Elsevier, 1983.

Gates, J. R., et al. Ictal characteristics of pseudoseizures. *Arch. Neurol.* 42:1183, 1985.

Gold, P. W., Goodwin, F. K., and Chrousos, G. P. Clinical and biochemical manifestations of depression. *N. Engl. J. Med.* 319:348, 1988.

Hyman, S. E., and Cassem, N. H. Pain. In E. Rubenstein and D. D. Federman (eds.), *Scientific American Medicine: Current Topics in Medicine.* New York: Scientific American, 1989. Pp. 1–17.

Kotila, M., and Waltimo, O. Epilepsy after stroke. *Epilepsia* 33:495, 1992.

Krauthammer, C., and Klerman, G. L. Secondary mania: Manic syndromes associated with antecedent physical illness or drugs. *Arch. Gen. Psychiatry* 35:1333, 1978.

Larson, E. W., and Richelson, E. Organic causes of mania. *Mayo Clin. Proc.* 63:906, 1988.

Lesser, R. P. Psychogenic seizures. *Psychosomatics* 27:823, 1986.

Masand, P., Murray, G. B., and Pickett, P. Psychostimulants in post-stroke depression. *J. Neuropsychiatry* 3:23, 1991.

Richelson, E. Pharmacology of antidepressants. *Psychopathology* 20(Suppl. 1):1, 1987.

Richelson, E. Synaptic pharmacology of antidepressants: An update. *McLean Hosp.* 13:67, 1988.

Schiffer, R. B., et al. Evidence for atypical depression in Parkinson's disease. *Am. J. Psychiatry* 145:1020, 1988.

Signer, S., Cummings, J. L., and Benson, D. F. Delusions and mood disorders in patients with chronic aphasia. *J. Neuropsychiatry* 1:40, 1989.

Starkstein, S. E., and Robinson, R. G. Affective disorders and cerebral vascular disease. *Br. J. Psychiatry* 154:170, 1989.

Starkstein, S. E., et al. Mania after brain injury: Neurological and metabolic findings. *Ann. Neurol.* 27:652, 1990.

World Health Organization. *The ICD-10 Classification of Mental and Behavioural Disorders.* Geneva: WHO, 1992.

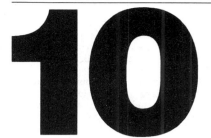

Stroke

Richard C. Hinton

Cerebrovascular disease usually may be distinguished from other neurologic disorders by the sudden or very rapid development of symptoms that are almost always focal. At times, however, other conditions such as seizure equivalents, hemorrhage into a tumor, or, rarely, demyelinating disease may be mistaken for cerebrovascular disease. A **completed stroke** is suspected when there is persistence of the neurologic deficit for longer than 24 hours. When the deficit completely disappears after a period of 24 hours or longer, the term **reversible ischemic neurologic deficit (RIND)** has been applied. A **transient ischemic attack (TIA)** refers to a transient neurologic deficit lasting less than 24 hours with complete return to normal. If appropriate therapy is to be administered, the precise **nature of the underlying cerebrovascular disease** must first be understood and clarified with the clinical examination and diagnostic studies.

Stroke can be conveniently divided into two categories: **ischemic strokes,** including embolic and thrombotic strokes, and **hemorrhagic strokes,** such as primary intracerebral hemorrhage and subarachnoid hemorrhage (usually the result of leakage from a cerebral aneurysm or vascular malformation). Successful prevention of stroke may be possible with the identification of important **risk factors,** such as hypertension, atrial fibrillation, smoking, and perhaps myxomatous degeneration of the mitral valve. Hyperlipidemia may also be a risk factor for cerebrovascular disease, although probably not as strong as in coronary artery disease. Antiphospholipid antibodies such as the lupus anticoagulant and anticardiolipin antibodies may also be risk factors for cerebrovascular disease, and deficiencies of clotting inhibitory factors such as antithrombin III, protein S, and protein C have also at times been implicated.

In this chapter, guidelines for treatment of the various types of stroke are presented. However, it should be stated that controversies exist among clinicians, particularly in the use of anticoagulants and antiplatelet agents for cerebral ischemia. Therefore, these guidelines must be applied with caution and tailored to the individual patient. Although a general orientation to the clinical picture for each variety of stroke is provided, a detailed description is beyond the scope of this manual.

I. **Ischemic strokes.** The clinician is most commonly confronted with two types of ischemic stroke: **primary thrombotic occlusion** of a vessel and occlusion of a vessel by material from a distant source **(embolism).** Primary thrombotic occlusion usually occurs in a vessel already partially occluded by atherosclerosis, for instance the carotid artery or the basilar artery. The heart is the most common source of embolic material (e.g., mural thrombus formation in the setting of atrial fibrillation or myocardial infarction, patent foramen ovale, prosthetic valves, septic and bland emboli in bacterial endocarditis, marantic [nonbacterial] endocarditis, Libman-Sacks endocarditis, and atrial myxoma). Less commonly embolism arises from ulcerated atherosclerotic plaque in the aortic arch or at the origin of the great vessels. Although the carotid arteries are subject to primary thrombosis, often symptoms are the result of embolism to the intracranial vessels, so-called local embolism. Rare causes of ischemic stroke include cerebral vein thrombosis, paradoxical embolism, polycythemia vera, meningovascular syphilis, arteritis secondary to tuberculosis, arteritis in association with collagen vascular disease, giant-cell arteritis, Takayasu's arteritis, moyamoya, fibromuscular dysplasia, subclavian steal, and dissecting aortic aneurysm.

A. **Description.** Although not invariable, the neurologic deficit associated with embolism characteristically begins suddenly, with a maximum deficit occurring at the onset; preceding TIAs may occur but are less common than in primary thrombosis Preceding TIAs are common with thrombotic strokes. This type of stroke also may progress over hours or days, and the neurologic deficit fluctuates or changes in a stepwise fashion with a series of sudden events, the so-called stroke-in-evolution.

1. **Middle cerebral artery syndrome.** Middle cerebral artery occlusions are usually embolic, and middle cerebral artery stenosis with or without thrombotic occlusion is less common. When the entire territory of the middle cerebral artery is affected, the resulting clinical picture includes contralateral hemiplegia and hemianesthesia; contralateral homonymous hemianopia with impairment of conjugate gaze in the direction opposite the lesion; aphasia with language-dominant (usually left) hemispheral involvement; and apractagnosia, asomatognosia, and anosognosia, with nondominant hemispheric involvement. When middle cerebral branch occlusions occur, which is often the case, incomplete syndromes result: nonfluent or Broca's aphasia with contralateral lower-face and arm weakness from upper-division middle cerebral artery occlusion, Wernicke's aphasia with lower-division middle cerebral artery occlusion, and others.

2. **Anterior cerebral artery syndrome.** Anterior cerebral artery occlusion, also usually embolic, may lead to **paralysis** of the opposite foot and leg, contralateral grasp reflex, gegenhalten rigidity, abulia, gait disorder, perseveration, and urinary incontinence. Occlusion of the stem of the anterior cerebral artery is often inconsequential because of collateral flow through the anterior communicating artery. However, when both anterior cerebral arteries arise from a common stem, occlusion can result in a severe deficit, involving the territories of both arteries.

3. **Carotid artery syndrome.** Carotid occlusive disease can produce symptoms in two ways: by **hypoperfusion** secondary to stenosis or occlusion, and, as already mentioned, by providing a source of embolic material (artery-to-artery emboli, or **local embolism**). Even when the artery is only mildly stenotic, ulceration of the atheromatous plaque can be a nidus for thrombus formation and thus a potential source for embolism. However, there is uncertainty whether there is a significant risk from these **ulcerated plaques** in the absence of severe stenosis of the vessel. While occlusion of the carotid artery is occasionally asymptomatic, symptomatic occlusion most commonly produces **deficits** that involve all or part of the **middle cerebral artery** territory, although other clinical presentations are possible:

   a. Because of variations in the origins of cerebral vessels, the territory supplied by the anterior cerebral artery and at times the posterior cerebral artery may be involved. When the internal carotid artery is severely narrowed and collateral flow is compromised, the most distal regions supplied by the middle cerebral, anterior cerebral, and at times the posterior cerebral arteries (the so-called border zones, or **"watershed"**) may be affected. These zones represent the areas of collateralization among the three arteries. The damage in this situation typically produces **weakness or paresthesias** in the **contralateral arm** and, if more extensive, the face and tongue.

   b. Carotid artery disease is responsible for approximately 50% of the cases of **transient unilateral loss of vision** (transient monocular blindness or amaurosis fugax). This is usually the result of platelet emboli from atheromatous plaques in the carotid system. Occlusion of the central retinal artery or one of its branches, with persistent total or partial loss of vision, is less commonly caused by carotid artery disease. Nevertheless, carotid artery disease should be excluded in this case.

   c. The presence of **prominent facial pulses, reversed flow in the ophthalmic artery, or low retinal artery pressure** by ophthalmodynamometry usually signifies severe stenosis or occlusion of the ipsilateral internal carotid artery.

4. **Posterior cerebral artery syndrome.** The posterior cerebral artery may be occluded by embolus or thrombosis, and this can result in various combinations of the following **neurologic signs:** contralateral homonymous hemianopia (often upper quadrantanopia), memory loss, dyslexia without dysgraphia, color anomia, mild contralateral hemiparesis, contralateral hemisensory loss, and ipsilateral

third-nerve palsy, with contralateral involuntary movements, hemiplegia, or ataxia.

5. **Vertebrobasilar artery syndrome.** While not as common as anterior circulation ischemia, the basilar and vertebral arteries are vulnerable to atherosclerosis and thrombosis as well as embolism.

   a. **Occlusion of branches of the basilar artery** usually results in unilateral pontine or cerebellar dysfunction or both. Depending on the level of involvement, clinical features include combinations of ipsilateral ataxia; contralateral hemiplegia with sensory loss; ipsilateral horizontal gaze palsy, with contralateral hemiplegia (the opposite of that seen in hemispheric lesions); ipsilateral peripheral seventh-nerve lesion; internuclear ophthalmoplegia; nystagmus, vertigo, nausea, and vomiting; deafness and tinnitus; and palatal myoclonus and oscillopsia.

   b. **Occlusion or severe stenosis of the basilar artery itself** usually gives rise to bilateral clinical signs, such as quadriplegia, bilateral conjugate horizontal gaze palsies, coma, or the de-efferented ("locked-in") syndrome. These same signs may be produced by bilateral vertebral artery disease or unilateral disease when one vertebral artery is the dominant source of blood supply.

   c. Damage to structures in the medulla may be the result of **occlusion or stenosis of the intracranial vertebral arteries or posteroinferior cerebellar artery.** This leads to various symptom complexes; the best known of these is the lateral medullary syndrome, consisting of nystagmus, vertigo, nausea, vomiting, dysphagia, hoarseness, impaired sensation on the ipsilateral side of the face, ipsilateral ataxia, ipsilateral Horner's syndrome, and impairment of pain and thermal sense over the contralateral side of the body.

6. **Cerebellar infarction.** Early in its course, cerebellar infarction usually produces dizziness, nausea, vomiting, direction-changing nystagmus, and ataxia. There is often heel-to-shin or finger-to-nose ataxia. Over 1–3 days, there may be resultant edema of the cerebellum manifested by such signs of brainstem compression as conjugate gaze palsy, ipsilateral fifth-nerve dysfunction, and ipsilateral facial nerve palsy. The disorder may then progress rapidly to coma and death. Patients with these clinical signs should always be evaluated thoroughly and observed for several days, since the complication of brainstem compression can be remedied by surgical decompression of the posterior fossa.

7. **Lacunar infarction.** A special type of vascular disease is characterized by hyaline thickening of the small penetrating arteries of the brain **(lipohyalinosis)** and is most commonly seen in patients with diabetes mellitus and hypertension. Occlusion of these vessels results in small, deep, often cystic infarcts referred to as **lacunar infarcts.** These infarcts are often asymptomatic but may **cause certain clinical syndromes,** such as pure motor stroke, pure sensory stroke, clumsy hand–dysarthria syndrome, homolateral ataxia and crural paresis, pure motor hemiparesis with contralateral paralysis of lateral gaze and internuclear ophthalmoplegia, sensorimotor lacune, ataxic hemiparesis, and others. This diagnosis may be suspected when the EEG is normal and the clinical symptoms fit one of these syndromes. While primary occlusion of these small arteries is the usual mechanism, the arteries may also be the target of embolism, and at times the origin of the affected small vessel is occluded by atherosclerotic plaque in the large vessel from which it arises.

B. **Diagnosis.** While careful history taking and physical examination may give a fairly accurate clinical impression, certain diagnostic tests are often necessary. For instance, **it is imperative to distinguish hemorrhage from infarction.** Therefore, diagnostic studies should be arranged early in the course to chart an appropriate course of therapy.

1. A **CT scan** is usually the first test to perform because it easily distinguishes hemorrhage from infarction in almost every case. It may occasionally fail to detect hemorrhagic infarction.

2. An **MRI** is even more sensitive than CT scanning in detection of early cerebral infarction. It is not as accurate as CT for the identification of acute hemorrhage

and thus not as useful as an emergency procedure. Special MR techniques are now generally available to image cerebral vessels (MR angiography). Although not as accurate as cerebral angiography, MR angiography nevertheless can be a valuable noninvasive technique in the evaluation of the cerebral vasculature, provided the clinician is aware of its limitations.

3. **Lumbar puncture (LP).** Examination of the cerebrospinal fluid (CSF) is important in the unlikely event that CT scan or MRI is not available, since blood appears in the CSF of most patients with intracerebral hemorrhage and all patients with subarachnoid hemorrhage. Small intraparenchymal hemorrhages that do not communicate with the subarachnoid space will not yield positive CSF early. The same is often true of hemorrhage into an area of infarction (hemorrhagic infarction), which is usually the result of an embolus. In these situations, the CSF may become hemorrhagic after 48 hours due to seepage of blood into the ventricular system or subarachnoid space. Diagnostic confusion may arise when bleeding into the CSF is induced by needle insertion at LP—the so-called traumatic tap. If four to six tubes of CSF are collected successfully, traumatic taps usually show a diminishing number of RBCs in each successive tube, whereas true hemorrhage produces a more uniform RBC count in each tube. Moreover, when blood has been present in the CSF for approximately 6 hours or longer, the supernatant CSF will appear xanthochromic after centrifugation.

4. **Noninvasive evaluation of the carotid arteries.** Several noninvasive tests are currently available to evaluate the carotid circulation, including oculoplethysmography, ultrasound carotid imaging, and Doppler evaluation. The most sophisticated of these, **Duplex scanning,** combines ultrasound real-time imaging with a Doppler probe. The newer machines provide a very sophisticated Doppler analysis and are rather accurate in detecting significant disease at the carotid bifurcation; these are less accurate with disease above this area and, of course, offer little in the evaluation of the vertebrobasilar system or intracranial circulation. A newer ultrasound technique called **transcranial Doppler** allows a Doppler spectral analysis of some of the intracranial arteries, thus providing an indirect assessment of the velocities in these arteries. This has some utility in the identification of intracranial stenoses and is of particular value in the evaluation of vasopasm secondary to subarachnoid hemorrhage. It is also under investigation for use in the evaluation of other conditions including cerebral death, migraine, and vascular malformations and in the detection of cerebral embolism.

5. **Digital subtraction angiography** uses a computerized subtraction technique that allows visualization of the arteries with either an intravenous injection of contrast material or a small dose of intra-arterial contrast. With the intravenous injection **(digitalized venous imaging),** the extracranial carotid images generally provide a high degree of correlation with those obtained using conventional carotid arteriography. Although the extracranial vertebral arteries and the intracranial vessels are seen, the detail necessary for an adequate evaluation of these arteries is lacking. Side effects of the intravenous procedure have included allergic reactions, pulmonary edema, and acute renal failure. The quantity of contrast medium for the intravenous injection is much greater than that needed for conventional arteriography; thus, digitalized venous imaging is relatively contraindicated in patients with renal insufficiency, particularly diabetics. The digital technique is also utilized for arteriograms **(digital intra-arterial angiography)** to reduce the amount of contrast required to obtain the images.

6. **Angiography.** Intra-arterial angiography is the most definitive test and is necessary at times, particularly when surgery is contemplated. In experienced hands, the associated risk is small, especially when the femoral or brachial approach is used. Nevertheless, there is always some potential risk of stroke or dissection of the catheterized artery, and this procedure must be utilized judiciously and only when the information obtained will be crucial in planning treatment.

7. The **EEG** is usually abnormal in cortical cerebral infarctions, with slowing over the area of infarction. When it is normal, it may support a clinical impression of lacunar infarction.

8. **Brain scan** often shows increased uptake in the area of infarction, but often it does not become positive for 4–5 days or longer. Moreover, the disphosphonate scan seems to give positive evidence of infarction more often than does the conventional technetium scan. In most circumstances, radionuclide brain scan is an outmoded procedure.

9. **Metabolic imaging studies.** Positron emission tomography (PET) and single photon emission computed tomography (SPECT) are methods for imaging and, in the case of PET, measuring various aspects of brain metabolism. These techniques are valuable in assessing a transient ischemic episode in which there is no anatomic lesion or in an early stroke prior to the development of an infarction, which is not visible by CT scan or MRI. Currently neither PET nor SPECT is widely available.

10. **Laboratory tests.** When cerebral embolism is accompanied by fever and an increased **sedimentation rate, infective endocarditis** or less commonly **atrial myxoma** should be considered. Serial blood cultures would be important when infective endocarditis is suspected.

11. **Echocardiography** is positive in virtually all patients with left atrial myxoma and is useful in the evaluation of valvular heart disease. However, in searching for an embolic source, a newer technique, **transesophageal echocardiography** is more accurate in the detection of mural thrombi and valvular vegetations. It is also very sensitive in the detection of patent foramen ovale when paradoxical embolism is suspected. Although some degree of patency of the foramen ovale is relatively common, whether a minor degree of patency represents a significant risk for stroke remains to be determined. Transesophageal echocardiography has also been useful in detecting embolic sources in the great vessels in the form of ulcerated plaque and mural thrombus.

12. When no source for embolism has been discovered, **Holter monitor** may at times reveal unsuspected intermittent atrial fibrillation.

C. **Treatment**

1. **General precautions**

   a. Rapid lowering of blood pressure should be avoided in the first 10 days unless it is critically high (persistent diastolic pressure > 120 mm Hg), and of course, hypotension should be reversed. The patient might be kept in the horizontal position for a few days, with the feet slightly elevated, especially for stenotic lesions.

   b. **Vomiting** is common in the early stages of some types of stroke, particularly vertebrobasilar strokes and hemorrhages. If vomiting occurs, nasogastric suction is instituted together with intravenous fluid and electrolyte maintenance; close attention must be given to the control of nasopharyngeal secretions. Patients who are dysphagic must also be maintained on intravenous fluids.

   c. **Intraveous solutions** that contain excessive amounts of free water (such as 5% D/W) may increase cerebral edema and are contraindicated. A solution of 5% dextrose and 0.45% normal saline is preferable.

   d. **Inactivity** can itself be a problem. Antiembolic stockings, although of doubtful efficacy in preventing thrombophlebitis, are usually worn, and a footboard is placed at the foot of the bed. Intermittent compression devices that promote venous flow in the legs are available and may be effective. With prolonged inactivity, the patient should be turned q2–3h to prevent decubitus ulcers.

   e. Within 24–48 hours of completion of the stroke, passive range-of-motion exercises are begun 3–4 times a day to prevent the development of **contractures.**

2. **Anticoagulants.** The most commonly used anticoagulants for cerebrovascular disease are the coumarin agents and heparin. These drugs should not be given to noncompliant patients or to those who cannot be followed closely with clotting tests. They are contraindicated in patients with bleeding diatheses, active peptic ulcer disease, uremia, or severe liver disease and in patients who are at risk of falling frequently.

   a. **Coumarin agents.** Either bishydroxycoumarin (average maintenance dose, 75 mg/day) or warfarin (maintenance dose, 2–15 mg/day) may be used for oral long-term anticoagulant therapy. These agents alter synthesis of the vitamin K–dependent clotting factors (II, VII, IX, and X) and result in production of biologically inactive forms.

(1) Although prolongation of the prothrombin time (PT) may be achieved in 48 hours or so, this is merely a reflection of the short half-life of factor VII, and the patient's intrinsic clotting mechanism is still very much intact. It is usually 5 days or longer before the other factors reach their lowest levels and adequate therapeutic anticoagulation is achieved. For this reason, a loading dose at the commencement of therapy is unnecessary, and a daily maintenance dose, such as warfarin, 10 mg/day, may be started. Daily PT determinations are made, and the dosage is adjusted to maintain the PT level at 16–19 seconds (although variations from one laboratory to another may dictate a different value).

(2) Once the PT has been controlled and the patient has been discharged from the hospital, the PT should be determined no less frequently than every 2–3 weeks. Other drugs that may augment or antagonize the effect of the coumarin agents are always kept in mind.

(3) **Coumarin effects can be reversed** in 6–12 hours after the intravenous injection of 50 mg of vitamin K, provided that the liver is functioning properly. Rapid reversal of coumarin effects can be achieved by administering fresh-frozen plasma IV, starting with 15–20 ml/kg, followed by one-third the dose at 8- to 12-hour intervals.

b. **Heparin** combines with a circulating plasma cofactor, antithrombin III, and neutralizes not only thrombin but also some other serine proteases of the coagulation system. When heparin therapy is indicated, two methods of administration can be used. An IV bolus of 5000–10,000 units may be given, followed by a **continuous infusion** by syringe pump of 800–1000 units/hour. The alternative method calls for an initial IV bolus of 5000–10,000 units, followed by **repeated bolus** injections of 5000–10,000 units q4h. Either the Lee-White whole-blood clotting time or the activated partial thromboplastin time (PPT) may be used to adjust the heparin dose to maintain the clotting time at approximately double that of the control. If the continuous-infusion method is used, the clotting tests can be performed approximately 4 hours after a bolus of heparin has been given. Coagulation tests are performed at least once a day. Hemorrhagic areas on the patient's skin or microscopic hematuria might indicate excessive anticoagulation.

In case of hemorrhagic side effects, **the effects of heparin can be reversed** in minutes by intravenous administration of **protamine,** given in a 2-mg/ml solution (5 ml of a 1% solution is mixed with 20 ml of saline). The protamine is injected slowly IV, with no more than 50 mg given in any 10-minute period. If the protamine is needed just after a dose of heparin has been given, the amount of protamine required may be calculated by assuming that 1 mg of protamine will neutralize approximately 90 USP units of heparin of beef lung origin or 115 USP units of heparin derived from intestinal mucosa; however, the package insert for heparin should be checked, since preparations vary. The quantity of protamine required to neutralize the heparin decreases rapidly after heparin administration. For instance, the requirements after one-half hour has elapsed are approximately half the amount required immediately after the heparin is given. If 4 hours or more have passed, no protamine is given, since an overdose of protamine may produce a hemorrhagic state. Side effects include hypotension, bradycardia, dyspnea, and flushing.

c. **Antiplatelet agents.** Many drugs interfere with platelet function and might serve as antiplatelet agents, but the experience is greatest with **aspirin, dipyridamole,** and **sulfinpyrazone.** A new antiplatelet agent, **ticlopidine,** is now available and has been demonstrated to be at least as effective as aspirin in preventing stroke in both men and women (aspirin does not appear to be as effective in women as in men). There is some suggestion that it might be more effective in general than aspirin, but this requires further clarification.

Because the risk of hemorrhagic side effects may be smaller with antiplatelet agents, they may be tried as alternative forms of therapy in patients in whom the coumarin agents and heparin are contraindicated.

- **(1) Dosage**
  - **(a)** Experimental evidence suggests that **aspirin** is more effective in lower doses because of a selective inhibition of thromboxane A_2. In the Dutch trial of aspirin in TIAs, 30 mg of aspirin daily was no less effective in the prevention of subsequent vascular events than 283 mg/day. Nevertheless, based on contrary results from earlier studies, some physicians still advocate a higher dosage of aspirin such as 325 mg/day or higher.
  - **(b) Dipyridamole** (Persantine), 50 mg PO tid, and **sulfinpyrazone** (Anturane), 200 mg PO tid, have not been demonstrated to be effective in the treatment of cerebrovascular disease either alone or in combination with aspirin.
  - **(c)** The usual dosage of **ticlopidine** (Ticlid) is 250 mg bid.
- **(2) Side effects**
  - **(a)** Although the side effects of **aspirin** are numerous, the major ones at this dosage are gastrointestinal (e.g., gastric irritation and aggravation of peptic ulcer disease).
  - **(b)** Side effects with **dipyridamole** are uncommon but include headache, dizziness, nausea, flushing, weakness or syncope, mild GI distress, and skin rash.
  - **(c) Sulfinpyrazone,** a uricosuric agent, can lead to urolithiasis and upper GI disturbances, with aggravation of peptic ulcer disease, skin rash, anemia, leukopenia, agranulocytosis, and thrombocytopenia. It may augment the effect of the coumarins.
  - **(d)** The most common side effects of **ticlopidine** are GI distress such as diarrhea, although neutropenia and aplastic anemia have been described; for this reason the manufacturer recommends a CBC determination every 2 weeks for the first 3 months of usage. Skin rash is another potential complication of ticlopidine.
- **d. Use of anticoagulants.** The choice of therapeutic agents in cerebral ischemia is a source of great controversy, partly because of the difficulties involved in conducting meaningful clinical trials. The thrombin inhibitors, such as the coumarin agents and heparin, have been used in numerous clinical trials, many of which have shown a beneficial effect of these drugs. In some, however, the hemorrhagic complication rate was high, and the earlier studies have been criticized for their small sample sizes as well as for other defects in study design. It is therefore difficult to draw any firm conclusions from these studies. (See **Selected Readings** for more extensive reviews.)
  - **(1)** A number of **clinical trials** with the antiplatelet agents have been completed. In the Canadian Cooperative Platelet-Inhibiting Drug Trial, aspirin, 1200 mg/day, was significantly effective in reducing the risk of continuing TIAs, stroke, and death, but only in men. Sulfinpyrazone had no therapeutic effect. In the Aspirin in Transient Ischemic Attack Study conducted in the United States, aspirin failed to achieve statistical significance against placebo in reducing subsequent continuing TIAs, cerebral or retinal infarction, or death, although it appeared superior to placebo in certain subgroups, such as those with multiple TIAs, and particularly in those with carotid lesions on the side appropriate to the symptoms. Prospective studies of healthy male physicians in both the United States and Britain failed to show a protective effect of aspirin for cerebrovascular events, and in fact in both studies there was an increased number of hemorrhagic strokes in the aspirin group. In a double-blind trial with dipyridamole in patients with TIAs, there was no beneficial effect over that of placebo with regard to subsequent TIAs, stroke, or death. So, as with the antithrombin agents, there is some uncertainty over the effectiveness of the antiplatelet agents in the treatment of

cerebral ischemia. Note that the dose of aspirin used in the Canadian trial was large (i.e., 1200 mg/day), whereas in vitro evidence suggests that lower-dose aspirin (i.e., 300 mg/day) may be more effective. As mentioned, in the Dutch trial of aspirin in TIAs, 30 mg/day of aspirin was no less effective than 283 mg/day.

(2) Although platelet aggregation may initiate the clotting process, theoretically inhibition of the thrombin system would seem to be of paramount importance in symptomatic individuals with severe arterial stenoses or other underlying risks for thrombus formation such as atrial fibrillation. In these situations, there is sludging and turbulence with accumulation of proaggregatory substances and thrombin, and the therapeutic effect of the antiplatelet agents may be overwhelmed in this setting. Furthermore, microscopic platelet plugs pose little threat to the brain, although the retina may be damaged. Macroscopic fibrin thrombi represent the greatest danger to the cerebral circulation and are responsible for the more serious types of stroke such as middle cerebral artery occlusion. For these reasons and based on prior experience, many clinicians still utilize anticoagulation with heparin and the coumarin agents at least in the acute setting.

(3) With these points in mind, the following **guidelines** are presented for medical management of cerebral ischemia, although they are by no means universally accepted. It should be emphasized that patients with severe and permanent deficits need not be treated aggressively, and the larger the area of infarction, the greater the danger of anticoagulants in making the ischemic area hemorrhagic.

(a) **Stenotic lesions.** Once a major stroke is complete, the patient is often severely incapacitated, and little can be accomplished with treatment. Therefore, early detection and treatment are critical. Ideally, cases are detected at the stage of TIAs. However, stroke-in-evolution may also respond very favorably to aggressive treatment. Likewise, if a completed stroke has taken place but only a minor deficit is present, the risk of a more serious stroke may still be present, and early treatment is very important. When a stenotic lesion is responsible in these situations, intravenous heparin is given according to the guidelines in sec. **I.C.2.b.** If surgery is indicated, heparin is continued until the time of surgery; carotid artery stenosis is a typical example of this type of stroke. If surgery is not indicated, heparin is continued for at least a few days, and the patient is gradually anticoagulated with one of the coumarin agents while the heparin dosage is tapered and discontinued. In severe stenosis of a surgically inaccessible artery (e.g., basilar artery stenosis), anticoagulation may be necessary indefinitely. With lesser degrees of stenosis, anticoagulation might be discontinued after several months and antiplatelet agents substituted.

(b) **Embolic lesions.** Transient ischemic attacks can occur in embolic disease, and the same guidelines apply as for stenotic lesions. When embolism results in a completed stroke, there is some risk of hemorrhagic infarction, and full-dose heparin is probably contraindicated. The larger the area of infarction, the greater the risk of this complication. When a minor deficit is present in the face of a significant embolic source such as valvular heart disease or myocardial infarction, there is risk of further embolism. In this situation, one might consider low-dose heparin (e.g., 5000 units SC q8h early in the course). If CT scan is negative after several days, it is safer to anticoagulate fully. Heparin is continued until the patient is adequately anticoagulated with one of the coumarin agents (as in stenotic lesions). When an ongoing risk for embolism is present (e.g., atrial fibrillation), it may be appropriate to continue anticoagulation indefinitely. In other cases in which the embolic source is unknown, the coumarin agent could be continued for several months and then perhaps replaced with an antiplatelet agent.

Because of the hemorrhagic risk, patients with embolic complications of infective endocarditis probably should not be anticoagulated.

3. **Surgery.** Carotid endarterectomy is the most commonly performed surgical procedure for ischemic cerebrovascular disease. Surgery also may be effective in the rare cases of symptomatic extracranial vertebral artery disease, subclavian steal, and aortic arch disease. As mentioned previously, posterior fossa decompression can be lifesaving in the case of massive cerebellar infarction and brainstem compression. The procedure of anastomosing the temporal artery to the middle cerebral artery has not been shown in a multicenter study to be any more effective than medical management for patients with such lesions as middle cerebral artery stenosis or intracranial carotid artery stenosis.

Carotid endarterectomy has now been shown to be superior to medical management in symptomatic patients with lesions of 70% or greater stenosis, provided there are no serious medical contraindications to surgery. It should be cautioned that some centers have reported unacceptably high morbidity and mortality figures with the procedure, and carotid endarterectomy can be recommended only in centers where low morbidity and mortality have been achieved. One source of morbidity with carotid endarterectomy is the **shunt,** which may dislodge a loosely adherent clot at the time of placement. Some centers feel this risk can be minimized with the use of intraoperative EEG monitoring; in this case the shunt is used only when EEG abnormalities persist after cross-clamping of the artery. Surgery for complete carotid occlusion must be performed within 24 hours or so if lasting patency is to be achieved.

a. **Transient ischemic attacks.** Carotid endarterectomy is indicated for hemispheric TIAs in the carotid territory in patients with severe stenosis of 70% or greater (usually corresponds to a lumen diameter of 2 mm or less). Some controversy exists among clinicians and surgeons regarding patients with lesser degrees of stenosis but with ulceration of the plaque seen on angiogram. In these patients, other potential sources of embolism, such as the heart or great vessels, must be considered.

b. **Completed stroke and stroke-in-evolution.** When carotid artery disease leads to massive infarction of a cerebral hemisphere, surgical results are poor. However, carotid endarterectomy is indicated when there is less than maximum damage and the potential for an acceptable recovery exists. Potential surgical lesions include severe stenosis of 70% or greater and possibly lesser degrees of stenosis with an ulcerated plaque. Although coexisting asymptomatic stenosis or occlusion of the contralateral carotid artery may be present, in most cases this would not alter the decision to operate on the symptomatic side.

The timing of the surgical procedure is another source of controversy. In the past, there was concern that sudden restoration of blood flow to an area of infarction might result in a more serious hemorrhagic infarct, and often surgery was delayed for days or weeks. However, many surgeons are comfortable with operating immediately, and early surgical intervention could potentially prevent a more serious stroke. If the blood pressure is maintained in the normal range at surgery and postoperatively, the hemorrhagic complication is rare.

c. **Asymptomatic stenosis.** Although some multicenter studies are in progress, the risk for stroke without warning in patients with asymptomatic carotid artery stenosis has not yet been determined. However, prophylactic carotid endarterectomy must be considered in a relatively young patient with severe asymptomatic carotid stenosis in centers that have achieved an acceptably low morbidity with the procedure (approximately 2–3%).

d. When a surgical carotid lesion is present but **severe coexisting medical illness** precludes an operation, anticoagulants or antiplatelet agents should be administered according to the guidelines in sec. **I.C.2.**

  e. For stenotic lesions not accessible by carotid endarterectomy (e.g., cavern
ous carotid stenosis), anticoagulants or antiplatelet agents would be selecte
on an individual basis according to the severity of the lesion and th
suitability of the individual patient for anticoagulation. However, in patien
in whom there is a major contraindication to anticoagulation or in whom TIA
occur despite adequate anticoagulation, an extracranial-intracranial bypas
graft could be considered.

4. Antiedema agents.

  a. Corticosteroids have not been shown to be effective in cerebral infarction c
cerebral hemorrhage, although there is some evidence that they are effectiv
in reducing cerebral edema in other conditions. In spite of this evidence, som
clinicians feel they should be given when there are signs of increase
intracranial pressure, such as obtundation, coma, or signs of herniation. I
this situation, dexamethasone is given in an initial bolus of 10 mg IV or IM
followed by 4 mg IV or IM q4–6h.

  b. Osmotic agents such as **mannitol** or **glycerol** are probably more effective i
reducing intracranial pressure. It is important to keep in mind that thes
agents may have only a transient benefit, and there is some evidence that
"rebound" increase in cerebral edema may occur when they are discontinued
particularly with mannitol. Mannitol is of particular value when an immedi
ate reduction in intracranial pressure is necessary. The dosage of mannitol i
usually 0.5–1.5 g/kg IV. The dosage of glycerol is 1 g/kg PO q6h.

  c. High-dose barbiturates have been administered in patients in whom all othe
measures have failed, although this treatment cannot be recommended base
on the available evidence at this point in time. Guidelines for barbiturat
coma are outlined in Chap. 1, sec. **VII.D.6.**

5. Anticonvulsants. Some patients with cerebral infarction develop seizures, bu
this often a late complication. Anticonvulsants are generally withheld unti
there is evidence of seizure activity.

6. Vasodilators. In spite of evidence that cerebral blood flow is increased by amy
nitrate, papaverine, isoxsuprine, acetazolamide, carbon dioxide, and othe
agents, these agents do not seem to alter the course of ischemic strokes favorably
Indeed, some physicians feel that the resultant vasodilation from these agent
reduces perfusion to the area of ischemia (so-called intracerebral steal).

7. Other therapeutic agents. Some agents such as clofibrate have been tried in brie
clinical trials in the treatment of stroke, but they have not been clearly shown t
be of value. Despite disappointing initial results with agents promoting fibrin
olysis such as streptokinase and urokinase, there has been recent renewed
interest in these agents as well as **tissue plasminogen activator.** Tissue
plasminogen activator may be more specific than the other agents, and its effec
on fibrinolysis seems limited to fresh thrombi in situ; currently multicenter
cooperative studies are under way to evaluate this agent. A large prospective
double blind placebo-controlled study of intra-arterial pro-urokinase, a new
more clot-specific genetically produced thrombolytic agent, is also underway
Prostacyclin, a potent platelet aggregator and vasodilator, has not been shown in
clinical trials to be of benefit. Clinical trials with volume expanders, such as
low-molecular-weight dextran or hydroxyethyl starch, have produced mixed
results, and a final verdict concerning these agents must await further clinical
trials. The same is true of pentoxifylline, which increases RBC deformability,
and naloxone, an opiate receptor antagonist. Clinical trials in stroke and cardiac
arrest with barbiturates have failed to show any beneficial effect. The influx of
calcium into ischemic neurons seems to be an important determinant in cell
death. Initial encouraging reports in the treatment of cerebral ischemia with
nimodipine, a calcium channel inhibitor, have not been confirmed in more recent
studies. Glutamate N-methyl-D-aspartate (NMDA) receptor antagonists have
been suggested as treatment for cerebral ischemia and are currently under
investigation.

8. In the recovery phase, in which some degree of improvement almost always
occurs, **speech, occupational, and physical therapy** are beneficial.

II. Hemorrhagic strokes. The most common varieties of hemorrhagic stroke are intracerebral hemorrhage secondary to hypertension or amyloid angiopathy and subarachnoid hemorrhage secondary to ruptured saccular aneurysm or arteriovenous malformation. Other, less common causes of hemorrhage are anticoagulants, bleeding diatheses, trauma, hemorrhage into a primary or metastatic brain tumor, idiopathic subarachnoid hemorrhage, and rupture of a mycotic aneurysm. Rare causes include carotid cavernous arteriovenous fistulas, hemorrhage after vasopressor drugs, hemorrhage on exertion, encephalitis, and pituitary apoplexy.

A. Intracerebral hemorrhage

  1. **Description.** It is the small penetrating arteries that are damaged by hypertension and give rise to hypertensive intracerebral hemorrhage. As a consequence, the hemorrhage almost always arises in the following locations in decreasing order of frequency: putamen, thalamus, pons, and cerebellum. Hemorrhage secondary to anticoagulants, bleeding diatheses, or trauma often involves other areas of the brain, such as the frontal, temporal, or occipital lobes—sites rarely involved with hypertensive hemorrhage.

     Amyloid angiopathy has recently been recognized as a relatively common cause of hemorrhage in the elderly; these hemorrhages tend to be **lobar** in location in contrast to hypertensive hemorrhages, and they may be recurrent or multiple. The onset of intracerebral hemorrhage is abrupt, and the stroke usually evolves gradually over minutes or hours without the stepwise progression seen in thrombotic strokes.

     a. **Putaminal hemorrhage.** When first seen, patients with putaminal hemorrhage often present a clinical picture that is almost indistinguishable from that of middle cerebral artery occlusion, with contralateral hemiplegia, hemianesthesia, homonymous hemianopsia, aphasia (if the dominant hemisphere is involved), and hemineglect, anosognosia, and the like, with nondominant hemispheral involvement. There is usually a greater alteration of the state of consciousness in patients with hemorrhage. Smaller hemorrhages produce more restricted deficits, while larger ones may produce coma and signs of herniation.

     b. **Thalamic hemorrhage** produces contralateral hemiparesis or hemiplegia with contralateral hemianesthesia. The sensory loss may be disproportionately greater than the motor deficit. Unusual eye signs provide a clue to the diagnosis of thalamic hemorrhage. Often there is restriction of upward gaze, at times with forced downward deviation of the eyes; skew deviation of the eyes is common. The eyes may even be deviated conjugately away from the side of the lesion (so-called wrong-going eyes). As in putaminal hemorrhage, massive hemorrhage in the thalamus leads to coma and signs of herniation.

     c. **Pontine hemorrhage** usually results in early coma, pinpoint pupils that react to light, and bilateral decerebrate posturing. The eyes are often in midposition, with impaired or absent response to caloric testing. More restricted hemorrhages in the pons, although uncommon, may produce deficits that resemble those seen in pontine infarction.

     d. **Cerebellar hemorrhage** may be diagnosed early with a careful clinical evaluation. Patients typically develop sudden dizziness and vomiting, along with marked truncal ataxia. On examination they are unable to stand or walk because of the ataxia. They are often perfectly alert early in the course. There frequently are signs of compression of the ipsilateral pons, such as paresis of lateral conjugate gaze to the side of the lesion, ipsilateral facial weakness, and diminished corneal reflex on the affected side. Untreated, they rapidly progress to coma and death from brainstem compression. It is critically important to make the diagnosis early, since surgical evacuation of the hematoma can be lifesaving.

  2. **Diagnosis.** Clinical guidelines for the diagnosis of intracerebral hemorrhage are provided in sec. II.A.1.

     a. **Lumbar puncture.** Almost all cerebellar and pontine hemorrhages produce bloody CSF, as do most hemorrhages in the putamen and thalamus. Some of the small hemorrhages in the putamen and thalamus may not show blood in the CSF early; however, as previously mentioned, the CSF is almost alway positive within 48 hours. Lumbar puncture is usually safe, but with mas effect there is always the threat of herniation, and this is a particular hazard in cerebellar hemorrhage. In this case lumbar puncture would be indicated only if CT scan was not available.

   b. A **CT scan** is usually available and is the procedure of choice to confirm the diagnosis of intracerebral hemorrhage and to determine the extent of damage Before the advent of CT scans, angiography would often show an avascular mass in the region of hemorrhage.

3. Treatment

   a. General measures. The same general measures listed for ischemic stroke (see sec. **I.C.1**) apply to the management of intracerebral hemorrhage with the exception of blood pressure control. In the patient with intracerebral hemorrhage, efforts are made to maintain the blood pressure in the normal range

   b. Antiedema agents. Patients with intracerebral hemorrhage may have considerable cerebral edema, and if drowsiness or evidence of herniation is present, antiedema agents, such as steroids, mannitol, or glycerol, are given in the dosages discussed in sec. **I.C.4.**

   As mentioned, steroids such as dexamethasone have not been shown to be effective in patients with intracerebral hemorrhage, and osmotic agents such as mannitol or glycerol are more effective in reducing cerebral edema. It is important to keep in mind that the osmotic agents are of transient benefit and when discontinued a rebound effect may ensue. They are of particular value when given just before decompressive surgery or as a last-resort effort to reverse herniation.

   c. Surgery. Evacuation of a hematoma in an accessible location, such as the cerebellum, putamen, thalamus, or temporal lobe may be lifesaving, and this type of emergency surgery must be considered if the condition of the patient does not stabilize and signs of herniation begin to appear. However, when the patient's condition is stable and the hemorrhage is not life-threatening, it is not clear that emergency evacuation of the clot is any more beneficial than conservative, nonsurgical management.

   d. Anticonvulsants may be withheld until there is evidence of seizure activity.

   e. Clotting abnormalities. In patients with hemorrhage secondary to clotting abnormalities or anticoagulant therapy, appropriate measures are taken to reverse the abnormality (e.g., platelets for thrombocytopenia, fresh-frozen plasma and vitamin K for coumarin agents, and protamine for heparin).

B. Subarachnoid hemorrhage

   1. Description

   a. Aneurysmal rupture. Subarachnoid hemorrhage is most commonly the result of rupture of a saccular aneurysm, which is a defect in the internal elastic lamina or the arterial wall that occurs at sites of arterial bifurcation or branching. The majority of patients who experience rupture are between the ages of 35 and 65 years. Associated conditions include polycystic kidneys and coarctation of the aorta. Another type of aneurysm occurs along the trunk of the internal carotid, vertebral, or basilar arteries, and these are described in terms of their morphology as fusiform, globular, or diffuse. These aneurysms may cause symptoms by compressing local structures or thrombosis, but they seldom rupture. A rare cause of subarachnoid hemorrhage is rupture of a mycotic aneurysm, the result of septic embolism. Unfortunately, aneurysms are usually asymptomatic until they rupture.

   (1) Typically there is a **sudden onset of severe headache,** usually the worst headache the patient has ever experienced. The patient may lose consciousness, and while this event may herald the onset of coma, the patient often reawakens somewhat confused. At times, the loss of consciousness is sudden and unaccompanied by headache. The event often occurs during physical exertion, such as during sexual intercourse. Although patients with ruptured cerebral aneurysms usually have supportive clinical signs, their examination may be perfectly normal early, and a high index of suspicion is in order for patients with severe headache of sudden onset.

(2) On examination, signs of **meningeal irritation** are common, as is **low-grade fever.**

(3) **Subhyaloid hemorrhages** are often seen on funduscopic examination.

(4) The hemorrhage may be only subarachnoid, or blood may dissect into the brain parenchyma itself, causing **focal neurologic deficits.**

(5) **Infarction** early in the course may also result from compromise of blood flow or thrombosis in the arteries involved by the aneurysm.

(6) **Clinical localization of the aneurysm** is usually difficult, although certain signs may be helpful: pain behind the eye and dysfunction of the second to sixth cranial nerves with cavernous carotid artery aneurysms; hemiplegia, asphasia, and so on with middle cerebral artery aneurysms; third-nerve palsy with aneurysm at the juncture of the posterior communicating and internal carotid arteries; abulia or weakness of the lower limb with anterior communicating artery aneurysms; and involvement of the lower cranial nerves with basilar and vertebral artery aneurysms.

(7) Focal neurologic deficits that occur a few days after the initial hemorrhage, either transient or permanent, are usually caused by **vasospasm** resulting from the presence of blood in the subarachnoid space.

(8) **Hydrocephalus** may occur as an early or late complication of subarachnoid hemorrhage and may require shunting.

b. **Arteriovenous malformations (AVMs)** are usually brought to clinical attention because of seizures or hemorrhage, although large ones may shunt enough blood to result in ischemia of the surrounding brain. Symptoms are most likely to occur in childhood or young adulthood. Since AVMs commonly extend from the surface into the brain parenchyma, hemorrhage from these malformations is often a combination of intracerebral and subarachnoid hemorrhage. A chronic headache is a common complaint prior to hemorrhage, and the presence of a bruit over the eyeball, carotid artery, or mastoid of a young patient strongly suggests the presence of a cerebral AVM. Other vascular malformation may occur including telangiectasias, cavernous angiomas, and venous angiomas. MRI is particularly useful in separating these types of malformations, and this has some clinical importance since hemorrhage with venous angiomas and possibly telangiectasias is probably rare. However, it has recently become apparent that cavernous angiomas pose some risk of hemorrhage, although not as great as in the case of AVMs, and these malformations have a characteristic appearance on MRI.

In any large series of patients with subarachnoid hemorrhage, a considerable number will have no demonstrable lesion. At least some of these result from rupture of so-called cryptic AVMs, which are too small to be detected angiographically. Spinal AVMs must be considered in young patients with subarachnoid hemorrhage and no demonstrable cerebral lesion. Also, a bruit may sometimes be heard over the spine in these patients.

2. **Diagnosis**

a. Whenever a subarachnoid hemorrhage is suspected, a **CT scan** is the diagnostic procedure of choice. In most, but not all cases, the subarachnoid blood is seen on CT. The CT scan can also provide information about cerebral edema, parenchymal hemorrhage, ventricular hemorrhage, and hydrocephalus. The finding of a large, localized collection of subarachnoid blood may identify the site of hemorrhage.

b. **Examination of CSF.** An LP is indicated only if the CT scan is not available or is nondiagnostic. The risk of herniation or of inducing rehemorrhage by the LP must be considered. Bloody CSF on LP examination will always be found with subarachnoid hemorrhage. Traumatic tap can usually be ruled out according to the guidelines in sec. **I.B.3.**

c. **Skull x rays** may show calcification in an AVM and occasionally in an aneurysm but are not routinely ordered.

d. **Angiography.** Many physicians would perform angiography shortly after admission, since early surgery (in the first 24–48 hours) is now probably the treatment of choice for ruptured cerebral aneurysms in patients with minor neurologic impairment. For more severely impaired patients, angiography might be delayed, unless diagnostic confusion exists between ruptured aneurysm or AVM and hypertensive intracerebral hemorrhage and particularly when any type of decompressive surgery is necessary.

e. If no lesions are demonstrated by cerebral angiography and no localizing neurologic signs are present, an aneurysm is not completely ruled out, since at times these lesions are obliterated initially by thrombosis only to appear on angiography at a later time as the clot dissolves. For this reason, a repeat angiogram is usually performed after a few weeks. A rare cause for subarachnoid hemorrhage is a spinal AVM, and if there are any clinical findings consistent with this such as a bruit over the spine or localized collections of blood along the spine on imaging studies, spinal angiography might be indicated, although these lesions may also be demonstrated by MRI.

3. Treatment. Surgery is the treatment of choice for suitable patients whose aneurysms are surgically accessible. In the preoperative period, therapeutic efforts are directed toward prevention and treatment of the two most important complications: **recurrent hemorrhage** and **vasopasm.** Arteriovenous malformations may or may not be amenable to surgery. Since there is risk of recurrent hemorrhage from AVMs, although less than that for aneurysms, the following preoperative measures apply in the early period after bleeding.

a. Preoperative measures

   (1) General precautions

   (a) Elevation of blood pressure is avoided if possible. If hypertension exists, antihypertensive drugs are used to maintain the blood pressure in the normal range.

   (b) Sedation with phenobarbital or diazepam is instituted to prevent excitement and elevation of the blood pressure.

   (c) Seizures are a complication and raise the blood pressure, so prophylactic **anticonvulsants** are given. Phenobarbital is an effective anticonvulsant (starting dosage, 30 mg PO tid) and may serve a dual purpose, as sedative and anticonvulsant.

   (d) To prevent straining with bowel movements, **stool softeners** are given, such as dioctyl sodium sulfosuccinate (Colace), 100 mg PO tid.

   (e) The room is darkened and **noise minimized.**

   (f) While hypertension is to be avoided preoperatively, if there is evidence of reduced intravascular volume, **volume expansion** is probably important and can be accomplished according to the guidelines in sec. II.B.3.a.(4)(b). **Caution** is in order **preoperatively,** as the artificial colloids such as hetastarch may alter the coagulation mechanism with prolongation of the PT, PTT, and the bleeding time.

   (2) Antifibrinolytic agents. It is thought that lysis of the clot formed at the point of bleeding is partly responsible for recurrent hemorrhage from aneurysms and AVMs. This provides some rationale for the use of antifibrinolytic agents; indeed, most studies suggest considerable efficacy of these agents in preventing rebleeding. However, clinicians are now trying to avoid using these agents because of a higher risk of both venous and arterial thrombotic complications. Nevertheless, in the case of ruptured aneurysm when surgery must be delayed for a prolonged period of time, their use must be considered.

   Epsilon-aminocaproic acid (Amicar), 30–36 g/day, may be given IV. This is usually prepared by mixing 30–36 g in 1 liter of 5% dextrose and 0.45% normal saline or a similar solution. The mixture is infused over 24 hours with a microdrop apparatus. Alternatively, the drug may be administered in a dosage of 4 g PO q3h. The drug is continued until the time of surgery or for 6 weeks if surgery is contraindicated. Complications include nausea, cramps, diarrhea, dizziness, tinnitus, conjunctival suffusion, nasal stuffiness, headache, skin rash, thrombophlebitis, and pulmonary embolus.

(3) **Antiedema agents.** Corticosteroids, mannitol, or glycerol may be given if there are signs of increased intracranial pressure, as discussed in sec. **I.C.4.**

(4) **Management of vasospasm.** Vasopasm may be responsible for drowsiness or focal neurologic signs, but these signs do not usually occur until 2–3 days after the initial hemorrhage and peak in occurrence at about 7 days. The spasm is thought to result from the release of vasoactive compounds such as serotonin, catecholamines, peptides, and endothelin.

(a) Intravenous **isoproterenol** and **nitroglycerin** have been used in an effort to dilate the cerebral vessels. Both have produced variable results.

(b) **Volume expansion** as a measure to increase cerebral perfusion may be the most effective therapy for vasospasm. Hypervolemic volume expansion is accomplished by administering 5% albumin or other plasma fraction solutions IV. As an alternative, artificial colloids such as hetastarch may be given IV. A word of caution is in order when administering the artificial colloids preoperatively because they may alter the coagulation mechanism with transient prolongation of the PT, PTT, and bleeding time. This therapy is relatively contraindicated in patients with reduced cardiac output or congestive heart failure. The therapy is monitored via a central venous catheter, adjusting the central venous pressure to 8–12 mm Hg or the pulmonary capillary wedge pressure to 12–16 mm Hg. Hypervolemia may be combined with phlebotomy and hemodilution to achieve a hematocrit of 30–35%. If spasm is still a problem even after hypervolemia, the blood pressure can be raised with hypertensive agents such as intravenous dopamine, phenylephrine, and dolbutamine. This therapy is much safer once the aneurysm has been clipped, since the risk of rebleeding is probably increased as the blood pressure is raised.

(c) Recently, dilation of vasospastic segments of cerebral vessels has been successfully performed using balloon angioplasty.

(d) Slow-channel calcium inhibitors have been proposed for the treatment of vasospasm, and one such agent, **nimodipine,** is available for this purpose. It appears to have some effect in reducing vasospasm if given early before vasospasm appears. The dosage is 30–60 mg PO q4h. The most undesirable side effect is hypotension, and this is of course to be avoided in the presence of vasospasm.

b. **Surgery.** Patients who undergo surgery for ruptured aneurysms generally fare somewhat better than those who are treated medically because of the sharp reduction in the incidence of rebleeding with surgery. The decision to operate is made with the guidance of the neurosurgeon and depends to a certain extent on his or her preferences. However, certain generalizations can be made.

(1) **Contraindications.** Surgery is not usually performed on patients in coma or with severe neurologic deficits because of the high mortality and low potential for recovery.

(2) **Timing.** In the past, surgery was usually delayed for 10 days or so after the hemorrhage, provided that significant vasospasm was not present. Recently, multicenter studies have reported encouraging results with early aneurysm surgery in the first 24–48 hours for patients not severely impaired. It appears that surgery can be performed at this stage without worsening vasospasm, since vasopasm is usually a later development. With early surgery, the subarachnoid space is irrigated to remove the blood, and this is felt to reduce the threat of vasospasm; some centers are even instilling tissue plasminogen activator to dissolve the adherent clot after the aneurysm is securely clipped.

(3) **Procedures.** Various procedures have been devised for dealing with aneurysms surgically (e.g., clipping the neck of the aneurysm, wrapping it with muscle, coating it with plastic, and occluding the internal carotid

artery in the neck), the most common of which is **clipping the neck of the aneurysm.**

(a) **Block resection or ligation** of the major arteries is done for AVM, although the importance of the involved vessels in supplying blood to critical areas of the brain often precludes this form of therapy. When this is the case, embolic procedures may be used, employing such material as Gelfoam and Silastic balls.

(b) **Balloon occlusion.** Giant aneurysms of the intracranial carotid artery are usually not amenable to surgery. Angiographic techniques now allow balloon occlusion of the aneurysm in many patients. At times the neck of the lesion can be occluded, sparing the parent vessel. In other patients, the carotid artery must be occluded. In such cases a test occlusion is performed with the patient awake. If any signs of ischemia develop, the procedure is stopped. An extracranial-intracranial bypass procedure is done, and the occlusion can safely be performed a few days later.

(c) **Radiotherapy.** Conventional x-ray irradiation of AVMs in an attempt to induce hyalinization and occlusion of the involved vessels has been used in the past with little success. However, radiotherapy using a proton beam has enabled more accurate focusing of the beam and has produced more satisfactory results. A new procedure that has also been effective for this purpose, the gamma knife, allows precise focusing of gamma rays from a cobalt source.

(d) **Shunt.** Hydrocephalus can occur as an early or late complication of subarachnoid hemorrhage and may require a shunt procedure.

(e) **Embolization.** In patients in whom surgery for aneurysm is contraindicated, embolization procedures are sometimes employed in an effort to induce thrombosis, using such material as horse hair or fine coils. When surgery is contraindicated, the preoperative measures already listed as continued for approximately 6 weeks, after which time activity is gradually increased.

Selected Readings

Ackerman, R. H. Non-invasive Diagnosis of Carotid Disease. In R. G. Siekert (ed.), *Cerebrovascular Survey Report for Joint Council Subcommittee on Cerebrovascular Disease: National Institute of Neurological and Communicative Disorders and Stroke and National Heart and Lung Institute.* Rochester, N.Y.: Whiting, 1980. P. 190.

Ackerman, R. H. Non-invasive diagnosis of carotid disease in the era of digital subtraction angiography. *Neurol. Clin.* 1:263, 1983.

Allen, G. S., et al. Cerebral arterial spasm: A controlled trial of nimodipine in patients with subarachnoid hemorrhage. *N. Engl. J. Med.* 308:619, 1983.

American College of Physicians. Indications for carotid endarterectomy. *Ann. Intern. Med.* 111:675, 1989.

Barnett, H. J. M. Aspirin in stroke prevention: An overview. *Stroke* 21 (Suppl. IV): IV–40, 1990.

Bousser, M. G., et al. "AICLA" controlled trial of aspirin and dipyridamole in the secondary prevention of athero-thrombotic cerebral ischemia. *Stroke* 14:5, 1983.

Canadian Cooperative Study Group. A randomized trial of aspirin and sulfinpyrazone in threatened stroke. *N. Engl. J. Med.* 299:53, 1978.

Candelise, L., et al. A randomized trial of aspirin and sulfinpyrazone in patients with TIA. *Stroke* 13:175, 1982.

Cerebral Embolism Study Group. Immediate anticoagulation of embolic stroke: A randomized trial. *Stroke* 14:668, 1983.

Cerebral Embolism Study Group. Brain hemorrhage and management options. *Stroke* 15:779, 1984.

Curling, O. D., et al. An analysis of the natural history of cavernous angiomas. *J. Neurosurg.* 75:702, 1991.

The Dutch TIA Trial Study Group. A comparison of two doses of aspirin (30 mg vs. 283 mg a day) in patients after a transient ischemic attack or minor ischemic stroke. *N. Engl. J. Med.* 325:1261, 1991.

Feussner, J. R., and Matchar, D. B. When and how to study the carotid arteries. *Ann. Intern. Med.* 109:805, 1988.

Fields, W. S., et al. Controlled trial of aspirin in cerebral ischemia. *Stroke* 8:301, 1977.

Fields, W. S., et al. Controlled trial of aspirin in cerebral ischemia: II. Surgical group. *Stroke* 9:309, 1978.

Genton, E., et al. Platelet-inhibiting drugs in the prevention of clinical thrombotic disease. *N. Engl. J. Med.* 293:1174, 1975.

Genton, E., et al. Report of the Joint Committee for Stroke Facilities: XIV. Cerebral ischemia: The role of thrombosis and of antithrombotic therapy. *Stroke* 8:150, 1977.

Hass W. K., et al. A randomized trial comparing ticlopidine hydrochloride with aspirin for the prevention of stroke in high-risk patients. *N. Engl. J. Med.* 321:501, 1989.

Hinton, R. C. Treatment of cerebral ischemia. *Compr. Ther.* 7:24, 1981.

Kistler, J. P., Ropper, A. H., and Heros, R. C. Therapy of ischemic cerebral vascular disease due to atherothrombosis (first of two parts). *N. Engl. J. Med.* 311:27, 1984.

Kistler, J. P., Ropper, A. H., and Heros, R. C. Therapy of ischemic cerebral vascular disease due to atherothrombosis (second of two parts). *N. Engl. J. Med.* 311:100, 1984.

NACENT Collaborators. Beneficial effects of carotid endarterectomy in symptomatic patients with high-grade carotid stenosis. *N. Engl. J. Med.* 325:445, 1991.

Nibbelink, D. W., Torner, J. C., and Henderson, W. G. Intracranial aneurysms and subarachnoid hemorrhage: A cooperative study. Antifibrinolytic therapy in recent onset subarachnoid hemorrhage. *Stroke* 6:622, 1975.

Origitano, T. C., et al. Sustained increased cerebral blood flow with prophylactic hypertensive hypervolemic hemodilution ("Triple-H" Therapy) after subarachnoid hemorrhage. *Neurosurgery* 27:729, 1990.

Petty, G. W., et al. Complications of long-term anticoagulation. *Ann. Neurol.* 23:570, 1988.

Sandok, B. A., et al. Guidelines for the management of transient ischemic attacks. *Mayo Clin. Proc.* 53:665, 1978.

Sorenson, P. S., et al. Acetylsalicylic acid in the prevention of stroke in patients with reversible cerebral ischemic attacks: A Danish cooperative study. *Stroke* 14:15, 1983.

Steering Committee of the Physicians' Health Study Research Group. Final report on the aspirin component of the ongoing physicians' health study. *N. Engl. J. Med.* 321:129, 1989.

Swedish Cooperative Study. High dosage acetylsalicylic acid after cerebral infarction. *Stroke* 18:325, 1987.

Thompson, J. E., Austin, D. J., and Patman, R. D. Carotid endarterectomy for cerebrovascular insufficiency: Long-term results in 592 patients followed up to 13 years. *Ann. Surg.* 172:663, 1970.

Neoplasms

Howard D. Weiss

I. Introduction

A. Classification. Figure 11-1 presents a classification of the most common neoplasms of the CNS and their sites of predilection.

B. Prevalence. Brain tumors are not rare. New brain tumors are diagnosed in over 35,000 adult Americans each year. Primary brain tumors are the second most common form of cancer in children. There are approximately 8500 deaths each year in the United States due to malignant primary brain tumors and many more due to cerebral metastases.

C. Genetic syndromes. Specific genetic disorders that are associated with brain tumors include

1. **Neurofibromatosis** with spinal neuromas, acoustic neuromas, meningiomas, and gliomas.
2. **Tuberous sclerosis** with astrocytomas.
3. **Von Hippel–Lindau disease** with hemangioblastomas.

D. Symptoms. Cerebral neoplasms produce subacute and **progressive** neurologic signs and symptoms. The patient's symptoms depend on the size, location, rate of growth, and amount of edema surrounding the tumor.

1. **Increased intracranial pressure** occurs with many cerebral neoplasms and will cause headache, at times with nausea and vomiting. The headaches may be mild and are often bilateral or diffuse, without localizing value. The "early morning headache" usually thought to be associated with increased intracranial pressure is a pattern seen in only a small proportion of patients. Recurrent headache in an adult not previously prone to headaches should always raise the suspicion of an intracranial mass lesion.
2. **Focal clinical manifestations** (e.g., hemiparesis, ataxia, aphasia, visual loss) depend on the location of the lesion and the extent of the surrounding brain edema. Tumors in relatively "silent" regions of the brain commonly present with changes in personality and behavior rather than "focal" signs or symptoms (Table 11-1).
3. **Seizures.** Generalized convulsions or focal seizures (or both) occur in about one-third of patients with tumors in the supratentorial compartment. Seizures are more likely to accompany slower-growing tumors than highly malignant ones.
4. Occasionally, **hemorrhage** into a highly vascular tumor can produce a sudden change in neurologic status that can be mistaken for a stroke syndrome. Glioblastoma multiforme and metastatic brain tumors from choriocarcinoma, melanoma, and anaplastic lung cancer are the tumor types most likely to bleed spontaneously.

E. Diagnosis. Once a brain tumor is suspected on clinical grounds, brain imaging studies are undertaken to confirm its presence and exact location.

1. **CT scan** reveals most brain tumors and also allows assessment of accompanying cerebral edema, midline shift, and ventricular compression or obstructive hydrocephalus. The sensitivity of CT scan for brain tumors is greatly increased by obtaining scans with **intravenous contrast.** CT scan may fail to detect certain types of intracranial tumors, especially small posterior fossa tumors, some isodense infiltrating gliomas, and meningeal carcinomatosis.

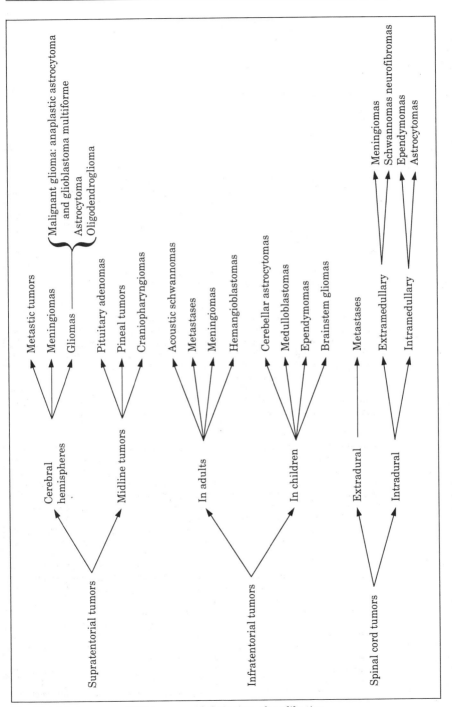

Fig. 11-1. Most common CNS tumors and their sites of predilection.

Table 11-1. Tumors that can present without conspicuous focal signs on routine neurologic examination

Anterior frontal lobe tumors
Nondominant temporal lobe tumors
Gliomas of corpus callosum
Posterior fossa tumors
Colloid cyst of third ventricle
Multiple (bilateral) metastases
Meningeal carcinomatosis

2. **MRI** has technical advantages over CT scans because of its greater resolution and lack of artifact from the temporal bones. MRI is particularly useful in visualizing the brainstem and other posterior fossa structures. The MRI contrast agent, gadolinium, helps differentiate between the borders of tumor and edema. Some meningiomas are isodense with the surrounding brain on MRI and can only be clearly seen after gadolinium enhancement.
3. **Differential diagnosis.** Enhancing cerebral infarcts, brain abscesses, large demyelinating plaques, and intracranial granulomas can easily be mistaken for neoplasms on CT or MRI. Brain imaging studies cannot predict the histopathology of brain tumors with complete accuracy and do not obviate the need for tissue diagnosis in most patients.
4. **Cerebral angiography** has become less important in the diagnosis and localization of intracranial tumors since the development of the CT scan and MRI.
5. **Lumbar puncture (LP)** may reveal increased opening pressure or other nonspecific findings such as elevated cerebrospinal fluid (CSF) protein. LP is potentially dangerous in patients with intracranial mass lesions and is not part of the routine preoperative evaluation of patients with CT scan or MRI evidence of brain tumor. The major exception to this dictum is in patients suspected of having meningeal carcinomatosis or meningeal leukemia. In these patients, the diagnosis can be confirmed only by demonstrating malignant cells on cytologic examination of the CSF, and one or more LPs are mandatory.

II. **Treatment**
A. **Tumor-related brain edema**
1. **Corticosteroids.** Steroid therapy is initiated prior to tissue diagnosis in symptomatic patients with CT or MRI studies revealing an intracranial mass lesion with surrounding edema. High-dose corticosteroids can reduce tumor-associated cerebral edema, thereby lowering intracranial pressure and paliating focal deficits. The use of corticosteroids has had a major beneficial impact on the preoperative and postoperative management of patients with brain tumor.
   a. **Mechanism of action.** Most brain tumors (primary or metastatic) cause edema in the surrounding brain parenchyma. If the edema is considerable or widespread, it can produce a marked increase in intracranial pressure, causing neurologic deficits by compressing nearby structures. The symptoms of many patients may be more a reflection of cerebral edema than destruction of the brain by tumor. The mechanism by which steroids act to reduce cerebral edema is probably related to stabilization of the capillary endothelial junction and reduction of cerebrovascular permeability.
   b. **Clinical effects.** Improvement in focal neurologic signs and symptoms of intracranial hypertension begins within 24–48 hours of starting steroids in most patients with brain tumors, whether primary or metastatic. The maximum degree of improvement is usually obtained by the fourth or fifth day, although improvement may continue for several weeks.
   c. **Choice of corticosteroid.** Response is independent of the corticosteroid selected (e.g., dexamethasone, methylprednisolone, prednisone, hydrocortisone), provided that equivalent doses are used. Dexamethasone has been the

most widely used steroid for treating cerebral edema, due to its relatively low mineralocorticoid (salt-retaining) side effects.

d. Initial dosage. The use of steroids in brain tumor patients was derived from empirical observations, and most clinical studies have employed different dosages in steroid administration. Although the information regarding optimal dosage is largely anecdotal, several guidelines have been established:

  (1) There is a clear dose dependency of clinical response to corticosteroids. The great majority of patients with brain tumors who respond favorably to steroids do so with dexamethasone, 4–6 mg given PO or parenterally qid. This is a large dose of steroid (dexamethasone, 20 mg/day, is roughly equivalent to prednisone, 130 mg/day). There is no advantage to starting therapy at lower dosages, since the drug toxicity is similar, whereas the therapeutic benefit may be greatly diminished.

  (2) Administering dexamethasone in daily divided doses seems to be necessary because some patients begin to suffer recurrent symptoms if there is a prolonged interval between doses.

e. Dosage increases. Critically ill patients or patients who do not have a favorable response to the "standard" dexamethasone dosages (4–6 mg qid) should be treated with even more massive dosages (e.g., 25 mg qid). The risk of serious side effects is increased with these dosages, but in seriously ill patients the favorable response may be lifesaving and allow time for more definitive therapies (e.g., surgical decompression or radiotherapy) to be undertaken.

f. Side effects. The complications and side effects of steroid therapy in brain tumor patients are similar to those that occur in any other group of patients (e.g., opportunistic infection, hypothalamic-pituitary-adrenal axis suppression, carbohydrate intolerance, Cushing's syndrome, and "steroid psychosis"). However, fear of inducing side effects is seldom a good reason for withholding steroid therapy from patients seriously ill with brain tumor.

g. Duration of treatment. Steroid doses are slowly tapered after "definitive therapy" (i.e., surgical decompression, radiation therapy) is completed. The duration of a favorable steroid response or whether the patient will tolerate tapering dosages is often unpredictable. Steroids can be successfully tapered and discontinued without recurrent neurologic symptoms in patients who have responded well to definitive therapy. Unfortunately, many patients with incompletely treated tumors will experience recurrent cerebral edema and clinical deterioration when the dosage is tapered below a critical level. Higher steroid dosages should be reinstituted in these patients, and most will improve again, although some will never return to their previous level of function. Many patients with malignant primary or metastatic brain tumors become "steroid dependent" to maintain some degree of neurologic function during their last months of life.

2. Osmotic agents for lowering intracranial pressure acutely. Patients with brain tumor may experience life-threatening intracranial hypertension with imminent cerebral herniation and death. Situations in which a very rapid reduction in intracranial pressure is needed are indications for therapy with osmotic agents such as mannitol.

  a. Rapid infusion of hypertonic solutions of mannitol quickly reduces brain water by creating an osmotic gradient between the brain and plasma. When mannitol, 1 g/kg, is given over 10–15 minutes (e.g., 250 ml of a 20% solution in an average adult), a reduction of intracranial pressure of 30–60% can be expected for 2–4 hours. It is important to administer mannitol with a filter in the IV apparatus to prevent undissolved crystals from entering the circulation. At the same time, steroid therapy should be started for its longer-term antiedema effects.

  b. A massive osmotic diuresis will follow mannitol therapy, so all patients should have a bladder catheter inserted and careful monitoring of fluid and electrolyte balance. Smaller doses of mannitol (i.e., 0.25–0.50 g/kg) may be repeated every few hours thereafter, if needed, to control intracranial pressure.

    c. Mannitol gradually diffuses from the vascular compartment into the CNS. This can cause a rebound increase in intracranial pressure. Thus, hyperosmolar therapy is useful only in the short term until more definitive therapy such as surgery and steroids, can be instituted.

B. Surgical therapy of intracranial tumors. Many factors influence the decision for advising surgical intervention.

    1. Histologic confirmation. Despite the recent advance in radiologic diagnostic techniques, there is still no absolutely reliable substitute for histologic diagnosis. Patients who are suspected of harboring an untreatable malignant glioma are still occasionally found to have an occult metastasis, treatable meningioma, lymphoma, or brain abscess. Direct histologic confirmation provides the basis for determining the prognosis and need for radiotherapy or chemotherapy.

    2. Restoration of impaired neurologic function. If the preoperative neurologic deficit is due to direct infiltration and destruction of brain tissue by tumor, surgical resection cannot be expected to improve the situation. Conversely, to the extent that the deficits are linked to pressure-related phenomena, they may be surgically reversible. Surgical resection can be palliative, even in patients in whom total resection is not possible, by providing an "internal decompression." Patients with benign brain tumors that cannot be totally resected may be given many additional years of productive life by repeated decompressions at appropriate intervals.

    3. Possibility of cure. The complete removal of the brain tumor and permanent prevention of tumor recurrence can be achieved in many extra-axial tumors (e.g., meningiomas, schwannomas, pituitary adenomas). Very few intra-axial tumors can be resected completely or cured surgically.

    4. Surgical risks. The patient's general condition and the presence of concurrent systemic illness (e.g., heart disease, pulmonary disease, disseminated cancer) will influence the risks of anesthesia and neurosurgery for brain tumor. The major neurosurgical consideration for operative risk is the location of the tumor. Deliberate resection or inadvertent compression, retraction, or devascularization of the brain can produce irreversible deficits. Adverse anatomic location can render surgical removal of benign tumors hazardous and complete resection impossible. This is particularly true for tumors in the hypothalamic and third-ventricle region, brainstem tumors, tumors of the clivus and foramen magnum, and tumors that are intimately involved with major vascular channels (e.g., carotid artery or sagittal sinus). Conversely, tumors in relatively silent areas (e.g., anterior frontal lobe, cerebellar hemisphere, anterior temporal lobe) can be widely resected with relatively little risk of iatrogenic neurologic impairment. The size of the tumor also affects the anticipated operative risk. Resection of large tumors requires more extensive manipulation of adjacent normal structures, thereby increasing the risk of an adverse outcome.

    5. Operative techniques. The use of intraoperative magnification and the operating microscope allows stereoscopic visualization of otherwise inaccessible structures and has played a major role in reducing the morbidity and mortality of brain tumor surgery.

        a. The most common approach to tumors in and around the hemispheres is a **craniotomy.** A portion of skull overlying the tumor is removed en bloc, thereby allowing adequate access to the intracranial compartment. The bone flap is then replaced at the end of the procedure for protective and cosmetic reasons.

        b. Newer CT-monitored techniques have increased the safety of **stereotactic biopsy** of brain lesions without craniotomy or direct tumor exposure. Stereotactic biopsy is indicated for deep mass lesions inaccessible to surgical resection or when no preoperative neurologic symptoms are present and the risks of craniotomy outweigh the benefits. Many primary brain tumors are quite nonhomogeneous, and stereotactic biopsy may yield tissue samples that are not representative of the tumor as a whole.

        c. Whenever possible, **extensive tumor resection** is the surgical procedure of choice, as it lowers intracranial pressure (often with improved postoperative neurologic status) and enhances the likelihood that adjunctive therapies such as radiation or chemotherapy will be effective.

6. Operative complications

a. Hemorrhage. Intracerebral hemorrhage can occur in or away from the operative field, often due to traction of an adjacent artery or vein. Postoperative hemorrhage is usually venous in origin and extrinsic to the brain itself (subdural or extradural). Evacuation of the extracerebral collections may be necessary if hemorrhage produces obtundation or focal deficit.

b. Brain edema usually is present prior to surgery and may be severely aggravated during surgery by mechanical retraction, venous compression, brain manipulation, and overhydration. Patients should receive corticosteroids for several days prior to craniotomy to reduce preoperative cerebral edema. Intraoperative use of osmotic agents such as intravenous mannitol may be necessary to reduce cerebral edema.

c. Infection. The risk of wound infection is increased in lengthy operations and procedures in which foreign materials (e.g., shunt tubing) are implanted. Most infections are by airborne contaminants (e.g., gram-positive cocci, most notably staphylococci). The routine use of prophylactic antibiotics in brain tumor surgery is not recommended.

d. Seizures. Supratentorial operations carry a risk of causing focal or generalized seizures. The likelihood of seizures depends on the location and histology of the tumor as well as operative complications. When postoperative seizures develop, they usually do so within the first month after surgery. The following guidelines seem appropriate:

(1) All patients with a history of seizures prior to surgery should be maintained on a proper anticonvulsant regimen during and after surgery.

(2) Prophylactic anticonvulsant therapy is not routinely warranted in patients undergoing surgery for intraparenchymal brain tumors. Most studies of prophylactic anticonvulsant therapy have shown postoperative seizure rates to be similar for treated and untreated patients. There is an increased incidence of side effects due to anticonvulsant therapy in patients undergoing radiation therapy.

(3) Falx and parasagittal meningiomas carry the highest risk of postoperative seizures. In these cases, prophylactic anticonvulsant therapy should be given before surgery and continued at least 4 months thereafter.

e. Communicating hydrocephalus. The spillage of blood into the CSF pathways during surgery can result in impairment of CSF absorption in the arachnoid villi, producing a communicating hydrocephalus. This is usually a self-limited problem and only seldom requires surgical relief by a shunt.

f. Neuroendocrine disturbances

(1) The syndrome of inappropriate antidiuretic hormone (SIADH) secretion will occasionally occur after any type of brain surgery. Electrolytes should be monitored in the postoperative period, as the retention of free water results in hyponatremia and severe cerebral edema. Rigorous fluid restriction will correct the fluid and electrolyte disturbance. Inappropriate ADH secretion seldom lasts for more than a week or two postoperatively.

(2) Surgery in the region of the hypothalamic-pituitary axis can result in various degrees of panhypopituitarism, diabetes insipidus, or both.

III. Brain tumors in adults

A. Malignant glioma

1. Incidence. The most common primary brain tumor in adults is malignant glioma, which includes anaplastic astrocytoma and glioblastoma multiforme. The histologic distinction is based largely on the absence or presence of tumor necrosis.

There are approximately 5000 new cases of this disorder each year in the United States. The age of peak incidence is 45–55 years, and men are more frequently afflicted than women, in a ratio of 3 : 2. The tumor may arise in any portion of the cerebral hemispheres, the frontal and temporal lobes being the most frequent sites. The cerebellum, brainstem, and spinal cord are rare sites for malignant glioma in adults.

2. **Prognosis.** Malignant gliomas are rapidly growing anaplastic tumors, with a uniformly fatal prognosis. Although these tumors are highly invasive within the CNS, they do not metastasize outside of the nervous system. Survival at 24 months is 40% in patients with anaplastic astrocytoma and only 10% in patients with glioblastoma multiforme. Age is an important prognostic indicator. Patients younger than 45 survive significantly longer than patients over 65, regardless of therapy. Patients presenting with personality change or impaired functional status have a worse prognosis than patients without these findings.

3. **Surgical therapy.** The surgical treatment of choice is **craniotomy** followed by **extensive resection** of the largest volume of tumor possible. This is the most reliable method for obtaining adequate histologic samples and results in internal decompression of the swollen brain. Patients with malignant gliomas treated with extensive surgical resection do better postoperatively and survive longer than patients who have undergone only partial excision or biopsy.

   Although malignant gliomas often appear relatively well circumscribed on CT or MRI examination, the tumor invariably infiltrates into adjacent lobes or across cerebral commissures. Therefore, although the neurosurgeon may optimistically report "gross total removal of the tumor," malignant gliomas will always recur, usually within months. Therefore surgery is never curative in these cases.

4. **Radiation therapy**

   a. **Dosage and fields.** Malignant glioma is not a radiosensitive tumor. Nevertheless, studies performed in the 1970s showed that patients who received 5500–6000 cGy postoperative whole-brain radiation therapy given over 5–6 weeks survived significantly longer than patients who received less than 5000 cGy. The median survival following surgery and radiation therapy for glioblastoma multiforme is approximately 40 weeks. Current practice is to administer part of the radiation to the whole brain (e.g., 4000 cGy) plus additional coned-down radiation to the tumor bed (e.g., 2000 cGy) to spare as much normal brain as possible from the adverse effects of radiation. Tumor doses less than 6000 cGy probably yield inferior survival rates, while higher doses increase neurotoxicity without improved survival.

   Brachytherapy using stereotactically placed interstitial radionuclide implants can deliver very high radiation doses to the tumor with a much lower dose to the surrounding brain. The role of brachytherapy has not been defined, but this technique may prolong quality survival in selected patients whose tumors have recurred after traditional radiation therapy.

   b. **Complications of radiation therapy**

   (1) The incidence of radiation-induced brain damage is thought to be small if standard doses are used. However, as many as 40% of malignant glioma patients who survive for more than 18–24 months after whole-brain radiation therapy develop **progressive cognitive impairment, cerebral atrophy,** and **white matter changes** on CT or MRI as a delayed complication (see sec. **VI.A**). These observations have led to the use of lower doses to the whole brain with additional booster doses to the tumor bed.

   (2) Radiation may cause an **increase in cerebral edema.** Steroids are continued throughout radiation therapy and can be slowly tapered during the last few weeks of treatment if the patient's condition is clinically stable.

   (3) All patients suffer **loss of hair** as a result of therapy, although in many instances the hair regrows over the next few months.

   (4) **Time required for treatment.** Perhaps the greatest morbidity that most patients suffer as a result of cranial irradiation is the extra 5–6 weeks during which they must either remain in the hospital or return each day for treatment. In view of the poor prognosis of glioblastoma, this is an important consideration.

   c. **Value of radiotherapy.** Although radiation is not curative, it does ameliorate symptoms and lengthen short-term survival. These modest benefits justify the continued routine use of postoperative cranial irradiation in malignant glioma (Table 11-2).

Table 11-2. Results of various treatment programs for malignant glioma

Therapy	Median survival (weeks)	2-Year survival (%)
Surgery alone	17	0
Surgery plus semustine	24	8
Surgery plus radiotherapy	38	10
Surgery plus semustine and radiotherapy	42	12
Surgery plus carmustine and radiotherapy	51	15

Key: Radiotherapy = 6000 rad over 6 weeks; semustine dose = 200 mg/sq m every 6–8 weeks; carmustine dose = 80 mg/sq m IV for 3 successive days every 6–8 weeks.
Source: Data adapted from the Brain Tumor Study Group—M. D. Walker, et al., Randomized comparisons of radiotherapy and nitrosoureas for the treatment of malignant glioma after surgery. *N. Engl. J. Med.* 303:1323, 1980.

5. **Chemotherapy**
   a. **Early drug trials.** The failure of surgery and radiation therapy to alter the grim prognosis has led to clinical trials of antineoplastic agents in malignant glioma. As with other solid tumors, the progress in finding effective chemotherapy has been disappointingly slow.
   b. **Lipid-soluble drugs—the nitrosoureas.** Small, lipid-soluble molecules that can cross the normal blood-brain barrier, such as the nitrosoureas, may have the best chance of attaining sufficient concentration for chemotherapeutic effectiveness in all areas of the tumor. To date, the only large controlled studies that confirm efficacy of chemotherapy in the treatment of gliomas involve the use of the nitrosoureas. A large randomized study demonstrated statistically significant increases in median survival (from 36 to 51 weeks) and long-term survivors (24% at 18 months) for patients receiving intravenous carmustine **(BCNU)** in addition to surgery and radiation therapy.

   BCNU is currently the most effective cytotoxic agent against malignant glioma. Intravenous BCNU (200 mg/m² body surface area) is administered every 8 weeks, depending on the recovery of the patient's blood counts. Leukopenia and thrombocytopenia usually occur 2–4 weeks after each treatment. Myelosuppression is cumulative with repeated courses of BCNU. Other major side effects include potential hepatic dysfunction and pulmonary fibrosis.
   c. **Other agents,** including **procarbazine,** oral lomustine **(CCNU),** and **streptozocin,** are probably as effective as BCNU.
   d. **Recommendation for chemotherapy.** Chemotherapy (e.g., BCNU, CCNU) is not recommended routinely for all patients with malignant glioma. The data indicate that these treatments are only marginally effective, and the additional morbidity of chemotherapy is justified only in younger patients with minimal neurologic deficits.
   e. **Immunotherapy** offers the theoretic promise of specific antitumor cytotoxicity with little or no damage to normal brain. Studies involving active immunization with irradiated autologous tumor cells, adoptive immunotherapy (intratumoral or intravenous injection of immune cells), humoral immunomodulators (e.g., interferons), and monoclonal antibody therapy are all in the experimental stage.
   f. **Recurrent glioma.** Weeks to months after treatment with surgical resection, radiation therapy, and chemotherapy, patients will develop worsening neurologic symptoms and CT or MRI evidence of recurrent glioma. The tumors tend to recur at or within a few centimeters of their original site. Metastases to other parts of the CNS are uncommon. Metastases outside the CNS are

rare. A "second look" surgical procedure and reinstitution of high-dose steroids can reduce mass effect and lower intracranial pressure. Unfortunately, these measures only extend survival by 3–4 months. Additional external beam radiation is of little value at this point and would exceed the tolerance of normal brain.

g. Referral for research protocols. Many medical centers are actively studying new cytotoxic drugs and other experimental approaches for recurrent malignant gliomas (e.g., interstitial brachytherapy, hyperthermia, immunotherapy). Patients in relatively good neurologic condition who request that "everything possible" be done should be referred to one of these research centers. The prospective data gathered at these institutions will one day result in an improved outlook for patients with malignant glioma.

B. Supratentorial astrocytomas and oligodendrogliomas
1. **Description.** Astrocytoma, grades 1 and 2 (the so-called low-grade astrocytomas) and oligodendroglioma of the cerebral hemisphere occur less commonly in adults than malignant glioma and account for only 10% of adult primary brain tumors. Patients with these tumors will typically present with a transient neurologic event (e.g., a seizure), a normal neurologic examination, and brain imaging studies revealing a nonenhancing supratentorial lesion with minimal mass effect.
2. **Surgery.** Since these tumors may remain clinically dormant for many years, some experts advocate waiting until the lesion has progressed or focal deficits occur before advising any treatment other than anticonvulsants. Most would agree that the treatment of choice is biopsy and extensive surgical resection if the lesion is in an area that is surgically accessible. These tumors have an infiltrative growth pattern, and only rarely can complete excision be achieved.
3. **Postoperative radiation therapy** (5500 cGy to the tumor bed) may modestly delay tumor recurrence, but it is unclear whether long-term (10-year) survival is increased or whether the benefit outweighs the risk of delayed postradiation cognitive impairment (see sec. VI.A). Prospective studies are under way to determine whether radiation therapy should be routinely administered.
4. The **prognosis** for supratentorial astrocytoma and oligodendroglioma is highly variable. Statistics taken from a large heterogeneous series of cases suggest a median survival of over 5 years after surgery, and the range in survival time is quite great. Some patients die within the first year, whereas a small number survive over 10 years without further symptoms. The vase majority of patients eventualy suffer recurrence and progressive neurologic symptoms. In many patients, this represents a malignant dedifferentiation of the tumor to glioblastoma multiforme.

   Patients in whom the recurrent tumor is in a surgically accessible location often benefit substantially from repeated craniotomy and tumor resection. Antineoplastic chemotherapy has not been shown to be of great benefit in these patients.

C. Primary CNS lymphoma
1. **Epidemiology.** Primary CNS lymphomas are non-Hodgkin's lymphomas, usually of B-cell origin, occurring in the absence of systemic lymphoma. These tumors were formerly quite rare, accounting for only 1% of primary brain tumors. In the past 15 years, however, primary CNS lymphoma has tripled in frequency in the nonimmunosuppressed population. Furthermore, there is an increasing risk of these tumors in patients with immunosuppression of inherited (e.g., Wiskott-Aldrich syndrome) or acquired (e.g., AIDS patients, organ transplant recipients) origin. Three percent of AIDS patients will develop primary CNS lymphoma either prior to AIDS diagnosis or during their subsequent course. The incidence of primary CNS lymphoma will continue to increase during the 1990s.
2. **Description.** There are four distinct clinical presentations of primary CNS lymphoma.
   a. Solitary or multiple discrete intraparenchymal brain tumors are the most common clinical presentations. The tumors are multifocal in nearly half the cases.

    b. Diffuse meningeal or periventricular infiltration is the second most common clinical presentation. This can occur simultaneously with discrete intraparenchymal mass(es).

    c. Retinal or vitreous infiltration can antedate (or follow) the development of brain or meningeal lesions. Slit-lamp examination should be a routine part of monitoring patients with primary CNS lymphoma.

    d. Involvement of the **spinal cord** with discrete intramedullary tumor nodules can rarely occur.

  3. Diagnosis. Surgical biopsy and excision are indicated for patients with solitary parenchymal lesions. Unfortunately, surgical cure is not possible for a tumor characterized by invasion and multicentricity. Stereotactic biopsy or CSF cytology (including immunocytoloic studies) are diagnostic procedures of choice in patients with multifocal or diffuse meningeal disease. In AIDS patients, it is important to distinguish between primary CNS lymphoma and other multifocal diseases, such as cerebral toxoplasmosis and brain abscess.

  4. Treatment. Partial regression of clinically and CT/MRI evident lesions after institutions of high-dose steroids (e.g., dexamethasone, 6 mg qid) reflects not only anticerebral edema effects but also glucocorticoid cytotoxicity for lymphoid cells. Treatment also involves the use of radiation therapy approaches tailored to each clinical situation and the extent of disease (e.g., tumor bed, whole-brain, and/or spinal irradiation). The lack of efficacy of radiation alone has led to trials of pre- and post-irradiation chemotherapy. Intrathecal methotrexate is used to treat patients with diffuse meningeal disease (see sec. **III.G.2**).

  5. Prognosis. Mean survival times after corticosteroids and irradiation are 12–24 months in nonimmunosuppressed patients and much shorter in AIDS patients. Neuraxis dissemination ultimately occurs in 60% of patients and systemic lymphoma in 10% of patients who survive over 1 year. These features suggest that systemic chemotherapy should be used as primary treatment for this disease. Administration of nitrosoureas, high-dose methotrexate with leucovorin rescue, or combination chemotherapy regimens may prolong survival in primary CNS lymphoma.

D. Meningiomas

  1. Biology. Meningiomas are histologically benign tumors that arise from arachnoidal cells. They are the second most common primary intracranial tumors in adults. Their peak incidence is in the fourth and fifth decades, and unlike other primary brain tumors, meningiomas occur more commonly in women than in men (in a ratio of 2 : 1). Cytogenetic analysis has demonstrated multiple deletions on chromosome 22 in most patients with meningioma. Progesterone receptors are present in many meningiomas and may have fuctional importance in the growth of these tumors.

  2. Location. Meningiomas can arise wherever arachnoidal cells are present, but the chief sites of origin are over the cerebral convexity (50%—parasagittal, falx, or lateral convexity) or base (40%—olfactory groove, sphenoid wing, or suprasellar). Meningiomas of the foramen magnum, posterior fossa, or ventricular system are relatively uncommon.

  3. Surgery. Meningiomas are well-circumscribed, slow-growing tumors. They may infiltrate the dura, dural sinuses, or bone but generally do not invade the underlying brain parenchyma. Complete surgical removal and surgical cure are often possible in cases of meningioma. This is not true of the tumors previously discussed.

  4. The **prognosis** is generally favorable, and prolonged survival after surgical resection is the rule rather than the exception. Nevertheless, the rate of tumor recurrence and life expectancy may vary, depending on the location of the tumor and whether complete surgical resection is possible.

    In a large series of patients with meningioma, a macroscopically complete removal of the tumor was achieved in about 60% of cases. Meningiomas over the convexity of the brain, parasagittal region, lateral sphenoid wing, and olfactory groove were generally more accessible to complete resection than tumors at the base of the brain. The vast majority of patients with convexity meningiomas were permanently cured. There was a 10% rate of tumor recurrence in the patients with "complete tumor removal," probably due to residual untreated nests of tumor, and the average time that elapsed between primary operation and confirmation of recurrence was 4–5 years (range, 1–13 years). Many of these patients benefited from a second tumor resection. In the group of patients in whom the resection of intradural tumor was frankly incomplete, there were clinical recurrences in about 40% of cases. However, there were many satisfactory results even in this group: 25% survived more than 10 years after only partial resection.

5. **Histology.** The major histologic subtypes of meningiomas are endotheliomatous, transitional, and angioblastic. The prognosis of these tumors is the same. The rare hemangiopericytoma and malignant meningioma recur with significantly higher frequency and after shorter intervals than the other types of meningiomas.

6. **Radiation therapy** may be indicated for some patients with progressive neurologic deficits due to recurrent meningioma in whom further surgical therapy is inadequate or contraindicated. Retrospective studies have suggested prolonged survival and delayed recurrence rates for selected patients with subtotally resected meningioma who have undergone local radiation therapy.

7. **Incidental meningioma.** With the advent of CT and MRI, meningiomas are being discovered serendipitously in patients who are being evaluated for unrelated problems (e.g., head trauma, stroke). The size and location of the tumor, the presence or absence of mass effect and edema, and the age of the patient help determine proper management. Meningiomas with considerable surrounding edema can justifiably be removed after the first evaluation. Small asymptomatic tumors without mass effect can be followed clinically and with serial CT scans. Surgical resection is not indicated unless there is evidence of progression.

E. **Acoustic schwannoma**

1. **Incidence.** Schwannomas, tumors of the Schwann cells of peripheral nerves, commonly occur in the intracranial cavity, originating from the acoustic nerve at the cerebellopontine angle. Schwannomas are the most common cerebellopontine angle tumors, but meningiomas, gliomas, and cholesteatomas also may occur in this location.

   Acoustic schwannomas account for 8% of all brain tumors. They occur mainly in middle adult life and are rare in childhood. About 5–10% of patients with acoustic schwannoma have the central form of von Recklinghausen's neurofibromatosis. In these patients, the acoustic tumors are often bilateral and may be associated with multiple cranial and spinal schwannomas, meningiomas, and gliomas.

2. **Diagnosis.** The earliest symptoms of acoustic schwannoma are caused by impairment of the acoustic nerve (deafness, tinnitus, and unsteadiness), with trigeminal dysfunction (loss of corneal reflex, facial numbness), facial weakness and ataxia occurring later. The clinical features are described in more detail in Chap. 4. An MRI with contrast enhancement is the diagnostic procedure of choice and can detect even small intracanalicular tumors.

3. **Treatment**
   a. **Surgery**
      (1) Schwannomas are slow growing, and symptoms are usually present for months to years before the diagnosis is made. The tumors are usually encapsulated and compress but do not invade the adjacent neural tissue. Tumors less than 2 cm in diameter can usually be completely removed. Complete removal is seldom possible with large tumors. Thus, complete surgical excision and cure are often possible with early diagnosis (see Chap. 4).
      (2) Serious surgical morbidity also has been directly related to the size of the tumor, being less than 5% for tumors smaller than 2 cm in diameter and more than 20% for tumors greater than 4 cm in diameter. If left untreated, these tumors ultimately cause increased intracranial pressure and fatal brainstem compression. This underscores the importance of early diagnosis and treatment to reduce the morbidity and mortality of this disease.

(3) The surgical approach varies with the size of the tumor, the presence or absence of functional hearing, and the expertise of the surgical team. Recent advances in diagnostic and surgical techniques have resulted in improved ability to resect these tumors completely. Anatomic preservation of the adjacent facial nerve is usually possible, although permanent facial paralysis occurs postoperatively in many patients. Preservation of functional hearing after surgery can be expected in only a small proportion of cases.

b. Standard radiotherapy has **not** been of value in the treatment of incompletely resected acoustic schwannomas.

c. Stereotactic radiosurgery (the "gamma knife"—multiple highly collimated beams of gamma irradiation focused on the tumor) shows promise for treating elderly patients or patients with serious medical conditions that would increase the risk of surgery.

F. Pituitary adenomas

1. Classification. Pituitary adenomas can be classified on a functional (endocrine) or anatomic basis.

a. Functional classification

(1) Nonfunctioning (null-cell) adenomas.

(2) Hypersecreting adenomas (prolactin, adrenocorticotropic hormone [ACTH], or growth hormone). The prolactin-secreting and nonfunctioning adenomas are by far the most common pituitary tumors.

b. Anatomic classification

(1) Microadenomas (< 10 mm in diameter).

(2) "Diffuse adenomas" (surrounded by dura but with some suprasellar or parasellar extension).

(3) "Invasive adenomas" (infiltrating dura, bone, or brain).

2. Clinical features

a. Microadenomas will be asymptomatic unless they are hypersecreting tumors.

(1) Hyperprolactinemia can be determined by measurement of morning basal prolactin levels. Levels greater than 100 ng/ml (normal value is < 15 ng/ml) almost always indicate a tumor. Levels between 15 and 100 ng/ml can be due to a pituitary tumor but are more often caused by medications (e.g., phenothiazines, antidepressants, estrogens, metoclopramide) or disorders that interfere with normal hypothalamic inhibition of prolactin secretion.

(2) Hyperprolactinemia sometimes will cause no symptoms. In women it usually causes amenorrhea or galactorrhea (or both). Perhaps one-fourth of all women with secondary amenorrhea and galactorrhea have prolactin-secreting pituitary tumors. In men, the earliest symptoms of hyperprolactinemia are impotence and loss of libido. Gynecomastia and galactorrhea are much later manifestations in men.

b. Macroadenomas. Larger tumors compress the adjacent normal pituitary gland and can produce variable degrees of hypopituitarism; gonadotropin deficiency is usually seen before the development of corticotropin deficiency. Extension of tumor above the sella turcica will compress the optic chiasm. This causes progressive visual loss that often starts as a bitemporal superior quadrantanopia. Advanced cases will invade the cavernous sinus, third ventricle, hypothalamus, or temporal lobe. Most macroadenomas come to medical attention because of visual loss, while in 20% headache is the intital symptom.

c. Tumors that secrete ACTH or growth hormone are usually diagnosed while they are relatively small in size, since the striking endocrine disturbances (Cushing's disease or acromegaly) lead to early detection.

3. Diagnosis. High-resolution enhanced and nonenhanced CT scans with axial and coronal views can visualize the mass and the bony anatomy of the sella and sphenoid sinus. An MRI provides sagittal as well as coronal and axial views. The bony anatomy is not as well seen as on CT, but MRI provides images of the arteries adjacent to the pituitary to rule out an aneurysm mimicking a tumor.

4. **Treatment** of pituitary adenomas depends on the size of the tumor and the associated endocrine or visual disturbances (or both).

a. **Surgery.** Signs of significant extrasellar extension, such as involvement of the optic chiasm or cranial nerves, are indications for surgery. Since the introduction of the dopamine agonist **bromocriptine,** many patients with prolactin-secreting tumors who previously might have required surgery have been treated successfully medically (see sec. **III.F.4.c).**

(1) Transsphenoidal surgery has a much lower operative morbidity and mortality than the transcranial approach. With the use of the operating microscope, it is possible to dissect and remove both microadenomas and larger tumors while preserving a normal pituitary gland.

(2) Modern microsurgical technology has reduced the risk of operative morbidity in patients with pituitary tumors to 1%. After surgical decompression and tumor resection, visual improvement occurs in about 70–80% of patients, and vision may return to normal in up to 50%. The prognosis for visual recovery is best when the history of impairment has been brief. The endocrine status after surgery is also improved occasionally (e.g., fertility may return in 70% of patients).

(3) During surgery for pituitary tumors, patients are treated with corticosteroids as prophylaxis against adrenal insufficiency. The degree of pituitary impairment is reassessed postoperatively so that appropriate replacement therapy can be administered if it is indicated. Diabetes insipidus can occur after surgery, but it is usually transitory.

(4) Despite meticulous effort, it is often impossible to completely remove pituitary adenomas that have extended beyond the sella turcica; in such cases, the tumor probably will recur.

b. **Postoperative irradiation.** Radiation therapy has proved to be a useful adjunct in significantly reducing the rate of postoperative recurrence in patients in whom complete resection is not possible. In one series of patients, the recurrence rate was decreased from 42% to 13% by postoperative irradiation. Current practice is to administer 5000–6000 cGy over 5–6 weeks. The field size is determined by the radiographic and surgical findings. Stereotactic radiosurgery may have a role in treating small tumors (particularly those causing acromegaly or Cushing's disease) that have recurred despite microsurgery.

c. **Medical treatment with bromocriptine.** Dopamine is the hypothalamic neurotransmitter that normally inhibits prolactin secretion from pituitary cells. Bromocriptine is a synthetic dopamine agonist that causes a marked fall in prolactin levels in normal patients and patients with prolactin-secreting pituitary tumors.

(1) Pharmacologic therapy with bromocriptine should be the initial treatment for patients with a prolactinoma. Most prolactinomas can be successfully managed with bromocriptine (usual dosage, 2.5–5.0 mg tid) without surgery. In hyperprolactinemia with amenorrhea and galactorrhea, the symptoms are reversed in over 80% of women treated with bromocriptine, and fertility is restored.

(2) Patients with infertility must use barrier contraception during treatment. If pregnancy is desired, contraception is eliminated and the bromocriptine should be discontinued when menses are delayed by 48 hours. There is some apprehension about letting a patient with a prolactinoma become pregnant for fear of precipitating symptomatic tumor growth (during normal pregnancy, pituitary volume may double). Fortunately, this complication is uncommon, occurring in only 1% of women with microadenomas and 25% with macroadenomas. Bromocriptine appears to be safe in pregnancy and can be reinstituted if pregnancy occurs. Nevertheless, surgery is usually recommended for patients with macroadenomas who desire pregnancy.

(3) Large "diffuse" or "invasive" prolactin-secreting tumors may shrink dramatically during bromocriptine therapy, with resolution of visual field

and endocrine disturbances. Although in most centers surgery remains the primary treatment of choice in these patients, bromocriptine is a useful adjunct and may be the only treatment needed in many patients.

(4) Bromocriptine has also been used in addition to, or instead of, radiation therapy after subtotal removal of large tumors. Some nonfunctioning adenomas as well as growth hormone–secreting tumors also may respond favorably to bromocriptine, but this is less predictable. The somatostatin analogue octreotide may decrease the size of growth hormone–secreting pituitary tumors.

G. **Cerebral metastases.** Metastasis to the brain or meninges (or both) is a common complication of systemic cancer. Approximately 15–20% of patients dying of cancer will have brain metastases at the time of autopsy. The frequency of brain metastases varies considerably with the histology of the cancer. Bronchogenic carcinoma, breast carcinoma, and malignant melanoma are the cancers most likely to metastasize to the brain, but any malignant neoplasm may potentially involve the brain. When neurologic signs and symptoms develop in a patient with cancer, a variety of potential diagnoses in addition to cerebral metastasis must be considered (Table 11-3).

There are two major patterns of cerebral metastasis: the formation of a solid tumor mass lesion within the CNS parenchyma, and diffuse, sheetlike infiltration of the leptomeninges by tumor cells (meningeal carcinomatosis). These two entities may sometimes coexist in an individual patient, but their clinical picture and therapy differ considerably, so they are considered separately.

1. **Intraparenchymal metastases**
    a. **Diagnosis.** The formation of a solid mass lesion is the most common type of cerebral metastasis. Metastases reach the brain by hematogenous spread. The frequency of metastasis in these structures is roughly in proportion to the blood flow to the region (cerebral hemispheres > cerebellum > brainstem). These lesions cause symptoms through increased intracranial pressure, destruction of brain tracts, cerebral edema, or seizures (similar to primary brain tumors). Headaches, intellectual or behavioral changes, focal weakness, and unsteadiness are the most common presenting signs. In about 40% of cases of brain metastasis, a **solitary** lesion will be seen on CT scan; in the remaining 60%, **multiple** tumors are seen. MRI is more sensitive for demonstrating small tumors and may show multiple lesions when only one is seen on CT.
    b. **Cancer presenting as brain metastasis.** In patients with a known history of malignancy, the development of neurologic signs or symptoms prompts immediate investigation for evidence of CNS metastases. Occasionally a

Table 11-3. Common neurologic complications of cancer

Complications due to metastasis
   Intraparenchymal brain metastases (solitary or multiple)
   Meningeal carcinomatosis
   Spinal cord compression by epidural tumor
   Compression of nerves, roots, and plexuses
Nonmetastatic complications
   Metabolic encephalopathy (e.g., organ failure, hypercalcemia, electrolyte imbalance, drug-induced, sepsis)
   Infections (e.g., opportunistic CNS infections in an immunosuppressed host: fungal, viral, or bacterial)
   Vascular disorders (e.g., cerebral vein thrombosis, embolism from marantic endocarditis, coagulopathy, hemorrhagic diathesis)
   Complications of therapy (e.g., vincristine neuropathy, radiation myelopathy or plexopathy, cerebral radionecrosis)
   "Paraneoplastic syndromes" (e.g., Eaton-Lambert syndrome, carcinomatous cerebellar degeneration, polyneuropathy, limbic encephalitis)

brain metastasis will be the initial clinical manifestation of a systemic cancer The possibility of metastasis from an occult primary tumor therefore must be considered in every patient with brain tumor.

Thorough general physical examination and routine screening tests (e.g. urinalysis, stool guaiac, CBC, liver function tests, chest x ray) always should be performed before craniotomy for a (presumed) primary brain tumor. Since virtually all parenchymal brain metastases are hematogenous in origin, the lung is likely either the site of the underlying tumor or involved metastati-cally. Chest CT scan is the most useful diagnostic test in patients suspected of having a brain metastasis of unknown origin in whom the routine laboratory tests and chest x ray are negative. Further search for a primary tumor is seldom fruitful if there are no other clues on history or physical examination

c. **Corticosteroids.** High-dose corticosteroids are useful in palliating symptoms from cerebral metastases by reducing brain edema. Steroids should be started if the CT or MRI scan shows mass effect or edema and should be continued through the course of surgery or radiation therapy. "Mega-doses" of dexa-methasone (e.g., 25 mg q6h) may palliate intractable headaches or progressive deficits when "standard" doses (4–6 mg q6h) fail (see sec. **II.A.1**).

d. **Surgery for solitary metastasis.** If the brain metastasis is solitary and is in a relatively accessible location (e.g., frontal lobe, nondominant temporal lobe, cerebellum), total surgical excision is sometimes possible. The tumor resection is then followed by radiotherapy of the whole brain (2500–4000 cGy over 2–4 weeks) to suppress any residual tumor or micrometastases that escaped detection.

Surgery should be reserved for patients with a solitary metastasis who do not have extensive systemic disease or for patients in whom the histology of the CNS abnormality is in serious doubt. Recent randomized studies reveal that surgery provides symptomatic relief and longer survival in patients with solitary metastasis compared to radiation therapy alone.

e. **Radiotherapy.** Patients with multiple cerebral metastases and patients with solitary metastases who are not candidates for surgery should undergo cranial irradiation. This is one of the few instances in which radiotherapy is justified without a histologic diagnosis of the lesion. The presence of intra-cerebral metastases is documented on CT scan before starting radiotherapy. The radiation dosage is generally 2500–5000 cGy, delivered to the whole brain over 2–4 weeks.

The response to therapy varies somewhat with the histology of the under-lying tumor. For example, metastases from breast cancer and lung cancer generally respond better than metastases from melanoma or sarcomas. These patients are quite ill, and 20–30% may die within 1 month of radiotherapy or before therapy is completed. Nevertheless, most patients who complete the course of cranial irradiation experience at least some relief of symptoms. The 6-month survival rate in this group is 33%; the 1-year survival rate is 10%. Death is usually due to disseminated metastases rather than to brain disease itself. Patients who suffer recurrent cerebral metastasis after standard radiotherapy will experience limited if any benefit from a second course of treatment.

f. **Stereotactic radiosurgery** using a **linear accelerator** or a **gamma knife** unit may have a role in the initial management of small brain metastases, as a boost to whole-brain radiotherapy, and for treatment of recurrent tumors. Stereotactic radiosurgery refers to a single-fraction high-dose external irradi-ation administered to a very limited target volume of tissue. A single high-dose treatment can be tolerated provided that the volume of irradiated tissue is small and that dose falls off rapidly with distance from the target to avoid radionecrosis of normal brain. The indications, relative risks, and benefits of these techniques compared to traditional treatments have not been clearly defined.

g. **Systemic chemotherapy** (e.g., with methotrexate, 5-fluorouracil, nitrogen mustard, vincristine, and cyclophosphamide) has not proved useful in the treatment or prevention of cerebral metastases. For example, brain metastases often continue to grow despite shrinkage of pulmonary or hepatic metastases in patients undergoing chemotherapy. The difficulty has probably been related to the inability of most drugs to cross the blood-brain barrier. Although the nitrosourea derivatives, BCNU and CCNU, can cross the blood-brain barrier in therapeutic concentrations, few solid tumors are sensitive to the nitrosoureas. Thus, to date, these drugs have not been of great value in treating patients with brain metastases.

2. Meningeal carcinomatosis and meningeal lymphoma

a. Incidence. Infiltration of the leptomeninges by neoplastic cells (meningeal carcinomatosis), once believed to be rare, is now recognized as a common complication of career. Meningeal carcinomatosis occurs most often in patients with non-Hodgkin's lymphoma, small-cell lung cancer, breast cancer, malignant melanoma, GI neoplasms, and acute leukemias. Meningeal involvement is so common in acute lymphoblastic leukemia and transformed cell lymphomas that patients with these neoplasms are given prophylactic CNS treatment.

b. Descriptions. The neurologic signs of meningeal carcinomatosis are caused by focal infiltration of cranial or spinal nerves (e.g., radicular pain and weakness, facial palsy, oculomotor palsy) or cerebral symptoms (headache, change in mental status). This clinical picture is different from that generally associated with intraparenchymal metastases, in which tract findings (e.g., hemiparesis, hemianopsia) are common. Approximately one-third of patients with meningeal carcinomatosis will have concomitant parenchymal brain metastases.

c. Diagnosis

(1) The diagnosis of meningeal carcinomatosis is confirmed by demonstrating **malignant cells in the CSF.** In some patients, multiple CSF specimens must be examined cytologically before malignant cells are successfully identified. Malignant cells are not found in the CSF in tumors that are strictly intraparenchymal, but only when the meninges are invaded.

(2) The **CSF protein** is often elevated and the **CSF glucose** is often diminished in meningeal carcinomatosis, but these are nonspecific abnormalities. The CSF may show a modest pleocytosis or be relatively acellular.

(3) **MRI or CT scan** of the brain can be helpful in suggesting the diagnosis of meningeal carcinomatosis if contrast enhancement of the basal cisterns is seen. In most patients, however, CNS brain imaging studies are unrevealing or just show mild hydrocephalus. An MRI with gadolinium of the lumbar spine or myelography may reveal tumor nodules in the nerve roots of the cauda equina in many patients with meningeal carcinomatosis.

(4) The clinician must keep a high index of suspicion and obtain one or more CSF cytology specimens to make an early diagnosis of meningeal carcinomatosis.

d. Treatment. Since the tumor is seeded throughout the meninges, treatment must encompass the entire neuraxis.

(1) Craniospinal irradiation (e.g., 4000 cGy to the brain and 3000 cGy to the spine) might successfully control the disease. However, most cancer patients do not have adequate bone marrow reserve to tolerate such extensive radiotherapy. Even in those patients with adequate bone marrow reserve, craniospinal irradiation limits their ability to tolerate future systemic chemotherapy, so this treatment is not recommended. Since the tumor is located in the meninges, this is the one situation in which injection of antineoplastic drugs directly into the subarachnoid space makes therapeutic sense.

(2) Intrathecal chemotherapy. The current approach to treatment of meningeal carcinomatosis is local irradiation delivered to areas of focal disease (e.g., local irradiation for a facial palsy or cauda equina syndrome), and frequent intrathecal injections of **methotrexate, cytosine arabino-**

side, thiotepa, or combinations of these agents. Most patients requir whole-brain irradiation, especiallly when a concomitant intraparench; mal metastasis is suspected. Typical doses for intrathecal treatment a methotrexate, 12 mg; cytosine arabinoside, 50 mg; or thiotepa, 10 m; These agents are administered biweekly. Intrathecal methotrexate enter the systemic circulation and can cause severe mucositis and myelosup pression. This can be prevented by oral administration of citrovoru factor. Chemotherapeutic agents for intrathecal use must be injecte using preservative-free diluents. The preservatives in bacteriostatic d luents can cause severe CNS complications.

Pharmacokinetic studies have recently shown that smaller doses give at more frequent intervals increase the duration of CSF exposure to dru while avoiding excessively high peak concentrations that may contribut to neurotoxicity. One milligram of methotrexate given every 12 hou; may be as effective as 12 mg given biweekly but with a total lower dos and fewer side effects.

(3) Duration of treatment. When clinical and CSF cytologic improvemer occur, the response is generally seen after the first two to four doses intrathecal chemotherapy. Intrathecal therapy is then continued unt; the CSF is devoid of malignant cells, after which two or more "booste doses" are given. Monthly maintenance therapy is subsequently given fc 6 months to 1 year (or until time of relapse).

(4) Method of subarachnoid injection. After multiple LPs, the openin; pressure is often very low (due to CSF leakage), and it is often difficult t determine whether the drug is actually administered into the subarach noid space. Also, the distribution of drug throughout the CSF is ofte; erratic, even when lumbar subarachnoid injection is successful. Intraven tricular administration through an indwelling **Ommaya reservoir i** considered superior, since the drug reliably reaches the subarachnoi; space, there is better drug distribution after ventricular injection com pared with lumbar injection, and chemotherapy can be administered an; CSF sampled without the discomfort of multiple LPs. In inexperience; hands, however, the morbidity associated with the Ommaya reservoi (e.g., infection, misplaced ventricular cannula) can be prohibitive.

Flow imaging of the CSF using 111-indium DTPA injected through th; Ommaya reservoir allows detection of ventricular outlet obstruction o abnormalities of flow in the spinal canal or over the convexities.

(5) Technique for making intraventricular injections using the Ommay; reservoir

(a) The patient should be placed in a slight Trendelenburg position t; facilitate gravitational force for specimen collection.

(b) The scalp is shaved over the reservoir and the surrounding ski; carefully cleaned and draped to maintain sterility.

(c) The reservoir is punctured obliquely with a small-bore (23- or 25; gauge) butterfly needle to facilitate self-sealing. Local anesthesia i; not necessary and should not be used.

(d) A sample of CSF is obtained by gravity for cell count, cytologi; examination, culture, and so on.

(e) Using sterile technique, the syringe containing the medication i; attached. The drug is slowly injected over several minutes. The volume of fluid injected should be less than the volume removed.

(f) The reservoir capacity is 1.4 ml, and it should be flushed with 2–3 m; or CSF or preservative-free normal saline.

(g) With proper handling, well over 100 punctures can be made into the Ommaya reservoir without evidence of leakage. The procedure i; relatively painless, although transient dizziness, headache, or nause; can occur after injections. Tenderness, fever, meningismus, or persis tent headache should be properly evaluated to rule out infection of th; device.

(6) **Side effects.** Neurotoxicity is the major side effect of intraventricular chemotherapy, especially when combined with whole-brain radiotherapy. Many patients who survive for a year will develop a leukoencephalopathy with cognitive dysfunction.

(7) **Prognosis.** Early and vigorous treatment is often successful in reversing neurologic symptoms and prolonging life in patients with leukemia, lymphoma, or breast cancer. Approximately 50% of patients with meningeal carcinomatosis from breast cancer and over 80% of patients with meningeal lymphoma or leukemia show considerable clinical improvement. Patients with lung cancer or melanoma seldom have a favorable clinical response. A course of intrathecal chemotherapy and radiotherapy involves considerable patient morbidity. This treatment should therefore be reserved for patients whose general condition and prognosis warrant very aggressive therapy. The disease is inexorably progressive and leads to death within weeks from neurologic dysfunction in patients who are untreated or fail to respond to treatment.

IV. **Central nervous system tumors in children.** Cancer is the second leading cause of death in children between 1 and 15 years of age. Brain tumors are the second most common type of cancer in children. The majority of childhood brain tumors arise in the posterior fossa or sellar region. Early diagnosis may be difficult because tumors in these locations produce relatively nonfocal neurologic signs and symptoms.

A. **Cerebellar astrocytoma**

1. **Incidence.** The most common brain tumor in childhood is cerebellar astrocytoma. These tumors generally are slow growing and may have an excellent prognosis.

2. **Description.** Cerebellar astrocytomas occur most frequently in children between 5 and 10 years of age. In younger children, the only signs may be irritability, vomiting, and an enlarging head (due to obstructive hydrocephalus). More commonly, the presenting symptoms include those of a cerebellar hemisphere lesion, namely incoordination and ataxia.

3. **Surgery.** Cerebellar astrocytomas occasionally occupy the vermis, but most often they are located in the cerebellar hemisphere. At least one-half of these tumors have an associated cyst, and the neoplastic mass is sometimes confined inside a relatively small mural nodule. When this occurs, surgical excision of the nodule is curative.

4. **Recurrence.** Subsequent tumor recurrence is uncommon in patients who have gross total tumor removal, even after decades of follow-up. Thus, successful removal of an astrocytoma of the cerebellum often results in a complete and permanent cure. These patients require follow-up clinical evaluation and serial MRI or CT scans to promptly identify evidence of tumor recurrence. Further surgery or radiation therapy may be indicated in patients with recurrent tumor.

5. **Radiotherapy.** Some cerebellar astrocytomas have relatively little potential for sustained growth, and even incomplete removal can be followed by an apparent tumor arrest and prolonged survival. More commonly, however, incomplete removal of cerebellar astrocytoma is followed by regrowth that can be fatal. There is some evidence that radiotherapy prolongs survival in patients in whom additional surgical resection is not feasible.

B. **Medulloblastoma**

1. **Incidence.** Medulloblastoma is the second most common brain tumor in childhood. The tumor occurs mainly between the ages of 2 and 10 years. However, about 30% of cases of medulloblastoma occur during adolescence and early adulthood.

2. **Descriptions.** Medulloblastomas arise from primitive neuroectodermal cells in the cerebellum, and the majority of tumors originate in the midline of the cerebellum, occupying the vermis and fourth ventricle. Initial clinical features therefore are often due to noncommunicating hydrocephalus and increased intracranial pressure. In older (over age 6) age groups, medulloblastoma is more likely to occupy a lateral lobe, and signs of cerebellar involvement (staggering gait, ataxia) are more prominent.

3. **Metastasis.** Medulloblastomas that arise from the vermis often fill the cavity of the fourth ventricle and infiltrate into the brainstem. The tumor may also spread

en plaque over the surface of the cerebellum. Infiltration of the subarachnoid space, with metastatic spread of medulloblastoma through the CSF pathways (to the spinal cord, base of the brain, or cerebral hemisphere) is present in 25% of cases at the time of diagnosis.

4. **Surgery.** Because of the unfavorable location, invasiveness, and metastatic potential of medulloblastoma, complete surgical resection with cure is rarely achieved. Nevertheless, surgery is indicated in all patients to provide the correct histologic diagnosis, to resect the tumor mass to the greatest extent possible, and to reestablish the patency of the CSF pathways. In some patients, a ventricular shunt may be necessary for decompressive purposes.

5. **Radiotherapy.** Unlike most other primary brain tumors, medulloblastoma is a highly radiosensitive neoplasm. It is now recognized that irradiation of the entire neuraxis (spine and brain) is necessary in all patients, due to the marked propensity of medulloblastoma to metastasize by way of CSF. The current trend in treatment has been to increase the radiation to the maximum tolerable dose: 5000–6000 cGy to the local tumor and 3600 cGy to the brain and spinal cord, with reduced doses for children under 3 years of age.

6. **Prognosis.** Patients with localized disease and extensive surgical resection have a 5-year disease-free survival rate of 60% after craniospinal irradiation. The majority of patients in the latter category have presumably been permanently cured of medulloblastoma. Over 80% of the long-term survivors have no serious neurologic disability and lead normal lives. Patients with disseminated disease have a survival rate of less than 40% at 5 years after craniospinal irradiation.

7. **Chemotherapy.** Medulloblastoma has biologic features that make the tumor susceptible to chemotherapy: The tumor is rapidly growing and highly radiosensitive. The use of adjuvant chemotherapy with CCNU, vincristine, cyclophosphamide, procarbazine, mechlorethamine, or cisplatin can substantially improve the survival in patients with disseminated disease at the time of diagnosis. Multicenter trials are now under way to determine optimal chemotherapy regimens, whether all children with medulloblastoma should receive adjuvant chemotherapy, and management of patients with recurrent tumor.

8. **Neurocognitive sequelae** of craniospinal irradiation can be significant, particularly for younger children. Adjuvant chemotherapy may allow the doses of craniospinal irradiation to be reduced, thereby decreasing the incidence of side effects.

C. **Ependymoma**

1. **Description.** Ependymomas, tumors derived from ependymal cells, are a common brain tumor in childhood. About 70% of childhood ependymomas arise in the fourth ventricle, 20% in the lateral ventricles, and 10% in the region of the cauda equina. The median age of onset in these sites is 2, 6, and 13 years, respectively. Ependymomas also occasionally occur in adults, the spinal cord and lateral ventricles being the sites of predilection. The majority of ependymomas are histologically benign, although a few cases have an anaplastic histology picture and are designated as **malignant ependymomas** (ependymoblastomas).

2. **Surgery.** The treatment of ependymoma begins with the most extensive surgical resection possible. Unfortunately, ependymomas in the fourth ventricle are often attached to the floor of the medulla, making total removal impossible. These tumors often have produced ventricular obstruction and hydrocephalus by the time of diagnosis and a ventricular shunt may be necessary.

3. **Radiotherapy.** Ependymomas almost invariably recur after surgery, regardless of their initial site or "completeness" of excision. Postoperative radiation therapy (4500–6000 cGy over 4–6 weeks) prolongs survival significantly.

4. **Prognosis.** The 5- to 10-year survival rates after surgery and radiotherapy are around 70% for histologically benign ependymomas that have been "totally resected." Subtotally resected tumors have a poorer prognosis (30–40% at 5 years).

5. **Metastasis.** Like medulloblastomas, the **malignant ependymomas** have a tendency to **metastasize through the CSF.** In these cases, irradiation of the entire neuraxis may reduce the risk of tumor-seeding elsewhere in the CNS and

thereby improve the survival rate. For histologically benign ependymomas, the risk of metastasis through the CSF is minimal, and local irradiation to the primary tumor site is sufficient. The quality of life in the surviving patients is generally good and justifies an aggressive approach to diagnosis and treatment. Multicenter treatment trials are under way to determine whether pre- or postradiation chemotherapy can improve the prognosis in patients with ependymoma.

D. Brainstem glioma
   1. **Incidence.** Intrinsic brainstem gliomas occur most frequently in the first decade of life and account for nearly 15% of childhood brain tumors.
   2. **Diagnosis.** The **pons** is the site of predilection for brainstem gliomas. The typical clinical presentation of these tumors consists of progressive cranial nerve impairment (particularly of the sixth, seventh, ninth, or tenth cranial nerves), ataxia, hemiparesis, and headache. High-resolution CT scan or MRI can often visualize the tumor.
   3. **Surgery.** In the majority of patients, surgical verification of the diagnosis is neither indicated nor attempted, due to the inaccessible location of the tumor within the brainstem parenchyma. The diagnosis therefore rests on the characteristic clinical and radiologic picture.
   4. **Radiotherapy** to the brainstem (4000–6000 cGy over 4–6 weeks) results in significant clinical improvement in about 70% of patients with presumed brainstem gliomas; perhaps 25–30% of these patients will survive longer than 5 years without recurrent neurologic symptoms. The results are difficult to interpret, since histologic verification of tumor is lacking in most cases. Furthermore, the natural history of brainstem gliomas can be highly variable. The majority of patients with brainstem glioma suffer recurrence of progressive neurologic deficits within 18 months of radiotherapy.
   5. High dose **corticosteroids** will reverse many of the signs and symptoms, perhaps for a few weeks or months, but will not alter the fatal outcome.
E. Craniopharyngioma
   1. **Incidence.** Craniopharyngioma is a tumor that originates from squamous cell nests in the region of the pituitary stalk. This tumor occurs in both childhood and adulthood and accounts for about 3% of all brain tumors.
   2. **Description.** Craniopharyngiomas can cause symptoms by compressing the optic chiasm or tracts, by depressing pituitary or hypothalamic function, by increasing the intracranial pressure, or all of these. **Calcification** is seen in or above the sella turcica in more than 80% of children and 40% of adults with craniopharyngioma.
   3. **Surgery.** Craniopharyngiomas are biologically and histologically benign, but their intimate relation to vital neural and neuroendocrine structures presents a formidable obstacle to complete surgical resection. With the use of the operating microscope, some tumors can be completely removed. However, the realities of unavoidable operative morbidity and almost certain postoperative dependency on exogenous hormones detract from the success of surgical cure. Even when the surgeon believes that the tumor was completely removed, recurrent tumor will develop in 20–30% of patients within a few years of surgery. Many craniopharyngiomas can be only partially resected; after this, recurrence will be very likely.
   4. **Radiotherapy.** Postoperative radiation therapy can substantially delay (and in some instances eliminate) tumor recurrence in cases of incomplete surgical resection. Recent series report greater tumor control (of more than 10 years' duration in the majority of patients) after subtotal resection and postoperative radiotherapy.
F. Tumors of the pineal region
   1. **Description.** Tumors that arise in the pineal region occur mainly during adolescence and early adult life. These tumors usually produce symptoms by compressing the midbrain tectum (causing Parinaud's syndrome) or obstructing the aqueduct of Sylvius (causing noncommunicating hydrocephalus). Pineal tumors can also encroach anteriorly to involve the hypothalamus (diabetes insipidus, precocious puberty) or optic pathways.

2. **Histology.** Several biologically and histologically distinct tumors can arise from the pineal region to produce this clinical picture.

   a. The **germinoma** (also referred to as **pinealoma** or atypical **teratoma**) is the most common pineal tumor, accounting for more than 50% of cases. Germinomas arise from primitive midline germ cells in the pineal or hypothalamic regions.

   b. Other germ cell tumors, including **teratomas** and **embryonal carcinoma,** occasionally occur in this region.

   c. Tumors of the pineal parenchyma (the **pineocytoma** and **pineoblastoma),** glial tumors **(astrocytoma, ganglioneuroma),** and **epidermoid cysts** account for the remainder of these tumors.

3. **Treatment.** Ventricular shunting is usually the initial treatment for the signs and symptoms of increased intracranial pressure due to obstructive hydrocephalus. Cerebrospinal fluid **alpha-fetoprotein** and plasma beta–human chorionic gonadotropin levels may be elevated in patients with germ cell tumors. In this situation, radiation may be considered empirically, since germ cell tumors are highly radiosensitive. Otherwise, surgical exploration and complete resection of the tumor should be attempted if possible.

4. **Metastasis.** Malignant pineal region tumors can metastasize through the CSF. Cytologic examination of the CSF is important in planning treatment. Spinal irradiation is administered in addition to cranial irradiation if there is evidence of spinal seeding. Chemotherapy may have a role in the palliation of tumors that have recurred after surgery and radiation therapy.

V. **Spinal cord tumors.** Tumors occur much less commonly in the spinal region than in the brain in both adults and children, accounting for only 10% of all primary tumors of the CNS. These tumors are seldom fatal, unlike their intracranial counterparts, but they are extremely disabling. Prompt recognition and treatment can do much to relieve the morbidity.

A. **Spinal neoplasms**

   1. **Description.** If the lesion is extramedullary (e.g., not growing within the spinal cord parenchyma), the tumor will often produce symptoms by compression or destruction of nerve roots or bone before the spinal cord itself becomes involved. Intramedullary tumors often produce manifestations of disturbed spinal cord function from the outset. The clinical picture in individual patients depends on the transverse level of the tumor (cervical, thoracic, lumbar, sacral, or cauda equina), the topography of the tumor, peculiarities in the local blood supply to the spinal cord, and the speed of compression.

   2. **Diagnosis**

      a. The diagnosis of intraspinal tumor is suggested by **radiologic evidence** of bony erosion of the pedicles and intervertebral foramina (e.g., by a schwannoma) or bony destruction (e.g., by metastatic cancer or lymphoma).

      b. An **MRI** with surface coils and contrast enhancement has become the noninvasive modality of choice for evaluation of the spinal cord, epidural space, and paraspinous structures.

      c. **Myelography,** using a water-soluble agent, combined with high-resolution **CT** imaging of the spine provides detailed anatomic information. These studies localize the tumor and enable the physician to deduce whether the tumor is intramedullary, extramedullary-intradural, or extradural. Myelography is occasionally followed by rapid clinical deterioration due to increased spinal cord compression. Fortunately, with the advent of MRI, myelography is often not necessary in detecting spinal tumors.

B. **Primary intraspinal tumors.** The relative incidence of primary intraspinal tumors by histologic type differs quite markedly from that of intracranial tumors (Table 11-4).

   1. **Schwannoma**

      a. **Description.** The most common primary intraspinal tumor is the schwannoma. Schwannomas are extramedullary-intradural tumors composed of Schwann's cells, which can arise from spinal nerves at any level (cervical, thoracic, lumbar, or cauda equina) and most often arise from a posterior

Table 11-4. Relative incidence of primary intraspinal neoplasms

Tumor	Percent of total
Schwannomas	30
Meningiomas	26
Gliomas (ependymomas)	23
Sarcomas	11
Hemangiomas	6
Other	4

(sensory) nerve root. The most common initial symptom therefore is **pain** in a radicular distribution. Schwannomas grow slowly, and pain may be present for years before the correct diagnosis is made, especially when the schwannoma is in the relatively spacious lumbosacral region. Schwannomas of nerve roots in the relatively tight cervical region compress the spinal cord early in their course, however.

   b. **Treatment.** Spinal schwannomas usually can be completely excised and cured by **surgery.** In some patients, the tumor grows through the intravertebral foramen to form an extraspinal mass **(dumbbell tumors),** and a second operation is often necessary to remove the extraspinal portion of these tumors. Fortunately, a high degree of clinical recovery can be expected because the diagnosis is generally made before the spinal cord has been extensively damaged by pressure.

   c. **Recurrence** of schwannoma is likely only in cases in which total extirpation is impossible, as in very large tumors or tumors with extradural extension.

2. **Meningiomas**

   a. **Description.** Meningiomas are the second most common primary intraspinal tumor. Spinal meningiomas have a marked propensity to occur in the **thoracic spinal cord,** and they are rare below the midlumbar level. Like schwannomas, meningiomas ae slow-growing extramedullary-intradural tumors. The clinical picture usually evolves slowly over months to years before the diagnosis is made.

   b. **Treatment.** Spinal meningiomas usually can be completely **removed surgically.** The neurologic deficits are at least partially reversible, and the patient is thus cured of the disease. However, complete resection is often technically quite difficult to achieve without damaging the spinal cord, especially in tumors located anterior to the cord. In these cases, it may prove impossible or unwise to attempt complete tumor removal.

   c. **Recurrence** is likely in patients with partially resected tumors, but it does not become clinically evident for months or years.

3. **Astrocytomas and ependymomas**

   a. **Description.** The most common intramedullary spinal tumors are the gliomas, which comprise mainly ependymomas and astrocytomas. The ependymomas predominate in the cauda equina and lumbar region; the astrocytomas, in the cervical region. The clinical syndrome produced by these tumors is usually indistinguishable from that produced by extramedullary tumors. Spinal gliomas are slow-growing tumors, and a history of deficits of several years' duration is common.

   b. **Surgery.** Most spinal gliomas are invasive as well as expansive; unfortunately, complete surgical resection is possible in less than 20% of cases. Most intramedullary spinal tumors can be **"decompressed"** by means of a laminectomy, partial resection, and opening of the dura mater. Moreover, approximately 60% of intramedullary spinal tumors are also associatd with **syringomyelia;** in these cases, its cavity should be opened to allow drainage.

   These procedures are likely to produce some recovery of neurologic function if the tumor has not caused irreversible damage to the spinal cord. The prognosis depends on the growth rate of the tumor, and in many patients, th deficits progress slowly over several years.

   c. **Radiotherapy.** Postoperative radiotherapy to the spinal cord is thought t delay the onset of recurrent neurologic symptoms and is therefore recom mended for patients with partially resected intraspinal glioma. The spina cord tolerance to irradiation is less than that of the brain, and the maximur permissible tissue dose is 3500–4500 cGy, depending on the field size.

C. Metastatic spinal tumors

1. **Biology.** Metastatic tumors can reach the spinal cord by direct spread from a involved vertebra, by extension of tumor through an intervertebral foramen, o (uncommonly) by direct hematogenous spread to the extradural fat. Therefore metastatic neoplasms of the spine are almost always contained in the extradura space. The tumors that are most likely to spread to the spinal canal are **multipl myeloma, lymphomas,** and **cancers of the lung, breast, prostate, kidney, an sarcomas.** A favorable outcome depends on early diagnosis and treatment.

2. **Description**

   a. **Prodromal phase.** Perhaps 80% of patients with cancer who develop spina cord compression pass through a prodromal phase, which is characterized b severe **back pain, radicular pain,** or both. This pain precedes the onset o spinal cord compression by weeks to months in nearly all cases.

   b. **Stage or pain without neurologic deficit**

     (1) Unremitting **back pain** is always considered a serious symptom in cancer patient. Although cancer patients may have pain of benig musculoskeletal origin, this symptom is often the first indication o metastasis to a vertebral body or the epidural space.

     (2) Evidence of metastatic tumor (e.g., lytic or blastic **lesions in the vertebrae** a **paravertebral soft-tissue mass,** or a **positive bone scan**) should b sought diligently in cancer patients with back pain or radicular pain o both. If a tumor is found, a course of local radiotherapy, chemotherapy, o both, depending on the histology of the primary neoplasm, might effectivel relieve the pain and prevent eventual spinal cord compression.

   c. The **stage of spinal cord compression** usually begins with subtle **weaknes and/or numbness in the legs.** Hesitancy or urgency may lead to painles **urinary retention** with overflow. The tempo of neurologic progression i usually quite rapid, and over the next few days the patient becomes completel **paraplegic.** Metastic lung cancers, renal carcinoma, and lymphomas are sai to produce the most rapid progression to paraplegia. Thus, spinal cor compression is an **emergency.**

3. **Diagnosis.** The earliest signs and symptoms of spinal cord compression shoul promptly lead to spinal **MRI with gadolinium enhancement** or, if not available **myelography** combined with high-resolution spinal CT.

4. **Treatment**

   a. **Steroids.** There is experimental and clinical evidence that very high doses o corticosteroids relieve local spinal edema and, in some instances, may have significant oncolytic effect. Current practice is to start very large doses o corticosteroids (e.g., dexamethasone, 25 mg q6h) as soon as the diagnosis o spinal cord compression from metastatic tumor is suspected. This very larg dose is continued for several days and then reduced, often allowing the clinician to buy time while awaiting results of more definitive therap (radiotherapy or surgery).

   b. **Surgery and radiotherapy**

     (1) **Posterior decompression.** The majority of epidural metastases arise from the vertebral body and remain chiefly anterior to the spinal cord. The traditional surgical approach to the spine posteriorly via laminectom does not allow resection of major portions of most epidural metastases Postoperatively, local radiotherapy is administered to arrest furthe tumor growth (e.g., 3000 cGy given over 3 weeks, beginning about 6 day after surgery).

       Unfortunately, the results of this combined surgery and radiotherap approach are usually unsatisfactory. Surgical mortality and morbidity (e.g., poor wound healing, postoperative infection, worsening of neurologic deficits) are considerable. Retrospective studies of large series reveal that only 30–50% of patients with metastatic cancer of the spine have significant neurologic improvement (e.g., regain ambulation) after surgical decompression via laminectomy. The remainder are left with a stable deficit (about 40%) or continue to deteriorate (about 20%).

(2) Anterior decompression. New surgical approaches to decompress and stabilize the spine anteriorly rather than by traditional laminectomy are the optimal way to excise tumor and reduce mechanical distortion of the neural tissues. Initial reports of anterior decompression in patients with significant neurologic deficits are quite encouraging. This is the optimal avenue of therapy for patients with spinal cord compression whose overall medical condition and oncologic prognosis warrent aggressive intervention.

c. Radiotherapy alone. Most oncologists have realized that spinal epidural compression by radiosensitive tumors such as lymphomas can be managed effectively by radiotherapy without surgery. Recent data reveal that radiotherapy alone is as effective (or ineffective) as decompressive laminectomy followed by radiotherapy in treating epidural spinal compression, regardless of the underlying histology (e.g., prostate, lung, breast, or renal cancer). After both forms of treatment, the overall improvement rate was 40–50%, and the duration of clinical remission was similar. Patients with rapidly progressing neurologic deficits (weakness evolving over 48 hours) did as well or better when treated with irradiation alone as laminectomy-treated patients. Direct (anterior) resection and/or procedures to stabilize the spine are the only beneficial surgical procedures for most epidural metastases.

d. Prognostic features. The stage of underlying malignancy determines the patient's overall prognosis, and in some patients with widespread systemic cancer, it is appropriate not to treat spinal espidural compression at all.

(1) When the pretreatment neurologic deficit is complete (absolutely no motor, sensory, or sphincter function below the level of the cord lesion), the likelihood of significant recovery with any form of therapy is remote. Therefore, if treatment is to be undertaken, it should be initiated as soon as spinal epidural compression is detected clinically and confirmed radiographically.

(2) Patients with multiple myeloma, lymphoma, and breast cancer have a greater likelihood of responding favorably to treatment (whether radiation alone or surgery) than have patients with other cancers. Some patients will remain ambulatory for 1 year or more following radiotherapy for spinal epidural metastasis.

VI. Neurologic complications of radiation therapy

A. Delayed cerebral radiation necrosis can occur following radiation therapy to intracranial as well as extracranial neoplasms (e.g., nasopharyngeal or sinus cancers). This complication is related to the radiation dose, fraction size, and duration of therapy. Delayed radiation necrosis usually occurs within the portals of radiation, with most cases occurring within 6 months to 3 years of the last dose of radiation. Interstitial brachytherapy carries a high risk of radiation necrosis in the surrounding brain.

1. Cerebral necrosis after radiotherapy is being recognized more commonly now than previously estimated, particularly as the number of patients surviving more than a year or two after treatment increases.

2. Diagnosis. The symptoms of cerebral radionecrosis are those of an expanding mass. An MRI or CT scan cannot always differentiate between recurrent tumor and radiation necrosis. Positron emission tomography is very helpful in distinguishing tumor recurrence from necrosis but is not generally available.

3. Treatment. High-dose steroids can temporarily palliate the symptoms of delayed cerebral radiation necrosis. Surgical exploration and removal of the enlarging necrotic mass are necessary in many patients.

B. Symptomatic communicating hydrocephalus. A syndrome of progressive demen
tia, gait disturbance, and incontinence of urine can occur in patients who hav
received whole-brain irradiation for brain metastasis. A CT scan or MRI revea
ventricular dilatation, cerebral atrophy, and periventricular white-matter abno:
malities without a recurrent tumor. The symptoms begin 6–36 months (median 1
months) after treatment. Although the total dose of radiation therapy may not b
high in this group, patients with brain metastasis are often given relatively hig
daily fractions of radiation. This practice should be avoided in the safe an
efficacious treatment of low-risk patients with brain metastasis. High-dose steroi
and ventricular shunting offer significant but incomplete improvement in patient
with this syndrome.

C. Radiation-induced myelopathy
1. **Lhermitte's sign.** A sudden "electric shock" sensation precipitated by nec
   flexion commonly occurs after radiation therapy for neck or upper respirator
   tract tumors. This usually begins a few months after treatment and graduall
   abates within several months. Lhermitte's sign is **not** the harbinger of subse
   quent progressive spinal cord dysfunction following radiation therapy.
2. **Chronic progressive radiation myelopathy**
   a. **Description.** A chronic progressive myelopathy, with ascending paresthesia:
      predominantly spinothalamic sensory loss, spastic paresis, and sphincte
      dysfunction, can occur between 6 and 36 months (mean 12 months) afte
      radiation therapy to the mediastinum, cervical, or head and neck region.
   b. High radiation doses and overlapping ports increase the risk of radiatio
      induced myelopathy. The spinal cord is much more sensitive to the toxi
      effects of radiation than the brain. Individual variations in susceptibility t
      radiation damage may also be a factor.
   c. **Diagnosis.** The differential diagnosis includes spinal epidural tumor, a
      intramedullary spinal metastasis, meningeal carcinomatosis, necrotizin
      carcinomatous myelopathy (a paraneoplastic syndrome), and radiation mye
      opathy. Myelography and MRI in radiation myelopathy may be normal c
      show an atropic or swollen spinal cord. The CSF is usually normal.
   d. **Treatment.** There is no known effective therapy for chronic progressiv
      radiation myelopathy. A course of high-dose steroids is often administere
      particularly if the spinal cord appears swollen, but this produces transier
      benefit, if any.
D. Radiation-induced brachial plexopathy can occur following radiation therapy fc
breast cancer or Hodgkin's disease. Radiation with large doses per fraction (e.g
4500 cGy in 15 fractions) is more likely to cause this problem than treatment wit
small doses per fraction (e.g., 5400 cGy in 30 fractions).
1. **Description.** Tingling and numbness in the fingers and weakness in the hand o
   arm are the initial symptoms, beginning 1–5 years after radiotherapy to th
   region of the brachial plexus. The signs are usually referable to the uppe
   brachial plexus (C5–C6 dermatomes). Pain evolves only later in the course an
   is seldom the predominant symptom. The symptoms and signs slowly worser
   rendering the hand useless in many patients.
2. **Differential diagnosis.** Radiation-induced plexopathy must be distinguishe
   from metastatic tumor infiltrating the brachial plexus. Tumor infiltratio
   usually presents with severe pain followed by weakness and sensory loss in
   lower brachial plexus distribution (C7–C8–T1 dermatomes). A CT scan or MRI c
   the brachial plexus is useful but cannot always distinguish radiation fibrosi
   from tumor infiltration.
3. **Treatment.** Surgical exploration of the brachial plexus is necessary in som
   patients for diagnosis and treatment. Neurolysis or neurolysis plus omenta
   grafting does not stop the progression of deficits in radiation-induced brachia
   plexopathy but may produce pain relief.

Selected Readings

REVIEW ARTICLES

Black, P. M. Brain tumors. *N. Engl. J. Med.* 324:1471, 1991.

Clouston, P. D., et al. The spectrum of neurologic disease in patients with systemic cancer. *Ann. Neurol.* 31:268, 1992.

MALIGNANT GLIOMA

Committee on Health Care Issues, American Neurological Association. Chemotherapy for malignant gliomas. *Ann. Neurol.* 25:88, 1989.

Kornblith, P. L., and Walker, M. C. Chemotherapy for malignant gliomas. *J. Neurosurg.* 68:1, 1988.

PRIMARY CENTRAL NERVOUS SYSTEM LYMPHOMA

Hochberg, F. H., and Miller, D. C. Primary central nervous system lymphoma. *J. Neurosurg.* 68:835, 1988.

MENINGIOMAS

Black, P. M. Meningiomas. *Neurosurgery* 32:643, 1993.

PITUITARY ADENOMAS

Klibanski, A., and Zervas, N. T. Diagnosis and treatment of hormone-secreting pituitary tumors. *N. Engl. J. Med.* 324:822, 1991.

CEREBRAL METASTASIS

Patchell, R. A., et al. A randomized trial of surgery in the treatment of single metastasis to the brain. *N. Engl. J. Med.* 322:494, 1990.

Vecht, C. J., et al. Treatment of single brain metastasis: Radiotherapy alone or combined with surgery? *Ann. Neurol.* 33:583, 1993.

MENINGEAL CARCINOMATOSIS

Wasserstrom, W. R., Glass, J. P., and Posner, J. B. Diagnosis and treatment of leptomeningeal metastases from solid tumors. *Cancer* 49:759, 1982.

PINEAL REGION TUMORS

Edwards, M., et al. Pineal region tumors in children. *J. Neurosurg.* 68:689, 1988.

SPINAL TUMORS

Byrne, T. N. Spinal cord compression from epidural metastasis. *N. Engl. J. Med.* 327:614, 1992.

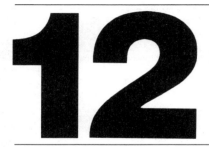

Trauma

Robert L. Martuza and
Mark R. Proctor

Severe Head Injury

I. **Background**
   A. **Severe head injury** is a problem of enormous magnitude. In adults, automobile and work-related accidents and, in children, accidents at play and falls account for most cases. Although methods of treating head injury have improved (e.g., nursing care, intracranial pressure [ICP] and vital sign monitoring techniques, control of brain edema, and expeditious imaging of intracranial mass lesions) and mortality has decreased, a substantial number of patients are left with varying degrees of disability. Even patients with only mild to moderate head injuries may have significant physical or neuropsychological deficits. Since many of these patients are unable to return to work, the economic consequences of head injury are staggering.
   B. **Classification.** Brain injury can be categorized as primary or secondary. Primary brain injury is damage that occurs as a result of the initial insult and is pathologically described as **diffuse axonal injury.** Secondary injury compounds primary injury and occurs as a result of intracranial complications (e.g., intracranial hematoma, brain edema, infections) or extracranial complications that affect delivery of oxygen and nutrients to the brain (e.g., pneumonia, pulmonary thromboembolism, hemodynamic instability). Each of these sequelae can alone or in combination lead to the demise of the patient. These complications must be diagnosed and treated vigorously, since the additive effect they have on the primary brain lesion increases the neurologic damage and resultant disability.
   C. **Initial management.** The final outcome following head trauma is related to the extent of parenchymal injury, the age of the patient, and the neurologic function at the time definitive therapy is instituted. Since only the last parameter is under partial control of the emergency room physician, it is essential that expeditious treatment be planned from the time of the accident and that evaluation and treatment proceed rapidly. Treatment should begin with a well-trained emergency medical team that is responsible for transporting severely injured patients. Whenever possible, the physician should be in contact with the emergency medical team to provide guidance regarding the need for intubation, intravenous volume expanders, or mannitol prior to the injured patient's arrival at the hospital. On arrival to the emergency room, the patient's respiratory pattern, skin color, pulse, pupil size, and level of consciousness should be quickly determined. This requires no diagnostic equipment and should take only a few seconds. The clinical tempo of the neurologic examination should be assessed, as deterioration during transport from the scene will mandate an especially efficient, rapid evaluation. The primary physician should determine how many doctors, nurses, and other personnel are available to help and assign appropriate tasks.
II. **Diagnosis**
   A. **History.** The ambulance team may provide information about the accident. Occasionally, a neurologic event such as a seizure, stroke, or subarachnoid hemorrhage may be witnessed to precede a motor vehicle accident, and the diagnostic possibilities will differ from the usual head injury. The neurologic state of the patient when first found is important to determine the rate and direction of change of neurologic

function. Such details and the current state of the neurologic examination in the hospital will determine the pace of the remaining evaluation.

B. **Neurologic evaluation.** If the patient is rapidly deteriorating, the neurologic evaluation should take only a few minutes; if the patient is stable, a more detailed examination is possible. It is useful to summarize the patient's presenting clinical status in the form of the **Glasgow Coma Scale (GCS) score** (Table 12-1). This simple score can be used quickly to define the severity of the injury and to estimate prognosis. Prior to assessing neurologic function, however, the basics of life support and resuscitation must be performed.

III. **Initial medical management for trauma patients**

A. **Airway.** An adequate airway is the first priority. It is essential for life. Additionally, hypoxia suppresses cerebral function and hypercarbia increases ICP. Together, these two factors make the neurologic examination prognostically inaccurate. If a patient is responsive and can protect his or her own airway, nothing further need be done. But the patient who is deteriorating or who is unresponsive will need to be intubated. When in doubt, it is best to intubate the patient, as hypocarbia is the most effective way to decrease ICP rapidly, thereby preventing secondary brain injury. Additionally, neuronal oxygenation is required to help prevent further cell injury or death. Generally, endotracheal intubation is used. With severe head injury there is a very high incidence of associated cervical spine injury. If the patient is hemodynamically and neurologically stable, it is wise first to do a lateral cervical spine radiograph with someone pulling the arms downward to exclude a cervical spine fracture; all seven cervical vertebrae and the cervicothoracic junction must be visualized. If a fracture is present, hyperextension of the neck, which is often necessary for intubation, can cause spinal cord damage, and nasotracheal intubation or fiberoptic intubation (if readily available) is preferred. If the patient is unstable and there is no time for a cervical spine x ray, a spine fracture should be assumed to be present until proved otherwise, and nasal intubation should be utilized. A word of caution is in order: In the presence of severe facial or basal skull fractures, nasal passage of any tubes may be difficult or dangerous. In emergency situations, it is sometimes necessary to perform a tracheostomy or a cricothyroidotomy, the latter technique having the advantage of speed and less blood loss.

B. **Breathing.** Once the patient is intubated, it is reasonable initially to use 100% oxygen at a volume and rate that will achieve hyperventilation. For the average

Table 12-1. Glasgow Coma Scale*

Best motor response	
6	Obeys commands
5	Localizes to pain
4	Withdraws to pain
3	Abnormal flexion
2	Abnormal extension
1	No movement
Best verbal response	
5	Oriented and appropriate
4	Confused conversation
3	Inappropriate
2	Incomprehensible sounds
1	No sounds
Eye-opening	
4	Spontaneous
3	To speech
2	To pain
1	No eye opening

* Glasgow Coma Scale (GCS) score equals the sum of the scores from each of the three groups.

adult, a rate of 12–14 breaths/min at a volume of 750–1000 ml is sufficient. Arterial blood gases should be checked as soon as possible.

C. Circulation. Severe head injury is often associated with loss of cerebrovascular autoregulation. Hypotension becomes equivalent to hypoxia, and brain function cannot be adequately assessed. It is essential to replace blood volume and to maintain an adequate blood pressure. An attempt is made to place a large-bore IV catheter in a nontraumatized extremity (an IV line placed into a severely injured limb will result in extravasation of replacement fluid into the soft tissues). If a peripheral IV is not easily placed, a subclavian or jugular vein catheter is placed, or an expeditious cutdown is performed. Generally, a subclavian catheter is preferable to a jugular line because it is less likely to interfere with further diagnosis and treatment of cervical spine or neck injuries. Blood is removed and sent for the following studies: CBC, prothrombin time, partial thromboplastin time, platelets, BUN, blood sugar, toxic screen, and clot to the blood bank for typing and cross matching.

The loss of cerebral autoregulation and the normal blood-brain barrier makes the brain more susceptible to edema, especially in the face of fluid resuscitation. Once the intracranial capacity to accommodate an increase in volume due to edema is overcome, ICP will quickly rise. For this reason, careful fluid resuscitation is crucial. If the patient has no evidence of hemodynamic instability, an attempt is made to maintain a normovolemic state. Although traditionally these patients were kept at two-thirds maintenance fluid, recent evidence suggests that euvolemia may provide better perfusion pressures to the brain while not increasing ICP. If hypotension is a problem, cautious volume reexpansion should be performed. If systemically indicated, packed RBCs are given. It is most advantageous to keep the hematocrit greater than 30 percent for neuronal oxygenation. If blood products are not required, the debate still exists as to whether to supply crystalloid salts or colloids. Recent evidence indicates that crystalloid fluids are adequate and should not unduly increase ICP.

D. Shock. If shock is present, its cause must be found in concert with volume administration.

1. Hemorrhagic shock. Even the most severe head injury only rarely is the cause of hemorrhagic shock. Such cases may be seen with serious transections of major scalp arteries, with penetrating lesions of the major cerebral venous sinuses, or rarely in infants with open cranial sutures where a significant percentage of blood volume can collect intracranially. However, it must be emphasized that these circumstances are unusual and the presence of shock suggests an associated injury with blood loss into the chest, abdomen, pelvis, retroperitoneum, or thigh. Physical examination and radiologic studies are needed, routinely including plain films of the chest, cervical spine, and pelvis. A bladder catheter is inserted. Peritoneal lavage or abdominal CT scan may be necessary to exclude intra-abdominal hemorrhage. Chest tube or chest CT scan may be necessary to rule out intrathoracic hemorrhage.

2. Spinal shock. Spinal injury must be excluded. Spinal shock is basically an acute sympathectomy and causes hypotension with a slow pulse rate. Intravascular volume expansion with or without the use of alpha-adrenergic agents or atropine is usually effective treatment.

E. Airway, breathing, and circulation (ABCs) are first priorities. Patients with mild injuries may require none of the previously mentioned treatments, whereas patients with severe injuries may require all of them. However, all trauma patients need consideration of these basics of care. If other physicians are present, they may attend to these matters while the neurologist or neurosurgeon is evaluating neurologic function. If the neurologist or neurosurgeon is the only physician present, the ABCs must be covered first; only then can a detailed neurologic evaluation be performed.

IV. Quick neurologic examination for the severely injured patient. A patient with an initial GCS of eight or less is defined as having a severe head injury. As indicated by the GCS, three parts of the physical examination are most useful for establishing rapid diagnostic and prognostic criteria. In true neurologic emergencies, this abbreviated examination may be all that is possible prior to operative intervention.

A. The level of consciousness is the most sensitive indicator of overall brain function.

and can be broken down into two components, alertness and content. Alertness reflects the level of brainstem ascending reticular activating system (ARAS) function, while content reflects the level of cortical function. It is a nonspecific indicator and can be severely altered by alcohol, toxins, hypotension, hypoxia, or trauma of the brainstem or cortex. The highest level of environmental awareness should be described. Brief descriptive phrases are more useful than terms such as "stupor" and "coma" and allow for comparison of serial examinations.

B. Eyes. Because the pathways involved in pupillary function and eye movements traverse large areas of the brain, eye signs are the second most important part of the neurologic examination.

   1. The size, shape, and reactivity of each **pupil** (direct and consensual) should be noted. Pupillary size is a balance between sympathetic pupillodilatory and parasympathetic pupilloconstrictor drives.

   a. A **sluggishly reactive or dilated pupil** suggests the possibility of cerebral herniation with compression of the third nerve on the tentorial edge. Because of their superficial location on the third nerve, parasympathetic pupilloconstrictor fibers are compromised before fibers controlling medial rectus function. This can be helpful in distinguishing compression due to herniation from associated local ocular trauma in which pupil and oculomotor function are equally affected. Progression from a normal pupillary examination to a unilaterally sluggish or dilated pupil is a cardinal indicator of herniation and mandates prompt aggressive intervention.

   b. **Pinpoint pupils** that are still reactive may occur with pontine lesions by segmentally compromising sympathetic tone. A unilateral **Horner's syndrome** can result from interruption of the sympathetic system anywhere along its course and in the setting of trauma should raise suspicion to the possibility of carotid artery dissection or cervical spine injury. The presence or absence of facial anhydrosis can help to localize the injury relative to the level of the carotid bifurcation. Toxins and metabolic insults only rarely affect pupillary function.

   2. Spontaneous **eye movements** should be noted. If they are full, further testing is not necessary. Conjugate lack of movement to one side may represent a visual field defect, parietal neglect, or an injury to a cortical brainstem gaze center. Unilateral lack of movement implies nerve damage intracranially or intraorbitally or an orbital fracture with muscle entrapment. If spontaneous eye movements are not full and the patient is unresponsive, the doll's-head maneuver, ice water calorics, or both are performed (see Chap. 1). In the traumatized patient, a cervical fracture must be excluded with a full cervical spine series before performing the doll's-head maneuver, and otoscopy should be done before caloric testing.

   3. The **corneal reflex** (afferent fifth cranial nerve, efferent seventh cranial nerve) is tested on each eye with a wisp of cotton. This reflex is often preserved even in rather deep levels of coma. A unilateral facial palsy may obscure the reflex, but the eye will roll superiorly **(Bell's phenomenon)** or a contralateral blink will be noted. Loss of this reflex carries serious prognostic implications, especially when associated with other signs of brainstem dysfunction.

C. Motor function. Mortality figures based on the GCS have been shown to correlate particularly well with best motor response. In the severely injured patient, fine testing of various muscle groups is not the immediate objective. Spontaneous movements of each limb are noted. If none are present, movements are elicited verbally or with the application of noxious stimuli to the chest or proximal limb, and the highest level of response is recorded. Purposeful movement is considered a coordinated response to a verbal command or noxious stimuli. Flexor posturing **(decorticate)** generally implies injury to the cerebral hemisphere or their peduncles. Extensor posturing **(decerebrate)** generally implies unopposed spinocerebellar tone secondary to injury between the pontine and midbrain levels. Flaccid extremities suggest intoxication, drug overdose, or medullary spinal cord injury. Focal weakness may represent local extremity or nerve injury, whereas a hemiplegia more likely reflects spinal, brainstem, or higher cortical dysfunction.

D. Changes in the examination suggesting any of the four types of **herniation**

syndromes must be recognized. When attributable to a discrete mass lesion, each these herniation syndromes may represent a true neurosurgical emergency. Eac syndrome can be associated with systemic hypertension, bradycardia and irregula respirations **(Cushing's response)**, a nonspecific indicator of increased ICP.

1. The **uncal herniation syndrome** of rostrocaudal deterioration is caused masses that compress the hemisphere laterally and push the inferomedial part the ipsilateral temporal lobe (uncus) through the tentorial incisura, compressin the midbrain. Progressive agitation may be a subtle sign of herniation, but it nonspecific. The ipsilateral oculomotor nerve is compressed early, giving rise pupillary dilation and fixation. Complete ophthalmoplegia follows along wit **contralateral** hemiparesis, due to pressure on the ipsilateral cerebral pedunci Consciousness deteriorates, often precipitously, secondary to compromise of th midbrain ARAS. Another neighboring anatomic structure that may be affecte is the posterior cerebral artery, compression of which gives rise to hemorrhag infarction of the posterior temporal and occipital lobes. Less commonly (abo 10%), the contralateral peduncle is crowded against the opposite tentorial edg producing a hemiparesis ipsilateral to the lesion and initial pupillary chang (Kernohan's notch phenomenon). If herniation is prolonged for more than a fe minutes, irreversible brainstem damage occurs due to pressure on and stretchin of the vasculature with consequent hemorrhagic infarction (Duret hemorrhages

2. **Central herniation syndrome.** Like the uncal herniation syndrome, centr herniation involves a transtentorial descent of brain matter with herniatic rostrocaudally through the incisural notch. Clinically, it may be difficult interpret, as it has few localizing signs other than progressive loss of consciou ness. Unlike in uncal herniation, the entire diencephalon (including the thala mus, hypothalamus, and basal nuclei) is the region at risk, and it may actuall buckle up against the midbrain. Hemorrhage and edema of the diencephalon ar classic, with vascular compression of the posterior cerebral and anterior choro dal arteries. High ICP is almost certain, with compression of subarachnoi cisterns and the cerebral aqueduct preventing egress of CSF. This tends worsen herniation.

3. **Cerebellar herniation syndrome.** Lesions in or around the cerebellum compres the pons from the rear or distort the medulla as the cerebellar tonsils are force downward through the foramen magnum. The heralding features of this ofte rapidly progressing syndrome are cerebellar ataxia, unilateral or bilateral sixt cranial nerve dysfunction (lateral gaze), diminishing level of consciousness, an the presence of Babinski's signs. A gaze palsy to the side of the offending mas followed by small but reactive pupils (pontine pupils), loss of all horizontal ey movement, and tetraparesis may then occur. Medullary failure with disordere respirations and apnea soon follow. This syndrome can progress very rapidly, sinc the amount of excess space in the posterior fossa is less than in the supratentoria regions; thus, expanding masses are not well tolerated in this region.

4. **Subfalcial (cingulate) herniation.** Expanding lesions in one frontal lobe ma herniate under the rigid falx cerebri. This herniation usually has no clinica expression and is noted only on CT scan or at autopsy, unless the herniatin mass compromises the anterior cerebral arteries and produces unilateral o bilateral leg weakness and abulia from inferior medial frontal lobe damage.

E. Once the quick neurologic examination of the severely injured patient is completec a decision must be made whether to proceed to surgery (e.g., persistent shock fror continuing abdominal hemorrhage), to CT scanning or other diagnostic tests, or t a more detailed neurologic examination. Although further examination is desirable the overall stability of the patient must be considered, and careful prioritizing i mandatory for the patient's well-being.

In the absence of other extracranial life-threatening injuries, surgical interven tion without first obtaining a **CT scan** is rarely indicated. The availability c extremely rapid new-generation CT scanners, coupled with the possibility of a fals or incompletely localizing neurologic examination, usually warrants temporizin with hyperventilation, mannitol, and diuretics long enough to obtain a scan. W generally prioritize a CT section through the level of suspected injury and the proceed to the operating room while awaiting reconstruction of the remaining images. One instance where it may be justified to proceed directly to surgery is in the patient with a rapidly progressing uncal herniation syndrome localizing to the side of a squamous temporal bone fracture that traverses the middle meningeal groove.

V. Detailed neurologic evaluation

A. Cerebral hemispheres. Once the level of consciousness is determined, a comprehensive mental status examination should be performed. Evaluation of new memory formation and recall of recent and past events is particularly important. Amnesia is a common sequela of head injury and may be retrograde (loss of recall of events immediately preceding the injury) or antegrade (loss of recall of events after the injury).

B. Cranial nerves

1. **Olfactory.** Testing of the sense of smell requires patient cooperation. A response to alcohol or ammonia reflects irritation of the nasal mucosa (trigeminal nerve). Although the olfactory bulb or nerve may be injured in ethmoid or orbital fractures, it is most frequently affected in patients with severe concussion. Up to one-third of patients recover the sense of smell spontaneously.

2. **Optic nerve and chiasm.** Visual acuity, visual fields, and visual neglect should be tested. Ophthalmoscopy should evaluate the cornea, lens, media, retina, and optic disk. Papilledema is uncommon in the acute setting. Subhyaloid hemorrhage may be due to nontraumatic subarachnoid hemorrhage. Retinal vein stasis suggests intracranial hypertension. Optic nerve and (more rarely) chiasmal lesions occur in approximately one-half of orbit fractures. The nerve most often is affected at the level of the optic foramen. Chiasmal damage usually follows serious trauma; however, optic nerve damage may be caused by more trivial injuries. Chiasmal lesions are sometimes associated with hypothalamic damage, which can cause diabetes insipidus. Unilateral, optic nerve damage results in deafferentation of the pupillary light reflex. This engenders a defective direct light reflex, but an intact consensual reflex (the so-called Marcus Gunn, or deafferented, pupil). Visual-evoked responses may be used to evaluate optic nerve function as well.

   Surgery is sometimes helpful in decompressing the optic nerve from bone fragments. Ophthalmologists also frequently advocate the use of high-dose methylprednisolone for optic nerve injury. The prognosis for return of vision is poor.

3. **The oculomotor, trochlear, and abducens nerves** may be affected within the orbit or at the superior orbital fissure in sphenoidal fractures. The sixth (abducens) nerve may be affected by a fracture at the apex of the petrous bone or by torsion, secondary to increased ICP, at the level of its passage into the cavernous sinus (Dorello's canal). Due to its long intracranial course, the sixth nerve is frequently affected by intracranial trauma. Pupillary and extraocular movement abnormalities may be produced by brainstem, particularly midbrain, contusion, and diplopia may be caused by orbital trauma and consequent misalignment of the visual axis.

4. **Trigeminal nerve.** The skin in each of the three divisions should be tested with a pin to differentiate a peripheral branch injury from a more central lesion. In most cases, the trigeminal nerve is affected in its extracranial course, the maxillary branch being the most frequently damaged. The gasserian ganglion can be damaged in basilar skull fractures or penetrating injuries. In the presence of trigeminal nerve injury, other neighboring structures (cavernous sinus; third, fourth, and sixth cranial nerves; and the carotid artery) are usually affected.

5. **Facial nerve.** An injury of the motor cortex or internal capsule produces a contralateral lower facial palsy sparing the frontalis muscle, which has bilateral cortical innervation. A brainstem injury, however, produces an ipsilateral palsy of the entire face and is usually associated with an alteration of consciousness and other brainstem signs. A peripheral facial nerve injury also causes an ipsilateral palsy but without other central signs. Although the facial nerve can be injured extracranially, it is more frequently damaged in its intrapetrosal course. Paresis (incomplete lesion) has a better prognosis than paralysis because

the latter often reflects anatomic transection of the nerve. Delayed onset may be a result of hemorrhage or edema within the canalicular portion of the nerve, and it may be amenable to treatment. Whether to decompress the nerve surgically is controversial; medical treatment with glucocorticoids has been suggested. To differentiate physiologic nerve impulse blockage from actual axonal degeneration, electric testing is required.

    a. Percutaneous nerve excitability testing may be done at the bedside and is simple to perform. It can detect evidence of axonal degeneration earlier than can electromyography.

    b. Electromyography is a useful tool for detecting evidence of axonal regeneration. It is important to determine whether the lesion is situated proximally or distally to the geniculate ganglion because the surgical approach is easier in the latter case.

    c. Evoked responses can be used to evaluate the blink reflex. This can be done using visual stimuli (afferent limb, second cranial nerve; efferent limb, seventh cranial nerve) or tactile stimuli (afferent limb, fifth cranial nerve; efferent limb, seventh cranial nerve—which is the corneal reflex). The integrity of the facial nerve and its brainstem connections can be evaluated in this way without the necessity of patient cooperation.

    d. Schirmer's test is based on the fact that the greater petrosal nerve leaves the facial nerve at the level of the geniculate ganglion. Thus, a strip of filter paper is left in the lower conjunctival sac, and the wetting by tears is compared between the two sides. Normally, the lacrimal gland can wet a minimum of 2–3 cm of the paper in 5 minutes, whereas the denervated gland will wet only a few millimeters.

  6. Vestibulocochlear nerve

    a. Vestibular branch. Posttraumatic dizziness and vertigo are discussed in Chap. 4.

    b. The **cochlear branch** often is damaged in temporal bone fractures, usually in conjunction with the vestibular branch, and is heralded by the presence of cerebrospinal fluid (CSF) otorrhea or hemotympanum. Whenever such a lesion is suspected, **audiometry** should be performed as soon as the patient's condition permits. **Brainstem auditory-evoked responses** may be used to evaluate the cochlear nerve and its CNS connections in patients who are unable to cooperate.

      (1) Posttraumatic tinnitus may result from injuries to the cochlear nerve, labyrinth, and blood vessels supplying the inner ear. There is no reliable treatment for traumatic tinnitus.

      (2) Hearing loss is usually mixed at the onset, with both conductive and sensorineural components.

        (a) In **conductive** hearing loss, the sound is impeded from reaching the receptor organ due to tympanic rupture, hemorrhage in the middle ear, or disorganization of the ossicular chain. The conductive component tends to resolve spontaneously in many patients by resorption of edema and hemorrhage, except in cases of ossicular chain disruption. An otology consultation is indicated.

        (b) Sensorineural hearing loss results from direct injury to the receptor organ, the cochlear nerve, or its neural connections. The prognosis in this type of hearing loss is poor.

  7. Injury to the **glossopharyngeal, vagus, spinal accessory, and hypoglossal nerves** is usually associated with severe basilar skull fracture. Most patients do not recover from this type of injury.

C. Cerebellar testing. Unilateral dysmetria or ataxia may indicate cerebellar injury. Nystagmus may also be present, but associated vestibular injury can be confusing. A worsening level of consciousness in the presence of cerebellar signs or a gaze palsy may indicate an expanding posterior fossa mass. The potential for apnea and death are ever present, and an expeditious CT scan is indicated.

D. Motor testing. The quick neurologic evaluation may miss an associated spinal, brachial plexus, or peripheral nerve injury. Detailed testing of all muscle groups should exclude these problems. Additionally, neurologic worsening from the time of the initial examination may be detected. Muscle strength should be graded as follows:

5 Normal
4 Overcomes gravity plus some resistance
3 Overcomes gravity but not added resistance
2 Moves horizontally but cannot overcome gravity
1 Trace movement
0 No movement

   E. Sensory testing. Pin, light touch, and position sense should be tested to anatomically localize any central or peripheral deficit. An injury initially thought to be a complete motor and sensory deficit on one or both sides may, on more detailed testing, demonstrate some preservation of light touch, vibration, or position sensibility, suggesting an anterior spinal cord syndrome.

   F. Reflexes. The presence of extensor plantar responses or ankle clonus suggests an upper motor neuron injury. Depressed reflexes are less specific and may be due to an overall depression of neurologic function, spinal shock, metabolic insults, or peripheral nerve damage.

   G. Traumatic carotid and vertebral artery dissection and/or thrombosis. Occasionally, the carotid artery is injured in the neck during trauma and may develop an intimal tear resulting in dissection, thrombosis, or both; an ipsilateral Horner's syndrome is often present. It may also be injured in or above the cavernous sinus. The vertebral artery may be damaged in a similar manner in fracture-dislocations of the neck. Physical examination may not be very sensitive for detecting arterial dissections, and cerebral angiogram or MR angiography may be necessary. The clinical syndromes associated with great-vessel thrombosis are covered in Chap. 10.

   H. Injury list. After the ABCs, the general examination, and either the quick or detailed neurologic examination, a list of definite and possible injuries should be made, with the most serious injury at the top. Ancillary studies should be planned to achieve a definite diagnosis for each problem, and the patient should generally be placed under the primary care of the specialist treating the most threatening organ injury.

VI. Ancillary tests
  A. Nervous system
    1. Cervical spine x rays. The lateral view is the most useful and should generally be taken with someone pulling the arms toward the feet to ensure that all seven cervical vertebrae and the cervicothoracic junction are visualized. The stiff cervical spine collar should not be removed until the cervical spine series is cleared. Fractures, displacement, and perispinal edema all suggest injury. Anteroposterior (AP) views may demonstrate a unilateral jumped facet not appreciated on the lateral view. The odontoid view is essential. With oblique views, the x-ray tube should be angled rather than the patient's neck turned. If an adequate set of cervical spine films cannot be obtained (especially in the unresponsive or unreliable patient, or the patient with neck pain), a spinal fracture must be assumed to be present until further studies are done. The CT scanning, intubation, and surgery may need to be done with the patient maintained in cervical immobilization.

    2. The **CT scan** has revolutionized trauma care and is the single most important neurologic study in the **acutely** head-injured patient. The CT scan is omitted only in mild head injuries where the history is not significant for loss of consciousness and there is no abnormality on neurologic examination. Rarely, in rapidly evolving deficits where surgery is immediately necessary and the neurosurgeon is nearly certain of the location of the lesion, the CT scan may be deferred. In this latter situation, a postoperative CT scan is obtained.

      a. Intracranial hematomas can be differentiated by their shape and location.

        (1) An **epidural hematoma** is biconvex and is bounded by the dural insertion at the cranial sutures. Only occasionally can high arterial pressures result in violation of the suture lines.

  (2) A **subdural hematoma** is not bounded by normal sutures and can cover most of the hemisphere but does not cross the interhemispheric fissure. Of note, it may not be radiographically possible to distinguish epidural from subdural hematoma.

  (3) Parenchymal hemorrhages can be at any location.

  (4) Subarachnoid hemorrhage is frequent in severe head injury and usually appears as a serpiginous density in the sulci, fissures, and basal cisterns and can track into the ventricular system.

 b. Contusions may appear as areas of increased, decreased, or normal density. They are most common at the temporal and frontal tips and may be associated with significant swelling.

 c. Increased ICP. Subfalcial herniation, obliteration of the basal cisterns with early temporal lobe herniation, or compressed ventricles suggest increased ICP.

 d. Intracranial air indicates a **sinus injury, penetrating wound,** or **compound fracture.** Foreign bodies should be noted. Associated orbital, facial, and soft-tissue injuries should be noted.

3. MRI

 a. Head injury. The MRI has replaced CT scanning as the study of choice for evaluating subacute and chronic head injury.

  (1) In **subacute injury,** MRI is superior for evaluating both hemorrhagic and nonhemorrhagic contusions, petechial shearing injuries commonly seen in the brainstem and white matter adjacent to the corpus callosum, and extra-axial fluid collections.

  (2) In **chronic injury,** parenchymal abnormalities, correlating with the patient's clinical state, are best visualized with MRI. Encephalomalacia is identified by increased signal on T2 resulting from increased tissue water content. Again, extra-axial fluid collections, such as **isodense chronic subdural hematomas** (isodense by CT criteria), are readily diagnosed with MRI.

  (3) In the **acute** setting, CT remains superior to MRI. Although MRI may give a better anatomic picture in some cases, it physically isolates the acutely traumatized patient from lifesaving modalities and personnel. However, MRI is utilized when the patient's clinical condition does not correlate with CT findings and for circumventing problems with bone artifact in the posterior fossa. The evolution of the MRI appearance of hemorrhage is characteristic and corresponds to the metabolic degradation of hemoglobin (Table 12-2).

 b. Spinal cord injury. With the advent of MRI-compatible halo tong systems, MRI is now the preferred method for evaluating acute, subacute, and chronic traumatic spinal cord injuries. Assessment of soft tissues by MRI is superior to both myelography and myelography/CT, while obviating the dangers of lumbar puncture in a patient who potentially has a spinal block or associated

Table 12-2. Evolution of the MRI appearance of hemorrhage

Metabolic change	T1	T2	Time from injury
Intact RBC with oxyhemoglobin	—	—	
Intact RBC with deoxyhemoglobin	—	↓	~8 hours
Intact RBC with methemoglobin	↓	↓	~3 days
Free methemoglobin	↓	↑	4–6 days
Hemosiderin/macrophages	—	↓	7–10 days
Edema	↑	↑	

Key: RBC = red blood cell; — = no change; ↓ = shortening (darker T2/brighter T1); ↑ = lengthening (darker T1/brighter T2).

intracranial mass lesion. Transport of a patient to MRI in the presence of an acute spinal cord injury is hazardous and should be supervised by a physician, preferably a neurosurgeon.

4. **Cerebral angiography** is indicated in the emergency evaluation of intracranial hemorrhage that could be due to an aneurysm or arteriovenous malformation, when there is the possibility that a penetrating injury has traversed a major cerebral artery resulting in a traumatic aneurysm, or when carotid or vertebral artery dissection is suspected. Cerebral angiography is rarely used when CT scanning is available for evaluating traumatic mass lesions, as it is more risky, time-consuming, and expensive while providing less information. If a CT scan is available at a nearby institution and the patient can be moved safely, this is often preferred.

5. **Skull x rays** are infrequently used to assess fracture of the cranial vault. A CT scan windowed appropriately for bone provides essential information regarding the possibility of fractures, while windowing for soft tissue demonstrates the integrity of the underlying parenchyma. Facial x rays, however, can be quite useful for assessing sinus injuries and orbital and facial fractures. If CT is not available, displacement of a calcified pineal gland or habenula on skull x ray may also provide evidence of an intracranial mass.

6. **Thoracic and lumbar spine x rays** are not done routinely. Their use is dictated by local pain or the presence of neurologic abnormality.

7. **Nuclear brain scanning, electroencephalography (EEG), and echoencephalography** have little use in the current management of head trauma. **Lumbar puncture** is generally contraindicated. Even if subarachnoid hemorrhage is suspected, a CT scan is the procedure of choice.

B. **Chest** injuries occur in 3% of all patients with severe head injuries. A chest x ray may reveal rib fractures, a pneumothorax, or a hemothorax. Neurogenic pulmonary edema can be caused by cerebral or spinal injuries. Thoracic spine fractures may be associated with a widened mediastinum, suggesting an aortic tear and requiring angiography.

C. **Abdomen.** Intra-abdominal injuries occur in 4% of patients with severe head injuries. A **KUB** (a plain film of the **k**idneys, **u**reters, and **b**ladder) and lateral decubitus film may show intra-abdominal air or fluid or retroperitoneal hemorrhage, but CT is much more accurate and reliable. Generally, IV and oral contrast are needed and should be given *after* a head CT has been performed, since contrast can confound the interpretation of hemorrhage.

D. **Kidneys.** Hematuria or retroperitoneal injury on abdominal films requires an intravenous pyelogram. Whenever possible, this should be done after the noncontrast head CT scan, since the contrast may make a cerebral contusion look like a consolidated hematoma.

E. **Extremities.** X rays should be taken of any limb where a fracture is suspected.

VII. **Emergency treatment**

A. **Severe head injuries should not be managed alone.** A neurosurgeon and other specialists should be involved as early as possible. A dedicated nurse should be with the patient at all times.

B. The **ABCs** must be instituted and monitored with frequent measurement of vital signs.

C. Deteriorating neurologic function despite adequate oxygenation and blood pressure suggests **elevated ICP** from a hematoma or cerebral edema. Treatment should include hyperventilation to achieve a PCO_2 of 28–30 mm Hg, elevation of the head to decrease venous pressure, and administration of mannitol (1 g/kg) as an IV bolus with furosemide (0.5 mg/kg). Prevent jugular kinking or compression, which can raise intracranial venous pressures. These measures are only temporary and will allow time either for CT scanning to achieve a definite diagnosis or to proceed to the operating room.

D. **Phenytoin** (Dilantin) may be given to prevent seizures. A loading dose of 15 mg/kg is given at a rate not in excess of 50 mg/min IV with appropriate cardiac monitoring.

E. **Disseminated intravascular coagulation** may occur in as many as half of patients with severe brain injuries, as the brain has very high levels of tissue thromboplastin. This is particularly serious in massive injuries associated with gunshot wound. Diffuse bleeding from puncture sites and lacerations may require the administratio of fresh-frozen plasma before the results of clotting studies are obtained. If sever units of fresh-frozen plasma do not permit clotting, 10 units of platelets empirically given. Coagulopathies may also account for a fraction of the "**spat hematomas** (late or delayed) seen in the head-injured patient.

F. **Steroids (dexamethasone).** The use of steroids in head injury is controversia Because steroids have not been shown to favorably alter outcome in head-injure patients and have associated potential deleterious side effects, they are used onl when specifically indicated. In selected patients, a 10-mg dose of dexamethasone administered initially, followed by 4 mg q6h. The source of therapy is brief, and th steroids are then weaned over several days.

VIII. **Neurosurgical treatment**

A. **Epidural hematoma**

1. **Description.** Epidural hematoma is a collection of blood situated between the sku and dura. It most commonly occurs in association with a temporal bone fractur that traverses the middle meningeal groove. Because the dura becomes adherer to the skull with age, epidural hematoma is seen rarely in the elderly. Earl recognition of this true neurosurgical emergency can lead to a lifesaving operatio

   a. **Lucid interval.** Classically, after an initial short period of unconsciousness o impact, there is a lucid interval followed by progressive impairment consciousness and contralateral hemiparesis. In more than 50% of patient: however, there is no lucid interval, and unconsciousness is present from th moment of the injury. Extreme headache is usual, resulting from th stripping of the dura from the inner table of the skull, and is usuall progressive when there is a lucid interval.

   The lucid interval suggests minimal initial parenchymal damage. Thi interval represents the time elapsed between the initial traumatic uncor sciousness and the beginning of diencephalic derangement produced b transtentorial herniation. The length of the lucid interval is variable. A absent or short lucid interval suggests that the bleeding is brisk and probabl arterial.

   b. **Hemiparesis.** The focal neurologic deficit generally is contralateral hemipare sis, due to the effect of the expanding mass on the origin of the corticospina tract. Hemiparesis ipsilateral to the clot may also occur due to compression c the contralateral cerebral peduncle against the tentorial edge (Kernohan' notch).

   c. **Seizures** can occur but are more common with parenchymal injuries.

   d. **Herniation.** Unilateral pupillary dilation is an indication of transtentoria herniation.

2. **Diagnosis.** The classic history of initial loss of consciousness, followed by a luci(interval and later by progressive obtundation and hemiparesis, is highly sug gestive of epidural hematoma. When a linear skull fracture is seen across th middle meningeal groove in plain skull x rays, a CT scan is the next step Sometimes, however, herniation has already begun by the time the patien reaches the emergency room and exploratory burr holes are necessary.

3. **Pathophysiology.** Epidural hematoma usually results from low-speed, blun head injury, as from falls or impacts with objects, and it is almost always associated with linear skull fracture. In the majority of patients, the bleeding vessel is the middle meningeal artery, vein, or both. The middle meningea vessels are injured when the fracture line crosses the middle meningeal groove ir the temporal squama. Classically, there is little associated underlying parenchy mal injury.

4. **Treatment.** In this situation, time should not be wasted on unnecessary tests

   a. In **herniating patients,** emergency treatment with intubation, hyperventila tion, and mannitol are instituted, and the patient is taken to **surgery.**

   b. If at all possible, and only if it can be done very quickly, a **CT scan** should be performed first to exclude other lesions instead of or in addition to an epidura hematoma.

B. Subdural hematoma
1. **Description.** Subdural hematoma is a collection of blood between the dura and the underlying brain and is present in 10–15% of patients with severe head injuries. Depending on the time interval between the injury and the onset of symptoms, subdural hematomas are clinically divided into acute (up to 24 hours), subacute (1–10 days), and chronic (more than 10 days). About one-half of cases (mostly the acute subdural hematomas) are associated with skull fracture. Subdural hematoma can be located anywhere within the cranial cavity, but it is most frequently over the convexity. About 20% are bilateral and may be caused by birth injury, bleeding diathesis, or blunt trauma without fracture.
2. **Pathophysiology.** Cortical veins going to the dura or dural sinuses, or vascular tears in contusions and lacerations, are the most common sites of bleeding. They are often associated with cerebral contusions and edema. The CT scan may show mass effect and midline shift in excess of the thickness of the hematoma due to the associated brain injury.
3. **Specific types of subdural hematomas**
   a. **Acute subdural hematomas** are frequently the result of high-speed impacts, such as automobile accidents. Associated severe primary brain damage is the rule. The ultimate outcome is related to age, neurologic function at the time of surgery, time course from injury to operation, and the amount of underlying parenchymal injury. Overall mortality is about 50%. Nonremitting coma from the moment of impact is suggestive of acute subdural hematoma. The distinction between an acute subdural hematoma and an epidural hematoma is often difficult or impossible to make on clinical grounds.
   b. **Subacute subdural hematomas** are suspected when, after several days of headache or diminished alertness, deterioration of consciousness develops. In all other respects, this type of hematoma resembles the acute variety.
   c. **Chronic subdural hematomas.** In contrast to the other hematomas, chronic subdural hematomas may follow trivial trauma, at times unnoticed by the patient or not witnessed by family or friends. A gradual drift into stupor or coma, occasionally preceded by headaches, is common. Mental changes may be prominent and simulate dementia, psychiatric disorders, or drug toxicity. In infants, chronic subdural hematoma is most common between 2 and 6 months of age and often is caused by accidental or inflicted head injury (i.e., "shaken baby syndrome"). In this age group, the clinical picture is one of increasing ICP with vomiting, lethargy, and irritability; an increasing head circumference; and a bulging fontanelle. Seizures are common as well. In cases of suspected abuse, one must look carefully for associated retinal hemorrhages and long-bone fractures. Rotational acceleration can easily tear the superior cortical veins as they enter the superior sagittal sinus. Brain atrophy associated with aging, prolonging the trajectory of these veins, probably makes them more susceptible to rupture. This would explain the significant proportion of cases of chronic subdural hematoma in elderly and alcoholic patients following minor degrees of head injury or with no antecedent trauma. In nonfatal cases, the evolution is toward encapsulation of the clot in a progressively more fibrous capsule, lined with vascular granulation tissue. The dural or parietal layer of this capsule is much thicker than the arachnoidal or visceral layer. The contents of the hematoma vary from thick and tarry dark fluid with fragments of dissolving clot at the onset to thinner and clearer fluid at later stages. These contents are thought to increase in volume due to transudation of plasma and small hemorrhages from the highly vascular lining membranes.
   As the interval lengthens from the time of injury, the CT density of the hematoma changes from hyperdense to isodense to hypodense relative to brain. At the isodense stage, a sizable hematoma may not be detected by CT scanning unless IV contrast is administered to enhance the vascular chronic membrane. This is one reason why **MRI** has supplanted CT as the study of choice for evaluating subacute and chronic subdural hematoma. If MRI is not available, contrast CT, nuclear brain scanning, or arteriography can help to secure the diagnosis.

4. Treatment

a. **Acute subdural hematoma.** Surgical treatment is usually necessary. Acute intraoperative and postoperative cerebral edema often requires ICP monitoring and aggressive treatment.

b. **Chronic subdural hematoma**

(1) In **reliable patients** for whom good follow-up is possible, small chronic subdural hematomas may be followed by serial neurologic examination and CT scans. Many such patients can be managed successfully without surgery, and the lesion resolves spontaneously.

(2) In **patients with severe or progressive deficits** or in individuals who cannot be followed reliably, **surgical treatment** is recommended. Burr holes under local or general anesthesia can be used for drainage of fluid when the CT scan shows a hypodense collection; this treatment often results in a permanent resolution of the hematoma. In a few patients, repeat drainage via burr hole(s) is necessary. In patients with hyperdense CT collections, or where burr hole drainage is ineffective, craniotomy and evacuation of the solid clot are needed.

(3) **Children with open fontanelles.** The head is shaved and prepared with iodine. An 18- to 22-gauge short-beveled subdural needle with a stylet is introduced at the lateral corner of the anterior fontanelle at least 3 cm from the midline. If the fontanelle is small, the needle is introduced through the coronal suture. The needle is advanced slowly until the dura is punctured, and it is secured by the examiner's finger against the scalp. The stylet is then removed and fluid is allowed to drain. **Suction should not be used on the needle.** Subdural taps are repeated as often as is necessary to relieve symptoms or signs of increased ICP. If repeated subdural taps have failed and further treatment is necessary, temporary shunting procedures and occasionally craniotomy may be indicated.

C. Intracerebral hematoma

1. **Description.** The term *intracerebral hematoma* refers to hemorrhage larger than 5 ml within the brain substance (smaller hemorrhages are called **punctate** or **petechial**). The symptoms vary with the location of the hematoma. In the absence of prolonged initial unconsciousness, there may be a lucid interval with progressive headaches, and progressive contralateral hemiparesis may occur if the hematoma is in the appropriate site. Stupor that progresses to coma will develop if the diencephalon is displaced by the mass effect. Occasionally, a lucid interval with later deterioration suggests a **spat (late) hematoma,** despite absence of evidence for hemorrhage on an earlier CT scan. Approximately 13% of spat hematomas occur because of a coagulopathy; the etiology of the remaining 87% is unclear.

2. **Diagnosis.** A **CT scan** is the most useful study for demonstrating acute intracerebral hematoma.

3. **Pathophysiology.** Intracerebral hematomas are frequently located in the temporal and frontal lobes. Traumatic cerebellar hematomas are rare.

4. **Treatment.** For small hemorrhages, treatment consists of observation and supportive measures. Careful attention to blood pressure should be maintained, as hypertensive episodes can lead to rehemorrhage. Large intracerebral hematomas in eloquent areas of the brain may be treated with hyperventilation, mannitol, and steroids with ICP monitoring in an effort to avoid surgery. Surgery is indicated for large accessible hematomas in patients with serious neurologic derangement and mass effect or in those with neurologic deterioration or ICP elevation despite medical therapy. Temporal lobe hematomas are especially dangerous, as uncal herniation can lead to rapid progression to coma and death.

D. Intraventricular hemorrhage

1. **Description.** Intraventricular hemorrhage may occur following trauma or subarachnoid hemorrhage. In most patients, the CT scan shows blood density in the occipital horns. In others, small amounts of blood may block the aqueduct or fourth ventricle, or larger amounts may occlude the lateral ventricles at the foramen of Monro, causing acute hydrocephalus.

2. **Pathophysiology.** If no parenchymal injury is present, intraventricular hemorrhage may be associated with headache but no neurologic dysfunction. The block of CSF outflow leads to increasing obstruction without lateralizing signs. Lateral rectus weakness or diminished upgaze may be noted. At this stage, deterioration can proceed rapidly to respiratory arrest and death.

3. Minor hemorrhage without hydrocephalus will resolve spontaneously; for larger hemorrhages, an external **ventriculostomy** is generally necessary and is usually placed under local anesthesia in one or both frontal horns. This allows for CSF drainage and ICP monitoring. After several days, when the blood clears, the ventriculostomies are removed, and in many patients, a permanent shunt is not necessary.

E. **Skull fractures without underlying hematomas** may be closed (skin intact) or open (laceration overlies fracture). Closed fractures usually need no further treatment unless they are depressed and represent a local mass lesion or represent a significant cosmetic defect. Surgical elevation is then necessary. In contrast, open fractures almost always need neurosurgical care, since the dura may be lacerated and bacteria, dirt, and other foreign substances may lead to delayed infection. A CT scan is done and neurosurgical exploration, debridement, and repair are performed. Prolonged antibiotics are generally not necessary.

1. **Description.** Basal skull fractures may be anterior, suggested by **raccoon eyes** or CSF rhinorrhea, or posterior, suggested by **Battle's sign** or CSF otorrhea. Skull x rays or CT scan may show an air-fluid level or opacification of the mastoid air cells or the frontal, ethmoidal, or sphenoidal sinuses. Anterior basal skull fractures involving the anterior or middle fossa often injure the olfactory nerve, while posterior fractures most often injure the facial and vestibulocochlear nerves as they course through the petrous bone. **Leakage of CSF** frequently accompanies basal skull fractures. To differentiate blood from bloody CSF rhinorrhea, one can perform the "halo" test (a drop of CSF on a cloth sheet should form a double ring resembling a halo). To differentiate CSF from mucus, one can check the fluid for glucose and chloride content. The CSF is normally hyperchloremic with respect to serum, and glucose should be about two-thirds of the simultaneous serum glucose.

2. **Treatment.** The presence of any skull fracture suggests a significant impact, and all patients should be admitted to the hospital. Uncomplicated patients are monitored and may be treated with analgesics (acetaminophen, 650 mg PO q4h, and/or codeine, 30–60 mg PO q4h; aspirin and other nonsteroidal anti-inflammatory drugs are avoided because of their potential inhibition of platelet function). They can be discharged the next day. More complicated patients are admitted for variable lengths of time. Most CSF leaks will stop spontaneously with head elevation. Profuse or persistent leaks require continuous lumbar drainage or surgical repair to prevent meningitis.

F. **Scalp lacerations** in the absence of an underlying fracture may be debrided, irrigated, and sutured. If a fracture is present, a penetrating injury must be excluded. Treatment for tetanus must be given (see Chap. 16). Prophylactic antibiotics are used for contaminated wounds.

IX. **Nonoperative injuries.** The initial concern of the physician dealing with head trauma is the exclusion of an expanding mass lesion such as an epidural or subdural hematoma. This concern is justified by their immediate threat to life and function and the availability of a specific treatment, namely surgery. Yet traumatic hematomas are present in the minority of cases of head injury. **The most common problems following head injury are concussion, contusion, and cerebral edema.**

A. **Concussion**

1. **Description.** A concussion is reversible physiologic change in nervous system function without a gross anatomic abnormality. The 10-second knockout punch in boxing is a classic example. Consciousness is lost or impaired, and retrograde or anterograde amnesia (or both) may occur. Generally, no focal deficit is present. More severe concussion, as from a high-speed motor vehicle accident, may be associated with neurologic impairment for more extended periods of time, with recovery evolving through a period of restlessness and agitated confusion to

gradually increasing periods of rational behavior until normality returns.]
children, the syndrome often consists of lethargy, irritability, pallor, a
vomiting.

2. **Pathophysiology.** Rotational acceleration, provoked by sudden head motio
   induces a swirling movement of the hemispheres around the relatively fix
   diencephalon. This instantaneously deranges the function of the ARAS ar
   results in loss of consciousness. Linear acceleration and deceleration, producir
   complex intracerebral pressure changes, also may be operative in certain case
   The typical concussion involves no grossly observable anatomic abnormalit
   The CT scan is normal, although subtle changes may be seen on MRI. Derang
   ments at a cellular level may be present, accounting for the immediate neur
   logic impairment, the potential for delayed cerebral edema, and the cumulati
   effects noted in boxing and the long-term effects seen in the "postconcussio
   syndrome."

B. Contusion

1. **Description.** The term *contusion* refers to bruised necrotic cortex and whi
   matter, with variable amounts of petechial hemorrhages and edema. Subarac
   noid bleeding of variable magnitude is common. The clinical state in brai
   contusion is similar to that of concussion, but brain contusion is usually mo
   severe and has associated focal neurologic deficits.

2. **Pathophysiology.** Contusion may result from direct bruising of the brain at th
   site of impact (coup), fragments of bone under depressed fractures, or injury a
   the pole opposite the impact (contrecoup). The orbital surface of the frontal lobe
   and the frontotemporal junction of the hemispheres often are affected due t
   violent displacements of the brain against bony irregularities of the orbital ro
   or the lesser sphenoid wing.

3. **Treatment.** Most contusions are amenable to medical treatment; however, i
   must be recognized that extensive contusions with edema may represent foc
   mass lesions, and surgery must be considered when a noneloquent damaged are
   (frontal or temporal tip) is a potential threat to life or other neurologic functior

C. Cerebral edema

1. **Description.** Edema represents an excess accumulation of water within the brai
   tissue and is seen on the CT scan as a hypodense area with associated mass effec
   Cerebral edema may be associated with any of the operative or nonoperativ
   posttraumatic lesions already discussed and often represents a cause of progres
   sive neurologic worsening or even death from uncontrollable elevated ICP.

2. **Pathophysiology.** Several hypotheses have been studied regarding the causes c
   cerebral edema and include
   a. Obstruction to venous outflow from mass lesions with elevated ICP.
   b. Cellular metabolic derangements associated with dysregulation of the norma
      sodium-, potassium-, and water-pumping mechanisms.
   c. Breakdown of the blood-brain barrier.
   In head trauma it is not certain which of these factors is the most critical, an
   all may be present to a variable extent.

X. Medical treatment.
Once a surgically treatable mass lesion has been excluded, medica
measures are instituted. The patient who is stunned for a few seconds but who has n
loss of consciousness and has a normal neurologic examination may be discharged i
the care of a reliable friend or relative who is willing to make frequent observations o
the patient over the next 24 hours. We discharge patients with a **"head trauma sheet"**
that describes potential signs and symptoms of delayed neurologic dysfunction. Th
patient with loss of consciousness (even if transient) or with severe headaches i
observed further in the hospital. Often an overnight stay will suffice. For those with
more severe and persistent impairment of neurologic function, admission to ar
intensive care unit is generally necessary, and the following measures are instituted

A. Airway.
Although the airway was initially considered when the patient first arrive
in the emergency ward, it must continually be assessed. The patient who did no
require intubation may become less responsive or may not be able to protect the
airway, and intubation may be needed. Soft-cuff endotracheal tubes may be left in
place for 1 week or more without difficulty. A nasotracheal tube is often better

tolerated. Frequent suctioning with sterile technique is essential. If intubation is required for a week or more, due to persistent coma or because of copious secretions or other pulmonary problems, tracheostomy is advisable.

B. Breathing. If the patient does not have evidence of elevated ICP, normal ventilatory levels are appropriate. Episodes of acute neurologic deterioration are most quickly treated by hyperventilation using a hand-controlled Ambubag. For patients with persistent elevation of ICP, hyperventilation may be necessary to achieve and maintain a normal ICP. Acutely lowering PCO_2 to below 25 mm Hg is avoided because a paradoxical rise in ICP secondary to tissue ischemia–induced vasodilation can result. Chronically lowering PCO_2 to less than 28 mm Hg is usually avoided. The PO_2 should be kept higher than 90 mm Hg. Positive end-expiratory pressure (PEEP) may be needed to normalize PO_2. If PEEP is kept less than 10 mm H_2O, it is generally safe, but rises in ICP can be produced even at these levels.

C. Circulation. An arterial line is helpful for the patient with persistent coma and provides continuous blood pressure monitoring and multiple intermittent blood gas determinations. In the presence of head trauma, normal mechanisms of cerebral autoregulation are often inoperable, and extremes of blood pressure should be avoided. Hypotension may cause worsening of neurologic function or even ischemic stroke. Systolic pressures less than 95 mm Hg require the placement of a central venous pressure catheter to guide volume replacement to avoid exacerbation of cerebral edema from fluid overload. In patients with a history of cardiac disease, a pulmonary artery catheter may be preferable. Phenylephrine (Neo-Synephrine), dopamine, or other appropriate pressors as a continuous IV drip may be necessary for blood pressure support. Hypertension is also potentially hazardous and can cause an elevation in ICP and hemorrhage into contused brain. A systolic pressure of greater than 170 mm Hg adds little to cerebral perfusion and should be avoided. If agitation is the cause, sedation may suffice. A new mass lesion or hydrocephalus should be excluded as the cause of new-onset hypertension. Labetalol, 5–10 mg IV, may be used. Nitroprusside or nitroglycerin should be infused IV only if ICP is not a problem or if it can be closely monitored, since either drug can elevate ICP. If intravascular volume expansion is required, colloid or crystalloid may be employed. Generally, an isotonic crystalloid salt solution is used for gentle rehydration, with bolus colloid infusion (i.e., blood or albumin) for acute hydration.

D. Intracranial pressure. Elevated ICP from cerebral edema, extensive contusion, or hematomas not amenable to surgery is the most common serious problem associated with severe head injury. Intracranial pressure monitoring devices allow the physician to react quickly to increased pressure in an attempt to prevent secondary tissue injury from pressure-induced ischemia. Patients who are responsive and can be followed adequately by the neurologic examination usually do not require ICP monitoring. Those in coma (GCS < 8), however, generally require some form of monitoring of ICP. A number of systems are available. An intraventricular catheter provides accurate pressure monitoring and allows CSF to be drained to relieve sudden episodes of elevated ICP. Disadvantages of the catheter include risk of hemorrhage from insertion through traumatized brain, the potential for worsening midline shifts, and the risk of ventriculitis. Both epidural and subdural monitors are also available. The simplest and most widely used are the fiberoptic subdural device, which once placed requires no further calibration, and the open bolt connected to a strain gauge. Newer strain gauge models are also currently in clinical trials, which may offer further advantages. Although small amounts of CSF may be drained through the open bolt system, the effect is usually negligible. Due to compartmentalization of the brain, it should be recognized that a fiberoptic or bolt ICP measurement in the frontal region can be normal, yet the patient may develop progressive temporal lobe herniation. Therefore, clinical evaluation should still predominate whenever possible.

Although transient ICP elevation may be associated with neurologic deterioration, persistent elevations about 18 mm Hg result in diminished cerebral perfusion pressure (CPP equals mean arterial blood pressure minus mean ICP; see Chap. 1) and may be associated with a worse neurologic outcome. Treatment should include the following sequential measures:

1. **Elevate the head of the bed.** This should be part of the general care of the head-injured patient. It promotes venous drainage and often will suffice to decrease the ICP. Avoidance of jugular compression also allows for improved venous drainage.

2. **Ventricular drainage.** If a ventricular catheter is present, the venting of a small amount of fluid is the quickest method to lower ICP. Too much drainage may cause ventricular collapse and catheter blockage. If the catheter is not present, it may be needed if other methods fail to decrease ICP.

3. **Hyperventilation** with an Ambu bag will quickly lower ICP and may suffice to stop a transient ICP elevation or will buy time to institute other measures. For chronically elevated ICP, longer-term hyperventilation with a PCO_2 of 28–30 mm Hg may be needed.

4. **Mannitol** appears to enhance circulation by decreasing ICP as well as by a direct effect on cerebral perfusion in the microcirculation. Acute elevations of ICP are effectively treated with 100–200 ml of 20% mannitol. The effect is not immediate but results are usually seen within 20 minutes and last for 2–6 hours. Some patients require 100 ml q4h to maintain an ICP less than 15–20 mm Hg, in which case serum electrolytes and osmolarity should be checked frequently and hyperosmolarity (> 310) mOsm) should be avoided.

5. **Furosemide** (0.5 mg/kg, or 20–40 mg for the average adult) can be given IV in concert with mannitol for acute episodes to hasten the reduction of ICP.

6. **Barbiturates.** If the listed measures have been ineffective, 50–100 mg of pentobarbital can be given as an IV bolus and repeated qh as needed to maintain ICP below 15–20 mm Hg. Arterial pressure, ICP, cardiac output, and pulmonary capillary wedge pressures should be monitored. The most common complication of barbiturate therapy is hypotension, which can occur despite maintenance of adequate blood volume and cardiac output. Lowering of systolic blood pressure below 80 mm Hg should be avoided and limits the usefulness of barbiturates in some patients. The major disadvantage of barbiturate therapy is that the neurologic examination is suppressed or even nullified. Indeed, pentobarbital-induced coma with a burst suppression EEG pattern is often the end point of barbiturate therapy. However, the pupils usually remain small unless herniation is present. Therapy is continued with daily laboratory examination of pentobarbital levels until the ICP has been kept below 15–20 mm Hg for 24 hours. The barbiturates are then weaned, which may require 1–2 days for full reversal of drug effect.

   In addition to the effect on ICP, barbiturates may provide cerebral protection by blocking free-radical production, thus decreasing brain damage caused by these agents, and by decreasing cerebral metabolic oxygen consumption.

7. If a sudden marked rise in ICP has caused neurologic deterioration or has required most or all of the above measures, a repeat **CT scan** should be done to exclude a newly developed hemorrhage or hydrocephalus.

8. **Steroids** have not been shown to favorably alter outcome in most head-injured patients and may in fact have a deleterious effect secondary to steroid-related side effects. Their use is controversial, and we opt to avoid their use in this setting unless specifically indicated.

E. **Urinary drainage.** In the acute setting with vascular instability or when osmotic diuretics are being used, a continuous bladder catheter is needed. This should be discontinued as soon as possible in favor of a condom catheter or intermittent catheterization to reduce urinary infection.

F. **A nasogastric tube** is useful to evacuate stomach contents in the acute setting and later to administer antacids, medicines, and nutrition.

G. **Nursing care** should include adequate hand and foot restraints to prevent self-injury or pulling out tubes, frequent turning (q2–3h) to prevent decubitus ulcers, and sterile endotracheal suctioning of secretions. Therapy to prevent flexion contractures is also crucial.

H. **Fluids and electrolytes.**

1. **Maintenance** intravenous administration of 0.45% sodium chloride in 5% D/W (or its equivalent) supplemented with potassium chloride, 20–40 mEq/liter, is

utilized with the rate dependent on the ICP and on frequent measurements of serum electrolytes, osmolarity, and BUN. It is desirable to keep osmolarity above 290 mOsm and sodium above 140 mOsm for the first week after a severe injury to prevent exacerbation of cerebral edema. For intravascular volume expansion, colloid or crystalloid may be utilized, and packed RBCs should always be considered if hematocrit is less than 30%.

2. **Diabetes insipidus** may result from acute transection of the pituitary stalk or from elevated ICP compromising the stalk or its vasculature. Diagnosis is made by documenting a high-volume, hyponatremic urinary output in the presence of serum hypernatremia and hypertonicity. It is necessary to exclude diuresis due to mannitol or other diuretics or to fluid overload. Treatment initially consists of adequate fluid replacement, followed by pitressin or desmopressin (DDAVP), a synthetic substitute with less effect on blood pressure.

3. **Inappropriate antidiuretic hormone secretion** may also be noted and may be due to hypothalamic injury. The ensuing hyponatremia in the presence of concentrated urine may aggravate cerebral edema, depress neurologic function, or precipitate seizures. Usually, restriction of free water will suffice for treatment. Occasionally, furosemide diuresis is necessary. Only in rare severe cases is hypertonic saline administration necessary.

I. **Nutrition.** In the acute setting, nutrition is not a consideration, but serious trauma increases metabolic needs and decreases the immune response so that total parenteral nutrition should be started as soon as is feasible. If GI function is adequate, a soft flexible nasogastric tube is used. If not, intravenous alimentation is given. The goal is an intake of 2500 kcal/day or approximately 150% of the patient's baseline needs.

J. **Seizures.** Prophylaxis of seizures in a patient who has not had a seizure is controversial; however, the development of a seizure can acutely elevate ICP, and seizure prophylaxis with phenytoin (5 mg/kg/day) is given at most centers. Acute seizures are treated as described in Chap. 6.

K. **Gastrointestinal ulceration** is common in patients with severe head trauma and may be aggravated by steroids. H_2 blockers, ranitidine (150 mg q12h) or cimetidine (300 mg qid), and antacids are utilized to neutralize gastric pH. Generally, ranitidine is preferable to cimetidine, as it has fewer encephalopathic side effects. Gastroprotective agents such as sucralfate, 1 g PO qid, may also be used.

L. **A bowel regimen** is required in comatose patients and should include stool softeners, rectal disimpaction if necessary, and enemas if required.

M. **Pneumatic compression boots (Airboots)** are used routinely in the immobilized patient in an attempt to protect against lower-extremity deep venous thrombosis and the associated risk of pulmonary thromboembolism.

XI. **Delayed complications of head injury**
  A. **Posttraumatic epilepsy**
    1. **Description.** A proportion of head-injured patients will develop posttraumatic seizures, which can be classified as **immediate** (occurring at the time of or within a few minutes of injury), **early** (occurring within the first week), or **late** (occurring after the first week). Care must be exercised to ensure that the process is truly epileptic, distinguishing it from other paroxysmal disorders such as vasovagal syncope and anxiety attacks. The incidence of posttraumatic epilepsy varies markedly with the mode of injury (i.e., whether the injury was penetrating or blunt).
      a. The overall incidence of posttraumatic epilepsy in **penetrating injuries** is about 50%. Factors that influence the likelihood of seizures are the **extent** of the lesion, as measured by neurologic deficit (e.g., hemiparesis), **infection,** and the **location** of the lesion (lesions around the rolandic region have the highest propensity for becoming epileptogenic).
      b. **Blunt injuries** are more common in nonmilitary settings. The incidence of posttraumatic epilepsy in this group is about 5%, with exacerbating factors including hemorrhagic contusion or dural tear from a depressed skull fracture.
    2. **Pathophysiology.** Immediate seizures do not necessarily predispose to subsequent seizures. They are generally a nonspecific reaction to head trauma but may

represent an intracranial hematoma. Early seizures reflect the initial brain damage and are more common in children, provided that the injury is relatively minor. Moreover, early seizures are a well-recognized antecedent of late seizures. In addition to the occurrence of early seizures, depressed skull fractures and intracranial hematomas are associated with a high incidence of late posttraumatic seizures.

3. **EEG.** In most cases of blunt head injury, the EEG cannot help to determine which individuals will develop posttraumatic epilepsy. However, its predictive capacity is much better following penetrating injuries. Early tracings habitually show alpha suppression and focal theta or delta slowing unilaterally or generally.

4. **Pattern of seizures.** Although some early seizures tend to begin focally, most seizures (early and late) are generalized from the onset. The epilepsy remits (the criterion of "remission" being the occurrence of a 2-year seizure-free period) in 50–75% of cases.

5. **Treatment**
    a. **When to treat.** If traumatic unconsciousness has been brief and there is no hematoma, parenchymal injury, or neurologic deficit, no treatment is given. In patients with cerebral contusion, prolonged unconsciousness, and hematoma, many clinicians administer phenytoin prophylactically for a 1-week period (loading dose of 15 mg/kg, or 1000 mg in adults, over the first 24 hours then a maintenance dosage of 5 mg/kg, or 300–400 mg, daily in adults IV or by means of a nasogastric tube). Blood levels should be checked periodically (see Chap. 6).
    b. **Length of treatment.** Current data do not support the prophylactic use of anticonvulsants for longer than a 1-week period in patients who have not experienced seizure activity. If immediate seizure activity was present or the patient is at high risk, a 1- to 3-month course of anticonvulsants may be continued. For patients who develop posttraumatic epilepsy, a carefully tailored regimen should be instituted with one or more of the many existing anticonvulsants. Although phenytoin is effective in reducing seizure activity in the immediate posttraumatic period, it is often not the most appropriate drug for prolonged use. It is also important to avoid stopping anticonvulsants abruptly, since this may be associated with the recurrence of seizures. Anticonvulsants may be discontinued gradually over 2–3 months.

B. **Postconcussion encephalopathy.** See Chap. 3.

C. **Infection.** Meningeal and encephalic infection may occur after head injury, especially after compound and basilar fracture. These are discussed in Chap. 8.

D. **Leakage of CSF** is a frequent complication of basilar skull fracture. It will often stop spontaneously. When it does not, continuous lumbar drainage may decrease the pressure sufficiently to allow the tear to seal. If this fails, the location of the dural tear must be found and surgically repaired. Radionuclide-labeled materials placed in the CSF may be used to help localize the site of the leak.

Spinal Cord Injury

Since World War II, the creation of centers that specialize in spinal cord injuries has improved their treatment.

I. **Mechanisms of injury**
    A. Automobile accidents, falls, sports (e.g., diving), industrial accidents, and gunshot and stab wounds are all causes of spinal cord injury. Most of the lesions are in the lower cervical cord (C4–C7, T1) and the thoracolumbar junction (T11–T12, L1). The thoracic spinal cord is less frequently affected.
    B. Factors that set spinal cord injuries apart from cranioencephalic injuries are
        1. The high concentration of important neural tracts and centers in a structure of relatively small diameter.
        2. The position of the cord within the vertebral column.
        3. Pecularities of the spine such as canal size.

    4. Presence of osteophytes.

    5. Variability of vascular supply.

  C. Table 12-3 demonstrates the anatomic relationships of the cervical spinal segments to the corresponding vertebral bodies, nerve roots, and neurologic functions. Note that roots C2–C7 exit superior to their respective vertebral bodies, while all other nerve roots of the spinal cord exit inferior to the vertebral body.

  D. The effects on neural tissue are most important in spinal injuries. The cord and roots are injured by the following four mechanisms:

    1. Compression by bone, ligaments, extruded disk material, foreign body, and hematoma. The most severe damage is caused by bony compression, compression from a posteriorly displaced vertebral body fragment, and hyperextension injuries.

    2. Stretching of tissues. Overstretching that causes disruption of tissue usually follows hyperflexion. The stretch tolerance of the cord may decrease with age.

    3. Edema. Cord edema appears soon and produces further impairment of capillary circulation and venous return, compounding the primary injury.

    4. Circulatory disturbances are the result of compression by bone or other structures of the anterior or posterior spinal arterial systems.

 II. Immediate care of the spinal cord–injured patient. The aim is to prevent further damage to the spinal cord by all possible means. A certain proportion of spinal cord injuries are worsened by improper handling of the patient in this stage or by the effects of hypotension or hypoxia on already compromised neural tissue.

  A. Move the patient carefully if a spinal lesion is suspected.

  B. Place the patient on a firm, flat surface for transport. If a cervical lesion is suspected,

Table 12-3. Relationship of spinal segments, vertebral bodies, nerve roots, and their functions

Spinal segment	Vertebral body	Nerve root	Muscle	Reflex	Sensory
C1	C1				
		C2			
C2	C2				
		C3			
C3	C3				
C4		C4			
	C4				
C5		C5	Deltoid		Shoulder
	C5				
C6		C6	Biceps	Biceps	Radial forearm, thumb, index fingers
	C6				
C7		C7	Triceps and wrist extensors	Triceps	Index and middle fingers
C8					
	C7				
		C8	Intrinsics		Little, ring ± middle fingers; ulnar hand
T1					
	T1				
		T1	Intrinsics		Ulnar arm

a person should be assigned to ensure ability of the patient's head during move
ments. Many sophisticated modalities now exist for transferring the patient wit
minimal spinal disturbance.

C. Pillows, rolled blankets, or sandbags may be used at the patient's sides to preven
lateral displacements.

D. Cover the patient with blankets to avoid loss of body heat.

E. Transfer the patient to an acute care hospital or to a center that specializes in spina
cord injuries.

III. Care of the neural lesion

A. Spinal cord concussion

1. **Description.** Spinal cord concussion is a state of transient loss of cord functio
   due to trauma with or without associated fracture or dislocation. Immediat
   flaccid paralysis occurs. Recovery is complete in a matter of minutes to hour:
2. **Pathophysiology.** Violent pressure waves propagated through deep tissues ar
   believed to transiently change the normal properties of tracts and neurona
   groups.
3. **Treatment.** Fracture or unstable dislocation must be excluded. If recovery i
   complete, no further treatment is necessary. If recovery plateaus with a persis
   tent deficit, a compressive lesion must be excluded.

B. Spinal cord contusion and transection. In these conditions, there is some discern
ible anatomic change of the spinal cord, although there may be functional
complete transection with few pathologic changes. The cord is rarely completel:
severed. Delayed loss of neurologic function can occur early or late. The early losse
are usually caused by spinal cord edema or by hemorrhagic necrosis of central gra:
matter. This can lead to a neurologic deficit extending to a higher level than th
initial injury. However, one must always exclude delayed hematoma, disk fragment
or an unrecognized fracture as other treatable causes. Because time is so crucia
immediate exploration for treatable lesions is mandatory. If complete paralysis an
sensory loss are present for longer than 48 hours, the chances for functiona
recovery are minimal, and the spinal cord changes are assumed to be anatomi
rather than physiologic.

1. In **cord contusion,** early changes include edema, petechial hemorrhages, neu
   ronal changes, and an inflammatory reaction. At later stages, the cord may b
   reduced to a fibrotic structure, and the pathologic changes may extend above an
   below the damaged segment. Late deficits are usually a result of the formation c
   intramedullary cysts or syringomyelic cavities. The neurologic syndromes tha
   result from spinal cord injury are varied, but a few are well established.
2. **Complete functional cord transection**
   a. **Spinal shock.** At first there is immediate flaccid paralysis and sensory los
      below the level of the lesion. In the immediate postinjury period of neurogeni
      shock, priapism is often present in males, and the bulbocavernosus reflex i
      lost. After this initial period of several hours, the bulbocavernosus reflex wil
      return, but most other reflexes remain absent through the period of spina
      shock. This state usually lasts 3–6 weeks, but sepsis, malnutrition, or othe
      complications may prolong it for months.
   b. **Increasing reflex activity.** Spinal shock is replaced by gradual return and a
      eventual increase of reflex activity. In cervical lesions there is an initia
      tendency to flexion that later is followed by extension. The presence o
      internal stimuli, such as urethritis, cystitis, and decubitus ulcers, provoke
      flexor spasms, which if repeated tend to fix the posture in flexion. The **mass
      reflex** is the most dramatic manifestation of increased flexion activity. I
      consists of contraction of the abdominal muscles, triple flexion of the lowe
      limbs, profuse perspiration, piloerection, and automatic urination in respons
      to stimuli below the lesion.
   c. **Sensation.** In incomplete lesions there is usually some recovery of sensatio
      after a variable interval of time. Complete lesions show no recovery.
   d. **Pains.** Radicular pain due to root involvement may be present for weeks o
      months. More frequently, however, a more severe type of pain, commonl:
      described as a dysesthetic burning, occurs below the lesion level. This pai

lasts longer and may be resistant to narcotics. Note that pain, whatever its nature, is markedly influenced by the patient's emotional state.

e. **Autonomic disturbances**

(1) **Temperature regulation.** Sweating is decreased or absent below the level of the lesion if it is above T9–T10. If the lesion is above C8, all thermoregulation is lost. It is not uncommon to see wide fluctuations of body temperature, especially in response to sepsis. The profuse sweats seen in these patients are reflex in nature and are triggered by impulses from the bladder or rectum (distention). Hyperhydrosis is another manifestation of this hyperreflexic state.

(2) **Blood pressure regulation.** Orthostatic hypotension is caused by a lack of reflex contraction of the capacitance vessels in response to postural changes. If the patient is tilted up, a precipitous drop in blood pressure occurs, which may lead to unconsciousness. Episodes of paroxysmal hypertension also occur, usually in response to a distended bladder or rectum.

(3) **Bladder regulation.** Disturbances of bladder function and its result, chronic renal failure, are the most frequent causes of death in these patients (for details on neurogenic bladder, see Chap. 17).

(a) **First stage.** Immediately following cord damage, reflex bladder function, as with other reflexes in spinal shock, is abolished. There is marked atony and overdistention of the bladder, and overflow voiding occurs. This stage may last days to weeks, depending on the same factors operative in spinal shock (e.g., age, associated diseases, malnutrition, sepsis).

(b) The **second stage** varies according to the location of the lesion. In lesions above the lumbosacral segments, reflex bladder function returns, and an automatic or reflex bladder develops. Initially, the detrusor contractions are weak, and the volume of urine voided is small, although subsequent emptying becomes more complete. Bladder distention may be heralded by flushing, headache, nasal congestion, and other signs the patient learns to recognize as bladder fullness.

The establishment of satisfactory reflex micturition depends on avoidance of both infection and overdistention during the initial stage of bladder atony. If the lesion is at the level of the conus medullaris or cauda equina, the bladder is called **autonomic** (i.e., deprived of voluntary and reflex activity). Detrusor contractions mediated by the intramural autonomic plexus are not effective, and voiding is never complete (as in the automatic or reflex type). Intravesical pressure is high, dribbling may occur, and there is a large residual volume. If the external sphincter is surgically severed, the bladder may be emptied by abdominal compression.

(c) In the **third stage** of reconditioning, the patient with an autonomic bladder, having learned the signals of bladder distention, is able to trigger micturition by such acts as abdominal pressure.

(4) **Bowel dysfunction** goes through the same three stages. Initially, the bowel is distended and atonic, and peristalsis is abolished. Return of bowel sounds and passage of flatus signal the beginning of the second stage. Once peristalsis begins, reflex or automatic evacuation may be accomplished if the stool is kept soft (by stool softeners, bulk-producing agents) and if there is no fecal impaction. Reflex evacuation may be triggered by abdominal compression or by the insertion of a suppository. In the autonomic type, the sphincter is patulous, and rectal incontinence develops. Reconditioning of the bowels is easier than reconditioning of the bladder.

Gastric atony and distention can be dramatic during the first stage of bowel dysfunction. To prevent overdistention and potential gastric perforation in the spinal cord–injured patient, who may not sense the overdistention, a **nasogastric tube** should be placed for drainage.

    f. Sexual dysfunction varies, depending on the severity of the process.

  3. Anterior cord syndrome is characterized by paralysis and loss of pain sensation below the level of the lesion; there is some preservation of touch, vibratory, and position sense, which run in the posterior columns of the spinal cord. An extruded anterior disk fragment is a treatable cause that must be excluded.

  4. Central cord syndrome is characterized by a greater motor deficit in the arms than in the legs, and there are variable sensory deficits. The greater predilection for the arms (versus the legs) may be explained by anterior horn cell damage in the cervical cord and by involvement of the more medially placed fibers of the corticospinal tract in the lateral columns. Anatomically, lumbar and sacral tracts run more laterally and are therefore relatively spared from a centrally placed lesion. This syndrome is most commonly seen in hyperextension injuries in patients with spondylosis, therefore being mainly a disease of the elderly. Recovery of hand function is usually incomplete.

  5. Brown-Séquard syndrome results from damage to one-half of the cord, with resulting ipsilateral weakness, proprioceptive and vibratory loss, segmental anesthesia at the level of the lesion, and contralateral loss of pain and temperature sensation. This syndrome is most common with penetrating spine injuries.

IV. Diagnosis of spinal cord injury

  A. Shortly after the patient's arrival at the hospital, a detailed **neurologic examination** is carried out and recorded (see **Severe Head Injury,** sec. **V**).

  B. The **spine** is examined carefully for deformities, swelling, tenderness, and limitation of movement, particularly in the neck. Be careful not to move the spinal elements unduly until fractures have been ruled out.

  C. Radiologic examination should include all areas of the spine where injury is questioned. Lateral and AP projections are performed. In the cervical region, an open-mouth view of the odontoid and oblique projections of the spine are necessary. Cautious, supervised flexion and extension views may be indicated. If the plain x rays do not adequately show a suspected lesion, CT scanning or polytomography may be necessary for clarifying bony injury. If a neurologic deficit is present, **MRI** is preferable to other diagnostic modalities, as it is superior for demonstrating both extrinsic and intrinsic spinal cord pathology. If MRI is not available, the instillation of contrast material (nonionic, water-soluble contrast media) by C1–C2 puncture should precede CT scanning.

V. Treatment. The best results have been achieved in special centers where large numbers of spinal cord–injured patients are seen. The treatment is determined by the interval of time that has elapsed since the injury, the presence of associated problems, the level and completeness of the injury, and the specific bony abnormalities present, if any. The need for an airway, ventilation, and treatment of associated injuries is self-evidence and is similar to the precautions noted in the discussion under **Severe Head Injury.** Although many medical treatments for spinal cord injury are currently in clinical trials, one treatment has become widely accepted. Based on the National Acute Spinal Cord Injury Study, a methylprednisolone protocol has been adopted at most centers. The administration consists of methylprednisolone, 30 mg/kg IV bolus dose over 15 minutes, followed by 5.4 mg/kg/hr maintenance dose to begin 45 minutes after the bolus and to continue for 23 hours. The infusion must be begun within 8 hours of injury to have a therapeutic effect on motor function. Prophylaxis for peptic ulcer disease is mandatory. On a cellular basis, methylprednisolone probably acts by inhibiting lipid peroxidation and secondary increase in arachidonic acid.

  A. Acute surgery. Posterior decompressive laminectomy is not advocated at the present time except in rare instances. Current indications for surgery are as follows:

    1. Open reduction of dislocation, with or without fracture in the cervical region, if traction and manipulation have failed.

    2. Cervical fractures with partial cord lesions, in which a bony fragment remains compressing the anterior aspect of the cord despite adequate traction.

    3. Cervical injuries with partial cord lesions, in which no bony fragment can be seen, but extruded disk material is suspected of compressing the cord. MRI, myelography, or CT scan may be necessary to demonstrate this condition.

    4. Depressed fragments of the neural arch.

5. **Compound injuries,** with foreign bodies or bone fragments in the spinal canal.
6. **Partial cord lesions, with gradual worsening** of the neurologic examination or worsening after initial improvement despite maximal conservative management. A hematoma must be suspected. Repeat MRI prior to surgery is advisable if quickly available.
B. **Treatment of the vertebral injury.** After achieving initial cardiorespiratory stability, the correct radiographic diagnosis is essential, and treatment is guided accordingly. When traction is needed, either cranial tongs or a halo-traction apparatus can be used to apply force along the longitudinal axis of the cervical spine. An MRI-compatible system should be employed, as MRI will often be necessary sometime in the treatment course of the patient. In general, greater amounts of weight are needed for lower cervical spine fractures. A useful guideline for the initial weight is to place 5 lb/level above the injury (e.g., for a fracture at C5, one would use 25 lb). Traction weights should be placed by an experienced person. Weight should be added under fluoroscopic guidance, or a lateral cervical spine x ray should be checked with each weight change. Attention to ligamentous instability is necessary to prevent overdistraction with subsequent cord stretching and injury. For thoracic or lumbar fractures, traction is usually not helpful.
  1. **Cervical injuries**
     a. **Atlantooccipital dislocation.** Injury at this level is usually fatal due to vertebral artery injury or direct medullary compromise. The rare patient who survives to reach the hospital may have little or no neurologic deficit. Traction can cause further distraction and neurologic deficit. If ventilation is compromised, tracheostomy may be required, since head manipulation is treacherous. Occipitocervical fusion is needed.
     b. A **Jefferson fracture** usually results from a blow to the vertex of the head, causing a bilateral fracture through the posterior arch of C1. Radiographically, the open-mouth view should be diagnostic. If the patient survives, pain may be present, but often there is no neurologic deficit, in part because the nature of the C1 disruption widens the spinal canal. In most instances, these fractures will heal with halo-vest fixation. Occasionally, an occipital–C1–C2 fusion is needed.
     c. **Atlantoaxial** injuries are conveniently divided into four groups.
        (1) **Ligamentous injuries.** Open-mouth views may show an intact odontoid, but lateral views demonstrate an abnormal separation of the odontoid from C1 anteriorly (normal predental space should be less than 3 mm in adults and 5 mm in children). Cautious flexion and extension views demonstrate hypermobility. Spontaneous healing will always be unstable, and early C1–C2 fusion is required.
        (2) **Odontoid tip fracture (type I).** Fracture through the bone will usually heal spontaneously following halo-vest stabilization.
        (3) Fractures through the **odontoid base (type II)** may compromise the blood supply to the odontoid, leading to nonunion. C1–C2 fusion is recommended in most cases.
        (4) Fractures involving the **C2 body (type III)** will usually heal adequately with halo-vest immobilization.
     d. A **hangman's fracture** refers to a bilateral pedicle disruption of the arch of C2 with associated C2–C3 dislocation. It is usually the result of a hyperextension injury, such as when a passenger in a motor vehicle accident strikes his or her chin on the dashboard. A surgical fusion is usually not required. Most heal following immobilization, but rarely an anterior C2–C3 fusion will be required.
     e. **Locked (or jumped) facets** may be unilateral or bilateral. Unilateral injuries often cause partial (<50%) compromise of the spinal canal. Root injury with or without cord injury may be seen. Locked facets are seen as a vertebral subluxation on the lateral x ray and are often first detected on the AP x ray by noting a rotation in the normal vertical alignment of the spinous processes. Oblique films confirm the facet dislocation. Traction frequently will relocate the unilateral locked facet, especially at higher cervical levels. For lower

cervical segments, surgical intervention may be needed. In contrast, bilateral jumped facets are usually associated with spinal injury and are more easily realigned with traction. Essentially all facet disruptions remain unstable due to associated ligamentous injury and often easily redislocate necessitating fusion.

    f. A flexion teardrop fracture refers to a wedge-shaped fracture of the edge of the anterior vertebral body. It is often associated with disruption of the interspinous and other posterior ligaments, causing instability. Frequently significant neurologic deficit is present from anterior impingement of the spinal cord by the disrupted body.

    g. Dislocations through the **disk space** are generally unstable and will not fuse spontaneously. Surgical fusion is needed. In contrast, dislocations caused by a fracture through the **vertebral body** will usually fuse after an adequate period of immobilization.

  2. Thoracic injuries. Because of the buttressing effect of the rib cage, most thoracic injuries are relatively stable. Traction is not helpful. Surgery is needed if misalignment is severe or if further future angulation is expected. However, less severe misalignment may be tolerated and will heal with bed rest and immobilization with a form-fitted plastic jacket.

  3. Thoracolumbar injuries are often associated with a burst of the vertebral body with significant bone displacement into the canal compressing the conus or cauda equina. If the deficit is incomplete, surgery to decompress the spinal canal and to promote realignment and fusion will often result in neurologic improvement.

C. General nursing care

  1. Bladder care. The aim of bladder care is to obtain a patient-controlled reflex bladder that is free of infection. To accomplish this, the technique of intermittent sterile, "no touch" catheterization has yielded the best results. Also, maintenance of an acidic urine with ascorbic acid, 1 g qid, helps prevent infection and urinary calculi.

    Although urine production is decreased for the first day or so after injury, we intermittently catheterize patients 2–3 times daily, depending on residual volumes, from the outset to decrease the risk of urinary infection (see Chap. 17 for details).

  2. Bowel care. The aim of bowel care is to obtain a patient-controlled reflex evacuation. The initial stage of bowel distention is treated by rectal tube or enemas. Later, when peristalsis returns, bulk-producing agents, such as psyllium hydrophilic mucilloid (Metamucil), or stool softeners, such as dioctyl sodium sulfosuccinate (Colace), are used. As the bowel becomes more active, enemas are replaced by suppositories. The patient should be examined frequently for fecal impaction.

  3. Skin care. Blankets and sheets are drawn tight and smooth, and the patient is put on a mattress or foam pad placed on a hard, flat surface. The patient should be turned q2h, day and night. In specialized centers, continuously rotating beds are utilized to protect pressure points and to facilitate care. In cases of vertebral injury, beds that do not offer spinal support should not be employed.

  4. Nutrition. A high-calorie, high-protein diet is essential. If the patient is unable to eat, supplements are given parenterally or by means of a nasogastric tube. Fluid and electrolyte balance should be watched closely.

  5. Pain control. If possible, narcotics are avoided because of their addictive potential. Aspirin, propoxyphene (Darvon), and, in rare cases, codeine are used. Sedative drugs (e.g., barbiturates, benzodiazepines) can be used to control anxiety. In patients with partial cord function, both barbiturates and benzodiazepines theoretically can interfere with function by enhancing gamma-aminobutyric acid–mediated inhibition. Phenytoin, carbamazepine, and amitriptyline have all been employed for dysesthetic pain associated with cord injuries.

  6. Psychiatric care. Early contact with experienced psychiatric health care personnel is arranged.

VI. Complications
  A. Urinary calculi are related to improper urinary drainage, infection, and hypercalciuria due to prolonged immobilization. Prevention is accomplished by acidifying the urine, promoting a high urine output, avoiding infection, and mobilizing the patient early.
  B. Decubitus ulcers are heralded by an area of redness in the pressure points. The incidence of decubiti has fallen dramatically since World War II, attesting to the better nutritional state and nursing care these patients receive. Body casts that cover pressure points are contraindicated unless applied by skilled therapists for the treatment of flexion contractures of the extremities. Small decubiti often heal spontaneously, provided that they are scrupulously cleansed and kept dry. Larger lesions may require plastic surgery (see Chap. 17, sec. **V**).
  C. Muscle spasms may be greatly diminished if their precipitating factors are kept to a minimum (e.g., urethritis, cystitis, decubiti, rectal or vesical distention). Also, they tend to ameliorate spontaneously after the second year.
    Drugs used for the treatment of spasticity include diazepam, baclofen, and dantrolene sodium. If drug treatment is ineffective, intrathecal injection of phenol may be necessary (for details, see Chap. 15, sec. **II.D.1**). Intrathecal baclofen pumps are becoming increasingly employed for the treatment of spasticity in patients with preserved voluntary muscle control. Rhizotomy is reserved for exceptionally severe cases and is rarely done.
VII. Rehabilitation
  A. Physiotherapy. Massage and passive movements are started as soon as possible. Later, special exercises are devised for the development of certain muscle groups necessary for independence. Specialists in rehabilitation medicine or spinal cord injury rehabilitation should be consulted for the design and maintenance of these programs.
  B. Vocational therapy prepares patients for future gainful employment, while at the same time shifting their attention away from the disability. Multiple devices are available that permit a wide range of activities for these patients.
  C. Sports. Wheelchair basketball, archery, bowling, road racing, swimming, and bag punching are available. Special hunting seasons are set for paraplegics.
  D. Psychiatric therapy is nearly always indicated and may be essential for suicidal or excessively depressed patients.

Selected Readings

Annegers, J. F., et al. Seizures after head trauma: A population study. *Neurology* (NY) 30:683, 1980.

Becker, D. P., and Gudeman, S. K. *Textbook of Head Injury*. Philadelphia: Saunders, 1989.

Bracken, M. B., et al. A randomized controlled trial of methylprednisolone or naloxone in the treatment of acute spinal cord injury. *N. Engl. J. Med.* 322:1405, 1990.

Bracken, M. B., et al. Methylprednisolone or naloxone treatment after acute spinal cord injury: 1 year follow-up data. *J. Neurosurg.* 76:23, 1992.

Ducker, T. B., et al. Complete sensorimotor paralysis after cord injury: Mortality, recovery, and therapeutic implications. *J. Trauma* 19:837, 1979.

Gomori, J. M., et al. Variable appearances of subacute intracranial hematomas on high-field spin-echo. MR. *A.J.N.R.* 8:1019, 1987.

Gonsalves, C. G., et al. Computed tomography of the spine and spinal cord. *Comput. Tomogr.* 2:279, 1978.

Goodnight, S. H., et al. Defibrination after brain tissue destruction: A serious complication of head injury. *N. Engl. J. Med.* 290:1043, 1974.

Guttman, L. The Conservative Management of Closed Injuries of the Vertebral Column Resulting in Damage to the Spinal Cord and Spinal Roots. In P. J. Vinken and G. W.

Bruyn (eds.), *Handbook of Clinical Neurology*. New York: American Elsevier, 197⬥ Vol. 26, pp. 285–306.

Hall, E. D., and Braughler, J. M. Glucocorticoid mechanisms in acute spinal cor injury: A review and therapeutic rationale. *Surg. Neurol.* 18:320, 1982.

Jennet, B., and Teasdale, G. Aspects of coma after severe head injury. *Lancet* 1:87⬥ 1977.

Johnson, R. M., et al. Cervical orthoses: A study comparing their effectiveness i restricting cervical motion in normal subjects. *J. Bone Joint Surg.* [*Am.*] 59-A:33⬥ 1977.

Kaufman, H. H., et al. Delayed and recurrent intracranial hematomas related t disseminated intravascular clotting and fibrinolysis in head injury. *Neurosurger* 7:445, 1980.

Levin, H. S., et al. Long-term neuropsychological outcome of closed head injury. *J Neurosurg.* 50:412, 1979.

Marshall, L. F., Smith, R. W., and Shapiro, H. M. The outcome with aggressiv treatment in severe head injuries. Part I: The significance of intracranial pressur monitoring. Part II: Acute and chronic barbiturate administration in the managemen of head injury. *J. Neurosurg.* 50:20, 1979.

Miner, M. E., et al. Disseminated intravascular coagulation fibrinolytic syndrom⬥ following head injury in children: Frequency and prognostic implications. *J. Pediatr* 100:687, 1982.

Peyster, R. G., and Hoover, E. D. CT in head trauma. *J. Trauma* 22:25, 1982.

Schmidek, H. H., et al. Management of acute unstable thoracolumbar (T11–L1 fractures with and without neurological deficit. *Neurosurgery* 7:30, 1980.

Schmoker, J. D., et al. An analysis of the relationship between fluid and sodium administration and intracranial pressure after head injury. *J. Trauma* 33:476, 1992

Simon, R. H., and Sayre, J. T. *Strategy in Head Injury Management*. Norwalk, CT Appleton & Lange, 1987.

Sonntag, V. K. H. Management of bilateral locked facets of the cervical spine *Neurosurgery* 8:150, 1981.

Temkin, N. R., et al. A randomized, double blind study of phenytoin for the preventior of post-traumatic seizures. *N. Engl. J. Med.* 323:497, 1990.

Tranmer, B. I., et al. Effects of crystalloid and colloid infusions on intracranial pressure and computerized electroencephalographic data in dogs with vasogenic brain edema *Neurosurgery* 25(2):173, 1989.

Wilkins, R. H., and Rengachary, S. S. (eds.). *Neurosurgery*. New York: McGraw-Hill, 1985. Vol. II, part VIII, pp. 1531–1766.

Youmans, J. R. (ed.). *Neurological Surgery*. Philadelphia: Saunders, 1982. Vol. IV, part VIII, pp. 1875–2532.

Young, B., et al. Posttraumatic epilepsy prophylaxis. *Epilepsia* 20:671, 1979.

Young, B., et al. Failure of prophylactically administered phenytoin to prevent early posttraumatic seizures. *J. Neurosurg.* 58:231, 1983.

13

Demyelinating Diseases

Daniel B. Hier

I. Multiple sclerosis (MS)

A. Diagnosis

1. No specific laboratory test is currently available to confirm the diagnosis of MS. The diagnosis generally rests on two features of the illness:

   a. A history of **fluctuations in the clinical course**—either well-defined exacerbations and remissions or lesser variations in a progressive downhill course.

   b. A physical examination consistent with that of **multiple lesions** in the white matter of the CNS.

2. The spinal fluid is abnormal in about 90% of patients, and about 50% of patients have a **cerebrospinal fluid (CSF) pleocytosis** with more than five lymphocytes. Pleocytosis tends to be more marked early and during acute exacerbations in the course of MS.

   a. Nearly 75% of patients have **elevated CSF gamma globulins** (with immunoglobulin G [IgG] making up more than 12% of the CSF total protein). Mild elevations of total CSF protein are common, but elevations over 100 mg/dl are unusual. A variety of CSF indices are useful in the diagnosis of MS, including the IgG-albumin ratio, the IgG synthetic rate, and the IgG index. Caution must be exercised in interpreting these IgG indices because they are abnormal in a large number of inflammatory diseases other than MS.

   b. By utilizing high-resolution electrophoresis of concentrated CSF, **oligoclonal bands of IgG** can be demonstrated in 85–95% of patients with definite MS. However, oligoclonal bands of IgG also occur in neurosyphilis, subacute sclerosing panencephalitis, fungal meningitis, and progressive rubella panencephalitis. Nevertheless, this test often is useful in confirming the diagnosis of MS, since it is frequently abnormal early in the course of the disease. The test is available from commercial laboratories.

   c. An increase in **CSF myelin basic protein** may confirm an acute attack of MS. Elevated values (> 9 ng/ml) suggest active demyelination. However, myelin basic protein levels may also be increased in transverse myelitis, optic neuritis, or radiation-induced demyelination. This test is not generally useful in confirming the initial diagnosis of MS. It is also available from commercial clinical laboratories.

   d. **Lumbar puncture** has not been shown to have any adverse effect on the course of the disease, and it should be performed diagnostically in all suspected cases.

3. **Pattern shift visual-evoked responses** are abnormal in approximately 80% of patients with definite MS and 50% of patients with probable MS. In as many as 50% of MS patients, visual-evoked responses reveal a clinically unsuspected lesion of the optic pathways.

4. **Brainstem auditory-evoked responses** are abnormal in about 50% of patients with definite MS and 20% of patients with probable MS. Unsuspected lesions of the auditory pathways are found in about one-thrid of MS patients.

5. **Somatosensory-evoked responses** are abnormal in about 70% of patients with either probable or definite MS. Clinically unsuspected lesions of the somatosensory pathways are detected in about one-half of patients with MS.

6. The **MRI** is more sensitive than CT scanning in detecting CNS demyelination. The MRI is more sensitive than evoked potentials and is probably as sensitive as

CSF examination in the diagnosis of MS. When the MRI shows white-matter lesions in the setting of abnormal CSF and evoked potentials, the diagnosis of MS is almost unequivocal.

a. **Normal MRI in suspected MS.** Although the brain MRI may be normal in MS this is an uncommon finding. In patients with an initial neurologic event consistent with CNS demyelination and a normal MRI, the 5-year risk of MS is less than 5%. Conversely, patients with a first neurologic event consistent with demyelination and multiple white-matter brain lesions on MRI have 5-year risk of MS of about 60%.

b. **The MRI as a marker of disease severity in MS.** The MRI burden (number and size of white-matter lesions on MRI) correlates weakly with clinical status in MS. The MRI also can detect attacks of demyelination that have no obvious clinical correlate. Nonetheless, MRI remains an excellent measure of disease severity and progression.

7. **Differential diagnosis.** Other diseases affecting CNS white matter may resemble MS clinically or radiologically. Care must be taken to exclude these conditions before confirming a diagnosis of MS:

a. Certain tumors (especially lymphomas and gliomas of the hemispheres brainstem, and spinal cord).

b. Certain malformations (Arnold-Chiari and platybasia).

c. Spinal cord compression due to spondylosis, herniated invertebral disk, and epidural tumor.

d. Degenerations including spinocerebellar, motor neuron disease, and subacute combined degeneration of the spinal cord.

e. Collagen vascular disease including polyarteritis, isolated angiitis of the nervous system, and systemic lupus erythematosus.

f. Behçet's disease.

g. Human T-cell lymphotropic virus type I–associated myelopathy.

h. Neurosarcoidosis.

i. Postinfectious and postvaccinial encephalomyelitis.

j. Human immunodeficiency virus (HIV) encephalopathy.

k. Vitamin B_{12} deficiency.

l. Adult-onset adrenoleukodystrophy.

8. If the neurologic symptoms in a case of suspected MS are limited to the spinal cord, brainstem, or posterior fossae, MRI is useful in excluding cord compression tumors, or malformations. Features that cast doubt on the diagnosis of MS include completely normal CSF, completely normal MRI of brain and spinal cord neurologic signs and symptoms that can be explained by a focal lesion, or absences of fluctuations in the clinical course.

9. **The hot bath test** is an antiquated procedure for diagnosis of MS. Persistent deficits have been reported in some patients after testing. We do not recommend use of this test.

B. **Prevalence and etiology.** Prevalence and incidence of MS vary with latitude increasing with distance from the equator. In industrialized northern hemisphere countries, the annual incidence of MS is approximately 3/100,000 with a prevalence of 60/100,000. Epidemiologic studies suggest that the prevalence of MS has been rising for the past 40 years. The cause of MS is unknown. One hypothesis is that some environmental factor, possibly a limited gorup of viruses, acts early in life to initiate the disease process in a genetically susceptible group of individuals.

C. **Prognosis.** After the patient has been diagnosed as having MS, the physician must correct any misconceptions the patient may have about the nature and prognosis of the illness. The course is highly variable.

1. A review of 146 persons treated at the Mayo Clinic over a 60-year period revealed a 25-year mortality of about 26% compared with 14% in the general population. After 25 years, two-thirds of the survivors were still ambulatory.

2. Approximately 20% of patients have "benign" MS, and an additional 20–30% have "remitting-relapsing" MS. Only about 50% develop "chronic progressive" MS. Poor prognostic signs include motor or coordination symptoms at onset or

older age at onset. Predominance of sensory symptoms is usually associated with a benign course.

3. A decreased risk of exacerbations has been found during **pregnancy**. However, exacerbations increase immediately post partum.

D. Treatment

1. Therapy aimed at halting the progression of MS

a. Ineffective treatments. Diets based on either restriction or supplementation with linoleic acid are not of proven benefit. Long-term therapy with adrenocorticotropic hormone (ACTH) or corticosteroids (intrathecally or systemically administered) does not alter the course of MS. Hyperbaric oxygen is of unproven benefit.

b. Treatments under investigation. Use of intravenous gamma globulins, plasmapheresis, cyclophosphamide, cyclosporine, oral tolerization using myelin, T-cell vaccination, or azathioprine remains investigational.

c. Interferon beta-1B (Betaseron) has been approved for the treatment of ambulatory patients with relapsing-remitting MS. Interferon beta-1B is a new drug so its full range of indications, its long-term efficacy, and long-term risks are not yet fully known. Changes in its use and dosing should be expected.

(1) Dosage. The recommended dosage of interferon beta-1B is 8 million IU SC every other day. Efficacy data beyond 2 years of treatment are not currently available. Safety data beyond 3 years are not currently available. Current recommendations are to treat patients for 2 years and then reevaluate therapy.

(2) Contraindications include hypersensitivity to interferon beta or human albumin.

(3) Efficacy. In a 2-year placebo-controlled study, interferon beta-1B reduced exacerbations by 31% compared to placebo. When compared to placebo-treated patients, patients treated with 8 million IU of interferon beta-1B had a longer duration to first study exacerbation, fewer severe exacerbations, and less progression on MRI. However, disability scores were not significantly different between the two groups.

(4) Adverse reactions to interferon beta-1B include injection site reactions (85%), injection site necrosis (5%), and flulike symptoms (76%). Flulike symptoms tend to abate with time. Depression, anxiety, confusion, and suicide attempts occurred in some of the interferon beta-1B trial patients. Neutropenia and elevation of liver transaminases occurred in some patients.

(5) Laboratory monitoring (CBC with differential, blood chemistries including liver enzymes, and platelet count) is recommended before onset of treatment and at 3-month intervals during treatment.

2. Treatment of acute exacerbations

a. Deterioration in the neurologic status of a patient with MS may be due to a new attack of demyelination or, less commonly, intercurrent infection (especially of the urinary tract), electrolyte imbalance, fever, drug intoxication, or conversion reaction. When doubt exists, demonstration of lymphocytes in the CSF may support the diagnosis of acute demyelination.

b. Intravenous methylprednisolone has largely replaced ACTH or oral prednisone as treatment for acute attacks of MS. Controlled studies have shown intravenous methylprednisolone to be superior to placebo for acute exacerbations of MS. Intravenous methylprednisolone is also probably more effective than either ACTH or oral prednisone for acute exacerbations.

(1) Response rate. More than 85% of patients with relapsing-remitting MS show improvement with intravenous methylprednisolone; less than 50% of patients with chronic progressive MS will improve with such treatment.

(2) Dosage. Methylprednisolone is administered intravenously at a dosage of 250–500 mg q12h for 3–7 days, followed by oral prednisone at a dosage of 60–80 mg daily for 7 days. The prednisone is then tapered 10 mg every 4 days over a 1-month period.

(3) Complications of methylprednisolone therapy

   (a) Fluid retention and **hypokalemia** may occur. Electrolytes are checked regularly. Potassium is replaced if necessary. Fluid retention and associated **hypertension** can be controlled with diuretics.

   (b) As prophylaxis against **gastric irritation** and **hemorrhage,** treatment with either antacids or cimetidine (Tagamet) is recommended.

   (c) Restlessness, anxiety, and **insomnia** generally diminish with chlor diazepoxide, 20–75 mg daily, or flurazepam, 15–30 mg at bedtime. Depression, psychosis, or euphoria may occur, especially in the presence of extensive cerebral lesions.

   (d) Psychosis is best managed with the assistance of a psychiatrist. A major tranquilizer (**haloperidol,** 10–40 mg daily, or **chlorpromazine,** 100–1000 mg daily), coupled with reduction of methylprednisolone dosage, is usually effective in controlling psychosis. Psychosis may require cessation of corticosteroids in some patients sensitive to these drugs. If these patients remain in relapse, they may require treatment with alternative immunosuppressant drugs such as **cyclophospha mide.**

   (e) Infection and **sepsis** are occasional complications and require prompt treatment with appropriate antibiotics. When the patient has a positive tuberculin test, concurrent treatment with an antituberculous drug is indicated.

   (f) Osteoporosis and vertebral body collapse do not generally complicate short courses of corticosteroids.

c. Oral corticosteroids may also be effective in shortening acute attacks of MS. Prednisone may be used in less severe exacerbations of MS when hospitalization is unnecessary. However, the decision to use oral prednisone in place of intravenous methylprednisolone must be made with some caution; in a placebo controlled study of optic neuritis, intravenous methylprednisolone followed by oral prednisone proved superior to either oral prednisone or placebo.

   (1) Dosage. The selection of dosage is somewhat arbitrary. An acceptable regimen is the following:

      Days 1–10 : prednisone, 60 mg daily.
      Days 11–13 : prednisone, 50 mg daily.
      Days 14–16 : prednisone, 40 mg daily.
      Days 17–19 : prednisone, 30 mg daily.
      Days 20–22 : prednisone, 20 mg daily.
      Days 23–25 : prednisone, 10 mg daily.
      Days 26–28 : prednisone, 5 mg daily.

   (2) Concurrent antacid or cimetidine therapy is recommended. Potassium supplementation and diuretic therapy are generally not necessary.

E. Complications of MS

1. Weakness. Physical therapy is of benefit when weakness is due to lack of use, but it does not strengthen muscles weakened by CNS demyelination. This therapy maintains range of motion, assists in gait training, and boosts patient fitness and morale.

2. Spasticity

   a. Physical therapy is of little benefit in diminishing spasticity.

   b. Baclofen (Lioresal) is the drug of choice in the treatment of spasticity due to MS. It is highly effective in reducing painful flexor and extensor spasms and is somewhat less effective in reducing baseline spasticity or hyperreflexia. Its major side effect is drowsiness, which generally diminishes with continued use. Confusion may occur at higher dosages, especially if cognitive impairment is present. Unlike dantrolene, use of baclofen is not associated with increased weakness. However, some very weak patients cannot tolerate the loss in spasticity that is important in permitting them to bear weight. The usual starting dosage is 5–10 mg tid, which may be gradually increased to 20 mg qid. Intrathecal baclofen is under investigation for intractable spasticity.

c. **Diazepam** (Valium) may reduce spasticity in some patients. Its mechanism of action is believed to be central. Side effects include drowsiness and fatigue. Usual effective dosage is 5–50 mg daily.

d. When diazepam and baclofen are ineffective, **dantrolene** (Dantrium) may be tried. Dantrolene always produces **increased weakness**, since its mechanism of action involves decoupling of excitation-contraction in muscle. The drug has proved useful in only a few patients with spasticity, but in responsive individuals the improvement can be dramatic. Dosage can be initiated at 25 mg daily and gradually increased to a maximum of 400 mg daily over several weeks. Dantrolene may produce **hepatitis**, and its use is contraindicated in the presence of hepatic disease. Thus, liver function must be monitored regularly. Other side effects include drowsiness, dizziness, and diarrhea. Because dantrolene is a potentially toxic drug, its use should be discontinued unless a therapeutic effect can be demonstrated.

e. **Intrathecal phenol, anterior rhizotomy,** and **peripheral nerve block** are considered only if spasticity or flexor spasms are refractory to drug treatment and make the patient uncomfortable. These procedures are reserved for patients with long-standing paraplegia, since relief of spasticity is accompanied by further paralysis.

   (1) **Intrathecal injection of 5–20% phenol** in glycerol has been used widely to relieve spasticity. The procedure can be performed easily without general anesthesia. A radiopaque dye is added to the phenol solution, and the procedure is done under fluoroscopic control on a myelography table. Spasticity is relieved by the production of a **flaccid paralysis** that lasts 3–12 months. **Sensory loss** usually accompanies the paralysis and can lead to pressure sores. Also, **bladder and bowel sphincter dysfunction** commonly occurs.

   (2) In patients with normal bowel and bladder function, **anterior rhizotomy** is probably the procedure of choice. Irreversible weakness is produced, but sensory loss and urinary retention are avoided. Alternatively, **peripheral nerve block** with phenol may relieve spasticity without risking bladder or bowel dysfunction.

3. **Tremor and ataxia.** About 70% of patients experience cerebellar intention tremor or ataxis at some time during their illness.

   a. Mild degrees of tremor or ataxia are often improved by **weighting** the affected limbs. Tremors of the head and trunk are particularly resistant to treament.

   b. **Thalamotomy** remains a rarely used procedure for cerebellar tremor.

   c. **Propranolol** (40–160 mg daily), **diazepam** (5–15 mg daily), **primidone** (500–1500 mg daily), or **clonazepam** (0.5–2.0 mg daily) may be tried for the tremor, although results are often unsatisfactory.

4. **Pain.** Shooting or lancinating pains that affect the pelvic girdle, shoulders, and face are common features of MS. Facial pain that is indistinguishable from **trigeminal neuralgia** occurs in about 3% of patients, and most **bilateral** trigeminal neuralgia is caused by MS.

   a. These neuritic pains, regardless of location, often respond to **carbamazepine**, 400–1200 mg daily.

   b. In drug-refractory cases, **surgical management** is recommended (see Chap. 9).

   c. **Baclofen,** 10–20 mg tid is also effective for the neuritic pains of MS and may be useful in refractory cases of trigeminal neuralgia.

   d. **Burning pains** or **uncomfortable dysesthesias** may improve with tricyclic antidepressants such as **imipramine**, 25–100 mg daily.

5. **Bladder, bowel, and sexual dysfunction** are common. In patients with either urinary retention of incontinence, correctable anatomic lesions must be excluded.

   a. Rational therapy of bladder dysfunction depends on urodynamic (cystometric) studies. Bladder dysfunction is often complex in MS. About 33% of patients have difficulty **retaining** urine, about 20% have difficulty **emptying** the bladder, and 50% have a mixture of retention and emptying difficulties.

   b. When failure to store urine is due to **uninhibited involuntary detrusor contractions, propantheline,** 7.5–15.0 mg qid, may abolish incontinence.

However, some of these patients may develop urinary retention that require intermittent catheterization.

  c. Failure to store urine associated with both involuntary detrusor contraction and **sphincter incompetence** may require either a urinary diversion procedure, an indwelling catheter, or an external drainage appliance (condom catheter).

  d. In patients with a failure to empty the bladder, anatomic obstructions should be corrected. In cases of **functional obstruction at the bladder neck**, alpha sympathetic blocking agents may be of value (**phenoxybenzamine** [Dibenzyline], 5–10 mg bid). If there are weak contractions of the detrusor muscle, **bethanechol** (Urecholine), 10–25 mg qid, may be of benefit. Other patients show improved voiding with either **Credé's** or **Valsalva's maneuvers**. The remaining patients will require either indwelling catheters, intermittent catheterization, or urinary diversion procedures.

  e. A penile prosthesis may restore potency in men whose **impotence** is secondary to MS.

6. Psychiatric complications include depression, euphoria, emotional lability, and psychosis.

  a. Reactive depressions that occur soon after diagnosis are often relieved by sympathetic, supportive psychotherapy.

  b. Depressions related to increasing disability are best managed by providing the patient with a positive therapeutic regimen, including physical therapy.

  c. Depression related to cerebral lesions may be resistant to treatment. However, antidepressant drugs are sometimes of benefit.

  d. Euphoria tends to occur late in the course of MS, and it is associated with signs of generalized intellectual deterioration and extensive cerebral demyelination. **Psychosis** is a relatively rare complication, usually related to high-dose corticosteroid therapy. Treatment with an appropriate major tranquilizer (haloperidol, 10–40 mg, or chlorpromazine, 100–1000 mg daily) is generally effective.

7. Fatigue is a common complaint in MS, affecting up to 90% of patients. Amantadine (Symmetrel), 100 mg PO bid, may relieve fatigue in some patients. Patients unresponsive to amantadine may respond to **pemoline** (Cylert), 37.5 mg PO every morning.

8. Heat sensitivity is common in MS. Neurologic deterioration may occur in hot weather or during febrile illnesses. Management consists of aggressive treatment of intercurrent illnesses and liberal use of air conditioning during hot weather.

9. Seizures occur in about 5% of patients with MS. They are generally easily controlled with either **phenytoin**, 200–400 mg daily, or **carbamazepine**, 600–1800 mg daily.

II. Optic neuritis

  A. Diagnosis. The term *optic neuritis* (ON) refers to the abrupt (usually over 2–3 days) loss of vision that results from optic nerve demyelination. When the optic nerve head is visibly inflamed or swollen, the term **papillitis** is used. Other cases are classified as **retrobulbar neuritis**, in which visual acuity is diminished in the affected eye. Pain in the eye is common. There may also be a central scotoma. Loss of color vision (achromatopsia) is frequent.

  1. Differential diagnosis. A variety of other illnesses may resemble the symptoms and clinical features of demyelinative ON:

  a. Vascular: giant-cell arteritis, temporal arteritis, retinal ischemia, central retinal artery occlusion, and ischemic optic neuropathy.

  b. Neoplastic: pituitary adenoma, intrinsic optic nerve tumors, and compressive tumors of the optic nerve.

  c. Hereditary: Leber's optic atrophy.

  d. Nutritional: vitamin B_1 and B_{12} deficiency.

  e. Inflammatory: retinitis, meningitis, encephalitis, and choroiditis.

  f. Toxic and drug-related optic neuropathy.

  g. Papilledema due to pseudotumor cerebri.

h. Pseudopapilledema due to tumor, vascular disease, inflammatory disease, metabolic disorders, and retinal lesions.

2. Laboratory tests. When the diagnosis is in doubt, a more extensive evaluation may be needed, including MRI of brain and orbits with gadolinium enhancement; cerebral angiography; CSF examination for infection, inflammation, or neoplasm; CT scan of orbits with contrast infusion; or fluorescein angiography of the retinal vessels.

3. When the authenticity of the patient's complaints are doubted (conversion reaction or malingering), the demonstration of **abnormal pattern shift visual-evoked potential** can be useful in confirming the diagnosis of ON.

B. Relation of ON to MS. In one longitudinal study, the risk of MS in patients with one attack of ON was 34% for men and 74% for women at 15 years. Early age of onset increased the risk of MS, but risk was not increased by multiple attacks. Forty percent of MS patients have at least one attack of ON. In 10–15% of MS patients, ON is the first symptom of demyelination. As with MS, **CSF pleocytosis and increased CSF IgG** may occur in ON, but with a lesser frequency.

C. The **prognosis** for spontaneous recovery of vision is quite good. About 50% of patients have recovery of vision within 1 month; 75%, within 6 months. Neither **pain** in the orbit (70% of cases) nor **papillitis** (20% of cases) alters the prognosis for recovery.

D. Treatment

1. Recent studies indicate that oral prednisone, retrobulbar injection of corticosteroids, and injection of ACTH are not effective treatments for ON. In a placebo-controlled study, intravenous methylprednisolone followed by prednisone speeded recovery of vision when compared to placebo. At 6 months, however, vision was only marginally better than in the placebo group. Oral prednisone alone was not superior to placebo.

2. Indications. Despite the generally favorable prognosis for spontaneous recovery of vision, some neurologists continue to choose to treat ON with intravenous methylprednisolone. Others reserve treatment for either bilateral ON or unilateral ON with poor vision in the contralateral eye. Current guidelines suggest administering intravenous methylprednisolone at a dosage of 250 mg q6h for 3 days, followed by oral prednisone at a dosage of 1 mg/kg for 11 days.

3. Patients must be carefully observed for **complications,** which include gastrointestinal hemorrhage, infection, hypertension, fluid retention, hypokalemia, and psychosis. Concurrent antacid therapy is recommended.

III. Acute disseminated encephalomyelitis

A. Description. Acute disseminated encephalomyelitis is an uncommon demyelinating disease of the brain and spinal cord. Pathologically, it closely resembles experimental allergic encephalomyelitis, with extensive demyelination and perivascular infiltrates of lymphocytes. Most cases develop 4–6 days after the viral exanthem of measles, chickenpox, smallpox, or rubella **(postinfectious encephalomyelitis)** or 10–15 days after vaccination against smallpox or rabies **(postvaccinial encephalomyelitis).** Acute disseminated encephalomyelitis in children must be distinguished from Reye's syndrome (a nondemyelinative postinfectious encephalopathy).

B. Diagnosis. Acute disseminated encephalomyelitis is a monophasic self-limited disease of varying severity. In mild cases, there may be only headache, stiff neck, fever, and confusion. In more severe cases, however, convulsions, quadriplegia, cerebellar ataxia, multiple cranial nerve palsies, sensory loss, and coma may occur in varying combinations. An MRI is useful in demonstrating widespread white-matter lesions. A CSF examination shows changes consistent with aseptic meningitis.

C. Prognosis. Mortality is 10–20% in postmeasles encephalomyelitis and as high as 30–50% in postvaccinial encephalomyelitis. Approximately 25–50% of survivors are left with severe neurologic sequelae.

D. Treatment. Uncontrolled studies have shown that **corticosteroids** reduce the severity of the illness. Dosages of methylprednisolone similar to those used for acute MS are recommended. One protocol is to administer methylprednisolone, 500 mg IV q12h for 3 days, followed by oral prednisone, 60–80 mg/day for 7 days, followed by

a taper of 20 mg each week. Anticonvulsants may need to be administered to contr•
seizures. Mannitol may be administered for cerebral edema. Vigorous supportiv
measures are indicated, since many patients make good or excellent recoveries.

IV. Acute transverse myelitis

A. Description. Acute transverse myelitis is a common complication of MS. Transvers•
myelitis also occurs as an idiopathic illness, a postvaccinial illness, a postinfectiou
illness, or as a complication of HIV infection, systemic lupus erythematosu•
syphilis, or *Borrelia burgdorferi* infection. Most patients present with leg weaknes
associated with a sensory level and sphincter disturbance. Back pain is commo•

B. The **diagnosis** of transverse myelitis is largely clinical. Imaging of the cervical an
thoracic spinal cord is essential to rule out spinal cord compression, infarction, an
neoplasm. The spinal cord is best imaged by either MRI with gadolinium enhanc•
ment or myelography if MRI is unavailable. Brain MRI is useful in determining th
likelihood of coexisting MS. The CSF should be examined for changes to exclud
infection or neoplasm; however, CSF changes are similar in myelitis due to MS an
idiopathic transverse myelitis.

C. Prognosis. Idiopathic transverse myelitis and postvaccinial and postinfectiou
transverse myelitis are monophasic self-limited illnesses of varying severit•
Prognosis for recovery is often good.

D. Treatment. If transverse myelitis is due to an infection (e.g., *B. burgdorferi*, HIV
syphilis) or a connective tissue disease (e.g., systemic lupus erythematosus), the
treatment is that of the underlying condition. If the transverse myelitis is due to M•
or is idiopathic, postvaccinial, or postinfectious, then the attack is treated as if •
were an attack of acute MS with intravenous methylprednisolone followed by or•
prednisone (see sec. **I.D.**).

Selected Readings

DIAGNOSIS AND PROGNOSIS OF MULTIPLE SCLEROSIS

Berger, J. R., and Sheremata, W. A. Persistent neurological deficit precipitated by hc
bath test for multiple sclerosis. *J.A.M.A.* 249:1751, 1983.

Chiappa, K. H. Pattern shift visual, brainstem auditory, and short-latenc
somatosensory-evoked potentials in multiple sclerosis. *Neurology* (Minneapolis) 30:11•
1980.

Clark, V. A., et al. Factors associated with a malignant or benign course of multipl•
sclerosis. *J.A.M.A.* 248:856, 1982.

Koopmans, R. A., et al. Benign versus chronic progressive multiple sclerosis: Magneti•
resonance imaging features. *Ann. Neurol.* 25:74, 1989.

Miller, D. H., Morrissey, S. B., and McDonald, W. I. The prognostic significance of brai•
MRI at presentation with a single episode of suspected demyelination: A five yea•
follow-up study. *Neurology* 42:427, 1992.

Nelson, L. M., et al. Risk of multiple sclerosis exacerbation during pregnancy an
breast-feeding. *J.A.M.A.* 259:3441, 1988.

Paty, D. W., et al. MRI in diagnosis of MS: A prospective study with comparison •
clinical evaluation, evoked potentials, oligoclonal banding, and CT. *Neurology* 38:18•
1988.

Percy, A. K., et al. Multiple sclerosis in Rochester, Minn.: A 60-year appraisal. *Arch
Neurol.* 25:105, 1971.

Rudick, R. A., et al. Multiple sclerosis: The problem of incorrect diagnosis. *Arch
Neurol.* 43:578, 1986.

Spencer, W. Suspicion of multiple sclerosis: To tell or not to tell? *Arch. Neurol.* 45:441
1988.

Troiano, R., et al. Effect of high-dose intravenous steroid administration on contrast
enhancing computed tomographic scan lesions in multiple sclerosis. *Ann. Neuro•
15:257, 1984.

Willoughby, E. W. Serial magnetic resonance scanning in multiple sclerosis: A second prospective study in relapsing patients. *Ann. Neurol.* 25:43, 1989.

Wolinsky, J. S. Multiple sclerosis. *Curr. Neurol.* 13:167, 1993.

DRUG THERAPY OF MULTIPLE SCLEROSIS

Chrouso, G. A., et al. Side effects of glucocorticoid treatment: Experience of the optic neuritis treatment trial. *J.A.M.A.* 269:2110, 1993.

Compston, A. Methylprednisolone and multiple sclerosis. *Arch. Neurol.* 45:670, 1988.

Duquette, P., et al. Interferon beta-1B is effective in relapsing remitting multiple sclerosis: Clinical results of a multicenter, randomized, double-blind, placebo-controlled trial. *Neurology* 43:655, 1993.

Hauser, S. L., et al. Intensive immunosuppression in progressive multiple sclerosis: A randomized, three-arm study of high-dose intravenous cyclophosphamide, plasma exchange, and ACTH. *N. Engl. J. Med.* 308:173, 1983.

Kappos, L., et al. Cyclosporine versus azathioprine in the longterm treatment of multiple sclerosis: Results of The German Multicenter Study. *Ann. Neurol.* 23:56, 1988.

Killian, J. M., et al. Controlled pilot trial of monthly intravenous cyclophosphamide in multiple sclerosis. *Arch. Neurol.* 45:27, 1988.

Menken, M. Consensus and controversy in neurologic practice: The case of steroid treatment in multiple sclerosis. *Arch. Neurol.* 46:322, 1989.

Weiner, H. L., and Hafler, P. A. Immunotherapy of multiple sclerosis. *Ann. Neurol.* 23:211, 1988.

CEREBROSPINAL FLUID IN MULTIPLE SCLEROSIS

Caroscio, J. T., et al. Quantitative CSF IgG measurements in multiple sclerosis and other neurological diseases: An update. *Arch. Neurol.* 40:409, 1983.

Farlow, M. R., et al. Multiple sclerosis: Magnetic resonance imaging, evoked responses, and spinal fluid electrophoresis. *Neurology* (Minneapolis), 36:828, 1986.

Farrell, M. A., et al. Oligoclonal bands in multiple sclerosis: Clinical-pathologic correlation. *Neurology* (Minneapolis) 35:212, 1985.

Gerson, B., et al. Myelin basic protein, oligoclonal bands, and IgG in cerebrospinal fluid as indicators of multiple sclerosis. *Clin. Chem.* 27:1974, 1981.

Johnson, K. P. Cerebrospinal fluid and blood assays of diagnostic usefulness in multiple sclerosis, *Neurology* (Minneapolis) 3:106, 1980.

Schapira, K. Is lumbar puncture harmful in multiple sclerosis? *J. Neurol. Neurosurg. Psychiatry* 22:238, 1959.

WEAKNESS AND SPASTICITY IN MULTIPLE SCLEROSIS

Coffey, R. J., et al. Intrathecal baclofen for intractable spasticity of spinal origin: Results of a long-term multicenter study. *J. Neurosurgery* 78:226, 1993.

Duncan, G. W., Shahani, B. T., and Young, R. R. An evaluation of baclofen treatment for certain symptoms in patients with spinal cord lesions. *Neurology* (Minneapolis) 26:441, 1976.

Gelenberg, A. J., and Poskanzer, D. C. The effects of dantrolene sodium on spasticity in multiple sclerosis. *Neurology* (Minneapolis) 23:1313, 1973.

Lenman, J. A. R. A clinical and experimental study of the effects of exercise on motor weakness in neurological disease. *J. Neurol. Neurosurg. Psychiatry* 22:182, 1959.

Levine, I., et al. Diazepam in the treatment of spasticity: A preliminary quantitative evaluation. *J. Chronic Dis.* 22:57, 1969.

Liversedge, L. A., and Maher, R. M. Use of phenol in relief of spasticity. *Br. Med. J* 2:31, 1960.

Selker, R., Greenberg, A., and Marshall, M. Anterior rhizotomy for flexor spasms and contractures of the legs secondary to multiple sclerosis. *Ann. Surg.* 162:298, 1965.

BLADDER, BOWEL, AND SEXUAL DYSFUNCTION IN MULTIPLE SCLEROSIS

Betts, C. D., Dmellow, M. T., and Fowler, C. J. Urinary symptoms and the neurological features of bladder dysfunction in multiple sclerosis. *J. Neurol. Neurosurg. Psychiatry* 56:245, 1993.

Blaivas, J. G. Management of bladder dysfunction in multiple sclerosis. *Neurology* (Minneapolis) 30:12, 1980.

Massey, E. W., and Pleet, A. Penile prosthesis for impotence in multiple sclerosis. *Ann. Neurol.* 6:451, 1979.

Peterson, T., and Pedersen, E. Neurodynamic evaluation of voiding dysfunction in multiple sclerosis. *Acta Neurol. Scand.* 69:402, 1984.

Tarabulcy, E. Bladder disturbances in multiple sclerosis and their management. *Mod. Treat.* 7:941, 1970.

Vas, C. J. Sexual impotence and some autonomic disturbances in men with multiple sclerosis. *Acta Neurol. Scand.* 45:166, 1969.

PSYCHOLOGICAL AND NEUROPSYCHOLOGICAL COMPLICATIONS
OF MULTIPLE SCLEROSIS

Beatly, W. W., et al. Anterograde and retrograde amnesia in patients with chronic progressive multiple sclerosis. *Arch. Neurol.* 45:611, 1988.

Krupp, L. B., et al. Fatigue in multiple sclerosis. *Arch. Neurol.* 45:435, 1988.

Peyser, J. M., et al. Cognitive function in patients with multiple sclerosis. *Arch. Neurol.* 37:577, 1980.

Rosenberg, G. A., and Appenzeller, O. Amantadine, fatigue, and multiple sclerosis. *Arch. Neurol.* 45:1104, 1988.

Schiffer, R. B. The spectrum of depression in multiple sclerosis. *Arch. Neurol.* 44:596, 1987.

Weinshenker, B. G., et al. A double-blind, randomized, crossover trial of pemoline in fatigue associated with multiple sclerosis. *Neurology* 42:1468, 1992.

TREMOR AND ATAXIA IN MULTIPLE SCLEROSIS

Cooper, I. S. Relief of intention tremor of multiple sclerosis by thalamic surgery. *J.A.M.A.* 199:689, 1967.

Goldman, M. S., and Kelly, P. J. Symptomatic and functional outcome of stereotactic ventralis lateralis thalamotomy for intention tremor. *J. Neurosurgery* 77:223, 1992.

Hewer, R. L., Cooper, R., and Morgan, H. An investigation into the value of treating intention tremor by weighting the affected limb. *Brain* 95:579, 1972.

PAIN IN MULTIPLE SCLEROSIS

Albert, M. Treatment of pain in multiple sclerosis: A preliminary report. *N. Engl. J. Med.* 280:1395, 1969.

Chakravorty, B. Association of trigeminal neuralgia with multiple sclerosis. *Arch. Neurol.* 14:95, 1966.

Moulin, D. E. Pain syndromes in multiple sclerosis. *Neurology* (Minneapolis) 38:1830, 1988.

OPTIC NEURITIS

Beck, R. W., et al. A randomized controlled trial of corticosteroids in the treatment of optic neuritis. *N. Engl. J. Med.* 326:581, 1992.

Bradley, W. G., and Whitty, C. W. M. Acute optic neuritis: Prognosis for development of multiple sclerosis. *J. Neurol. Neurosurg. Psychiatry* 31:10, 1968.

Compston, D. A. S., et al. Factors influencing the risk of multiple sclerosis developing in patients with optic neuritis. *Brain* 101:495, 1978.

Feinsod, M., and Hoyt, W. F. Subclinical optic neuropathy in multiple sclerosis. *J. Neurol. Neurosurg. Psychiatry* 38:1109, 1975.

Jacobson, D. M. Optic neuritis in the elderly: Prognosis for visual recovery and long-term follow-up. *Neurology* (Minneapolis) 38:1834, 1988.

Miller, D. H., et al. The early risk of multiple sclerosis after optic neuritis. *J. Neurol. Neurosurg. Psychiatry* 51:1569, 1988.

Rizzo, J. F., and Lessell, S. Risk of developing multiple sclerosis after uncomplicated optic neuritis: A long-term prospective study. *Neurology* (Minneapolis) 38:185, 1988.

ACUTE DISSEMINATED ENCEPHALOMYELITIS

Alvord, E. C. Acute Disseminated Encephalomyelitis and "Allergic" Neuroencephalopathies. In P. J. Vinken and G. W. Bruyn (eds.), *Handbook of Clinical Neurology.* Amsterdam: North-Holland, 1970. Vol. 9, pp. 500–571.

Johnson, R. T., Griffin, D. E., and Gendelman, H. E. Post-infectious encephalomyelitis. *Semin. Neurol.* 5:180, 1985.

Kesselring, J., et al. Acute disseminated encephalomyelitis: MRI findings and the distinction from multiple sclerosis. *Brain* 113:291, 1990.

Pasternak, J. F., deVivo, D. C., and Prensky, A. L. Steroid-responsive encephalomyelitis in childhood. *Neurology* (Minneapolis) 30:481, 1980.

Scott, T. F. Post-infectious and vaccinial encephalitis. *Med. Clin. North Am.* 51:701, 1967.

Selling, B., and Meilman, E. Acute disseminated encephalomyelitis treated with ACTH. *N. Engl. J. Med.* 253:275, 1955.

TRANSVERSE MYELITIS

Ropper, A. H., and Poskanzer, D. C. The prognosis of acute and subacute transverse myelopathy based on early signs and symptoms. *Ann. Neurol.* 4:51, 1978.

Tyor, W. R. Post-infectious Encephalomyelitis and Transverse Myelitis. In R. T. Johnson and J. W. Griffin (eds.), *Current Therapy for Neurologic Disease* (4th ed.). St. Louis: Mosby-Yearbook, 1993.

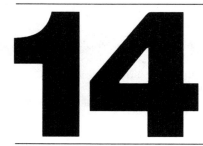

Toxic and Metabolic Disorders

Stephen M. Sagar

I. Liver disease

A. Hepatic encephalopathy is an acute, reversible global derangement of mental function that occurs in the presence of portosystemic shunting. The syndrome is marked by depressed mental status, asterixis, and EEG slowing. Elevated blood ammonia concentrations may be a pathogenic factor.

1. Elimination of predisposing factors

a. Avoid use of sedatives, tranquilizers, and analgesics.

b. Correct fluid and electrolyte derangements.

   (1) Hypokalemia and **alkalosis** increase renal ammonia production and may worsen hepatic encephalopathy. These conditions should be corrected promptly, and potassium-wasting diuretics should be avoided.

   (2) Intravascular volume must be maintained to prevent prerenal azotemia and to maintain adequate liver perfusion.

   (3) Hyponatremia associated with hepatic encephalopathy must be treated promptly but cautiously, as the overly aggressive correction of hyponatremia can lead to **central pontine myelinolysis** (see secs. **V.C** and **V.D**)

c. Infection anywhere in the body is a common precipitant of hepatic encephalopathy. Moreover, the patient may fail to manifest fever or other systemic signs of sepsis. Therefore, a careful search for occult infection, in particular peritonitis, should be conducted.

d. Acute **inflammation** (e.g., pancreatitis) and **trauma,** including surgery, may also precipitate hepatic encephalopathy.

2. Supportive measures

a. Patients in coma require an indwelling urinary catheter, skin care, and careful attention to fluid balance.

b. Deeply comatose patients may require tracheal intubation to protect the airway.

3. Dietary protein restriction

a. When the diagnosis of hepatic coma is first made, the patient should be placed on a **protein-free diet** until neurologic function shows definite improvement.

   (1) The patient may be fed by mouth, nasogastric tube, or parenterally depending on the mental status.

   (2) Enough calories (at least 500 kcal/day in adults) should be provided to inhibit proteolysis; 1500 ml of 10% D/W provides 600 kcal. If possible, a nasogastric tube is used for feedings, in which case a mixture of 10% or 20% D/W and lipids may be administered in sufficient quantity to provide 1500–2000 kcal/day.

   (3) The administration of standard, commercially available **hyperalimentation mixtures** containing amino acids is **contraindicated** in hepatic encephalopathy. Experimental regimens of special amino acid mixtures or of alpha-keto precursors of essential amino acids (HepatAmine) are of no proven benefit.

b. Cathartics are used to eliminate dietary protein in the gut on admittance. Magnesium citrate, 200 ml of the commercial solution, or sorbitol, 50 g in 200 ml of water, may be administered PO or through a nasogastric tube.

c. Gastrointestinal bleeding may deliver a large protein load to the gut and thereby precipitate hepatic coma.

(1) The gastrointestinal bleeding is treated as vigorously as possible; one should bear in mind the high surgical mortality of patients with severe liver disease.

(2) Blood in the stomach is aspirated continuously through a nasogastric tube.

(3) The gut is purged with an enema followed by cathartics. Repeated doses of sorbitol, 50 g in 200 ml of water, are given to produce at least one loose bowel movement q4h as long as the bleeding persists.

d. Adequate **vitamin supplementation** is provided, with daily doses of folate, 1 mg; vitamin K, 10 mg; and multivitamins.

e. As the patient improves, a diet of 20 g of protein per day is provided, and the daily protein intake is then increased by 10 g every 2–3 days until the patient's maximum protein tolerance is reached. In outpatients, it is impractical to maintain a protein intake of less than 50 g/day.

4. Decrease gut ammonia absorption. Bacteria in the large bowel produce a significant quantity of nitrogenous products.

   a. Neomycin, a poorly absorbed antibiotic, will decrease the number of bacteria in the gut. The dosage for adults is 1 g qid given PO or by retention enema if necessary. With chronic administration, neomycin may produce hearing loss and renal impairment. Colitis, overgrowth of the bowel by *Candida,* and malabsorption are other possible complications of neomycin therapy.

   b. Lactulose (a synthetic disaccharide that cannot be digested in the upper gastrointestinal tract), 30–50 ml (0.65 g/ml) tid PO, by gastric tube, or by retention enema, will acidify the stool and minimize ammonia absorption from the gut. Lactulose may be used in patients who are unable to tolerate neomycin, and it may also be used on a chronic basis. Some patients will respond to neomycin but not to lactulose, and occasionally, some will respond to lactulose but not to neomycin.

   c. Flumazenil (Romazicon), an inverse agonist of the benzodiazepine receptor, 1–3 mg, by intravenous infusion, may temporarily reverse some of the neurologic effects of hepatic encephalopathy, but is not a cure for the disease.

5. L-Dopa has not proved of long-term benefit in patients with acute hepatic encephalopathy and is not recommended.

6. Monitoring therapy

   a. Clinically

   (1) Hepatic encephalopathy can be divided into four stages:

   (a) Stage 1 (precoma). Mild confusion and mental slowness without asterixis or EEG abnormalities.

   (b) Stage 2 (impending coma). Disorientation, drowsiness, asterixis, and possible mild EEG slowing.

   (c) Stage 3. The patient is asleep most of the time and is confused when aroused; there is asterixis and EEG slowing.

   (d) Stage 4 (coma). The patient responds only to pain; there is hypotonia and marked EEG slowing.

   (2) In mild stages of encephalopathy, a handwriting chart and tests of constructional ability (e.g., drawing a clock or constructing a star with match sticks) are sensitive indicators of clinical status.

   b. Blood ammonia levels. In a given patient, blood ammonia concentration correlates well with clinical status. Arterial levels correlate better than venous levels, but many patients with hepatic encephalopathy have coexistent coagulation defects that contraindicate repeated arterial punctures.

   c. EEG. In deeper stages of hepatic encephalopathy, the degree of EEG slowing has an excellent correlation with the patient's clinical status. Abnormalities of the visual-evoked response have also been shown to have a similar correlation.

   d. Cerebrospinal fluid (CSF) glutamine concentrations correlate with the presence and degree of hepatic encephalopathy and may be useful diagnostically. However, there is no indication for performing serial lumbar punctures to monitor therapy.

7. Chronic management

   a. Low-protein diet. Dietary protein is limited to the lowest practical and tolerable level (usually 50 g/day). **Vitamin supplementation** is provided wit folate, multivitamins, and vitamin K.

b. The patient should have at least one **bowel movement** each day.

c. Chronic use of **neomycin** is limited by its toxicity, but 500 mg PO bid–qid ca usually be tolerated for a few weeks or even months. The patient must b followed closely for evidence of diminished hearing or impaired renal functior **Lactulose,** 10–30 ml PO tid, is safer than neomycin and is equally effective i most cases. However, it is unpalatable to many patients.

d. As a last resort, **surgical exclusion of the colon** from the bowel may be don However, the operation carries a high morbidity and mortality.

B. Acquired chronic hepatocerebral degeneration (ACHD)

1. Description. The cardinal features of ACHD are dementia, dysarthria, cerebella ataxia, tremor, spastic paraparesis, and choreoathetosis. It develops in patient who are subject to hepatic encephalopathy, and it is often superimposed o recurrent bouts of that disease.

2. Treatment

a. There is no specific treatment for ACHD, and it is preventable only throug appropriate management of the underlying liver disease. It is possible, bu has not been proved, that prevention of bouts of hepatic encephalopathy ma prevent the progression of irreversible CNS damage.

b. The choreoathetosis may respond to neuroleptics (see Chap. 15), and th behavioral abnormalities may respond to protein restriction.

c. The dopamine receptor agonist **bromocriptine** has been claimed to be o benefit in ACHD. It is administered PO at an initial dosage of 2.5 mg/day i three or four divided doses. The dosage may be increased by 2.5 mg abou every 3 days until toxicity supervenes or until a dosage of 15 mg/day i reached. The major benefit is reported to be in mental status.

C. Acute liver failure. With acute hepatocellular failure, there is a severe CN dysfunction. Unless the liver disease reverses itself, coma and death occur. Effort to decrease blood ammonia concentrations, including protein restriction and admin istration of neomycin or lactulose, are commonly employed but have not been showr to improve the outcome. Elevated intracranial pressure (ICP) may be life threatening in fulminant hepatic failure and may be treated with mannitol (se Chap. 12, sec. **X.D**). In addition, hypoglycemia may contribute to the encephalopa thy and must be vigorously treated with intravenous dextrose.

D. Hepatolenticular degeneration (Wilson's disease) is an autosomal recessive disorde of copper metabolism. It leads to cirrhosis of the liver and cerebral dysfunction movement disorders, tremor, and personality changes are the usual neurologi manifestations. The therapy is discussed in Chap. 15, sec. **IV.E.1.c.**

E. Reye's syndrome

1. Description

a. Epidemiology. Reye's syndrome is an increasingly rare multisystem di sease that occurs almost exclusively in children between the ages of 2 and 1 years. It is associated with viral infection, and the majority of cases are related to either influenza B or chickenpox. Salicylate use has been cir cumstantially associated with Reye's syndrome; consequently acetamin ophen or ibuprofen is preferred over aspirin as an antipyretic in childhood infections.

b. Clinical course. Reye's syndrome is characteristically preceded by a relatively benign viral illness. Typically, as the viral illness is resolving, there is an abrupt onset of vomiting and lethargy. This is followed to varying degrees by agitation and delirium, which may progress to coma within hours. Mild cases occur, without profound changes in mental status. At the other extreme, death can result from brain swelling.

c. Clinical stages

(1) Stage 1. Drowsiness and vomiting with or without hyperventilation.

(2) Stage 2. Delirium with hyperventilation.

(3) Stage 3. Delirium recedes, and there is increasing lethargy, progressing to coma; dilated, reactive pupils; and decorticate posturing (i.e., the flexor posture of the upper extremities and extensor posture of the lower extremities).

(4) Stage 4. Coma with unreactive pupils and decerebrate posturing (i.e., extensor postures of both upper and lower extremities).

(5) Stage 5. Brain death.

  d. **Laboratory abnormalities**

  (1) Liver function abnormalities

    (a) SGOT and SGPT are elevated at least three to four times above normal.

    (b) Bilirubin is either normal or only mildly elevated.

    (c) The prothrombin time (PT) is moderately prolonged.

    (d) Blood ammonia is very high (up to 1000 µg/dl) during the early stages of the illness, but then it falls to normal values whether or not the coma resolves.

  (2) CSF

    (a) There are no cells, and the protein is normal.

    (b) After coma develops and the brain swells, the CSF pressure becomes elevated.

  (3) Hypoglycemia is frequent in children under 5 years of age.

  (4) Acid-base disturbances

    (a) Respiratory alkalosis is frequent.

    (b) Metabolic acidosis, with an anion gap and elevated lactate levels, develops in severe cases.

  (5) Muscle enzymes. Creatine kinase (CK) and aldolase are elevated, with CK fractionation yielding primary muscle (MM) and heart (MB) isozymes.

2. Diagnosis

  a. The diagnosis is generally made on the basis of the stereotypical clinical presentation and pattern of laboratory findings.

  b. Routine liver biopsy is not necessary, but it confirms the diagnosis in questionable cases. The pathognomic finding in the liver is **microvesicular fatty infiltration.**

  c. The **differential diagnosis** includes salicylate intoxication, hepatic encephalopathy from any cause, CNS infection, and, in young infants, inborn metabolic errors involving amino acid, organic acid, and carnitine metabolism.

  d. Because Reye's syndrome is now so rare, all patients presenting with a Reye's-like illness should be screened for **inborn errors of metabolism.** Green and colleagues (*J. Pediatr.* 113:156, 1988) present a useful scheme for screening and workup of these children. The following situations are especially suggestive of underlying metabolic disease:

  (1) Children younger than 3 years of age, especially if there has been developmental delay or failure to thrive.

  (2) Children of any age who have experienced a prior Reye's-like episode.

  (3) A family history of a similar illness.

  (4) A history in the patient or family of near miss or actual sudden infant death.

  (5) Unexplained lactic acidosis.

  e. **Inborn errors of metabolism that can mimic Reye's syndrome** include

  (1) Disorders of fatty acid oxidation, especially **medium-chain acyl–coenzyme A dehydrogenase deficiency.**

  (2) Organic acidurias.

  (3) Disorders of the urea cycle.

  (4) Carnitine deficiency.

  (5) Disorders of pyruvate metabolism.

  (6) Glycerol kinase deficiency.

  (7) Disorders of fructose metabolism.

3. Prognosis

  a. The chance of surviving Reye's syndrome diminishes progressively with an increasing depression of the mental status. The mortality of those in coma has been reported to range from 10–80%.

  b. The maximum elevation of blood ammonia is a good prognostic indicator. If ammonia does not rise above 300 µg/dl, the survival rate is virtually 100%.

4. Laboratory evaluation

a. Patients with Reye's syndrome should have the following tests on admittance

(1) Blood glucose.

(2) CBC and differential cell count.

(3) BUN or creatinine and urinalysis.

(4) Electrolytes, including calcium and phosphorus.

(5) Arterial blood gases and pH.

(6) Complete liver function tests, including SGOT (or SGPT), lactic acid dehydrogenase (LDH), alkaline phosphatase, total and direct bilirubin, total protein, and albumin.

(7) PT.

(8) Blood ammonia.

(9) Salicylate level and screening of blood and urine for toxic substances unless drug ingestion can be absolutely ruled out by history.

(10) Lumbar puncture is best performed early, prior to elevation of ICP.

(11) All children, especially those under 2 years of age and those with recurrent symptoms, should have serum and urine amino acid profiles performed and urine screened for organic acids.

b. If the diagnosis is confirmed, the hemoglobin, PT, and blood sugar must be followed q4–8h during the first 72 hours. Ammonia, SGOT, and electrolytes must be followed at least daily. Arterial blood gases are drawn as indicated.

c. There is no therapeutic indication for attempting to identify the associated virus.

5. Acute management

a. **Maintain vital functions.**

(1) **Vital signs** are monitored closely, and complications of coma are avoided. Reye's syndrome is a prime indication for placing the patient in an intensive care unit.

(2) The **airway** is protected with a cuffed endotracheal tube if the patient is stuporous or comatose. Respirator support may be required. The arterial PO_2 is kept above 100 mm Hg, a value higher than is usually required because of abnormalities of mitochondrial respiration that occur in Reye's syndrome.

(3) **Maintain body temperature** below 37°C (98.6°F) with a cooling blanket. Do not use salicylates.

b. Treat possible **hypoglycemia.**

(1) A **blood glucose** is drawn before administering IV fluids; the blood glucose is followed closely and maintained between 150 and 200 mg/dl.

(2) In children under 5 years of age and in all patients in coma, glucose, 1–2 ml/kg of 50% D/W, is given on admittance.

(3) A constant infusion of a glucose-containing solution (e.g., 10% dextrose in 0.45% saline) is maintained.

(4) The addition of **insulin** to intravenous glucose solutions in the ratio of 1 unit of insulin to 10 g of glucose is used in some centers in an attempt to inhibit mobilization of free fatty acids. There are no studies demonstrating benefit from this regimen, and blood insulin levels are known to be greatly elevated in patients with Reye's syndrome without the exogenous administration of insulin. If insulin is given, however, **albumin** should be added to the solution to prevent the insulin from sticking to glass. Alternatively, insulin may be administered as an IV bolus q4h, with careful monitoring of blood glucose with Dextrostix immediately before and 30 minutes after each insulin dose.

c. Treat complications of the **abnormal liver function.**

(1) **Hypoprothrombinemia** may lead to hemorrhagic complications and requires vigorous treatment. Vitamin K (10 mg IM) may have to be given as often as q6h. If the PT cannot be corrected to within 2 seconds of control with vitamin K, the administration of fresh-frozen plasma in sufficient quantities is required.

(2) Hyperammonemia is treated with measures similar to those used in hepatic encephalopathy.

    (a) No protein is administered for the first 72 hours of the illness.

    (b) If **gastrointestinal bleeding** occurs, the gut is kept free of blood by gastric lavage and catharsis.

    (c) After about 72 hours, the ammonia level will return to normal, whether or not the patient's mental status improves.

d. Treat brain swelling.

    (1) Fluids are restricted to 1200 ml total fluids/day/m^2 body surface area. The urine output, urine specific gravity, electrolytes, and serum osmolality are monitored at least daily.

    (2) Monitoring devices for ICP are useful in patients in stage 3 or worse and in patients who are rapidly deteriorating. The use of these devices allows the precise and continuous monitoring of ICP during the first 2–4 days of illness, when the patient is at high risk from brain swelling. They are used in conjunction with an arterial catheter to monitor systemic blood pressure, and an intense effort is made to maintain cerebral perfusion pressure (mean arterial blood pressure minus ICP) greater than 50 mm Hg.

    (3) For acute increases in ICP, **controlled hyperventilation** is often effective. The PCO$_2$ is generally maintained at 30 mm Hg and the patient hyperventilated to 25 mm Hg for a rise in ICP. Hyperventilation should be implemented at the first sign of a pressure wave and continued until the CSF pressure falls. Paralysis with pancuronium bromide (Pavulon), 0.1–0.2 mg/kg IV, will help control the PCO$_2$ and thus ICP. For paralyzed patients, continuous EEG monitoring will monitor for seizure activity.

    (4) If hyperventilation fails to provide adequate control of ICP, **mannitol,** 0.25 mg/kg, is given by IV infusion over 20 minutes and repeated as necessary. The serum osmolality should be maintained in the range of 300–320 mOsm/liter to prevent large "rebound" rises in ICP following each mannitol dose.

    (5) When all other measures to control CSF pressure fail and the patient is progressing to stage 4 (i.e., the onset of decerebrate posturing), barbiturate coma using **phenobarbital** may be used according to the protocol in Chap. 1, sec. **VII.D.6.**

    (6) The role of **corticosteroids** in Reye's syndrome has not been defined. There is no firm evidence for their clinical benefit, but many centers use high doses of dexamethasone to attempt to control the brain swelling associated with Reye's syndrome.

e. Treat **seizures.**

    (1) Prophylactic anticonvulsant therapy is recommended for all patients with Reye's syndrome who have significant mental status depression.

        (a) Phenytoin (Dilantin) is preferred over phenobarbital because large loading doses have less effect on mental status and respirations.

        (b) Dosage. Therapy is initiated with a **loading dose** of approximately 15 mg/kg given IV or PO. If given IV, the usual precautions necessary for the intravenous administration of phenytoin are followed (Chap. 6). The maintenance dosage is 5 mg/kg/day IV or PO. Anticonvulsants are continued until the patient's mental status returns to normal.

    (2) The therapy of seizures, once they occur in Reye's syndrome, follows the principles listed in Chap. 6.

f. Hemodialysis, peritoneal dialysis, and exchange transfusion have all been tried for the treatment of Reye's syndrome. None is recommended.

II. Endocrine disorders. Virtually all hormone disorders have associated neurologic signs and symptoms, often as the cardinal features of the syndrome. In most of these disorders, the therapy is correction of the underlying endocrine disorder. The exceptions are hyperthyroidism and pheochromocytoma, for which beta and alpha blockers, respectively, are used to control the manifestations of the autonomic nervous system while definitive therapy is being pursued.

III. Renal failure
A. Uremic encephalopathy
   1. **Description.** The clinical features of uremic encephalopathy are nonspecific a⬛ cannot be distinguished from those of other metabolic encephalopathies. There a global defect of cerebral function, beginning with difficulty in concentrati⬛ and subtle personality changes, progressing to confusion and then to drowsine⬛ stupor, and coma. Asterixis is prominent when higher cortical function becom⬛ affected and before coma supervenes. Generalized major motor (grand m⬛ seizures may occur during the stages of stupor and coma.
   2. **Diagnosis**
      a. The **EEG** shows low-voltage slowing in early stages, with the development generalized paroxysmal slowing in late stages.
      b. The **CSF** is normal, with the possible exception of a mild elevation of t⬛ protein.
      c. The more rapid the progression of the renal failure, the greater the severi⬛ of the encephalopathy for a given BUN or creatinine level.
   3. **Treatment**
      a. The underlying renal disease is treated.
      b. Incapacitating mental changes or the development of asterixis is an indicati⬛ for **dialysis.**
B. Seizures
   1. **Etiology.** In renal failure, generalized seizures may occur as a result of any ⬛ several mechanisms:
      a. Uremic encephalopathy.
      b. Water intoxication with hyponatremia.
      c. Hypocalcemia.
      d. Hypomagnesemia.
      e. Hypertensive encephalopathy.
      f. Dialysis disequilibrium syndrome.
   2. **Treatment**
      a. Treatable underlying metabolic problems are managed appropriately.
      b. Seizures that result from uremic encephalopathy are in themselves a⬛ indication for **dialysis.**
      c. Seizures that do not respond to metabolic correction or dialysis are treated i⬛ the same manner as seizures in other situations. As a general rule, anticor⬛ vulsants are metabolized in the liver, so dosages for dialysis patients ar⬛ similar to those for patients with normal renal function. However, some extr⬛ precautions may be necessary.
         (1) **Phenytoin** dosages do not have to be modified in the presence of ren⬛ failure, but absorption of oral phenytoin may be erratic. Consequentl⬛ the patient must be observed frequently for signs of clinical toxicity. Bloo⬛ levels of phenytoin may be helpful, but the percentage of phenytoin n⬛ bound to plasma proteins is higher in renal failure than in normal ren⬛ function. Therefore, in severe uremia the therapeutic range of plasm⬛ phenytoin concentration is 5–10 μg/ml. Measurements of free (unbound⬛ phenytoin concentration or salivary concentration are helpful (therapeu⬛ tic range, 1–2 μg/ml). Also, the half-life of phenytoin may be shortened i⬛ renal failure, so a tid dosage schedule is recommended.
         (2) **Phenobarbital** can be used in diminished dosages in renal failure. Th⬛ blood level must be measured frequently to adjust the dosage, and ⬛ supplemental dose following dialysis may be required.
         (3) **Diazepam** (Valium), up to 10 mg IV, or **lorazepam,** 2–4 mg IV, may b⬛ used for emergency seizure control when seizures threaten vital functio⬛ or when status epilepticus occurs. Benzodiazepines have only a temporar⬛ effect (20–30 minutes), so more definitive therapy must be undertake⬛ during this time to provide long-lasting seizure control (see Chap. 6, sec⬛ **V.C.5.c[6]**).
         (4) **Valproic acid** may be given in the usual dosages to uremic patients and i⬛ particularly useful in the control of generalized myoclonic and tonic-cloni⬛

seizures. The therapeutic range of plasma concentration in uremia is somewhat lower than in normal renal function, although the exact range has not been established.

(5) Carbamazepine (Tegretol) may be used in renal failure in the usual dosages, and the therapeutic range of plasma concentration (4–12 μg/ml) is the same as in normal renal function.

(6) Ethosuximide (Zarontin) may also be used in the usual dosages and with the usual therapeutic range (40–100 μg/ml). It is dialyzable, however, so a supplemental postdialysis dose is necessary.

d. Hemodialysis patients may have seizures during or up to 8 hours after dialysis, due to the disequilibrium syndrome.

(1) The risk of seizures may be reduced by decreasing the rate and duration of dialysis and increasing its frequency.

(2) Hemodialysis patients should be on prophylactic anticonvulsants. Phenytoin, 100 mg tid, is the usual regimen in adults.

C. Uremic neuropathy

1. Description. Uremia causes a distal sensorimotor neuropathy that affects the legs before the arms. The neuropathy is often painful, with "burning feet," and can be incapacitating.

2. Treatment

a. The only effective treatment known is correction of the underlying renal disease. A functioning renal transplant virtually always relieves neuropathic symptoms. Chronic hemodialysis is much less effective than renal transplantation.

b. There is some evidence that **carbamazepine,** 400–600 mg/day PO in divided doses, may reduce the pain of uremic neuropathy. *Clonazepam* (Clonopin) may also be tried, beginning with a dosage of 0.5 mg PO tid and increasing in 0.5-mg increments every 2–3 days until relief is obtained, toxicity supervenes, or a total dose of 20 mg/day is reached.

D. Neurologic complications of hemodialysis

1. Seizures and the disequilibrium syndrome are discussed in sec. **III.B.**

2. Subdural hematoma

a. There is an increased incidence of subdural hematoma among patients undergoing chronic hemodialysis. Possible predisposing factors are anticoagulation, rapid shifts in brain size, hypertension, and minor head trauma. In dialysis patients, subdural hematomas are frequently bilateral.

b. The treatment of subdural hematoma is **surgical drainage.** Because of the osmotic and volume shifts that occur between body compartments during hemodialysis, it is not safe to defer surgical treatment and follow the patient clinically (as one might do with other patients with chronic subdural hematomas). During the postoperative period, the patient is managed with peritoneal dialysis to minimize rapid osmotic shifts and to avoid systemic anticoagulation.

3. Headache

a. Migraine may be made worse by **hemodialysis.** Its treatment in the presence of renal failure is **ergot,** which is given in the same dosage as for other migraine headaches (see Chap. 2, sec. **II.B.2.a**).

b. The **dialysis disequilibrium syndrome** produces headache during and for up to 8 hours after dialysis. Ergots may be tried in the same manner as for migraine therapy.

c. Persistent headache suggests the presence of **subdural hematoma.**

4. Vitamin deficiency

a. All chronic hemodialysis patients should be on supplemental multivitamins, including folate, thiamine, and pantothenic acid.

b. Attempts to treat uremic neuropathy with various vitamins have been unsuccessful.

5. Dialysis dementia (progressive dialysis encephalopathy)

a. Description. A syndrome of subacutely progressive mental deterioration occurs in some patients on hemodialysis. Its incidence seems to vary widely among different dialysis centers; this suggests that toxins in the local water supply, most likely aluminum, are responsible. The course is one of relentless progression to death.

b. Treatment

(1) Response to **benzodiazepines,** either diazepam or clonazepam, is variable in this condition.

(2) The condition of some patients stabilizes after successful **renal transplantation,** although benefit is not universal.

(3) A controversial subject is the role of **aluminum** in the pathogenesis of dialysis encephalopathy. Improvement has been reported in some patients who reside in regions with high aluminum content of the tap water with the use of a deionizer to maintain the aluminum concentration of the dialysate at less than 10 μg/dl. Moreover, some nephrologists recommend the discontinuation of aluminum-containing gels used to prevent osteodystrophy in these patients.

6. Muscle cramps during or immediately following hemodialysis may cause severe pain. Quinine sulfate, 320 mg PO at the beginning of each dialysis, has been reported to be beneficial and safe.

E. Neurologic complications of renal transplantation

1. CNS infections (see Chap. 8).

2. CNS malignancy, including primary CNS lymphoma (see Chap. 11).

3. Cyclosporine neurotoxicity. Of patients taking cyclosporine, 15–20% develop an action tremor, which is generally not troublesome. A small percentage, however, develop some mixture of encephalopathy, cerebellar signs, and spinal cord dysfunction. Some of these patients have a leukoencephalopathy on imaging studies or pathology. The syndrome is usually reversible with discontinuation of cyclosporine or a reduction in dosage. Seizures, sometimes in association with hypomagnesemia, have been associated with cyclosporine use and cease with a reduction in dosage.

IV. Pulmonary disorders. Both hypercapnia and hypoxemia are associated with encephalopathy. The treatment is the same as for underlying lung disease.

V. Hyponatremia

A. Description

1. Sodium is the primary extracellular cation and the chief determinant of the osmolarity of the extracellular fluid, including the blood plasma. Consequently hyponatremia and hypoosmolarity generally coexist. Exceptions include the circumstances in which the sodium concentration is artifactually lowered (hyperlipidemia and hyperproteinemia) or in which an osmotic agent other than sodium makes up a significant portion of the serum solute content, producing hyponatremia with normal or elevated serum osmolality (e.g., hyperglycemia or the exogenous administration of osmotic agents, such as mannitol and glycerol).

2. In the absence of exogenously administered osmotic agents:

$$\text{Serum osmolarity (mOsm/liter)} = 2 \times (\text{sodium [mEq/liter]} + \text{potassium [mEq/liter]}) + \text{BUN (mg/dl)}/3 + \text{blood glucose (mg/dl)}/18$$

3. The hypoosmolar state may be asymptomatic, or it may cause a metabolic encephalopathy: confusion and agitation, progressing to lethargy and then to seizures and coma. Psychosis with hallucinations can occur, and asterixis may be seen.

4. Symptoms usually do not appear unless the serum sodium is lower than 125 mEq/liter; seizures generally occur only when the sodium level drops lower than 115 mEq/liter. The more rapid the development of the hyponatremia, the more severe the symptoms for a given sodium concentration.

B. Differential diagnosis

1. Loss of sodium out of proportion to water

a. Renal sodium wasting

(1) Salt-losing nephropathy.

(2) Diuretics.

(3) Hypoadrenocorticism.

b. "Cerebral salt wasting" after subarachnoid hemorrhage or head trauma.

2. Retention of water out of proportion to sodium
    a. Syndrome of inappropriate antidiuretic hormone (SIADH) secretion
      (1) Bronchogenic oat-cell carcinoma and other malignant tumors with ectopic vasopressin (antidiuretic hormone) production.
      (2) CNS disease: stroke, head trauma, infection, tumors, acute intermittent porphyria, and hydrocephalus.
      (3) Pulmonary disease: tuberculosis, pneumonia, lung abscess, and chronic obstructive airway disease.
      (4) Unknown etiology.
      (5) Drugs: chlorpropamide, vincristine, cyclophosphamide, phenothiazines, barbiturates, tricyclic antidepressants, clofibrate, acetaminophen, carbamazepine. In the elderly, tricyclic antidepressants and carbamazepine are frequent offenders.
      (6) Guillain-Barré syndrome.
    b. Beer drinking.
    c. Oliguric renal failure with overhydration with hypotonic fluids.
    d. Edematous states
      (1) Hepatic cirrhosis.
      (2) Congestive heart failure.
    e. Psychogenic polydipsia.
    f. Hypothyroidism.
3. Shifts in water between body compartments
    a. Hyperglycemia.
    b. Exogenous administration of osmotic agents: mannitol, glycerol.
    c. Hypoadrenocorticism.
    d. "Sick cell" syndrome.
4. Pseudohyponatremia
    a. Hyperlipemia
    b. Hyperproteinemia.
C. Correction of hyponatremia
    1. Acute hyponatremia is potentially life-threatening and needs to be treated vigorously. On the other hand, the overly rapid correction of hyponatremia, especially chronic hyponatremia, is associated with **central pontine myelinolysis.** The optimum rate of correction in various clinical circumstances is not entirely clear, but several guidelines can be suggested.
    2. Chronic asymptomatic hyponatremia is surprisingly well tolerated. The serum osmolality should be corrected at a rate of 5 mEq/liter/day or less, relying on water restriction as the major mode of therapy.
    3. In **chronic symptomatic hyponatremia** in which seizures occur, the sodium should be corrected to 120 mEq/liter at a rate no more rapid than 12 mEq/liter/day. At that point, slower correction should be undertaken.
    4. In **acute hyponatremia,** whether symptomatic or asymptomatic, the serum sodium should be corrected to 120 mEq/liter at a rate of 12 mEq/liter/day. Further correction should be no more rapid than 6 mEq/liter/day.
    5. In all situations, one must be careful not to overcorrect to serum osmolalities above normal.
D. Specific situations
    1. Dilutional hyponatremia occurs in patients, especially in women postoperatively, who are volume depleted and who are given access to hypotonic fluids. This is a common iatrogenic disease.
      a. The **clinical picture** is one of volume depletion with a low urine sodium concentration.
      b. The **treatment** consists of the replacement of volume and sodium deficits. A water diuresis will then ensue, and the serum sodium will return to normal. In mild cases, a liberalization of the sodium content of the diet or a reduction of dosage in a diuretic agent may be adequate therapy. Only when the patient is symptomatic or the serum sodium is less than 120 mEq/liter is intravenous isotonic saline given.

2. Water retention

a. Patients may retain water out of proportion to sodium in oliguric renal failure, hypothyroidism, and, very rarely, psychogenic polydipsia.

   (1) The treatment in most cases is to restrict the water intake to the amount of calculated insensible losses (800 ml/day in a normothermic adult) until the sodium is within the normal range.

   (2) In rare circumstances in which the patient has symptoms of severe water intoxication, it may be necessary to administer hypertonic saline in the form of 3% sodium chloride to raise the serum sodium to a level greater than 125 mEq/liter. This should generally be done with the aid of a central venous pressure (CVP) line; **furosemide** (Lasix) may be administered if volume overload occurs.

b. SIADH

   (1) Description. SIADH occurs in a variety of circumstances (see sec. **V.B.2.a**). The pathophysiology of the hyponatremia involves both water retention with volume expansion and sodium wasting. The patient is normovolemic or mildly hypervolemic but is not edematous.

   (2) Diagnosis. The following criteria must be met to verify the diagnosis:

   (a) Serum hyponatremia and hypoosmolality.

   (b) Renal sodium wasting. Generally, with a normal sodium intake, the urine sodium concentration is greater than 25 mEq/liter in the presence of SIADH. Occasionally, when the patient is sodium restricted and a steady state has been reached, the urine sodium may be lower.

   (c) The urine osmolality is inappropriately high for the serum osmolarity.

   (d) The patient is not volume depleted.

   (e) Normal renal function.

   (f) Normal adrenal function.

   (3) In **asymptomatic and mildly symptomatic cases,** water restriction is the treatment of choice. The patient's daily fluid intake is restricted to calculated insensible losses until the serum sodium is within normal limits. The water intake may then be limited to daily maintenance levels.

   (4) In **severe hyponatremia from SIADH,** the serum sodium can be corrected to 120 mEq/liter within 12–24 hours by the infusion of hypertonic saline.

   (a) A catheter to monitor CVP is placed, and an infusion of 3% saline is begun at a rate of about 100 ml/hour.

   (b) The CVP is carefully monitored and doses of furosemide, 1 mg/kg IV, are administered to control intravascular volume and prevent congestive heart failure.

   (c) Serum sodium and potassium and urine potassium are monitored hourly. Potassium chloride is added to the saline infusion to replace diuretic-induced potassium losses.

   (5) The **inciting cause of SIADH** should be eliminated if possible (i.e., offending drugs are discontinued, bulk tumor is removed if possible, or CNS or pulmonary infections are treated appropriately).

   (6) Chronic SIADH

   (a) The therapy of chronic SIADH is **water restriction.** However, water restriction is extremely unpleasant for the patient, so various means may be used to allow a more liberal water intake.

   (b) Dietary sodium supplementation allows greater water intake, but it may lead to congestive heart failure in the presence of compromised cardiac or renal function.

   (c) Lithium carbonate is effective, but alternative therapies offer fewer side effects.

   (d) Demeclocycline, 300 mg PO tid, will cause a partial renal diabetes insipidus and allow liberalized fluid intake.

   (e) Phenytoin acts centrally to inhibit ADH release, but in practice it has been of no benefit in the management of SIADH of CNS origin.

(f) Oral **furosemide,** 40 mg qd, has been reported effective in the chronic treatment of SIADH.

(g) Oral **urea** (30 g/day) as a single daily dose is effective but should be avoided in patients with peptic ulcer disease.

c. Subarachnoid hemorrhage. Many patients develop hyponatremia, often with volume contraction, after subarachnoid hemorrhage. Efforts to define the etiology of this condition have failed. The term *cerebral salt wasting* has been applied, as some patients undergo natriuresis. However, SIADH also contributes in some patients. Whatever the etiology, fluid restriction is dangerous in patients with subarachnoid hemorrhage, and these patients should be treated with infusions of isotonic saline to maintain plasma volume.

VI. Acute intermittent porphyria (AIP)

A. Description. Acute intermittent porphyria is an autosomal dominant disease of porphyrin metabolism manifested by recurrent attacks of abdominal pain and neurologic dysfunction. It results from a deficiency of porphobilinogen (PBG) deaminase (formerly called uroporphyrinogen I synthetase).

1. Symptoms rarely appear until puberty, and in most cases they begin in the second to fourth decade of life. Females outnumber males in symptomatic cases, and asymptomatic carriers of the defect exist.

2. Acute attacks are usually heralded by abdominal pain and constipation followed by neurologic disease. Peripheral neuropathy (which may progress to quadriplegia and respiratory paralysis), cranial nerve palsies, psychosis, depression, confusion, coma, and seizures may all occur during an acute attack. Attacks may leave the patient with residual peripheral nerve or psychiatric dysfunction. Even with optimum management, a severe acute attack of AIP carries a significant mortality.

B. Diagnosis. During acute attacks of AIP, and usually between attacks as well, patients have elevated urinary excretion of delta-aminolevulinic acid (delta-ALA) and PBG. The latter can be detected by the **Watson-Schwartz test.** The definitive test for this disease is to compare the activity of PBG deaminase in the patient's erythrocytes with that of relatives. Family members with this disease have enzyme levels that are about half those of unaffected family members. No definite sporadic cases of AIP have ever been documented.

C. The neurologic manifestations of **hereditary coproporphyria** and **variegate porphyria** and their treatment are similar to AIP, although their chemical manifestations differ.

D. Prophylaxis against acute attacks. The mainstay of management of this disease is the avoidance of factors known to precipitate acute attacks. Asymptomatic family members are identified by erythrocyte PBG deaminase levels, so appropriate measures can be taken to keep them in the asymptomatic class.

1. Drugs. The most common precipitant of an acute attack of AIP is the administration of a drug that induces hepatic delta-ALA synthetase activity. Drugs may be divided into the following four classes, according to their ability to induce delta-ALA synthetase.

a. Drugs that are definitely known to precipitate attacks and must be avoided in porphyrics whenever possible:

(1) Anticonvulsants: barbiturates, phenytoin, methsuximide (Celontin), primidone, trimethadione.

(2) Tranquilizers: chlordiazepoxide (Librium), meprobamate (Miltown), isopropyl meprobamate (Soma).

(3) Sedatives: barbiturates, glutethimide (Doriden), methyprylon (Noludar).

(4) Antibiotics: sulfonamides, griseofulvin (Fulvicin, Grifulvin), dapsone.

(5) Alcohol.

(6) Others: ergots, dichloralphenazone (Midrin), pyrazolone compounds (aminopyrine, antipyrine, isopropyl antipyrine, dipyrone), imipramine (Tofranil), eucalyptol, tolbutamide (Orinase), chlorpropamide, synthetic estrogens and progestins.

b. Drugs that have been shown experimentally to induce delta-ALA synthetase and that should be avoided whenever possible:

      (1) **Anticonvulsants:** mephenytoin (Mesantoin), phensuximide (Milontin) valproic acid.

      (2) **Antibiotic:** chloramphenicol, rifampin.

      (3) **Other:** 2-alkyloxy-3-methylbenzamide, clonidine.

    c. Drugs demonstrated to be safe in AIP:

      (1) **Analgesics:** salicylates, opiates (morphine, methadone, codeine, propoxyphene [Darvon], meperidine [Demerol]), acetaminophen.

      (2) **Sedatives:** chloral hydrate, bromides.

      (3) **Autonomic drugs:** atropine, hyoscine.

      (4) **Antihypertensives:** reserpine, guanethidine, propranolol.

      (5) **Antihistamines:** diphenylhydramine (Benadryl), meclizine (Bonine, Antivert), promethazine (Phenergan).

      (6) **Tranquilizers:** phenothiazines including chlorpromazine (Thorazine).

      (7) **Antibiotics:** penicillins, streptomycin, tetracycline, nitrofurantoin (Furadantin), mandelamine.

      (8) **Other:** ascorbic acid, B vitamins, digoxin, neostigmine (Prostigmin), succinylcholine, ether, nitrous oxide, corticosteroids.

    d. For drugs not listed, there is inadequate evidence on which to base a judgment.

  2. Hormones. Estrogen, progesterone, and testosterone have been shown to induce delta-ALA synthetase activity.

    a. Pregnancy has been reported to precipitate acute attacks and therefore carries an increased risk in the presence of AIP.

    b. Exogenous administration of estrogens and oral contraceptives has been reported to precipitate acute attacks and, with the exception discussed in sec. **VI.D.2.c,** should be avoided in these patients.

    c. Some women with AIP experience regular, cyclic attacks, usually mild, during the few days immediately preceding menstruation. **Oral contraceptives** have been successfully used to prevent these cyclic attacks and should be tried in women with this syndrome. Oral contraceptives do not prevent attacks and are contraindicated in patients who do not have this rare cyclic syndrome. A long-acting luteinizing hormone–releasing hormone agonist has been reported to prevent attacks in a single patient with this syndrome.

    d. Corticosteroids can be used safely.

  3. Infections. Although fever and leukocytosis may occur as a manifestation of an acute attack of AIP, they are more often manifestations of infection. Infections in these patients must be diagnosed and treated promptly.

  4. Starvation and dieting. A high-carbohydrate intake can suppress the induction of liver delta-ALA synthetase activity. Conversely, delta-ALA synthetase activity rises during periods of low-carbohydrate intake, and starvation may precipitate an acute attack. Thus, these patients should be maintained on a relatively high-carbohydrate diet, ingesting over half their calories as carbohydrates.

E. Treatment of the acute attack

  1. Suppression of porphyrin synthesis

    a. High-carbohydrate intake. The patient is provided with 450–600 g of carbohydrate daily, either PO or parenterally, during the attack. Especially if parenteral glucose solutions are used, the serum electrolytes are followed closely because of the frequent association of SIADH with porphyria.

    b. Hematin, like carbohydrate, lowers hepatic delta-ALA synthetase levels experimentally. In several reports, it has shown promising results when administered parenterally to patients with attacks of AIP. A freshly prepared hematin solution is administered IV at a dosage of 80–100 mg daily in adults. To avoid phlebitis, hematin should be administered through a central venous catheter or infused into a large peripheral vein slowly over 15–20 minutes.

  2. Management of complications of the acute attack

    a. Abdominal pain

      (1) **Chlorpromazine** is highly effective for the abdominal pain. It probably works through the autonomic nervous system to control the disordered

intestinal motility. Doses must be titrated for the individual patient to avoid oversedation. A dose of 50 mg IM may be repeated q3–4h as needed.

    (2) Opiates may be added to chlorpromazine as necessary. One must be careful not to depress respiration excessively in patients with severe neuropathies and respiratory compromise.

    (3) Fecal disimpaction is frequently necessary.

  b. Respiratory failure and **bulbar paralysis** may require tracheal intubation, respiratory support, or gastric feeding.

  c. Psychosis. Chlorpromazine or other phenothiazines may be used safely to control the psychiatric manifestations. Acute and chronic depression may occur; patients should be evaluated for suicide risk.

  d. Seizures. Because of the many drugs that cannot be used in these patients, including barbiturates, hydantoins, and succinimides, the treatment of seizures may be extremely difficult.

    (1) If the seizures are associated with an acute attack, **diazepam,** 5 mg IV, or **lorazepam,** 2–4 mg IV, may be sufficient, although repeated intravenous doses may be required until the attack is aborted.

    (2) Clonazepam in low doses (i.e., 0.5–1.0 mg PO tid) is probably safe for chronic administration, although high doses may exacerbate AIP. Blood levels therefore should be closely monitored and maintained in the middle of the therapeutic range.

    (3) Triple bromides are the only other alternative. Bromide has a narrow therapeutic index. Serum levels should be maintained in the range of 60–90 mg/dl. The effective dosage is in the range of 3–5 g/day.

    (4) Hyponatremia, hypocalcemia, and **hypomagnesemia** should be diagnosed and treated promptly.

  e. Labile hypertension or postural hypotension may accompany the autonomic nervous system disorders associated with AIP. The labile hypertension usually requires no treatment, although both reserpine and guanethidine are known to be safe if needed. Postural hypotension requires careful maintenance of intravascular volume.

3. Chemical abnormalities. Several endocrinologic abnormalities occur in association with AIP.

  a. The **oral glucose tolerance test** frequently is abnormal during an acute attack, but it usually requires no treatment.

  b. The **free thyroxine** and **protein-bound iodine** may be elevated, but these do not require specific therapy.

  c. Patients often have **type IIA hyperlipoproteinemia** that persists between attacks and, in the absence of information to the contrary, may be treated like any other case of hyperbetalipoproteinemia.

VII. Heavy metal poisoning

  A. Lead

    1. Sources of exposure. The most common cause of lead poisoning in children is residential remodeling. Inorganic lead is present in paints—both interior paints, which still line the walls of many older buildings, and modern exterior paints. The organic lead compound tetraethyl lead is a gasoline additive, which is present in high concentrations in the atmosphere around tanks used to store gasoline and in dirt collected from urban areas near heavily traveled intersections or expressways.

    2. Clinical manifestations of lead toxicity

      a. Encephalopathy

        (1) Epidemiology. Lead encephalopathy occurs in children who ingest large amounts of lead salts. It occurs only rarely in adults and only in those exposed to tetraethyl lead, which is lipid soluble and reaches high levels in the CNS. In children, it is usually accompanied by pica, and it is most frequent between the ages of 1 and 3 years. For unexplained reasons, lead encephalopathy is more common in summer than in winter.

        (2) Signs and symptoms. The usual symptoms of lead encephalopathy are personality change, lethargy, and irritability progressing to somnolence and ataxia, and finally, seizures, coma, and death. In children, acute episodes of lead encephalopathy may recur, superimposed on a state of chronic lead intoxication.

(3) Prognosis. The mortality of acute lead encephalopathy is less than 5% in the best of hands, but 40% of victims are left with permanent and significant residual neurologic deficits, which may include dementia, ataxia, spasticity, and seizures.

b. Lead colic is the most frequent manifestation of lead poisoning in adults. The patient is anorectic and constipated and often has nausea and vomiting. There is abdominal pain but no tenderness. Characteristically, the patient presses on the abdomen to relieve the discomfort. Lead colic generally accompanies lead encephalopathy in children.

c. Neuromuscular form. Slowing of motor nerve conduction velocity is an early sign of lead poisoning in children; symptomatic neuropathy is rare. In adults, however, symptomatic neuropathy is frequent in lead poisoning. Typically, lead neuropathy produces weakness, but paresthesias and sensory changes may occur. Extensors are weakened before flexors, and the most-used muscle groups (usually the extensors of the wrist) are involved earliest.

d. It is suspected that **chronic low-level lead exposure** in children causes an attention deficit disorder with hyperactivity.

3. Diagnosis

a. Physical examination. The only characteristic physical finding of lead poisoning is the presence of lead lines around the gum margins. These occur in a minority of cases and only in patients with poor dental hygiene.

b. Blood smear. In chronic lead exposure, there is usually a microcytic anemia that may be superimposed on an iron deficiency anemia. Basophilic stippling is seen in a minority of cases, and the bone marrow may show ringed sideroblasts.

c. Urine. There is proximal renal tubular dysfunction associated with lead toxicity, with glycosuria, phosphaturia, and amino aciduria.

d. X rays. Lead lines may be seen in the long bones. In children who have recently ingested lead-containing paint, radiopaque flecks may be seen in the abdomen.

e. Laboratory evidence of increased body lead burden

(1) The serum lead level is the most useful screening test, although it does not reflect the total body lead burden accurately. Lead levels that are measured on capillary blood (obtained from a finger stick) are subject to contamination by lead on the skin. Consequently a cleanly obtained venous specimen is preferred. The 24-hour urinary lead excretion test has the same limitations as the serum lead level test.

(2) An **ethylenediamenetetraacetic acid (EDTA) test** measures total body lead burden more accurately than does a single serum or urinary level test. However, this test is dangerous in children with high lead burdens because EDTA may mobilize lead from the tissues and precipitate encephalopathy. Therefore, it should not be performed in a child who has a serum lead level higher than 70 µg/dl or who has symptoms of early encephalopathy.

The test is performed by administering calcium EDTA in either one or three doses of 25 mg/kg IV at 8-hour intervals. A 24-hour urine specimen is collected, and the total lead excreted in 24 hours is measured. A positive test consists of greater than 500 mg of lead excreted per 24 hours, or greater than 1 mg of lead excreted per 24 hours per milligram of EDTA administered.

(3) Several tests measure the toxic effects of lead on porphyrin metabolism. These tests are generally the most sensitive measures of lead toxicity.

(a) Delta-ALA dehydratase activity in erythrocytes is the most sensitive test of lead poisoning, but it is not readily available.

(b) Urinary or serum delta-ALA levels higher than 20 mg/dl are indicative of lead toxicity.

    (c) **Urinary coproporphyrin excretion** greater than 150 mg/24 hours is indicative of lead toxicity.

    (d) **Erythrocytic protoporphyrin (EP)** levels higher than 190 μg/dl of whole blood are diagnostic of lead poisoning in the absence of either iron deficiency or erythropoietic protoporphyria, both of which may also elevate EP levels.

4. Treatment

  a. Encephalopathy. For lead encephalopathy caused by the ingestion of inorganic lead, **chelation therapy** with EDTA and dimercaprol (or British antilewisite [BAL]) is instituted immediately.

    (1) The immediate medical needs of the patient, which may include seizure control and protection of the airway, are attended to.

    (2) A urine flow of 350–500 ml/m^2/day is established. Overhydration, especially with free water, endangers the patient with increased ICP and should be avoided.

    (3) Dimercaprol is given at a dosage of 500 mg/m^2/day by deep intramuscular injection in divided doses q4h for children under 10 years of age. The adult dosage is 3 mg/kg/day in divided doses q4h.

    (4) Beginning 4 hours after the initial dimercaprol injection, simultaneous injections of dimercaprol and EDTA are given into separate sites. The dosage for EDTA is 1500 mg/m^2/day IM in divided doses q4h for children under 10 and 12.5 mg/kg/day for adults. In adults, EDTA may be administered as a continuous IV infusion of a solution of EDTA in 5% D/W at no greater concentration than 0.5%. The maximum adult dose is 7.5 g/day.

    (5) The usual course of therapy is 5 days.

    (6) Because of the danger of vomiting with dimercaprol, food is withheld for the first 3 days and then is given only if the patient is fully alert and without gastrointestinal upset. Iron therapy is not administered simultaneously with dimercaprol. Electrolytes, including calcium and phosphate levels, are measured daily. SIADH is a frequent accompaniment of lead encephalopathy.

    (7) **Increased ICP** is managed with osmotic agents. The role of steroids is unclear. There is some evidence of an adverse interaction of EDTA and steroids, so some experts avoid their concurrent use.

    (8) **Side effects of chelation therapy**

      (a) **Dimercaprol** may produce lacrimation, blepharospasm, paresthesias, nausea, vomiting, tachycardia, and hypertension. Its use is contraindicated in the presence of glucose 6-phosphate dehydrogenase deficiency.

      (b) **EDTA** may produce renal injury, cardiac conduction abnormalities, and electrolyte disorders. Renal function, calcium, and electrolytes are followed daily, and urine output is carefully monitored and maintained.

      (c) The **intramuscular injection of EDTA** is painful. It is commonly mixed with procaine at a final concentration of 0.5%.

  b. Lead colic and lead neuropathy in adults

    (1) These conditions require immediate attention but are not emergencies. The cornerstone of therapy is removal of the patient from the offending environment and elimination of sources of future lead exposure.

    (2) In patients who are very symptomatic and in those with serum lead levels of 100 μg/dl or greater (or EP levels > 190 μg/dl of whole blood), a course of chelation therapy with dimercaprol plus EDTA is given and followed with a course of oral penicillamine or succimer (see sec. **VII.A.4.c**).

    (3) In mildly symptomatic patients without markedly elevated serum lead or erythrocytic protoporphyrin levels, a course of oral penicillamine or succimer is probably adequate.

    (4) Lead colic responds acutely to calcium gluconate, 1 g IV, repeated as necessary.

c. Long-term therapy

(1) A 5-day course of **dimercaprol plus EDTA** usually removes about 50% of the soft-tissue stores of lead and reduces the serum lead level by a corresponding amount. After chelation therapy is stopped, however, lead may be mobilized from bone, again raising the soft-tissue and serum lead concentrations. Consequently, the serum lead should be checked every few days after completion of a course of chelation therapy, and another course given if the serum lead rises above 80 μg/dl. Some patients may require three or four courses of chelation therapy.

(2) **Succimer** (dimercaptosuccinic acid) has been approved by the Food and Drug Administration (FDA) for the oral therapy of lead intoxication. The drug is administered at a dosage of 30 mg/kg/day or 1050 mg/m² in three divided doses for 5 days. The dosage is then reduced to 20 mg/kg/day or 700 mg/m² in two divided doses for 14 more days. It is important to treat concurrent iron deficiency. Adverse effects can include GI upset, allergic rashes, and elevated liver enzymes. The drug has a bad odor, which reduces patient compliance. The capsules may be opened and the drug sprinkled on juice or a food vehicle.

(3) **Penicillamine** is not approved by the FDA for use in lead poisoning, and its precise role is not well defined. It was widely used prior to the introduction of succimer to promote the further excretion of lead following a course of dimercaprol plus EDTA. Its use now is reserved for patients who require oral chelation therapy but who cannot tolerate succimer. It is administered PO at a dosage of 600 mg/m²/day in a single dose. It should be administered on an empty stomach, at least 2 hours apart from meals. The therapy must be continued for 3–6 months. Toxic reactions to penicillamine include nephrotic syndrome, optic neuritis, and blood dyscrasias.

d. Tetraethyl lead may be absorbed through the respiratory tract and, unlike inorganic lead salts, may produce encephalopathy in adults. The usual treatment is chelation therapy with dimercaprol plus EDTA, although there is not strong evidence of its effectiveness. Serum lead levels and EP concentrations are not helpful in treating acute poisoning with tetraethyl lead; both diagnosis and therapy must be based on clinical findings.

e. Asymptomatic lead exposure in children. The Centers for Disease Control recommends that children at high risk for lead poisoning be screened with serum lead levels every 6 months. The management is based on the serum lead level:

(1) Serum lead level less than 10 μg/dl requires only continued routine screening.

(2) Serum lead level of 10–20 μg/dl may require more frequent screening and discusion with the family about eliminating potential sources of environmental lead.

(3) Serum lead level of 20–45 μg/dl (the upper limit is set at 40 μg/dl in some clinics) demands an evaluation of the patient's medical status, with particular attention to nutrition and possible anemia or iron deficiency, and vigorous efforts to remove the patient from environmental lead exposure. Many clinics would institute a course of oral chelation therapy with succimer.

(4) Serum lead level of 45–69 μg/dl requires a full medical evaluation, removal from the source of exposure, and immediate chelation therapy with succimer or EDTA.

(5) Serum lead level of 70 μg/dl or greater requires immediate inpatient chelation therapy with EDTA plus dimercaprol.

B. Mercury

1. Sources of exposure

a. Mercury salts and mercury vapor are potential environmental toxins in the chemical, paint, and paper industries, especially in chlorine production. Mercury vapor and dusts are absorbed through the skin and lungs, and

ingested mercury salts are absorbed from the gut. Elemental liquid mercury is poorly absorbed from the gastrointestinal tract unless it is divided finely.
  b. Organic mercury compounds pose the greatest threat to the CNS.
   (1) Phenolic and methoxy methyl mercury are degraded to inorganic mercury in the body and are metabolized as inorganic mercury salts.
   (2) Alkyl mercury, primarily methyl and ethyl mercury, is produced as a waste product in the plastics and agricultural fungicide industries. It is well absorbed through skin and is highly lipid soluble, reaching high concentrations in the CNS.
2. Clinical manifestations
  a. Acute mercury poisoning from a brief exposure to a large amount of mercury produces stomatitis and a metallic taste; a sensation of constriction of the throat; ulcers on the tongue and palate; gastrointestinal upset with nausea, vomiting, and bloody diarrhea; abdominal pain; acute renal failure; and circulatory collapse. The CNS manifestations include lethargy, excitement, hyperreflexia, and tremor.
  b. Chronic inorganic mercury poisoning produces stomatitis and a metallic taste, loss of appetite, a blue line along the gingival margin, hypertrophied gums, tremor, chorea, ataxia, nephrotic syndrome, and erythrism, a syndrome of personality change, shyness, and irritability. Pink disease, or acrodynia, occurs in infants. It is characterized by irritability, insomnia, stomatitis, loss of teeth, hypertension, and erythema.
  c. Organic mercury intoxication produces fatigue, apathy, memory loss, emotional instability, ataxia, dysarthria, tremor, dysphagia, paresthesias, and, characteristically, constriction of the visual fields. This may progress to seizures, coma, and death. Organic mercury also crosses the placenta and may produce retardation and paralysis in the offspring of asymptomatic mothers. Renal lesions with proximal tubular dysfunction also occur.
3. Diagnosis and treatment
  a. Acute mercury poisoning must be diagnosed by the history of exposure and the clinical picture. The aims of therapy are to remove unabsorbed mercury from the GI tract, chelate mercury that has already been absorbed, and prevent acute renal failure.
   (1) Emesis or gastric lavage is used to empty the stomach, which is then rinsed with a proteinaceous solution (egg whites, albumin, or skim milk) or charcoal. Because of the locally corrosive nature of mercury salts, the trachea is intubated if the patient is not fully alert.
   (2) Sodium formaldehyde sulfoxylate may decrease mercury absorption by chemically reducing mercuric salts to the less-soluble form of metallic mercury; 250 ml of a 5% solution may be instilled into the duodenum.
   (3) Dimercaprol can be given at a dosage of 4–5 mg/kg q4h, with no dose exceeding 300 mg. After the first 24 hours, the frequency of doses is reduced to q6h for 2–3 days and then q8h for the remainder of a 10-day course. N-Acetyl-D, L-penicillamine may be the best chelating agent for mercury compounds, but it is not generally available.
   (4) Intravenous fluids are administered to maintain urine flow, and **mannitol,** 1 g/kg IV, is given if the patient is oliguric. Dialysis may be necessary if the kidneys have shut down and the patient is severely intoxicated. Electrolyte management may be difficult due to the diuresis induced by mercury salts, with sodium and potassium losses as well as volume depletion.
  b. Chronic inorganic mercury poisoning generally does not present the severe emergency that acute poisoning presents. Removal from exposure and a course of **dimercaprol** or **penicillamine** (see sec. **VII.B.3.a.[3]**) are the cornerstones of therapy. Total body sodium, potassium, and intravascular volume may need to be repleted.
  c. Alkyl mercury poisoning is most often a chronic process. There is an enterohepatic circulation of alkyl mercury, so excretion can be promoted by binding the mercury compound in the small intestine with an unabsorbable

resin. **Cholestyramine,** 16–24 g/day in divided doses, may be given togethe
with enough of an osmotic cathartic (e.g., sorbitol) to prevent constipatio
The dosage of cholestyramine in children has not been established.

C. Arsenic

1. **Sources of exposure.** The primary cause of arsenic poisoning today is pestici
   ingestion, either accidentally in children and agricultural workers or intentior
   ally through suicide or homicide. Arsenic-containing rat poison is no longer i
   widespread use, but it may still be stored in some homes and farms. Occasionally
   iatrogenic poisoning occurs from arsenic-containing antiparasitic agents used i
   the treatment of trypanosomiasis (e.g., tryparsamide, carbarsone, and senite

2. **Clinical manifestations**

   a. **Acute poisoning.** Acutely, arsenic produces capillary endothelial damag
   with leakage, especially in the splanchnic circulation. Nausea, vomiting
   abdominal pains, and muscle cramps also occur. With somewhat larger dose
   intravascular hemolysis may occur, which can lead to acute renal failur
   Abnormalities are present on the ECG, and stomatitis appears. With letha
   doses, a sequence of shock, coma, and death occurs in 20–48 hours.

   b. **Chronic poisoning.** Gastrointestinal symptoms are less prominent than wit
   acute poisoning, but weight loss, anorexia, nausea, and diarrhea or constipa
   tion may occur. Neurologic toxicity may be manifested by a sensorimoto
   neuropathy, excessive salivation and sweating, and encephalopathy. The last
   in its early stages, consists of fatigue, drowsiness, headache, and confusior
   but it may progress to seizures, coma, and death. Rarely, there may b
   increased CSF protein and a mild pleocytosis along with fever, so the pictur
   may be mistaken for an infectious process. Dermatologic signs can b
   diagnostic, with characteristic arsenical keratoses and transverse lines in th
   nails (**Mees' lines**). Hepatic and renal damage may occur.

3. **Diagnosis**

   a. **Acute arsenic intoxication** must be recognized by a history of ingestion an
   by the clinical presentation. In acute intoxication, the urinary arseni
   excretion may be extremely high.

   b. **Chronic arsenic poisoning**

   (1) Chronic arsenic poisoning is suggested by the clinical picture, especially
   the dermatologic manifestations.

   (2) The upper limits of normal urinary arsenic excretion are not sharply
   defined, but levels higher than 0.1 mg/liter are suggestive of abnormally
   high exposure. Concentrations of arsenic in the nails or hair that are
   greater than 0.1 mg/kg are indicative, but not diagnostic, of arseni
   poisoning. Apparently, some individuals who are chronically exposed t
   arsenic may harbor large amounts in their tissues and excrete large
   amounts without developing symptoms of toxicity.

   (3) With chronic arsenic ingestion, there is increased urinary coproporphyrin
   ogen III, but normal urinary delta-ALA excretion.

4. **Treatment**

   a. **Removal from exposure** and **elimination of unabsorbed arsenic** from the G
   tract by the use of emesis or gastric lavage and osmotic cathartics are the
   initial steps.

   b. **Dimercaprol** is an effective chelating agent for arsenic. The usual course
   consists of 4–5 mg/kg IM q4h for 24 hours, followed by the same dose q6h fo
   2–3 days, followed by tapering doses to complete a 10-day course. Neuropath
   may require months to resolve.

   c. **Fluid and electrolyte disturbances** must be rapidly repaired, and intravas
   cular volume must be protected with electrolyte and albumin solutions
   Pressors may be required in cases of acute poisoning.

   d. The abdominal pain of acute arsenic poisoning may be severe and require
   large doses of **narcotics.**

D. Antimony

1. **Sources of exposure.** Antimony poisoning is rare but may occur from ingestior
   of acidic food that is stored in improperly made enamelware or from parasiticida

drugs (e.g., tartar emetic) used in the therapy of leishmaniasis, schistosomiasis, and filariasis.

2. The **clinical manifestations** are similar to those of arsenic poisoning (see sec. **VII.C.2**).

3. The **treatment** is identical to that of arsenic poisoning, including use of dimercaprol (see sec. **VII.C.4**).

E. Thallium

1. **Sources of exposure.** Thallium is the primary ingredient of some depilatories and rat poisons. Poisoning usually occurs as a result of accidental ingestion of these materials.

2. **Clinical manifestations.** Alopecia is the hallmark of thallium intoxication. Neurologic manifestations are prominent: ataxia, chorea, restlessness, and hallucinations, progressing to coma and death. Blindness, facial paralysis, and peripheral neuropathy may occur. Nausea, vomiting, constipation, and liver and renal damage may also occur.

3. **Treatment**
   a. **Removal from exposure** and **elimination of unabsorbed thallium** from the GI tract with emesis or gastric lavage and catharsis are the primary modes of therapy.
   b. **Prussian blue** (potassium ferric hexacyanoferrate) may be introduced by tube into the duodenum and may decrease thallium absorption. The dosage is 250 mg/kg given over 24 hours in two to four divided doses.

VIII. Carbon monoxide poisoning

A. Clinical manifestations

1. Carbon monoxide is the most frequent cause of death by poisoning in the United States. The acute manifestations of carbon monoxide inhalation are those of hypoxia without cyanosis. The textbook "cherry-red" appearance is uncommon. The earliest neurologic dysfunction is lethargy, which may progress to coma. Retinal hemorrhages may occur. As hypoxia becomes more severe, brainstem functions fail. Cardiac ischemia and acute myocardial infarction may occur.

2. The patient may either recover completely from the acute episode, if rescued in time, or be left with residual neurologic dysfunction. Characteristically, the basal ganglia are the most vulnerable structures. The patient may also recover completely from the acute intoxication only to succumb to a massive subacute demyelination of the cerebral white matter that begins 1–3 weeks after exposure.

B. Diagnosis

1. The history is usually sufficient to give the diagnosis. The cherry-red appearance may also give a clue. Generally, if the patient has inhaled smoke or flame, rather than air contaminated by carbon monoxide, the damage to the respiratory epithelium by heat or oxides of nitrogen is of more immediate concern than carbon monoxide poisoning.

2. Many blood gas laboratories can measure carbon monoxide saturation of blood. (Note that venous blood is adequate for carbon monoxide determinations.) In the absence of lung disease or a right-to-left shunt, SaO_2, while the patient is breathing 100% oxygen, will give an estimate of the carbon monoxide saturation. The PaO_2 is of no use in estimating carbon monoxide saturation because it will not be affected by the combination of hemoglobin with carbon monoxide.

C. Treatment

1. The primary therapy for carbon monoxide intoxication is to remove the patient from exposure as rapidly as possible and to administer 100% **oxygen.** Any patient with symptoms of hypoxia or carbon monoxide saturation greater than about 40% should be observed in the hospital for at least 48 hours and maintained on supplemental oxygen until the carbon monoxide concentration falls below 20%. For severely poisoned patients, hyperbaric oxygen administration (if a chamber is available) or exchange transfusion may be of benefit.

2. Any maneuvers that reduce the tissue demand for oxygen should be undertaken. Patients are kept at rest and tranquilized if they are hyperactive from encephalopathy or other causes. Hyperthermia is treated vigorously.

3. Fire victims frequently inhale both carbon monoxide and cyanide (a product o combustion of many plastics and synthetic materials). Although methemoglobin forming agents, such as amyl nitrite and sodium nitrite, are routinely used t treat cyanide poisoning, they reduce the oxygen-carrying capacity of the bloo and should probably be avoided when carbon monoxide levels are high.
4. Residual movement disorders are common after severe carbon monoxide poison ing. Choreoathetosis, myoclonus, and a parkinsonian syndrome may occur. Thes disorders are treated symptomatically in the same manner as movement disor ders of other etiologies (see Chap. 15). For parkinsonism associated with carbo monoxide intoxication, direct-acting dopamine agonists (bromocriptine, per golide) may be more effective than L-dopa.
5. There is no known treatment for or specific means of preventing the delaye massive demyelination that may follow carbon monoxide poisoning.

IX. Acetylcholinesterase (AChE)–inhibitor poisoning

A. **Source of exposure.** The usual source of AChE inhibitors is organophosphoru insecticides. Acute poisoning may occur through ingestion, inhalation, or absorptio through the skin. Chronic poisoning produces chronic peripheral neuropathy. It only treatment is discontinuation of exposure to the toxin.

B. **Clinical manifestations** of acute AChE-inhibitor poisoning are a combination o local effects, systemic muscarinic and nicotinic effects, and CNS toxicity.

1. **Local effects**
   a. **Inhalation exposure** produces symptoms referable to the eyes, mucous mem branes of the nose and pharynx, and the bronchial smooth muscle. Pupillar constriction, conjunctival congestion, watery nasal discharge, wheezing, an increased respiratory secretions are all prominent.
   b. **Ingestion** of AChE inhibitors produces anorexia, nausea, vomiting, abdomina cramps, and diarrhea.
   c. **Skin exposure** produces localized swelling and muscle fasciculations.

2. **Muscarinic effects** include salivation, sweating, lacrimation, bradycardia, an hypotension. Severe poisoning produces involuntary urination and defecation

3. **Nicotinic effects** referable to the neuromuscular junction include muscle fatigue weakness, and fasciculations that progress to paralysis. The most immediat life-threatening effect of AChE-inhibitor intoxication is respiratory paralysis which is especially dangerous when combined with bronchospasm and copiou bronchial secretions.

4. **Toxicity of the CNS** is manifested by confusion, ataxia, dysarthria, and dimin ished deep tendon reflexes, which may progress to seizures and coma.

C. **Diagnosis**

1. The clinical presentation and a history of exposure are the key elements o diagnosis.

2. Some clinical laboratories are prepared to assay AChE activity in plasma an erythrocytes. Although the normal range for AChE activity is broad, patient with significant systemic AChE-inhibitor toxicity all have extremely low levels

D. **Treatment**

1. **Exposure is terminated** by removal of the patient from contaminated air washing the skin copiously with water, or gastric lavage as indicated.

2. The **airway** must be protected, especially if gastric lavage is required, an respiratory assistance must be provided if necessary. Frequent suctioning o respiratory secretions is required.

3. **Circulatory collapse** is treated with maintenance of fluid volume and pressors a necessary.

4. **Seizures** are treated by the usual methods (see Chap. 6).

5. **Muscarinic effects** may be blocked with **atropine** in large doses. Therapy shoul begin with 2 mg IV and then be repeated q3–5min until muscarinic symptom disappear and bradycardia is reversed. If the patient is alert, doses of atropine may then be given PO as required. Intravenous doses will need to be repeated every few hours in comatose patients.

6. Reversal of peripheral AChE may be achieved with **pralidoxime** for the propor tion of the enzyme that has not "irreversibly" bound the inhibitor. The initia

dose for adults is 1 g, infused IV over 2 or more minutes. If improvement is not noted within 20 minutes, the dose is repeated.

The earlier pralidoxime is administered in the course of intoxication, the greater its effect. It may need to be repeated q8–12h. Pralidoxime does not reach CNS AChE, and compounds that do so are not available in the United States.

X. Alcohol

A. Acute intoxication

1. Pharmacokinetics of ethyl alcohol

a. Ethanol is completely absorbed from the GI tract within 2 hours. It is absorbed less rapidly if there is food in the stomach at the time of ingestion.

b. Ethanol is metabolized by the liver, and it is more rapidly metabolized in those who drink regularly and heavily than in occasional drinkers.

c. The rate of ethanol metabolism is approximately 7–10 g/hour, which represents about 1 oz of 90-proof spirits or 10 oz of beer per hour.

d. The lethal blood level of alcohol is about 5000 mg/liter. In a 70-kg man, this represents about 1 pint of 90-proof spirits distributed throughout total body weight.

e. The toxicity from a given dose of ethanol depends on the maximum blood ethanol level obtained, the rapidity with which that level is obtained, the patient's prior experience with alcohol, and the presence of other drugs.

2. Management of acute alcohol intoxication

a. In **mild intoxication,** the most important aspect of management is to see that patients can get home safely, without endangering themselves and others by attempting to drive. Analeptics, such as caffeine, amphetamines, and theophylline, do not help "sober up" the patient or improve driving performance.

b. **Moderate intoxication** with alcohol poses no danger to patients if they are merely observed until ready to make their own way home. If there has been ingestion within the preceding 2 hours, emesis, gastric lavage, and catharsis may be used to prevent further absorption. As with mild intoxication, analeptics are of no use.

c. The chief danger in **severe ethanol intoxication** is respiratory depression. As long as adequate supportive care is provided before significant hypoxia occurs, the outlook is excellent. Within 24 hours, the alcohol will be metabolized.

(1) The blood alcohol level may be measured directly or estimated by measuring the serum osmolarity. Each 100 mg/liter of blood ethanol raises the serum osmolarity by approximately 2 mOsm/liter.

(2) Tracheal intubation and respiratory support are provided at the earliest sign of respiratory depression. Respiratory support should be continued until the patient is fully awake.

(3) Gastric lavage is performed if there is a possibility of alcohol or other drug ingestion within the preceding 2 hours. If the patient is not fully awake, the trachea is protected with a cuffed endotracheal tube before gastric lavage is undertaken.

(4) Frequently, life-threatening ethanol ingestion is accompanied by ingestion of other CNS depressants. This possibility should be considered if the patient's mental status is depressed out of proportion to the blood ethanol level or if unexpected neurologic signs are present.

(5) Fluids are given to maintain adequate blood pressure and urine output, but there is no need to induce a forced diuresis.

(6) If the patient is suspected of being a chronic alcoholic or of having severe liver disease, blood is drawn for determination of glucose and electrolytes, and thiamine, 50 mg IV and 50 mg IM, and glucose, 25–50 g by IV push, are administered immediately in the event of complicating Wernicke's encephalopathy or hypoglycemia.

(7) Chronic alcoholics are frequently potassium depleted and may require replacement with potassium chloride. Acid-base balance is maintained, and alcoholic ketoacidosis is either ruled out or treated appropriately with intravenous glucose and fluids.

(8) If the blood ethanol level is extremely high (> 7000 mg/liter), peritoneal dialysis or hemodialysis may be justified to reduce the ethanol level rapidly.

(9) Although fructose administration hastens ethanol metabolism, its risk does not justify the benefit obtained.

B. Ethanol withdrawal

1. Mild withdrawal syndrome

a. Clinical manifestations of mild ethanol withdrawal are anxiety, weakness, tremulousness, sweating, and tachycardia.

b. Treatment

(1) In the absence of other intercurrent illness, such as coronary artery disease or infection, these patients may be treated at home if the social situation is appropriate.

(2) Patients are given **thiamine,** 50 mg IM, and a prescription for **multivitamins** if they are malnourished. They are instructed to maintain adequate hydration and food intake during the period of withdrawal.

(3) A **benzodiazepine** tranquilizer minimizes the symptoms of withdrawal. In general, one may begin with chlordiazepoxide, 25–50 mg PO q4h for the first 48–72 hours, and then taper the dosage over 5–7 days. Diazepam is equally effective. The initial dosage is 5–10 mg PO q4–6h.

2. Moderate and severe withdrawal syndromes

a. Patients who are febrile, irrational, hallucinating, or extremely agitated must be hospitalized until the severe manifestations of ethanol withdrawal have resolved.

b. General medical therapy

(1) These patients frequently are dehydrated, and total body potassium is depleted. Those deficits are replaced with appropriate **electrolyte solutions.** Vascular collapse may occur, but it usually responds to rigorous volume replacement.

(2) Ethanol withdrawal is often precipitated by an **intercurrent illness,** often infection. Such illnesses must be detected and treated appropriately.

(3) Chronic alcoholics are subject to bleeding disorders from liver disease or thrombocytopenia. Consequently, **acetaminophen,** 600 mg or 1.2 g PO or per rectum, is preferred to aspirin to treat hyperthermia.

(4) The patient is usually magnesium depleted. There is no good evidence that replacing magnesium has any effect on the course of the withdrawal syndrome, but many physicians elect to administer magnesium if the patient is admitted early in the course of withdrawal. **Magnesium sulfate** may be given in a 50% solution, 1–2 ml IM, or the same amount may be mixed with IV electrolyte solutions.

(5) Severe liver disease may result in hypoglycemia, and starvation may result in ketoacidosis. Consequently, **glucose** is administered early, either as a bolus of 25–50 g (if the patient is comatose) or as a dextrose plus electrolyte solution.

(6) **Thiamine,** 50 mg IV and 50 mg IM, is always administered to chronic alcoholics prior to glucose because of the risk of Wernicke's encephalopathy.

c. Tranquilization. The benzodiazepines are the preferred drugs for sedation in alcohol withdrawal.

(1) **Diazepam** and **chlordiazepoxide** are essentially identical in their therapeutic effect when used in equipotent doses. Both have a prolonged duration of action (12–36 hours), are well absorbed PO, are erratically absorbed when administered IM, and have a rapid and predictable effect when given IV. The primary danger from both drugs is excessive CNS depression after repeated doses, due to the cumulative effect of successive doses given within 24 hours of each other. Respiratory arrest may occur occasionally with rapid intravenous injection of either drug, but the risk is minimized with small doses.

(2) **Dosages.** Diazepam may be administered IV in 2.5-mg or 5-mg doses q5min until the patient is calm, and then 5–10 mg PO or by slow intravenous injection q2–6h as necessary. Chlordiazepoxide may be used in an identical manner, chlordiazepoxide, 12.5 mg, being equivalent to diazepam, 2.5 mg.

(3) The most important aspects of managing alcohol withdrawal with intravenous benzodiazepines are frequent observation of the patient to prevent cumulative toxicity and avoidance of large doses (> diazepam, 5 mg, or chlordiazepoxide, 25 mg) in any one intravenous injection. It is essential that each patient be individually titrated with tranquilizer and repeatedly reevaluated rather than being put on a fixed dosage schedule.

d. Withdrawal seizures

(1) **Description.** Ethanol withdrawal seizures occur between 12 and 30 hours after cessation of regular ethanol ingestion, are generalized major motor convulsions, and are usually brief and one or two in number. Ethanol withdrawal seizures can be prolonged, however, and status epilepticus may occur. The interictal EEG is normal, and except for periods of drug withdrawal, the patient is not predisposed to unprovoked seizures.

(2) The **diagnosis** of ethanol withdrawal seizure can be made only if the seizure fits the typical clinical pattern and there is no other possible cause. Seizures from other causes are likely to be precipitated by ethanol withdrawal and should be treated appropriately (see Chap. 6).

(3) **Treatment**

(a) **Phenytoin** may partially protect against ethanol withdrawal seizures. Assuming patients have not been taking an antiepileptic, they can be given a 1-g loading dose, either IV or PO, divided into two or three doses given 1–2 hours apart. Then patients are maintained on 300 mg/day PO or IV for 3 days, and the dosage is tapered over about 1 week after the risk of withdrawal seizures has passed. Ethanol withdrawal seizures are not an indication for long-term anticonvulsant therapy.

(b) Experts differ over the **indications for phenytoin prophylaxis** of withdrawal seizures. Some would administer phenytoin to all patients seen during the first 24 hours of withdrawal from heavy ethanol use. Others would limit its use to those with a history of withdrawal seizures or with an underlying seizure disorder.

(c) If a patient is seen **after a withdrawal seizure** has occurred, it is reasonable merely to observe the patient without therapy as long as other causes (particularly head trauma, subdural hematoma, metabolic derangement, and CNS infection) for the seizure have been ruled out. The probability is high that the seizure either will not recur or, if it does recur, will be brief. Some would argue that the risk involved in phenytoin use is sufficiently low that it should be used in this situation until the patient is out of danger.

(d) If the patient is allergic to phenytoin, **carbamazepine** is the alternative. Barbiturates should be avoided, as they may potentiate the respiratory depressant effects of benzodiazepines used to treat withdrawal symptoms.

C. Wernicke's encephalopathy

1. Description

a. Wernicke's encephalopathy is a **thiamine-deficiency** disease that occurs in chronic alcoholics or patients with chronic malnutrition. It has an acute onset, and its cardinal manifestations are confusion and memory loss, nystagmus, extraocular movement deficits (most often unilateral or bilateral sixth-nerve palsies), and ataxia, occurring in any combination. Drowsiness, stupor, and even coma may occur.

b. With prompt treatment, the ocular abnormalities usually clear within days, but about one-fourth of patients will be left with **Korsakoff's psychosis,** which is characterized by a deficit in higher cortical function whereby the ability to form new memories is impaired far out of proportion to other functions. Any patient with an appropriate predisposition who has any sign of ataxia, confusion, or extraocular movement abnormality should be treated for Wernicke's encephalopathy.

2. The **diagnosis** is usually obvious clinically, but it can be confirmed with erythrocyte transketolase levels. The blood sample must be drawn before the administration of thiamine to be diagnostic.

3. The **treatment** is parenteral **thiamine.** The dosage required is not known, but it is customary to give 50–100 mg IV and IM immediately and then 50 mg/day PO or IM for 3 days thereafter. Except for extremely rare immediate hypersensitivity reactions to commercial thiamine preparations, the drug causes no toxicity.

4. The administration of **glucose** before thiamine in a severely thiamine-deficient patient **may precipitate Wernicke's encephalopathy.** It is therefore recommended that thiamine be given before glucose in any patient in whom thiamine deficiency is a possibility, including patients with coma of unknown cause.

5. Patients at risk for Wernicke's encephalopathy should be treated with **multivitamins,** including vitamin B complex, along with thiamine.

XI. Opiates

A. Overdose

1. **Description.** Depressed mental status, respiratory depression, and pinpoint pupils are the typical symptoms of acute opiate poisoning. The body temperature may be subnormal, the blood pressure may be low, and the limbs and jaw are generally flaccid. With very high doses, convulsions and pulmonary edema may occur.

2. Emergency **treatment** is directed at respiratory depression.

   a. Patients who are cyanotic, have a respiratory rate below 10/minute, or cannot protect their own airway are **intubated** with an orotracheal or nasotracheal tube and given respiratory assistance with **positive pressure ventilation.**

   b. **Naloxone** (Narcan), an opiate antagonist, is given in 0.4-mg increments by rapid intravenous injection until the patient is respiring normally or until a total of 10 mg has been given, at which point the diagnosis must be called into question. Several aspects of the pharmacology of narcotic antagonists should be kept in mind:

      (1) The duration of action of naloxone is only 1–4 hours, depending on the dose, which is shorter than the duration of commonly available opiates. Therefore, after the action of an opiate is reversed with naloxone, patients require close observation in the event that they relapse into coma. Repeated doses of naloxone may be required, especially in methadone intoxication, because of the long duration of action of methadone (24–36 hours).

      (2) Paradoxically, opiate addicts are more sensitive to narcotic antagonists than are patients who are not tolerant of opiates. Therefore, narcotic antagonists are administered in small intravenous doses (naloxone, 0.4 mg) repeated q2–3min until the desired effect is achieved or until a total of 10 mg has been given.

      (3) When given to opiate addicts, narcotic antagonists may precipitate severe acute withdrawal within minutes of intravenous injection if given in sufficient doses. Once the antagonist is administered, the withdrawal syndrome will be extremely resistant to reversal by the administration of opiates until the effect of the antagonist has waned.

      Furthermore, in narcotic addicts, one should not attempt to reverse all the narcotic effects immediately with naloxone. Rather, the aim is to return patients' spontaneous respirations and restore level of consciousness to the point where they can protect their own airway and make spontaneous postural adjustments in bed.

      (4) Narcotic antagonists, including naloxone, have an **emetic effect.** Therefore, in comatose patients, the trachea is protected by a cuffed endotracheal tube.

B. Acute opiate withdrawal

1. Although many of the symptoms of opiate withdrawal are dramatic, the only potentially dangerous manifestation is dehydration due to nausea, vomiting,

sweating, and diarrhea, combined with failure to take in oral fluids. Consequently, the essential aspect of management of severe narcotic withdrawal is the administration of appropriate **electrolyte solutions** to maintain intravascular volume and electrolyte balance.

2. At any point in the course of the syndrome, as long as a narcotic antagonist has not been administered, the symptoms may be rapidly relieved by narcotic administration. For example, **morphine sulfate** may be administered by intravenous injection in small incremental doses of 2–5 mg q3–5min until the desired effect is achieved.

3. **Clonidine,** an alpha-adrenergic agonist and antihypertensive agent, administered as a single dose of 5 μg/kg, will alleviate the symptoms of opiate withdrawal. The patient may then be treated with a 2-week course of clonidine, beginning with a dosage of 0.1 mg q4–6h, as necessary to prevent withdrawal symptoms; the dosage is adjusted to a maximum of 1.2 mg/day or until oversedation or hypotension supervenes.

XII. Barbiturates

A. **Acute intoxication.** Barbiturates do no direct damage to the nervous system, so every patient who reaches medical attention before the development of CNS damage from hypoxia or shock has the potential to recover completely with adequate supportive therapy.

1. **Initial evaluation of the patient**

   a. A **classification** of the level of barbiturate intoxication is useful in determining the prognosis.

      (1) **Class 0.** Patients who are asleep, but who can be aroused to purposeful activity.

      (2) **Class I.** Patients who are unconscious, but who withdraw from noxious stimuli and whose muscle stretch reflexes are intact (the corneal reflex may be depressed).

      (3) **Class II.** Patients who are unconscious and do not respond to painful stimuli, but who retain muscle stretch reflexes and have no respiratory or circulatory depression.

      (4) **Class III.** Patients who are unconscious with loss of some or all reflexes, but with spontaneous respirations and normal blood pressure.

      (5) **Class IV.** Patients with respiratory depression, cyanosis, or shock.

   b. A complete **history** of the events surrounding the ingestion is obtained. In particular, the ingestion of alcohol, other sedatives, or tranquilizers along with barbiturates is frequent, accounting for neurologic depression that is out of proportion to the dose or serum level of barbiturate taken.

   c. The initial **laboratory evaluation** of patients in classes III and IV should include

      (1) Hemogram (hematocrit, WBC count, and differential).

      (2) Creatinine, BUN, or both.

      (3) Electrolytes.

      (4) Glucose.

      (5) Chest x ray.

      (6) Urinalysis.

      (7) Arterial blood gases.

      (8) A screen of the serum and urine for toxic substances.

   d. **Serum barbiturate levels** are helpful, but they must be interpreted in the context of the clinical situation.

      (1) A high barbiturate level confirms the diagnosis of barbiturate intoxication.

      (2) Prognostically, the serum level correlates with the duration of coma (Table 14-1). However, the usual method of measuring barbiturates does not distinguish between the different varieties of barbiturates, so the level must be interpreted with a knowledge of the compound ingested.

      (3) The drug level may not correlate with the clinical status of the patient in several situations:

Table 14-1. Serum levels of commonly used barbiturates

Drug	Trade name	Hypnotic dose (g)	Fatal dose (g)	Fatal plasma concentration (mg/dl)
Long-acting (6 hr)				
Barbital	Veronal	0.1–0.2	10	15
Phenobarbital	Luminal	0.3–0.5	5	8
Intermediate-acting (3–6 hr)				
Amobarbital	Amytal	0.05–0.20		
Butabarbital	Butisol	0.1–0.2		
Short-acting (3 hr)				
Pentobarbital	Nembutal	0.05–0.20	3	3.5
Secobarbital	Seconal	0.1–0.2	3	3.5

Source: Data from L. W. Henderson and J. P. Merrill, Treatment of barbiturate intoxication. *Ann. Intern. Med.* 64:876, 1966.

      (a) In **mixed ingestions,** the patient's nervous system may be more depressed than would be predicted from the barbiturate level.

      (b) **Patients who take barbiturates habitually,** either therapeutically or as drugs of abuse, can tolerate much higher levels of barbiturates than those who have no tolerance for the drug.

      (c) **Central nervous system stimulants** (analeptic agents) may temporarily elevate a patient's mental status.

  2. Supportive therapy. The lowest mortality reported (0.8%) was achieved at a Scandinavian center that employed only supportive measures in the treatment of barbiturate intoxication.

    a. Respiration. Patients in class IV require immediate endotracheal intubation and respiratory assistance. Patients in classes 0–III require a cuffed endotracheal tube if gastric lavage is to be undertaken, if the cough reflex is absent, or if there is any doubt as to the adequacy of respirations.

      Arterial blood gases must be monitored closely to maintain the PO_2 greater than 80 mm Hg ($SO_2 > 94\%$). The minimum necessary concentration of inspired oxygen is used to prevent the development of oxygen toxicity. In the absence of underlying lung disease, room air should suffice. In class III patients, care must be exercised in administering oxygen without respiratory assistance because removal of the hypoxic drive to ventilation may lead to more pronounced hypoventilation.

    b. Cardiovascular. Hypotension occurs in barbiturate poisoning from decreased intravascular volume, from hypoxia with acidosis, and, at extremely high doses, from the direct myocardial depressant effects of barbiturates. The decreased intravascular volume is caused by dehydration and the escape of fluid from the capillaries because of increased capillary permeability, which results from both barbiturate toxicity and hypoxia. The venous pooling of blood that follows may impair cardiac output further.

      (1) The chief therapy of hypotension consists of **correction of hypoxia,** if it exists, and **replacement of vascular volume.** A CVP line is placed, and volume-expanding solutions are infused at about 20 ml/minute until the CVP reaches 2–6 cm H_2O.

        (a) The initial liter of volume replacement may be in the form of a **5% albumin solution** because it will not only expand intravascular volume rapidly, but it will also bind some of the circulating barbiturates. However, this latter effect is significant only for long-acting and intermediate-acting compounds.

        (b) An **isotonic electrolyte solution** may be used after the initial liter of albumin is infused.

(2) **Pressors** may be required in patients with severe intoxication in which the blood pressure does not respond to volume replacement. In general, the pressor chosen is infused at a rate that is sufficient to maintain . systolic blood pressure at about 90 mm Hg, but the urine output is the ultimate guide. In cases of ingestion of long-acting and intermediate-acting barbiturates, which are excreted primarily in the urine, **dopamine** is the pressor of choice.

c. **Other supportive measures**

   (1) Frequent turning, attention to skin care, and other supportive measures are necessary for comatose patients.

   (2) Frequent suctioning of intubated patients, pulmonary physical therapy, and prompt antibiotic treatment of respiratory infections are also required.

3. **Removal of unabsorbed drug** from the gastrointestinal tract is helpful only if the patient is seen within 3 hours of ingestion. The only exceptions are the rare patients who ingest large amounts of barbiturates and develop a resultant ileus. Because of their intestinal hypomotility, these patients retain unabsorbed drug in the gut for many hours.

a. **Emesis** should be induced only in patients with mild ingestion who are awake and able to protect their own airways from aspiration.

b. **Gastric lavage** may be undertaken in patients who are seen within 3 hours of ingestion, but it should be performed only with a cuffed endotracheal tube in place.

c. After the stomach is evacuated, if bowel sounds are present, an **osmotic cathartic** may be administered.

   (1) **Sorbitol,** 50 g mixed with about 200 ml of water, or **magnesium citrate,** 200 ml of the standard commercial solution, may be used.

   (2) **Activated charcoal** will bind barbiturates and may be given along with the cathartic; the usual dose is 30 g.

4. **Removal of absorbed barbiturate from the body**

a. Both forced diuresis and, in the case of phenobarbital, alkalinization of the urine hasten excretion of barbiturates. However, these methods pose risks of volume and sodium overload and have failed to improve outcome. Therefore, they are not generally recommended.

b. **Hemodialysis** is more effective for removing intermediate- and long-acting barbiturates than short-acting compounds. The indications for its use are

   (1) Renal or hepatic insufficiency severe enough to prevent the elimination of the drug.

   (2) Shock or prolonged coma that does not respond to conservative management.

   (3) Ingestion of a lethal dose of drug (3 g of a short-acting or 5 g of a long-acting barbiturate).

   (4) A serum drug level predictive of prolonged coma (> 3.5 mg/dl for short-acting barbiturates or > 8 mg/dl for phenobarbital).

5. **Complications** of barbiturate intoxication result primarily from prolonged coma, but pneumonia and bladder infections are encountered frequently. Acute renal failure due to acute tubular necrosis or to nontraumatic rhabdomyolysis can also occur.

6. **Psychiatric evaluation** and care are provided to all patients who ingest overdoses of drugs intentionally.

B. **Barbiturate withdrawal.** Acute barbiturate withdrawal presents a clinical picture that is strikingly similar to that of alcohol withdrawal, with tremor, delirium, and seizures being prominent. Symptoms may be aborted by the intravenous administration of barbiturates. Pentobarbital may be given in 25-mg increments q5–10min until symptoms abate.

In contrast to ethanol withdrawal, the seizures associated with withdrawal from short-acting barbiturates are often severe. Intravenous barbiturate is the treatment of choice. Diazepam is generally effective, but the combination of barbiturate and diazepam frequently produces respiratory depression. After the acute symptoms are under control, the patient may be withdrawn from barbiturates gradually. As with ethanol withdrawal, careful attention is directed toward fluid and electrolyte balance, antipyresis, and prevention of infectious complications.

XIII. Poisoning with nonbarbiturate CNS depressants

A. The **basic therapy** of acute intoxication with all CNS depressants is similar to that of barbiturate intoxication. The respiratory and cardiovascular systems must be stabilized, unabsorbed drug is removed by lavage and catharsis, and the elimination of the drug from the body is speeded by whatever techniques are feasible for each drug.

B. Individual drugs

1. Glutethimide

a. Description. Glutethimide (Doriden) overdose carries high mortality. The characteristic fluctuating course is probably caused by delayed absorption of drug as a result of paralytic ileus. The signs are similar to those of barbiturate intoxication, except that the drug also possesses anticholinergic activity, producing dilated pupils.

b. Treatment is primarily supportive, and elimination of the drug may be hastened by forced diuresis. Hemodialysis against a lipid-containing dialysis should be employed if the patient has renal failure, fails to respond to conservative measures, or has ingested a potentially lethal dose (> 10 g total or blood level > 3 mg/dl).

2. Chloral hydrate and ethchlorvynol

a. Description. Chloral hydrate (Noctec) and ethchlorvynol (Placidyl) intoxications resemble barbiturate intoxication, except that chloral hydrate may produce constricted pupils.

b. The **treatment** is identical to that of barbiturate overdose. Hemodialysis is effective in eliminating both drugs and should be used with the same indications as with barbiturate overdose. Lipid dialysis increases the rate of elimination.

3. Benzodiazepines

a. Description. Diazepam and chlordiazepoxide taken alone PO generally do not produce life-threatening intoxication in medically sound patients. Respiratory depression is of significance only in patients with intrinsic lung disease or in cases of mixed ingestions.

b. Treatment of benzodiazepine intoxication consists of eliminating unabsorbed drug from the gastrointestinal tract and supporting these patients until they awaken.

XIV. Amphetamines

A. Acute toxicity

1. Description. Acute amphetamine toxicity produces psychosis, hyperpyrexia, hypertension, dilated pupils, vomiting, and diarrhea. Life-threatening effects of severe intoxication include cardiac arrhythmias, seizures, coma, and respiratory arrest. The lethal dose in children is about 5 mg/kg; in adults, it is about 1.5 g. The serum half-life is a matter of days, so toxic symptoms may persist for longer than a week.

2. Treatment

a. Sedation with neuroleptics controls **psychotic manifestations. Chlorpromazine,** 50 mg PO or IM, may be given initially and q30min until the patient is calm. Then it is given q4–6h as necessary.

b. Hyperpyrexia can be controlled with a cooling blanket and vigorous wetting with towels soaked in tepid water.

c. Arrhythmias are treated with appropriate drugs.

d. Seizures are a short-term problem if no irreversible CNS damage occurs from hypoxia or cardiac arrest. They should be treated with the usual measures (see Chap. 6).

e. Unabsorbed drug is removed with emesis, lavage, catharsis, or all three, as appropriate. Lavage may be of benefit even several hours after ingestion.

f. Acidification of the urine hastens the excretion of amphetamines and should be employed in the event of severe intoxication. **Ammonium chloride** may be administered PO or IV at a total dose of 8–12 g/day, and the urine pH is checked frequently. Ammonium chloride is contraindicated in shock, systemic acidosis of any cause, and hepatic failure or portosystemic shunting.

  g. **Severe hypertension** is best treated with an alpha-blocking agent, such as phentolamine (Regitine). Moderate hypertension responds to chlorpromazine.

B. **Chronic amphetamine abuse** should be treated psychiatrically. Acute amphetamine withdrawal produces no medical complications, so there is no need to taper doses. After sudden cessation of habitual amphetamine ingestion, a prolonged sleep generally occurs, requiring only observation and maintenance of hydration.

C. **Cocaine intoxication** is clinically similar to amphetamine overdose, and the supportive treatment is identical. Cocaine has a much shorter half-life than amphetamines, and it is metabolized rapidly by the liver. Consequently, forced diuresis or acidification of the urine is of no benefit. Seizures, stroke, subarachnoid hemorrhage, and cardiovascular collapse may occur as a result of cocaine intoxication.

XV. **Polycyclic antidepressants**

A. The **acute toxic effects** of polycyclic antidepressants resemble atropine poisoning, with hyperpyrexia, dilated pupils, hypertension, tachycardia, and dryness of the skin and mucous membranes. The life-threatening manifestations are coma, seizures, cardiac arrhythmias, and cardiac conduction defects.

B. **Supportive therapy**

  1. The **initial emergency treatment** is the same as for any overdose: stabilization of respiratory and cardiac status and elimination of unabsorbed drug from the gastrointestinal tract.

  2. **Cardiac conduction defects and arrhythmias** are prominent in tricyclic intoxication. The patient should be on a cardiac monitor, a temporary transvenous pacemaker should be readily available, and the patient should be placed in an intensive or coronary care unit. Lidocaine is effective for ventricular arrhythmias. Propranolol should be used with extreme care if a conduction defect is present.

  3. **Hyperpyrexia** can be controlled with a cooling blanket or by vigorous rubdowns with towels soaked in tepid water. Chlorpromazine may increase the effectiveness of hypothermic methods.

  4. Severe **hypertension** responds to the administration of an alpha blocker such as phentolamine.

C. **Physotigmine** is reported to antagonize the CNS toxicity of tricyclics and other anticholinergics.

  1. **Physostigmine** injection may serve as a **diagnostic test** to confirm anticholinergic ingestion. Physostigmine, 1 mg, is injected SC, IM, or slowly IV, which will produce peripheral cholinergic signs within 30 minutes if no anticholinergics have been ingested. These signs include bradycardia, salivation, lacrimation, and pupillary constriction. In a patient who has ingested anticholinergics, the injection will produce no significant effect.

  2. For the **treatment** of anticholinergic overdose, 1-mg doses of physostigmine are injected IM or slowly IV at 20-minute intervals until 4 mg has been administered or cholinergic signs appear.

  3. **Indications.** Physostigmine is most effective against the toxic delirium of anticholinergic overdose. It will occasionally awaken a comatose patient. However, physostigmine is itself toxic, so its use should be reserved for patients with life-threatening complications of tricyclic overdose: respiratory depression, intractable seizures, or severe hypertension.

  4. **Side effects.** If excessive physostigmine is administered, cholinergic side effects may, in themselves, exert harmful effects. Excessive respiratory secretions, salivation, and bronchospasm may interfere with pulmonary function. Vomiting, abdominal cramps, and diarrhea may also occur. Excessive cholinergic effects may be counteracted with atropine (see sec. **IX.D.5**). Physostigmine at toxic doses or administered rapidly IV can cause seizures.

  5. The **duration of action** of physostigmine is only 1–2 hours, whereas tricyclics persist over 24 hours. Therefore, the patient must be monitored and repeated doses are administered as necessary.

D. Tricyclic antidepressants are cleared mainly by the kidneys, so **forced diuresis** is effective. Dialysis is of no additional benefit except in renal failure.

XVI. Salicylate intoxication

A. Description

1. In the United States salicylate is the medicine that most frequently produces clinically significant intoxication. The most common source is aspirin, but sodium salicylate and oil of wintergreen are also common causes.

a. Aspirin. Adult aspirin tablets contain 325 mg of aspirin, whereas children's tablets contain 80 mg. Some so-called extra-strength aspirin tablets contain as much as 750 mg.

b. Oil of wintergreen contains methyl salicylate in a concentration of about 0.7 g/ml. It is highly toxic, and 1 or 2 tsp may be a fatal dose for a small child.

2. The **toxic dose** of salicylate is about 250 mg/kg in a healthy person. Lower doses of both methyl salicylate and aspirin may be intoxicating in a person who is dehydrated or in renal failure.

3. Pharmacokinetics

a. Salicylates are well absorbed from the gastrointestinal tract, over 50% of a therapeutic dose being absorbed within 1 hour of ingestion. Poisoning has occurred from oil of wintergreen from cutaneous absorption.

b. Once absorbed, aspirin is rapidly hydrolyzed to salicylic acid.

c. Salicylic acid is variably bound to albumin. At toxic levels, the serum albumin binding sites are 100% saturated.

d. Salicylic acid is excreted both unchanged and as its glucuronidated product in the urine. Salicylic acid has a pK_a of about 3, so it can be "trapped" in the alkaline solution. Thus, alkalinization of the urine may increase salicylic acid excretion as much as fivefold.

4. Signs and symptoms of toxicity

a. Central nervous system abnormalities dominate the clinical picture.

(1) The earliest signs are tinnitus and impaired hearing.

(2) Agitation progressing to delirium, stupor, and coma results from severe intoxication.

(3) Seizures may occur as a direct effect of salicylate toxicity or as a secondary manifestation of hypoglycemia or effective hypocalcemia (see sec. **XVI.A.4.b**).

(4) Salicylates in toxic doses stimulate respiration and produce hyperpnea, usually with tachypnea and respiratory alkalosis.

(5) With extremely high doses, respiratory depression occurs.

b. Metabolic derangements

(1) Salicylates interfere with **carbohydrate metabolism.**

(a) Hypoglycemia may occur in young children.

(b) The brain uses glucose inefficiently and may experience a "**relative hypoglycemia,**" even with a normal blood glucose.

(c) Mild to moderate **hyperglycemia** is frequent.

(2) In severe intoxication, **metabolic acidosis** occurs with an increased anion gap and organic aciduria.

(3) The **organic aciduria,** with or without glycosuria, produces an osmotic diuresis, which in turn produces dehydration.

(4) The **respiratory alkalosis,** when prolonged, has secondary effects on electrolyte metabolism.

(a) There is **renal sodium and potassium wasting.** The hypokalemia renders the metabolic acidosis unresponsive to alkali therapy until the potassium is repleted.

(b) The respiratory alkalosis produces **decreased unbound serum calcium levels,** which can lead to tetany and seizures.

(5) SIADH has been reported in association with salicylate poisoning.

c. Effects on blood clotting

(1) Salicylate in toxic concentrations exerts an **antiprothrombin effect,** with prolongation of the PT and diminished factor VII activity.

      (2) Salicylates interfere with **platelet function,** even in nontoxic doses.

      (3) Salicylates are locally irritating to the gastric mucosa and may lead to **gastrointestinal hemorrhage.**

    d. **Hepatotoxicity** may elevate the liver enzymes, which can lead to confusion with Reye's syndrome in children or with hepatic encephalopathy in adults.

    e. **Noncardiac pulmonary edema** has been reported.

B. **Diagnosis**

  1. Salicylate intoxication occurs frequently in three groups:

    a. Children under 5 years of age, as a result of accidental ingestion.

    b. Adolescents and young adults, as a result of intentional ingestion.

    c. Unintentional overdose in patients taking salicylates for rheumatic disease.

  2. The diagnosis is obvious with an adequate **history** of ingestion; however, it is frequently masked by chronic therapeutic overdose if the physician is unaware that the patient is taking salicylates.

  3. The diagnosis is considered in patients with mental status changes, hyperpnea, and respiratory alkalosis, with or without superimposed metabolic acidosis.

  4. **Serum salicylate levels** confirm the diagnosis. A level higher than 30 mg/dl may produce early symptoms of salicylism; mental changes and hyperpnea occur at levels higher than 40 mg/dl. With chronic ingestion, blood levels correlate poorly with the clinical status of the patient but will nevertheless serve to make or to rule out the diagnosis.

  5. The **ferric chloride test** serves as a rapid screening test for the presence of salicylic acid.

    a. A few drops of a 10% solution of ferric chloride are added to 3–5 ml of acidified urine. A purple color indicates a positive result.

    b. The test is extremely sensitive, so a positive result is not diagnostic of salicylate intoxication.

    c. Ferric chloride reacts only with salicylic acid, not with aspirin. Therefore, it cannot be used to test for the presence of aspirin in gastric contents.

    d. Phenothiazines react with ferric chloride, but they tend to give a pink rather than a purple color.

    e. Acetoacetic acid, present in ketosis, will react with ferric chloride. Its presence may be excluded, however, if the urine is boiled and acidified before adding the ferric chloride.

  6. The **initial laboratory evaluation** of a patient with salicylate intoxication should include the following:

    a. Serum salicylate level is of prognostic importance and gives a baseline value with which to judge the effects of therapy.

    b. Patients with intentional overdoses should have blood or urine (or both) screened for the presence of other toxic substances.

    c. CBC, including platelet count.

    d. Stool and gastric contents are tested for the presence of occult blood.

    e. Arterial blood gases and pH.

    f. BUN (or creatinine), electrolytes, calcium, and phosphorus.

    g. Liver function tests, including SGOT, LDH, alkaline phosphatase, total bilirubin, total protein, and albumin.

    h. Prothrombin time and partial thromboplastin time.

    i. Chest x ray.

    j. ECG, giving particular attention to signs of hypokalemia or hypocalcemia.

    k. Urinalysis with specific gravity. If the serum sodium is low and SIADH is a possibility, urine sodium concentration and osmolality are measured.

C. **Acute management**

  1. **Routine emergency measures for the treatment of drug intoxications**

    a. Protect the **airway** and support respiration, if necessary.

    b. Empty the **gastrointestinal tract** of unabsorbed drug.

      (1) Forced **emesis** is used if the patient is alert.

      (2) **Gastric lavage** is performed after tracheal intubation with a cuffed endotracheal tube if patients are stuporous, in coma, or unable to protect their own airway.

(3) **Activated charcoal** is given as 200–300 ml of a thick suspension to bind unabsorbed salicylates.

(4) **Cathartics** are administered after the charcoal has been given.

2. **Fluid and electrolyte management** is used to treat shock, to maintain urine output, and to restore electrolyte and acid-base balance.

3. **Alkalinization of the urine** by the infusion of sodium bicarbonate hastens the excretion of salicylic acid. However, in practice the technique has no use.

   a. In elderly patients and those with abnormal hearts, the risks of increased sodium load are not justified by the expected benefits of alkalinization of the urine.

   b. In patients with metabolic acidosis, the urine cannot be alkalinized except with massive and dangerous quantities of alkali.

   c. In patients with respiratory alkalosis and alkalemia, the administration of alkali is contraindicated.

4. **Hypoglycemia**

   a. In young children, after blood has been drawn, 50% D/W (0.5 ml/kg IV) is administered immediately.

   b. Only glucose-containing fluids are used for maintenance.

5. **Hemorrhagic complications**

   a. In severe salicylate poisoning, **vitamin K,** 50 mg IV, is given after an initial PT has been measured. The vitamin K is repeated as necessary to maintain a normal PT.

   b. If bleeding occurs or if the PT is found to be longer than twice the control value, **fresh-frozen plasma** or **concentrates of clotting factors** (Konȳne) are given.

   c. **Platelet transfusion** may be required to achieve control of hemorrhage because the patient's own platelets will have a disordered function.

   d. In comatose patients, **antacids** may be given by nasogastric tube in an effort to prevent gastric hemorrhage.

6. **Tetany** may be treated with the intravenous infusion of calcium gluconate in 1-g doses, repeated as often as necessary.

7. **Seizures**

   a. Hypoglycemia and hypocalcemia are treated appropriately (see secs. **XVI.C.4** and **6**). Other metabolic causes of seizures, such as hyponatremia and hypoxia, must also be considered.

   b. Seizures that occur as a direct toxic effect of salicylate are a poor prognostic sign, generally indicating the necessity for hemodialysis to hasten elimination of the salicylate. Diazepam, given IV, or muscle paralysis and respiratory support may be used for the temporary control of seizures until the salicylate level is lowered.

8. **Fever** can be treated with tepid water baths.

9. **Methods to hasten the elimination of salicylates**

   a. Forced diuresis is of little benefit, and the patient should not be subjected to a larger fluid load than necessary to achieve a reasonable urine output.

   b. Alkalinization of the urine is discussed in sec. **XVI.C.3**. Despite its theoretic advantages, it has no practical use in salicylate poisoning.

   c. **Peritoneal dialysis** is about as efficient as the normal kidneys in eliminating salicylate from the blood. Its primary use is in the setting of renal failure. The addition of albumin to the dialysis solution hastens the elimination of salicylate, but there is no evidence that its benefit outweighs the expense and added complexity of the dialysis.

   d. **Hemodialysis** is the most efficient means available for the elimination of salicylate. The generally accepted indications for hemodialysis are

      (1) Salicylate level higher than 70 mg/dl or known absorption greater than 5 g/kg.

      (2) Profound coma with respiratory failure.

      (3) Severe metabolic acidosis.

       (4) Renal failure.

       (5) Failure to respond to conservative therapy.

XVII. Hyperthermia

  A. Pathophysiology. Rises in body temperature may be due to excessive heat gain, insufficient heat loss, or both.

    1. Excessive heat gain

      a. Exercise.

      b. High ambient temperatures.

      c. Increased metabolic rate.

      d. Release of pyrogens (e.g., by infection).

      e. Neuroleptic malignant syndrome (see sec. **XVII.B.4**).

    2. Defective heat loss

      a. Excessively warm clothing.

      b. Increased humidity.

      c. Low wind velocity.

      d. Advanced age.

      e. Anticholinergic drugs (e.g., phenothiazines, tricyclic antidepressants).

      f. Sympathetic autonomic failure with decreased or absent sweating due to

        (1) Elevated body temperatures.

        (2) Spinal cord transection above T1.

  B. Categories of heat disorders

    1. Heat cramps

      a. Description. Muscle or abdominal cramps associated with exercise in warm, ambient environments are commonly seen.

      b. Treatment. Rest and oral electrolyte replacement are usually adequate.

    2. Heat exhaustion (heat prostration, exertional heat injury)

      a. Description. Heat exhaustion is marked by moderately elevated body temperatures (i.e., 39.5–42.0°C) and a neurologic syndrome characterized by headache, piloerection, hyperventilation, nausea, vomiting, unsteady gait, and confusion. **Sweating remains intact** in patients with heat exhaustion, so the skin is wet and cool.

      b. Treatment. Patients should be admitted to the hospital for treatment, since some may progress to heat stroke. Rest and parenteral rehydration are usually adequate to reverse the syndrome.

    3. Heat stroke

      a. Description. When body temperatures rise high enough, CNS mechanisms for control of heat loss may fail. When this occurs, there is a very rapid further rise in body temperature, which is a life-threatening medical emergency. Such patients may be diaphoretic or may have hot, dry skin (sweating having failed) and elevated body temperatures (> 41°C, ranging as high as 43°C). The level of consciousness becomes deranged, often quite suddenly, so that patients may rapidly deteriorate from confusion or delirium to deep coma, often with seizures. Cerebral edema occurs, which may lead to widespread cerebral ischemia and eventually brain death. Other abnormalities include circulatory failure, disseminated intravascular coagulation, severe dehydration, and hepatic necrosis. Electrolyte abnormalities, most commonly respiratory alkalosis and hypokalemia, are frequent.

      b. Treatment

        (1) Surface cooling should be started immediately. The most effective means is to use evaporative cooling by spraying the naked patient with tepid water and using a powerful fan to maintain a flow of air over the patient's body. Alternatively, immersion in ice or cold water may be used.

        (2) Intravenous fluids should be administered with care, as typically the patient is normovolemic but has redistributed fluid to peripheral, vasodilated tissues. With cooling, fluid will redistribute and cardiac output will be restored.

        (3) A bladder catheter should be placed and urinary output carefully monitored.

    (4) Isoproterenol via constant infusion (1 μg/min) may be used to increase cardiac output.

    (5) Avoid alpha-adrenergic drugs (e.g., norepineprhine) that produce vaso-constriction and thus retard heat loss.

    (6) Avoid anticholinergic drugs (e.g., atropine) that retard the return of sweating.

    (7) Monitoring of ICP using a dural bolt may be necessary if consciousness does not return promptly.

    (8) Treat increased ICP as outlined in Chap. 1, sec. **VII.D.**

    (9) Seizures may be treated with **phenytoin** or **phenobarbitol** as outlined in Chap. 6.

    (10) If disseminated intravascular coagulation develops, heparin, 1000 units/hour by constant infusion, may be used.

4. Neuroleptic malignant syndrome (NMS)

  a. Description. NMS is characterized by hyperthermia, muscular rigidity, and altered mental status. It occurs in patients taking neuroleptic medications or, rarely, in association with withdrawal of L-dopa or other dopaminergic agonists.

    (1) Although a preponderance of reported cases have occurred with the use of potent neuroleptics such as haloperidol, the syndrome has been associated with virtually all dopamine-receptor antagonists and dopamine-depleting agents (e.g., reserpine).

    (2) NMS may occur immediately after the first dose of a neuroleptic or in a patient who has been taking neuroleptics for many years. Many cases are associated with a rapid increase in dose.

    (3) Laboratory abnormalities may include an elevated serum CK, elevated WBC, and abnormal liver function tests. The CSF is normal, and the EEG shows generalized slowing. The CT scan and MRI are normal.

    (4) Life-threatening complications of NMS include respiratory failure secondary to muscular rigidity and renal failure secondary to myoglobinuria.

  b. Prevention. NMS is commonly precipitated by dehydration, fever, or environmental exposure to high temperatures in patients taking neuroleptics. These precipitants should be especially avoided in patients taking neuroleptics or dopamine-depleting agents. In addition, withdrawal of dopamine agonists, including carbidopa–L-dopa (Sinemet), should be carried out gradually.

  c. Treatment

    (1) Immediate withdrawal of all neuroleptic medications (including those administered as antiemetics) or dopamine-depleting agents (e.g., reserpine, tetrabenazine) is essential at the earliest sign of NMS. In cases associated with withdrawal of dopamine agonists (e.g., L-dopa, bromocriptine, pergolide), reinstitution of dopaminergic therapy and more gradual withdrawal should be undertaken.

    (2) The mainstay of management is **supportive care.**

      (a) Rehydration and maintenance of adequate urine flow.

      (b) Lowering body temperature with antipyretics, cooling blanket, or tepid water bath as required.

      (c) Protection of the airway by endotracheal intubation as required.

      (d) In unusual cases, respirator support with muscular paralysis may be required to maintain ventilation in the face of extreme muscular rigidity.

    (3) The direct-acting muscle relaxant **dantrolene** is widely used in severe cases of NMS, although there are no systematic studies documenting its benefit. Muscle relaxation may facilitate nursing care and aid in lowering body temperature. In addition, to the extent that muscle rigidity contributes to muscle necrosis and myoglobinuria, muscle relaxation may help prevent renal failure. However, it is clear that muscular rigidity is not the only cause of muscle damage in NMS and that hyperthermia may persist in spite of muscle paralysis. Dosages of dantrolene employed have varied from 1–10 mg/kg/day IV or by nasogastric tube given in four divided doses. Hepatic toxicity occurs with dosages above 10 mg/kg/day.

  (4) The dopamine agonist **bromocriptine** has also been widely used and has theoretic support. However, there are no systematic studies documenting its benefit in NMS. Dosages employed have varied from 2.5–10.0 mg IV or by nasogastric tube q4–6h.

  (5) Electroconvulsive therapy has shown effectiveness in anecdotal reports. Its role in the treatment of NMS is undefined.

  d. Prognosis. Although mortality rates from NMS as high as 15–20% are quoted in the literature, it is clear that with adequate supportive care the mortality is much less than that figure. To prevent relapse of NMS, neuroleptic medications must not be reinstituted until the syndrome has completely resolved. Patients may require sedation with benzodiazepines in the meantime. After resolution of all clinical signs of NMS, neuroleptics may be cautiously reinstituted. NMS is not an allergic reaction to neuroleptics, and the occurrence of NMS is not an absolute contraindication to neuroleptic use.

XVIII. Nutritional deficiency and excess

  A. Vitamin deficiency

   1. Thiamine

    a. Description

     (1) Thiamine deficiency is associated with **chronic alcohol abuse** (see sec. **X.C**) and with **severe nutritional deficiency,** as occurs in patients on long-term parenteral nutrition.

     (2) The acute syndrome of thiamine deficiency in adults, known as **Wernicke's encephalopathy,** is characterized by nystagmus and limitations of extraocular movements, gait ataxia, and mental confusion.

    b. Prevention

     (1) Patients receiving parenteral nutrition should have thiamine supplementation of 2–10 mg/day, depending on carbohydrate intake.

     (2) Chronic alcoholics and other chronically malnourished patients should receive supplementation with thiamine, 50 mg PO daily, as well as with daily multivitamins.

     (3) Hemodialysis patients should all receive regular thiamine supplementation.

    c. Treatment

     (1) Acute **Wernicke's encephalopathy** is an emergency (see sec. **X.C**).

     (2) Patients are administered **thiamine,** 50 mg IV and 50 mg IM immediately. They then receive thiamine, 50 mg IM daily for 3 days, and long-term supplementation with thiamine, 50 mg IM or PO daily.

     (3) Patients should also be supplemented with **vitamin B complex,** either PO or parenterally as appropriate.

   2. Cobalamin (vitamin B$_{12}$) deficiency (pernicious anemia)

    a. Description

     (1) Cobalamin deficiency is usually associated with an acquired defect in intestinal absorption of the vitamin due to intrinsic factor deficiency. Rarely, patients on highly restricted diets (so-called vegans) develop cobalamin deficiency from inadequate intake of the vitamin. There are rare inborn errors of metabolism that affect cobalamin absorption or transport or the activity of its target enzymes that duplicate various aspects of cobalamin deficiency. These syndromes generally present in early childhood. Finally, the recreational use or occupational exposure to the anesthetic gas nitrous oxide can duplicate all of the clinical features of cobalamin deficiency.

     (2) The classic picture of cobalamin deficiency consists of megaloblastic anemia, subacute combined degeneration of the spinal cord (demyelination of the posterior columns and corticospinal tracts), optic neuropathy (termed "tobacco amblyopia," since it is more common in smokers) and mental status changes. Any of these may occur in isolation. There is increasing recognition that personality change and dementia may be the only manifestation of cobalamin deficiency, mandating more aggressive screening. The administration of folate to cobalamin-deficient patients may predispose to the development of neurologic signs prior to hematologic abnormalities.

b. Diagnosis

   (1) Serum cobalamin. Some patients become symptomatic even with serum cobalamin concentrations in the low normal range (150–250 pmol/liter).

   (2) Elevated **serum concentrations of methylmalonic acid** and **total serum homocysteine** help substantiate the diagnosis in questionable cases. These tests are expensive and only performed by a few commercial laboratories; their role in the screening of patients with nonspecific neuropsychiatric symptoms or signs and borderline or low normal serum cobalamin levels is undefined.

   (3) Intrinsic factor deficiency can be confirmed by a **Schilling test.** Some patients may absorb free cobalamin normally and have a normal standard Schilling test, but absorb cobalamin poorly from food. These cases can be diagnosed by administering the oral cobalamin with egg white (the **food Schilling test**).

   (4) The presence of **anti-intrinsic factor** or **antiparietal cell antibodies** confirms the diagnosis of pernicious anemia.

c. Treatment

   (1) All patients suspected of cobalamin deficiency should have therapy initiated immediately after drawing serum for determination of cobalamin concentration. Cobalamin administration does not invalidate the Schilling test.

   (2) Cyanocobalamin or **hydroxycobalamin,** 1000 µg IM, is administered daily for 5–10 days, then weekly for four dosages, and then monthly for the remainder of the patient's life. Lower doses may suffice, but clinicians generally use high doses for neurologically symptomatic patients. There is evidence that hydroxycobalamin is more effective than cyanocobalamin in patients with optic nerve involvement.

   (3) Hematologic measurements (hemoglobin, mean corpuscular volume, and reticulocyte count) and **serum cobalamin levels** are followed periodically to verify the therapeutic response.

   (4) Severely anemic patients may develop **hypokalemia** as the anemia is corrected; in these patients the serum potassium concentration should be measured regularly over the first 2 weeks of therapy.

   (5) Folate administration may cause neurologic deterioration in cobalamin-deficient patients. Therefore, **folate should be withheld** until cobalamin stores are repleted (1–2 weeks of daily cobalamin injections).

3. Pyridoxine (vitamin B$_6$)

a. Description

   (1) Pyridoxine deficiency syndromes are rare. They occur predominantly in adults administered drugs that antagonize the action of pyridoxine, most notably the antituberculous agent isoniazid. Other drugs that can induce pyridoxine deficiency include hydralazine, cycloserine, penicillamine, and pyrazinamide. Purely dietary deficiency of pyridoxine is extremely rare.

   (2) Pyridoxine deficiency produces a symmetric, distal sensory and motor neuropathy. Rarely, seizures and encephalopathy occur.

b. Treatment

   (1) Adults taking isoniazid, 300 mg daily, should be supplemented with pyridoxine, 50 mg daily.

   (2) Symptomatic pyridoxine deficiency due to isoniazid is treated with pyridoxine, 100–200 mg IM or PO daily for 2 weeks, followed by supplementation with 50 mg daily.

   (3) Nutritional pyridoxine deficiency, in the absence of pyridoxine antagonists, requires doses of 2.5–5.0 mg daily.

(4) The **excessive ingestion of pyridoxine** can produce a sensory neuropathy, so doses in excess of those necessary to correct the deficiency should be avoided.

(5) Pyridoxine is a cofactor for the decarboxylation of L-dopa, so pyridoxine supplementation of patients taking L-dopa will decrease the antiparkinsonian effect of the L-dopa. Pyridoxine-free multivitamin preparations are available for such patients. Patients taking L-dopa in combination with a decarboxylase inhibitor (e.g., Sinemet) may take pyridoxine if indicated, since the decarboxylase inhibitors block the action of pyridoxine on L-dopa metabolism.

4. Vitamin E (alpha-tocopherol)

a. Description

(1) Vitamin E is a fat-soluble vitamin; deficiency states therefore occur with chronic malabsorption syndromes. This can occur in association with hereditary disorders such as abetalipoproteinemia, with intestinal resections, and with hepatobiliary disease.

(2) Clinical manifestations include peripheral neuropathy, ataxia, and proximal muscle weakness. The syndrome resembles spinocerebellar degeneration.

b. Treatment

(1) Dosage. In adults, 60–75 units of vitamin E, PO or IM, generally suffices. Dosage should be adjusted to achieve plasma vitamin E levels within the normal range.

(2) Excessive doses of vitamin E have been reported to produce a reversible myopathy.

(3) It may be necessary to **supplement other fat-soluble vitamins** (vitamins A, D, and K) as well.

B. Hypervitaminoses

1. Description. The administration of excessive doses of vitamins therapeutically and the ingestion of "mega" doses of vitamins by food faddists have introduced syndromes of hypervitaminosis into medicine.

a. Pyridoxine toxicity produces a predominantly sensory neuropathy.

b. Hypervitaminosis E rarely produces myopathy.

c. Hypervitaminosis A is associated with benign intracranial hypertension.

2. The **treatment** of all these conditions is cessation of vitamin supplementation. The sensory neuropathy of pyridoxine intoxication and the myopathy of hypervitaminosis E are both reversible. Benign intracranial hypertension associated with hypervitaminosis A resolves over several weeks once the vitamin excess is corrected, although permanent visual loss can occur.

Selected Readings

HEPATIC ENCEPHALOPATHY

Green, A., and Hall, S.M. Investigation of metabolic disorders resembling Reye's syndrome. *Arch. Dis. Child.* 67:1313, 1992.

Green, C. L., Blitzer, M. G., and Shapira, E. Inborn errors of metabolism and Reye syndrome: Differential diagnosis. *J. Pediatr.* 113:156, 1988.

Morgan, M. Y. The treatment of chronic hepatic encephalopathy. *Hepatogastroenterology* 38:377, 1991.

Mullen, K. D., and Weber, F. L. Role of nutrition in hepatic encephalopathy. *Semin. Liver Dis.* 11:292, 1991.

Trauner, D. A. Treatment of Reye's syndrome. *Ann. Neurol.* 7:2, 1979.

RENAL AND ELECTROLYTE DISORDERS

Arieff, A. I. Hyponatremia, convulsions, respiratory arrest, and permanent brain damage after elective surgery in healthy women. *N. Engl. J. Med.* 314:1529, 1986.

Diringer, M. N. Management of sodium abnormalities in patients with CNS Disease *Clin. Neuropharmacol.* 15:427, 1992.

Stearns, R. H., Riggs, J. E., and Schochet, S. S. Osmotic demyelination syndrom following correction of hyponatremia. *N. Engl. J. Med.* 314:1535, 1986.

Wijdicks, E. F. M., et al. Atrial natriuretic factor and salt wasting after aneurysma subarachnoid hemorrhage. *Stroke* 22:1519, 1991.

ACUTE INTERMITTENT PORPHYRIA

Kappas, A., et al. The Porphyrias. In C. R. Scriver et al. (eds.), *The Metabolic Basis o Inherited Disease* (6th ed.). New York: McGraw-Hill, 1989. Pp. 1305–1365.

HEAVY METAL POISONING

Angle, C. R. Childhood lead poisoning and its treatment. *Annu. Rev. Pharmacol Toxicol.* 32:409, 1993.

Chao, J., and Kikano, G. E. Lead poisoning in children. *Am. Fam. Physician* 47:113 1993.

Mortensen, M. E., and Walson, P. D. Chelation therapy for childhood lead poisoning The changing scene in the 1990s. *Clin. Pediatr.* 32:284, 1993.

CARBON MONOXIDE POISONING

Ilano, A. L., and Raffin, T. A. Management of carbon monoxide poisoning. *Chest* 97:165 1990.

DRUG AND ALCOHOL INTOXICATION

Brust, J. C. M. *Neurological Aspects of Substance Abuse.* Boston: Butterworth-Heineman, 1993.

Brust, J. C. M. (ed.). Neurological complications of drug and alcohol abuse. *Neurol. Clin.* 11(3), 1993.

Charness, M. E., Simon, R. P., and Greenberg, D. A. Ethanol and the nervous system *N. Engl. J. Med.* 321:442, 1989.

HYPERTHERMIA

Caroff, S. N., and Mann, S. C. Neuroleptic malignant syndrome. *Med. Clin. North Am.* 77:185, 1993.

Rosebush, P., and Stewart, T. A. Prospective analysis of 24 episodes of neuroleptic malignant syndrome. *Am. J. Psychiatry* 146:717, 1989.

Tek, D., and Olshaker, J. S. Heat illness. *Emerg. Med. Clin. North Am.* 10:299, 1992.

NUTRITIONAL DEFICIENCY

Beck, W. S. Neuropsychiatric consequences of cobalamin deficiency. *Adv. Intern. Med.* 36:33, 1991.

Lindenbaum, J. Neuropsychiatric disorders caused by cobalamin deficiency in the absence of anemia or macrocytosis. *N. Engl. J. Med.* 318:1720, 1988.

Shevell, M. I., and Rosenblatt, D. S. The neurology of cobalamin. *Can. J. Neurol. Sci.* 19:472, 1992.

Victor, M., Adams, R. D., and Collins, G. H. *The Wernicke-Korsakoff Syndrome and Related Neurological Disorders* (2nd ed.). Philadelphia: Davis, 1989.

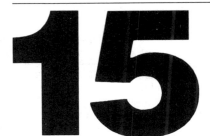

Movement Disorders

Robert D. Helme

I. **Motor control systems.** The rational management of movement disorders requires some understanding of the anatomic and physiologic substrate necessary for normal movement. Potential benefit from therapeutic maneuvers is often limited by our rudimentary, but improving, knowledge of human anatomy and physiology.

    A. **Pyramidal system.** The traditional concept of **motor** control is that of an upper motor neuron that arises in the precentral gyrus descends in the posterior limb of the internal capsule, cerebral penduncle, and pyramidal tract and then decussates in the medulla before entering the contralateral corticospinal tract to influence the lower motor neuron directly. To this pyramidal system are added local feedback systems in the spinal cord whereby the alpha motor neuron is influenced through the gamma loop and sensory input from the same and nearby segmental levels. This pyramidal system arises from much of the posterior frontal lobe, the sensory strip of the parietal lobe, and other areas of sensorimotor cortex. An important component of this system is the supplementary motor cortex where premovement signals are generated.

    B. A **parapyramidal system** also arises in part from the same motor areas as the pyramidal system and acts on the lower motor neuron through multisynaptic pathways through the red nucleus **(rubrospinal system)** and reticular formation of pons and medulla **(reticulospinal system).** The third major parapyramidal system is the **vestibulospinal system,** which has its major input from vestibular, reticular, and cerebellar sources. The neurotransmitters in these systems are not known.

    C. **The extrapyramidal system,** centered on the basal ganglia, influences motor control through these pyramidal and parapyramidal pathways, generally by means of input into the motor areas of the cerebral hemisphere via the thalamus and supplementary motor cortex (see sec. **IV**). The cerebellum influences the same pathways, especially through the vestibulospinal systems and through relays in the thalamus to the same motor areas of the cerebral hemisphere (see sec. **III**).

II. **Pyramidal and parapyramidal pathway dysfunction.** The clinical effect of lesions in the descending motor control system can best be summarized as paralysis and spasticity.

    A. **Paralysis** may be complete (plegia) or partial (paresis), and may be manifest only as loss of hand and foot dexterity. There is no chemotherapy that will improve paralysis. Physical therapy is of benefit because it provides retraining of the remaining neuromuscular apparatus and prevents contracture.

    B. **Spasticity** is characterized by increased limb tone of clasp-knife type, exaggerated tendon jerks and clonus, and Babinski's responses in the lower extremities. It may be manifested only as loss of dexterity. Flexor spasms are also a common manifestation of spasticity that largely result from unopposed stimulation of cutaneous afferent impulses to the spinal cord. The initial approach to patients with spasticity is to determine how much spasticity interferes with and contributes to their functional state. The presence of pain in association with flexor spasms also needs to be assessed. Basic management requires attention to positioning, avoidance of noxious stimulation, and a daily stretching program.

    C. **Chemotherapy of spasticity.**

        1. **Pharmacokinetics.** The major chemotherapeutic agents of use in spasticity are benzodiazepines, baclofen, and dantrolene (Table 15-1). The site of action of each has not been elucidated fully.

Table 15-1. Drugs useful for spasticity

Drug	Dosage	Major uses	Major side effects
Dantrolene sodium (Dantrium)	25 mg qd, slowly increased to 100 mg qd over 1 month	Wheelchair-bound paraplegic; spasticity of cerebral origin	Generalized weakness, nausea, diarrhea, drowsiness, hepatotoxicity
Baclofen (Lioresal)	10 mg qd, slowly increased to 30–100 mg qd in divided doses	Spinal cord lesions; flexor spasms; increased tone to passive movement	Nausea, drowsiness, depression, dyspepsia
Diazepam (Valium)	6 mg qd, slowly increased to 60 mg qd in divided doses	Spinal cord lesions; flexor spasms; increased tone to passive movement	Sedation, ataxia

a. **Benzodiazepines** appear to act in the spinal cord, enhancing postsynaptic effects of gamma-aminobutyric acid (GABA), which increases presynaptic inhibition. The site of action is a receptor near the GABA receptor. These drugs also act at brainstem sites. The major benzodiazepine drug used is **diazepam** (Valium).

b. **Baclofen** (Lioresal), an analogue of GABA, is thought to act through a bicuculline-insensitive GABA receptor to produce inhibition. It also reduces gamma efferent activity and thus reduces spindle bias.

c. **Diazepam** and **baclofen** are useful for reducing spasticity associated with primary afferent stimulation but are not of major benefit for functional activities that pass through pyramidal and parapyramidal pathways. These pyramidal and parapyramidal pathways probably utilize the excitatory neurotransmitters aspartate and glutamate or the inhibitory neurotransmitter glycine.

d. **Dantrolene sodium** (Dantrium) acts to suppress calcium release from the sarcoplasmic reticulum of the muscle fiber and thus interferes with excitation-contraction coupling. It follows that dantrolene sodium will produce benefit only in proportion to an increasing degree of weakness.

2. **Dosage.** Because the drugs act at different sites, it is possible to use combination therapy with doses low enough to avoid major side effects. In using these drugs one should realize that spasticity may be necessary for gait training in the rehabilitation of a patient with an upper motor neuron lesion. Without rigid legs, splinting may be useless. These drugs are not of proven benefit in treating the spasticity of motor neuron disease or stroke; trials have been done in patients with intrinsic spinal cord disease, multiple sclerosis, and cerebral palsy. Recommendations for use of the three major drugs are as follows:

a. **Diazepam** (Valium) is used in relatively high dosages, starting with 2 mg tid and increasing, as tolerated, to 60 mg/day. There is no absolute maximum dosage. Common side effects include weakness, sedation, and dizziness. Paradoxical insomnia, anxiety, and hostility may be serious long-term side effects and more often than not limit its use. Narrow-angle glaucoma is an uncommon contraindication. Alcohol use should be limited. Transitory hepatic dysfunction and blood dyscrasias have been encountered. Particular care is required in initiating and terminating therapy in patients on anticoagulant medication. Over the next several years, other benzodiazepines may be introduced for the treatment of spasticity in place of diazepam.

b. **Baclofen** (Lioresal) is used particularly in patients with painful flexor spasms. The starting dosage is 5 mg bid, which is increased as tolerated every 3 days to 80–120 mg/day. It is mostly excreted through the renal system. Recently intrathecal baclofen has been shown to be effective when administered in doses between 50 and 100 μg using a programmable drug pump. Epidural infusions have also been used successfully in limited studies. Common side effects of both oral and intrathecal medication are weakness, sedation, dizziness, GI symptoms, tremor, insomnia, headache, and hypotension. Serious side effects include personality disturbance and hallucinations. The drug should be withdrawn gradually. Epilepsy is a relative contraindication to its use. Alcohol use should be limited. Nocturnal dosage may be preferred. Hepatic dysfunction may occur. Intrathecal overdose may be managed by cerebrospinal fluid (CSF) drainage.

   c. Dantrolene sodium (Dantrium) produces weakness proportional to relief of spasticity and is therfore more useful in wheelchair-bound paraplegic patients. It may be more useful in spasticity of cerebral origin than the other drugs listed. Its use in ambulatory patients may cause unacceptable weakness. The starting dosage is 25 mg/day, which is increased as tolerated over about 4 weeks to 400 mg/day. Common side effects include weakness, sedation, dizziness, diarrhea, and reduced glomerular filtration rate. Nausea is generally transient. A serious side effect is hepatotoxicity, especially with dosages above 200 mg/day in older patients, and liver function must be monitored during treatment. Half of the drug's metabolism occurs in the liver by the hepatic microsomal mixed oxidase system. Use of the drug is therefore contraindicated in patients with preexisting liver disease. Care should also be used in prescribing the drug to patients with severe cardiac or pulmonary disease.

   d. Other chemical treatment modalities that may be useful in patients with spasticity who do not respond to the benzodiazepines, baclofen, and dantrolene are the following:

     (1) Tizanidine, an alpha-2 agonist, in dosages up to 36 mg/day, is equivalent in its antispastic effects to baclofen. Side effects include weakness, hypotension, sedation, and dry mouth. A slow-release form may allow once daily dosage. It is not available in the United States.

     (2) Clonidine (Catapres), either oral or transdermal, may benefit some patients.

     (3) A combination of **phenytoin** (Dilantin), 300 mg/day, together with **chlorpromazine** (Thorazine), 300 mg/day.

     (4) Vigabatrin, a new anticonvulsant drug, is said to be as useful as baclofen.

D. Other treatments

  1. Intrathecal treatments with alcohol or phenol may be useful in alleviating painful spasms in the lower extremities. However, this maneuver is likely to produce incontinence, so it can be utilized only in patients who have already lost bladder and bowel function. **Botulinum toxin** (Botox) may be used in some patients with spasticity that is producing proportionately more dysfunction than weakness (see sec. **IV.G**). It is likely to enhance nursing care. It can be used for conditions such as cerebral palsy, adductor spasm from multiple sclerosis, and stroke.

  2. Peripheral nerve blockade may be necessary for relief of severe spasticity in some patients. It is tried first with local anesthetic. If this is successful in relieving the spasticity, a permanent nerve block may be produced with alcohol or 5% phenol injection.

  3. Selective posterior rhizotomy has been used, usually in the context of spasticity associated with cerebral palsy. More major rhizotomies are occasionally indicated.

  4. Physical therapy is of paramount importance in the spastic patient in that contracture must be prevented if useful function is ever to be regained. Postural adjustments, topical cooling, close splinting ("second skin"), and range-of-motion exercises are the mainstay of treatment. Noxious stimuli of somatic and visceral structures should always be minimized.

5. **Transcutaneous electrical nerve stimulation** may occasionally be of benefit.
6. Cerebellar, dorsal column, and other forms of **electrical brain stimulation** are used in a few specialized centers, but there is no convincing evidence of benefit.
7. **Orthopedic procedures** are of benefit in selected patients.

III. **Cerebellar dysfunction**

A. **Description.** The anatomy and cellular physiology of the cerebellum are well known, largely because of its relatively simple design. Input comes from all levels of the CNS. Vestibular and spinal cord sensory input is especially important, as are descending frontal motor relays. Output is directed to the pyramidal system through the ventrolateral and ventroanterior nuclei of the thalamus and to the brainstem parapyramidal systems, especially the lateral vestibulospinal tract. Lateral regions of the cerebellum are involved with control of distal extremity coordination, and midline regions are involved with axial coordination and gait. Cerebellar or cerebellar tract dysfunction is evident clinically as **intention tremor dysmetria, dysdiadochokinesia,** and **hypotonia.** Other, nonmotor roles such as autonomic, sensory perceptual, emotional, and cognitive functions have been attributed to the cerebellum. The neurotransmitter systems in the cerebellar outflow systems are unknown, and medical therapy generally is ineffective in diseases involving the cerebellum, even if the cause is known.

B. **Treatment**
1. Therapy should first be directed toward the **underlying cause** of the syndrome if it can be identified.
2. **Physical therapy** is the mainstay of treatment. Frenkel exercises, isometric rhythmic stabilization, resistive gait and balance, and mobile walking aids have been utilized with partial success. Limb weights up to a few hundred grams may reduce the intention tremor of cerebellar disease.
3. **Scoliosis** may require orthopedic surgical intervention.
4. **Destructive lesions** of the ventrolateral thalamus (i.e., in the area of the thalamus that relays to cortical motor control systems) may alleviate cerebellar intention tremor and the so-called rubral or cerebellar outflow tremor (a tremor that combines the features of parkinsonian tremor and cerebellar tremor, which is thought to be due to lesions in the cerebellar outflow system).
5. **Medication**
   a. **Physostigmine,** administered as 1-mg tablets, has been reported to be of some benefit in some patients with inherited cerebellar ataxia at dosages approaching 8 mg/day.
   b. **5-Hydroxytryptophan,** 10 mg/kg/day, has recently been suggested to partially alleviate dysarthria and postural disequilibrium.
   c. The cerebellar syndrome may be associated with other abnormalities in motor control, which may be themselves amenable to treatment.

IV. **Basal ganglia dysfunction**

A. **Description**
1. The anatomic arrangement of the basal ganglia suggests that extrapyramidal function is mediated primarily through a series of closed loops (Fig. 15-1). Afferents come to the small neurons of the neostriatum (caudate and putamen) from the cerebral cortex, either directly or through connections with the centromedian nucleus of the thalamus. Efferent axons from the large meurons of the neostriatum pass to the cerebral cortex by way of sequential connections in the globus pallidus and ventroanterior and ventrolateral nuclei of the thalamus, influencing ipsilateral cortical motor centers and thus contralateral motor function. The neurotransmitters of these pathways are not all known, but it seems clear that GABA, acetylcholine, and glutamate are of major importance.
2. A number of other circuits influence the activity of the cholinergic and glutamate systems. Of primary importance is the nigroneostriatal system, which utilizes dopamine as an inhibitory neurotransmitter at terminals situated on dendrites of small, presumably cholinergic, neurons in the neostriatum. An understanding of the synthesis and metabolism of dopamine is essential to the successful management of extrapyramidal disorders (Fig. 15-2). The afferent systems that influence the perikarya of dopaminergic neurons in the pars compacta of the

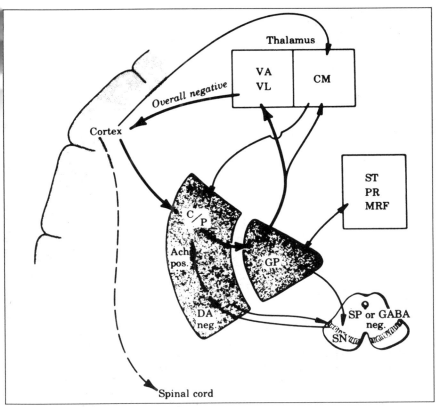

Fig. 15-1. Simplified outline of connections within the basal ganglia. C/P = caudate, putamen (neostriatum); CM = centromedian nucleus of thalamus; GP = globus pallidus; MRF
= mesencephalic reticular formation; PR = prerubal nucleus; SN = substantia nigra; ST
= subthalamus; VA = ventroanterior nucleus of thalamus; VL = ventrolateral nucleus of
thalamus. Presumptive neurotransmitters: DA = dopamine; Ach = acetylcholine; GABA
= gamma-aminobutyric acid; SP = substance P.

substantia nigra are not well documented, except for axons of descending
neurons located in the globus pallidus and neostriatum that contain GABA or
substance P as neurotransmitters. There may also be a striatonigral cholinergic
pathway. Other peptides such as somatostatin, leucine and methionine-
enkephalin, neurotensin, cholecystokinin, thyrotropin releasing hormone, vasoactive intestinal polypeptide, and angiotensin may also modulate neural activity
in the striatum. In addition, reciprocal connections exist between the striatum
and the subthalamus, prerubral nucleus, and the mesencephalon (part of which
contains 5-hydroxytryptamine as a neurotransmitter). From this outline, it is
clear that drugs that influence cholinergic and dopaminergic systems would be
expected to have an influence on motor control as effected by the basal ganglia,
although it is not clear why such effects are antagonistic.

3. The pathways for synthesis and metabolism of dopamine in the striatum are well
    characterized and summarized in Fig. 15-2. The important recent advances in
    our understanding of the biochemistry of dopamine in the basal ganglia relate to
    the neurotoxin 1-methyl-4-phenyl-1236-tetrahydropyridine (MPTP) and the po-
    tential for selective protection against this compound and other presumptive

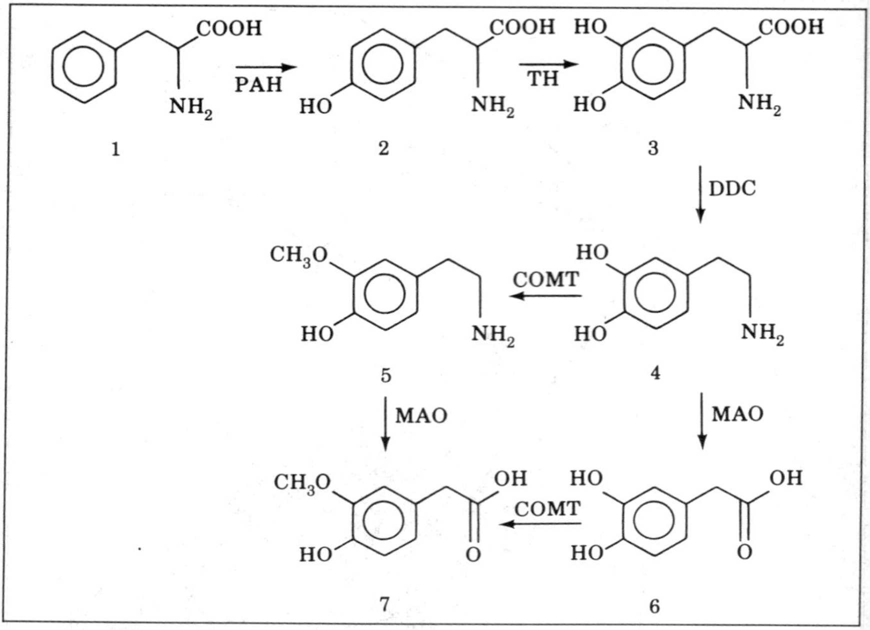

Fig. 15-2. Major synthetic and metabolic pathways for dopamine: PAH = phenylalanine hydroxylase; TH = tyrosine hydroxylase; DDC = dopa decarboxylase (actually L-aromatic aminoacid decarboxylase); MAO = monoamine oxidase; COMT = catechol-o-methyl transferase. The amino acids must compete with other neural amino acids for absorption at the level of the gastrointestinal epithelium and blood-brain barrier vascular endothelium. The peripheral circulation DDC inhibitors facilitate the use of lower L-dopa dosages, but it must be noted that conversion to dopamine requires active neuronal uptake in a reduced population of dopamine-containing neurons. There is an efficient reuptake mechanism for released dopamine that leads to intraneuronal metabolism of dopamine by MAO. Extraneuronal dopamine is metabolized by COMT. 1 = phenylalanine; 2 = tyrosine; 3 = dihydroxyphenylalanine (DOPA); 4 = dopamine; 5 = 3-methoxytyramine; 6 = dihydroxyphenylacetic acid; 7 = homovanillic acid.

neurotoxins such as 6-hydroxydopamine by monoamine oxidase B inhibitors. These factors are summarized in Fig. 15-3. The action of released dopamine on striatal neurons is mediated by at least two receptors known as D1 and D2. Activation of D1 receptors leads to production of cyclic adenosine monophosphate, whereas D2 receptor activation does not. D2 receptors probably exist in high and low affinity states on striatal neurons and terminals of corticostriatal afferents.

4. Movement disorders produced by dysfunction of the basal ganglia may be classified as those resulting in diminished activity (akinesia or bradykinesia), typified by Parkinson's disease and other causes of so-called parkinsonism, and those that result in overactivity (hyperkinesia or dyskinesia), typified by Huntington's chorea. Other abnormal movements produced by basal ganglia disorders include dystonias and tics. These are further described by specific examples in the text. There are a variety of disorders that may produce features of under- and/or overactivity also described in the text.

B. **Drug-induced extrapyramidal syndromes**
1. **Medications** can produce symptoms and signs of under- and/or overactivity of the basal ganglia.

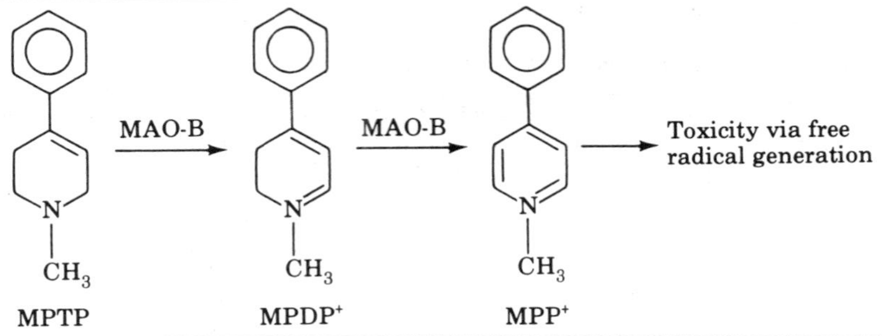

Fig. 15-3. MPTP (1-methyl-4-phenyl-1236-tetrahydropyridine) is converted to MPDP$^+$ (2,3-dihydropyridinium) and MPP$^+$ (1-methyl-4-phenyl-pyridinium) following astrocytic uptake. It is this product that is neurotoxic by generation of superoxide free radicals. Neurons containing neuromelanin appear to be selectively vulnerable to this process. MAO-B = monoamine oxidase B.

    a. With the introduction of the phenothiazines, drug-induced extrapyramidal symptoms became common. **Phenothiazines, butyrophenones,** and other more recently developed **neuroleptic drugs** act primarily as dopamine-receptor blockers, predominantly at D3 receptors in the limbic system, in the treatment of psychotic disorders. They produce a number of drug-induced extrapyramidal symptoms (Table 15-2).
    b. Similar drugs are also widely used as antinauseants including **prochlorperazine** (Compazine) and **metoclopramide** (Maxolon).
    c. Catecholamine analogues and depleting drugs such as **methyldopa, tetrabenazine,** and **reserpine** also produce extrapyramidal syndromes.
    d. **Long-term therapy with L-dopa** has also seen the introduction of another group of patients with drug-induced extrapyramidal syndromes of the dyskinetic type (see sec. **IV.C**).
  2. **Reversal.** Drug-induced movements are best reversed by stopping or reducing the dosage of medication.
  3. The **abnormal movements** produced include the following:

Table 15-2. Severity of induced parkinsonism and dystonic reactions with commonly used antipsychotic drugs

Antipsychotic medication	Drugs	Relative severity
Phenothiazines		
Aliphatic	Chlorpromazine (Thorazine)	+ +
Piperidines	Thioridazine (Mellaril)	+
	Pericyazine (Neulactil)	+
Piperazines	Perphenazine (Trilafon)	+ + +
	Trifluoperazine (Stelazine)	+ + +
	Fluphenazine (Prolixin)	+ + +
Thioxanthenes	Chlorprothixene (Taractan)	+ +
	Thiothixene (Navane)	+ +
Butyrophenones	Haloperidol (Haldol)	+ + +
Diphenylbutylpiperidines	Pimozide (Orap)	+ + +
Other	Clozapine	+

Key: + = mild; + + = moderate; + + + = severe.

a. Acute idiosyncratic dyskinesia and dystonia may occur within the first few days of treatment with neuroleptic medication.

   (1) Dyskinesia refers to rapid, brief involuntary movements that may take the form of chorea, athetosis, or ballismus (see sec. **IV.B.3.d**).

   (2) Dystonia may occur with the first dose of neuroleptic medication. It consists of long-duration, slow, contorting movements of axial, appendicular, or eye muscles **(oculogyric crisis)**. Muscles most commonly affected are those of the neck, trunk, and proximal extremities. Respiratory muscles may also be affected. Acute dystonia can be treated with a parenteral anticholinergic agent, such as **benztropine** (Cogentin), 1 mg IM or IV, or with **diphenhydramine** (Benadryl), 50 mg IV. In general, this should be followed by oral medication for the next 48 hours. Paradoxically, oral antihistamines have been documented as a cause of dystonic reactions. It is usually possible to stop the offending drug.

b. Parkinsonism. Dose-related akinesia, rigidity, and tremor (3–5 cps) may occur between a few days and 4 weeks after initiation of treatment. This state may persist for many months after cessation of therapy with antipsychotic medications. Treatment consists of

   (1) Decreasing the antipsychotic drug dosage **or**

   (2) Adding anticholinergic medication:

   (a) Benztropine (Cogentin), 0.5–4.0 mg bid.

   (b) Biperiden (Akineton), 1.0–2.0 mg tid.

   (c) Trihexyphenidyl hydrochloride (Artane), 1.0–5.0 mg tid.

   The half-life of benztropine is longer than that of biperiden, which has a longer half-life than trihexyphenidyl hydrochloride. The anticholinergic drugs may partially reverse the antipsychotic effects of the primary drug. They are not necessary for all patients and are rarely required for more than 2 or 3 months. **There is no indication for prophylactic use.** Theoretically, L-dopa and dopamine-receptor agonists should be of benefit, but they nearly always produce a coincident confusional state.

c. Akathisia is a dose-related side effect of antipsychotic drugs that usually occurs during the first few days of treatment and may be present in up to 20% of patients. The term refers to the restlessness seen in these patients. They are literally unable to sit still and appear intensely anxious. The etiology is obscure, and the treatment is withdrawal of antipsychotic medication. Initiation of treatment with the lowest possible dose of medication and recognition of the syndrome, thus preventing escalating doses of antipsychotic medication, are the two major factors in management. Anticholinergic medication is only partially effective. Other medications reported to be effective in alleviating symptoms include benzodiazepines, alpha antagonists, clonidine, and amantadine. Late-onset akathisia occurs rarely and is less responsive to medication.

d. Tardive (late) dyskinesias

   (1) Description. Tardive dyskinesias usually occur more than 1 year after continuous neuroleptic medication. The prevalence may be as high as 20% of patients and probably exceeds that figure in the elderly, especially women. Tardive dyskinesia is said to occur more frequently in patients who have manifested acute reactions to neuroleptic medications and who have an underlying affective disorder. Tardive dyskinesias may include facial and limb chorea, athetosis, dystonia, and akathisia. The involuntary movements of the tardive dyskinesias are often restricted to movements involving the head and neck, such as chewing and tongue-thrusting (orobuccal dyskinesia). The movements occasionally involve the muscles of respiration.

   (2) Treatment of tardive dyskinesias depends on either stimulating the cholinergic mechanism or decreasing dopaminergic activity. Another approach is the use of drugs active in the GABA system, which has a striatonigral projection. Further dopamine-receptor blockade achieved by increasing the dosage of antipsychotic drug may help the disorder in the short term, but eventual dosage reduction becomes necessary. It is important that antipsychotic medication be used in as low a dose as possible. Anticholinergic drugs should be used sparingly in patients with tardive dyskinesia, as they may exacerbate the problem, although they probably do not increase the initial risk of developing the signs of the disorder.

The symptoms may fluctuate and take months or years to resolve following drug withdrawal; approximately 50% are reversible within 5 years, but some may never resolve. Fortunately most do not continue to progress once a plateau of activity is reached. Treatment of tardive dyskinesia and dystonia is difficult, and many medicines have been advocated. Judicious use of drug holidays in the administration of neuroleptic medication has not proved beneficial and may be associated with increased risk.

(a) **Tetrabenazine** (Nitoman) depletes central biogenic monoamine stores. Treatment is started with one-half of a 25-mg tablet; this dosage is increased slowly to a maximum of 200 mg/day. Parkinsonism, drowsiness, and depression are common side effects. Anxiety, choking attacks, insomnia, and akathisia have been reported. Concurrent use of a monoamine oxidase (MAO) inhibitor is contraindicated. (Tetrabenazine is not yet licensed for use by the U.S. Food and Drug Administration.)

(b) **Reserpine** (Serpasil) depletes central biogenic monoamine stores much like tetrabenazine. Treatment is started with 0.25 mg PO daily and increased slowly to 2–4 mg/day. Orthostatic hypotension is a major problem, during which time the patient must be warned to rise slowly with careful monitoring of blood pressure. Tolerance will usually develop in 1–2 weeks.

(c) Other drugs that have been tried in this syndrome with variable sucess include baclofen, valproic acid, diazepam, alpha antagonists, amantadine, clonidine, and carbidopa–L-dopa.

C. Parkinson's disease

1. **Description.** Parkinson's disease is a movement disorder of unknown cause that primarily affects the pigmented, dopamine-containing neurons of the pars compacta of the substantia nigra. Recent experience with parkinsonism induced by neurotoxins, particularly MPTP, has implicated free radical generation in the pathogenesis of the disease (see Fig. 15-2). Familial cases do occur, which suggests that genetic predisposition to the effect of toxins may be a factor in pathogenesis. The lifetime risk for family members is raised approximately 10-fold. Clinically, Parkinson's disease is characterized by the slow development of **bradykinesia, increased tone,** and **resting tremor.** Slowness of voluntary movements is noted, particularly in the initiation of such movements as walking, rolling over in bed, and fine finger dexterity leading to micrographia. Patients have decreased facial expression, monotonous low volume speech, and decreased blinking. Posture is stooped, and gait is shuffling, with poor arm swing and reduced postural balance often associated with festination. The abnormal tone is referred to as lead-pipe and cogwheel rigidity. Most characteristic, and often present early in the course of the disease, is an asymmetric, coarse (3–7 cps) "resting" tremor characterized as pill-rolling. Tremor, however, disappears with complete muscle relaxation. A symmetric action tremor of 5–12 cps may also be present. The most useful classification of severity of Parkinson's disease is that introduced by Hoehn and Yahr (Table 15-3).

The presence of oculogyric crises is associated with postencephalitic Parkinson's disease and antipsychotic drug ingestion. It is often difficult to decide whether there is a concurrent dementia in long-term patients because of difficulty with communication. In one series, over 30% of patients were demented after 6 years of treatment. This is important in the assessment of individual patients because mildly demented patients are likely to have adverse side effects such as acute confusion when treated with medication. Other possible long-term

Table 15-3. Staging of Parkinson's disease

Stage	Clinical
1	Unilateral
2	Bilateral
3	Bilateral plus postural reflexes
4	Requires aids because of 3
5	Bedridden because of 3

Source: Adapted from M. M. Hoehn and M. D. Yahr, Parkinsonism: Onset, progression, and mortality. *Neurology* 17:427, 1967.

disabilities are increasing postural instability, unusual breathing patterns, and brief freezing patterns, all of which are essentially unresponsive to treatment. Before the advent of treatment with **L-dopa,** two-thirds of patients died within 7 years. The diagnosis is usually not a problem in the 50- to 60-year-old person with slow onset of the typical features. A history of encephalitis lethargica between 1919 and 1926 is always difficult to document and is now a very rare cause of newly diagnosed disease. The pathology in idiopathic cases consists of loss of neurons from the substantia nigra and other pigmented brainstem nuclei with consequent gliosis and the formation of Lewy bodies in remaining neuronal perikarya. Whether the disease is a generalized tissue defect is still uncertain.

2. **Differential diagnosis.** Atherosclerosis and syphilis are difficult to substantiate as the cause, and tumor is extremely rare. Other causes of parkinsonism, such as head trauma, drug ingestion, carbon monoxide, cyanide, and manganese poisoning, are usually obvious; normal-pressure hydrocephalus and Jakob-Creutzfeldt disease may not be. A vascular cause for Parkinson's disease is still disputed, although parkinsonism does occur. The degenerative diseases with parkinsonism as a major feature are usually known as "parkinsonism plus syndromes" and are listed in Table 15-4. It is not uncommon for these syndromes to be recognized after a course of **L-dopa** treatment has been shown to be ineffective, although patients with diffuse Lewy body disease may respond well initially. Treatment is symptomatic for the complications that may arise from associated system degeneration.

3. **Treatment** of Parkinson's disease is based on considerations of the dopaminergic-cholinergic balance discussed in sec. **IV.A,** as no drug therapy for peptide deficiencies has been described to date. The object is either to increase available dopamine or dopamine agonist in the neostriatum or to reduce cholinergic activity with anticholinergic agents. Choice of therapy depends on the age of the patient and the degree of disability. Indeed no therapy may be the best choice early in the disease. In general an **L-dopa** preparation is the treatment of first choice, although a case can be made for the use of **selegiline, bromocriptine,** or an **anticholinergic** in some younger patients.

   a. **L-Dopa** is active at D1 and D2 receptors and may down-regulate the latter early in the course of treatment. The major indication for use of L-dopa is the incapacity of bradykinesia. The drug is administered with a peripherally-acting dopa decarboxylase inhibitor to reduce side effects such as nausea and vomiting, cardiac arrhythmias, and postural hypotension. In the past, these side effects have often limited the rapid buildup to therapeutic efficacy. Some researchers have suggested that the introduction of L-dopa should be delayed as long as possible, but most physicians introduce L-dopa therapy when symptoms start to interfere with quality of life.

      (1) **Carbidopa–L-dopa** (Sinemet) (carbidopa, 10-mg, L-dopa, 100 mg; carbidopa, 25 mg, L-dopa, 100 mg; or carbidopa, 25 mg, L-dopa, 250 mg) has had the widest use. Carbidopa is a peripheral dopa decarboxylase inhibitor that increases the amount of L-dopa available for action within the CNS (see Fig. 15-3). The usual starting dosage is carbidopa, 25 mg, and L-dopa,

Table 15-4. Parkinsonism plus syndromes

Syndrome	Major added characteristics
Progressive supranuclear palsy (Steele-Richardson-Olszewski syndrome)	Loss of voluntary gaze (usually vertical initially), with preservation of oculocephalic reflexes, axial rigidity, progression to dementia within 5 years
Striatonigral degeneration	No tremor Late dementia
Corticobasal degeneration	Unilateral commencement of apraxia in combination with parkinsonism Late dementia Sensory-evoked myoclonus, dysarthria
Generalized Lewy body disease	Dementia prominent, early myoclonus L-Dopa sensitive
Shy-Drager syndrome	Autonomic insufficiency Variety with motor neuron and cerebellar signs
Olivopontocerebellar degeneration	Intention tremor Pseudobulbar signs
Parkinsonian–dementia–amyotrophic lateral sclerosis Complex of Guam	Dementia, motor neuron disease, source
Azorean motor system degeneration type 1	Autosomal dominant athetosis, spasticity Late sensorimotor neuropathy

100 mg, tid, given just after a meal to avert nausea. Thirty milligrams of carbidopa daily is ineffective as a peripheral dopamine decarboxylase inhibitor and precludes the use of Sinemet 10-100 as a starting dose if administered tid. The dosage is increased by 1 tablet/day, every 3 or 4 days, as tolerated, over about 4 weeks. The final dosage should be kept to a minimum compatible with a useful life for the patient. This is usually less than 1 g/day of L-dopa. If more L-dopa is required, dopamine agonist drugs should be considered as additional therapy. Improvement should be obvious 2 weeks after commencing treatment. A slow-release form of Sinemet (Sinemet CR) is available but is usually not needed until symptom fluctuation becomes apparent.

(2) Benserazide–L-dopa (Prolopa, Madopar) (benserazide, 50 mg; L-dopa, 100 mg) is administered in the same way as carbidopa–L-dopa. The greater amount of dopa decarboxylase inhibitor (i.e., 50 mg of benserazide versus 25 mg of carbidopa) may be better tolerated in some patients, especially if nausea is a problem. A slow-release form of Prolopa (Madopar HBS), in which the preparation floats on gastric contents, is used in some countries but is not available in the United States.

(3) Carbidopa and benserazide. In some countries, carbidopa and benserazide are available as separate preparations and may allow better individual dosage adjustment in terms of the L-dopa–decarboxylase ratio.

(4) Response to therapy. Approximately 80% of patients are improved significantly by L-dopa therapy, but there appears to be no way to predict which patients are responsive. Long-term studies suggest that there is a decline in benefit from L-dopa after the first 2–3 years of treatment, such that after 5 or 6 years, only 25–50% of patients have maintained their initial improvement. Wide swings in motor performance were not seen before the introduction of L-dopa therapy and are less frequent in patients with late-age–onset disease. Long-term treatment reduces mortality, although it appears that dementia often emerges as a problem in long-term survivors. One study reported that depression existed in over 20% of patients before treatment was begun. Latent depression may become overt as a patient begins to become more mobile with L-dopa therapy, and suicidal tendencies have been reported. Tricyclic medication, but not nonspecific MAO inhibitors, may be used concurrently with L-dopa to treat depression.

(5) Dose-related side effects

(a) Peak-dose dyskinesias. Fluctuations in motor performance early in the disease are less apparent than might be expected from the short half-life of the drug. This is probably because of storage and slow release from dopamine-containing neurons in the brain. However, high dosages of L-dopa preparations result in peak-dose dyskinesias, often near the end of the first year of treatment. These side effects become more severe and more generalized with time, and almost 75% of patients have them after 6 years of treatment. Peak-dose dyskinesias occur 20–90 minutes after taking medication and are clinically similar to the tardive dyskinesias seen with antipsychotic drug therapy. They are usually choreiform, although dystonic, ballistic, or myoclonic movements may occur. The abnormal movements respond to a gradual reduction in dosage over a few days, as do less troublesome side effects such as dry mouth, blurred vision, and postural hypotension. Vitamin supplementation in patients receiving L-dopa without a dopa decarboxylase inhibitor should not contain vitamin B_6 because this will counteract the beneficial effect of the drug.

(b) "End-of-dose" wearing-off phenomenon is another dose-related side effect that becomes more prominent in patients on long-term therapy. This effect may be correlated with low plasma concentrations of L-dopa. The usual approach to this problem is to administer smaller doses of L-dopa more frequently. Recent advances for "smoothing" the fluctuations in response to L-dopa have been the development of slow-release preparations. These agents appear to be moderately effective. As might be anticipated, they are associated with the slow onset of drug effectiveness in the morning and are used in conjunction with regular preparations, especially with the morning's first dose.

Another approach to the problem of dose-related side effects has been the use of a low-protein diet to diminish competition for absorption of phenylalamine and tyrosine, particularly at the blood-brain barrier. This is generally achieved with a diet containing 0.8 g of protein per kilogram of body weight, delivered at equal intervals through the day or concentrated in the evening meal. Many older people are already receiving a protein input at this level.

(c) Biphasic dose response. Some patients are aware of dyskinesias of brief duration that occur shortly after taking their first dose of medication in the morning, which resolves only to be followed 1–2 hours later by the onset of severe dystonic spasms, particularly in the lower extremities. These spasms can often be limited by a further dose of L-dopa. **Baclofen,** 5–40 mg/day, has also been used to treat this condition. These patients often progress to the "on-off" phenomenon.

(d) The most troublesome side effects are **nausea** and **vomiting,** even when the drug is administered in minimal doses with or after meals. Mild antinauseants such as **trimethobenzamide hydrochloride** (Tigan), 25 mg tid; **domperidone** (Motilium), 10–20 mg 30 minutes before L-dopa; anticholinergics; or antihistamines may be useful in this situation.

(e) Vivid dreaming is often reduced by avoiding the last dose of L-dopa preparation at night.

(f) Anxiety, agitation, confusion, delusions, visual hallucinosis, and **psychosis** usually respond quickly within a day or so to lowered dosage, although in rare cases it may take weeks to resolve completely. Euphoria, mania, and hypersexuality can also occur.

(g) Other side effects include flushing, orthostatic hypotension, and premature ventricular contractions. Orthostatic hypotension may be treated by elevation of the head of the bed, antigravity stockings, and 9-alpha-fludrocortisone, 0.1–0.2 mg/day. Hypertension can occur rarely. Minor transient changes can occur in liver function tests and hematologic parameters. Abrupt cessation of therapy should be avoided, as it may lead to a picture resembling neuroleptic malignant syndrome with fever, muscular rigidity, and coma.

(6) **Dose-unrelated side effects**

(a) The **"on-off" phenomenon** becomes a likely side effect with extended duration of therapy and is not seen in the absence of L-dopa therapy. This disability occurs in about 50% of patients treated for 5 or more years. This on-off effect consists of periods of unpredictable severe akinesia, hypotonia, and apprehension of rapid onset and termination, which last from 30 minutes to a few hours and which are unrelieved by further doses of L-dopa. The cause is unknown, although "off" episodes like "end-of-dose akinesia" have been correlated with low plasma concentration of L-dopa in some studies. However, maintaining constant L-dopa plasma levels with intravenous drug administration does not always abolish clinical fluctuations. Recently it has been proposed that L-dopa may itself have inhibitory effects on motor activity. Whether it is this function of L-dopa, accumulation of functioning dopamine metabolites, decreased storage capacity of the dopaminergic neurons, or pharmacodynamic fluctuations in receptor activity that underlies low dose-related side effects in advanced disease is currently unknown. Administration of an L-dopa preparation q2h may help to smooth out these effects. Sinemet, for example, can be cut in quarters with a razor blade to allow smaller doses to be administered. L-Dopa methylester is an experimental drug that may prove to be of benefit in this distressing condition. A drug holiday for up to 1 week has also been advocated in the past for treatment of on-off effects but is of little or no benefit. The initial dosage regimen of L-dopa appears not to affect the incidence of the on-off phenomenon or end-of-dose wearing-off effect but may be implicated in the development of peak-dose dyskinesia.

(b) **Treatment.** The main treatment of the on-off phenomenon is subcutaneous **apomorphine.** This medication is administered a few days after the introduction of **domperidone** (Motilium) to eliminate the inevitable vomiting that occurs without its use. The dose, initially commenced at 1.5 mg, is titrated for benefit up to 4.5 mg. A satisfactory result will produce a clinical improvement within 10 minutes that will last up to 50 minutes. The medication reduces the time a patient spends in the off state but does not reduce the frequency of on-off spells. Nasal and sublingual apomorphine have been of benefit in some patients.

(7) The **contraindications** to L-dopa therapy are relatively few. They include narrow-angle glaucoma (most glaucoma cases are of the chronic, wide-angle type), previous melanoma, although this has recently been questioned, and concurrent use of MAO inhibitors. Caution should be used in patients who have cardiac arrhythmias or recent myocardial infarction or for whom surgery is planned.

b. **Dopamine agonists**

(1) **Bromocriptine mesylate** (Parlodel) is a dopamine-receptor agonist predominantly active at D2 receptors. Ordinarily it is used to permit up to a 30% reduction of L-dopa dosage in difficult cases. These patients usually have dyskinesia, on-off, or wearing-off effects. Bromocriptine has effects at postsynaptic sites and modulatory effects on L-dopa–induced dopamine-receptor binding at presynaptic autoreceptors. Recent studies have used bromocriptine as initial therapy, but the benefit is less than that seen with L-dopa treatment alone. There are theoretic arguments that suggest that presynaptic (L-dopa) and postsynaptic (bromocriptine) effects may best be produced by simultaneous use of the drugs. The initial dosage of bromocriptine is 2.5 mg/day, and this is slowly increased over several weeks. Maximum therapeutic benefit is often of slow onset, and the dosage may be held at low levels (e.g., 12 mg/day) for several months before full effectiveness is noted. The maximum dosage is 30–50 mg/day usually given bid–tid. Extensive first-pass metabolism occurs in the liver. Side effects are more prominent at higher doses. Early side effects include nausea, which may be treated with **domperidone**, vomiting, and postural hypotension. They are less troublesome than with an L-dopa preparation, but late side effects are more troublesome, especially the acute confusional state that occurs with visual hallucinations. This may take several weeks to clear on cessation of the drug. Other psychogenic side effects are similar to those found with high-dose L-dopa. Ankle edema and erythromelalgia are less of a problem and clear rapidly when the drug is stopped. Pleuropulmonary fibrosis is rare.

(2) More recently developed ergot analogues have been shown to have a similar overall benefit as bromocriptine. **Pergolide mesylate** (Permax), active at D1 and D2 receptors, has undergone extensive evaluation. The mean effective dosage is usually about 2–4 mg/day. The starting dosage is 0.1 mg/day. It has been claimed that on-off phenomena may be less of a problem with this and other dopamine-receptor agonist drugs, but it has not yet been used for prolonged therapy in many patients. In addition, cardiac arrhythmias may be more prevalent with this drug. It must be used together with a small dose of L-dopa for maximum benefit. Hypersensitivity to this or other ergot derivatives is a contraindication to its use. The side effect profile is similar to that for bromocriptine.

c. **Combined therapy.** Many patients are now successfully manged by using an L-dopa preparation initially and then adding a dopamine agonist such as bromocriptine in low dosage. A typical regimen would be Sinemet 25-100 initially tid for 3 months and then adding bromocriptine, 2.5 mg/day, increasing over 3 months to 2.5 mg tid. Many other variations on this approach are in clinical use. The hope is that there will be fewer side effects with this strategy, particularly dyskinesias and motor fluctuations. Lowered mortality may also be possible.

d. **Anticholinergics** are said to be useful early in the disease when tremor is the most prominent problem. They are now being used less and less as first-line therapy.

(1) **Commonly used agents and the usual dosages** include
   (a) **Ethopropazine** (Parsidol), 10–20 mg tid.
   (b) **Benztropine** (Cogentin), 0.5–4.0 mg bid.
   (c) **Biperiden** (Akinetin), 1.0–2.0 mg tid.
   (d) **Trihexyphenidyl hydrochloride** (Artane), 1.0–5.0 mg tid.

(2) **The maximum dose** of these agents is determined by observation of the onset of side effects. The dosage is gradually increased to the tolerated maximum. For example, it may be possible to give up to 400 mg/day of ethopropazine.

(3) **Side effects.** Common, well-tolerated side effects of anticholinergic drugs include dry mouth, blurred vision, and dizziness. Other, often serious side effects are acute confusion, constipation, urinary retention, and precipitation of untreated glaucoma. The deleterious effects on cognitive function are reversed when dosage is reduced, but this must be done very slowly over several weeks. Abrupt cessation of anticholinergic medication can lead to worsening symptoms. This may mislead the clinician into thinking these drugs are of continuing benefit when, in fact, they are no longer necessary. It is not advisable to introduce a tranquilizer for cognitive side effects. Constipation responds to a gentle laxative. Bladder neck obstruc-

tion in men may require surgical intervention. If glaucoma is being managed appropriately, anticholinergic agents can still be used.

e. **Amantadine hydrochloride** (Symmetrel) and **amphetamines** may act by increasing endogenous dopamine release at the nerve terminal in the neostriatum.

    (1) **Amantadine hydrochloride** is used in an initial dosage of 100 mg/day and increased to 100 mg tid. The benefit obtained is short-lived, and intermittent use has been advocated. Prominent side effects are depression, congestive cardiac failure, pedal edema, livedo reticularis, urinary retention, and an acute confusional state, especially with visual hallucinations. The drug is excreted unmetabolized in the urine. This drug may also be effective through its anticholinergic properties.

    (2) **Amphetamine** has been used in the past for treatment of oculogyric crises. Side effects generally preclude its use. **Methylphenidate** is said to be helpful as an analgesic for sensory symptoms, which include headache, tingling, numbness, formications, and burning pain.

    (3) Subcutaneous **apomorphine** has D1 and D2 dopamine receptor and release activity. The drug is used with domperidone (10–80 mg/day) as antinauseant in the treatment of on-off effects (see sec. **IV.C.3.a.[6][b]**). Dyskinesia is common with this medication. Patients appear to adjust well to symptomatic self-administration.

f. **Selegiline** (Eldepryl), an MAO B inhibitor that also inhibits neuronal dopamine uptake, has also been shown to be useful in the treatment of Parkinson's disease as an adjunct to L-dopa therapy. Multiple potential modes of action, apart from MAO inhibition, have been shown for this drug, including that of protection from potential neurotoxins (see Fig. 15-2). This mechanism of action is based on the theory that free radical generation is important in the pathogenesis of the disease. Selegiline acts to induce superoxide dismutase and catalase, which increases free radical elimination. Selegiline has been used in a multicenter trial with the free radical scavenger vitamin E. The dosage of selegiline is 100 μg/kg/day after a loading dose of 10 mg daily for 1 week. The usual regimen is one 5-mg tablet in the morning and one 5-mg tablet at noon with meals. At 30 mg/day, the drug inhibits both MAO A and MAO B. It is metabolized to amphetamine, which may be responsible for part of the euphoric effect. Its place in the treatment of Parkinson's disease is still controversial, but it is probably best regarded as an L-dopa sparing agent that also prolongs the effect of L-dopa in patients with end-of-dose failure. The drug should not be used in combination with **meperidine,** other MAO inhibitors, or **fluoxetine.** Common side effects include increased dyskinesia, nausea, dizziness, and confusion.

g. **Propranolol** (Inderal) may on occasion be used for action tremor, a common accompaniment of Parkinson's disease. (See sec. **V.C.3.c.[1]** for dosage.) It is also said to be useful for pain that is not associated with dystonia.

h. **Botulinum toxin A** (Botox) has been used to treat equinovarus and claw dystonia in patients who have these conditions and where other medical therapies have not helped (see sec. **IV.G**).

i. Surgery

    (1) **Ventrolateral thalamotomy** has been used in patients with severe unilateral tremor, not controlled with drugs, who have the intellectual capacity for gainful employment. Bilateral thalamotomy has led to severe speech defects. **Pallidotomy** may be useful for bradykinesia and tremor and is coming back into favor in some centers. It has been claimed that prior surgery reduces the frequency of L-dopa–induced dyskinesias.

    (2) **Transplantation** of catecholamine-containing tissue from adult and neonatal sources into the basal ganglia of a few patients with Parkinson's disease resulted in major improvements and has led to the trial of this therapy in a number of coordinated centers. Tissues transplanted have included adrenal medulla (with very limited success) and neonatal substantia nigra. Reports to date suggest that any benefits from this procedure are unpredictable, and it is unlikely that it will become the preferred form of therapy in any but a very small number of patients.

j. **Nonpharmacologic treatment programs.** There is little direct evidence of the value of nonpharmacologic treatments apart from the value of socialization on psychological well-being. However, a general fitness program is wise for all older people. Speech therapy appears to be of limited benefit, although some patients speak more clearly if given cues such as a metronome. The occupational therapist can provide aids as required, and physical therapy can teach patients useful "tricks" to help initiate movement and gait; these all rely on noncontingent cueing.

4. **Nonmotor symptoms.** There are many nonmotor manifestations of Parkinson's disease, the most prevalent of which are listed in Table 15-5, together with their symptomatic treatment.

5. **Compliance.** The occasional patient appears to have no benefit from any medical therapy. It is usually wise to admit such patients to the hospital and begin therapy again under strict supervision. A review of the patient may also eventually reveal a parkinsonism plus syndrome.

D. **Huntington's chorea** (see also Chap. 3, sec. **III.A.4**)

1. **Description.** Huntington's chorea is an inherited, autosomal dominant, dementing disease for which, in adult-onset cases, the associated movement disorder typifies relative overactivity of the dopaminergic system. Hypotonia is a frequent concomitant of chorea. Chorea and athetosis may be considered together, since the two commonly coexist in this and in other extrapyramidal syndromes. Severe chorea is virtually indistinguishable from athetosis, and there does not appear to be a distinct anatomic substrate for each involuntary movement. **Chorea** refers to rapid, jerky, semipurposive movement, usually of the extremities; **athetosis** describes slower, less purposeful, continuous sinuous movements. Childhood onset of Huntington's chorea may be associated with parkinsonism. Dysarthria is frequently present. The other key features of Huntington's chorea are progressive emotional and personality changes and dementia. Depression is common, with suicide an outcome in approximately 5% of cases.

2. **Differential diagnosis.** Currently there is no single test for presymptomatic early detection of Huntington's chorea, although the genetic defect, a repeated replication sequence on chromosome 4, has recently been described. Other diseases of the basal ganglia that may result in similar movements are mercury poisoning; Sydenham's chorea of acute rheumatic fever and other acute infections including diphtheria, whooping cough, rubella, and encephalitis; oral contraceptives and, rarely, pregnancy; thyrotoxicosis; posthemiplegic athetosis; Lesch-Nyhan syn-

Table 15-5. Nonmotor manifestations of Parkinson's disease

Symptom	Symptomatic treatment
Sialorrhea	Local 1% atropine is partly effective Parotid irradiation
Seborrhea	None
Constipation	High-fiber diet Laxatives
Urinary dysfunction	Anticholinergics (may also exacerbate)
Visual blurring	None
Pain	Simple analgesics, adjuvant analgesics, propranolol, methylphenidate
Depression	Antidepressants (not MAO A) Electroconvulsive therapy
Dementia	None
Sleep disorders	Nonspecific

drome in childhood; kernicterus; senile chorea; drugs, particularly anticonvulsants, lithium, and antiemetics; and diseases that may present as parkinsonism or choreoathetosis (see sec. **IV.E**). Management of these movement disorders is the same, in principle, as for Huntington's chorea.

3. **Treatment** (Table 15-6). Pharmacologic treatment with dopamine depletion or receptor blockade is helpful in the early stages of Huntington's chorea.

   a. **Haloperidol** (Haldol), 1–4 mg qid. The side effects of neuroleptic medication, apart from those on movement at D2 receptors, should be borne in mind when using drugs of this class. They include postural hypotension and other anticholinergic side effects, sedation, and neuroleptic malignant syndrome.

   b. **Chlorpromazine** (Thorazine), 50 mg tid.

   c. **Tetrabenazine** (Nitoman). See sec. **IV.B.3.d.(2)(a)**.

   d. **Reserpine** (Serpasil), 0.5 mg qid, has been used in Sydenham's chorea.

   e. **Propranolol** (Inderal), in high dosage, may be useful for action tremor, which may be a component of the disorder.

   f. **Dantrolene sodium** (Dantrium) has been used for the chorea associated with hemiatrophy.

E. **Disease presenting with parkinsonism or choreoathetosis.** A group of uncommon diseases may manifest themselves with either choreoathetosis or parkinsonism as the primary movement disorder. At autopsy, these diseases demonstrate widespread pathology in the basal ganglia, usually in a distribution that does not clearly implicate any of the specific connections previously discussed. These diseases should be considered in the differential diagnosis of any patient having symptoms of parkinsonism or choreoathetosis alone. Management includes treatment of both the underlying disease and the movement disorder. However, it is intuitively apparent that parkinsonism secondary to a lesion of the neostriatum is unlikely to respond to L-dopa if the postsynaptic elements for neurotransmission in that system have been destroyed by the disease process.

1. **Wilson's disease**

   a. **Description.** Wilson's disease is a rare, inherited, autosomal recessive disorder that has its onset between the ages of 10 and 40 years. It is characterized by progressive liver and neurologic disease, Kayser-Fleischer rings of the cornea, and occasional renal dysfunction. The neurologic presentation has been subdivided into two major categories. Younger patients have rapid progression of either athetosis or rigidity and dystonia. Myoclonus also can occur, and this form of the disease is more difficult to treat. Adults are more likely to have a more benign course, with tremor (action and intention), dysarthria (which may have spastic, cerebellar, and hypokinetic components), and dysphagia as prominent symptoms. This form of the disease is more amenable to treatment. Asterixis (see sec. **VI**) may occur concomitantly with progressive hepatic dysfunction.

   b. The **diagnosis** is established by documenting the Kayser-Fleischer ring by slit-lamp examination, establishing disordered liver function, and evaluating copper metabolism. Useful screening tests include serum copper and ceruloplasmin levels (both are decreased in Wilson's disease) as well as urinary excretion of copper (increased). The cerebrospinal concentration of copper and urinary excretion of copper are useful tests for monitoring treatment. Liver biopsy may help to establish cirrhosis and may show an increased liver copper concentration.

   Heterozygotes are defined by measurement, over several days, of fecal excretion of intravenously administered radiolabeled copper or by demonstration of intermediate increases in liver copper concentration. CT scan lucencies in the basal ganglia may be observed but do not preclude a response to therapy.

   c. **Treatment**

      (1) ᴅ-**Penicillamine** (Cuprimine), 250 mg tid between meals, retards the progression of the disease in most patients with the late-onset form but may exacerbate symptoms when introduced. Medication is continued for life, but dosage may be reduced during pregnancy. Total drug withdrawal

Table 15-6. Drugs commonly used for movement disorders

Drug	Availability	Frequency of administration	Comments
Amantadine hydrochloride	100-mg capsules; 10-mg/ml syrup	bid	Excreted unchanged in urine; initial effect reached 48 hr after administration; half-life, 2–4 hr; adjunct to main therapy; initial dosage, 100 mg daily.
Baclofen (Lioresal)	10-mg tablets	tid	Begin with 10 mg daily and gradually increase to 30–100 mg daily.
Benztropine mesylate (Cogentin)	0.5-, 1.0-, and 2.0-mg tablets; injectable, 1 mg/ml	bid	Initial effect of PO dose requires 24 hr; if given parenterally, effect takes only min; cumulative action; initial dosage, 0.5 mg bid; half-life, 12–24 hr.
Biperiden (Akineton)	2-mg tablets; injectable, 5 mg/ml	tid	Initial effect of PO dose requires 24 hr; if given parenterally, effect takes 1 hr; cumulative action
Botulinum toxin (type A)	100-unit vials	prn	Diluted in saline before injection under EMG control; 2 days for effect; weakness invariable.
Bromocriptine mesylate (Parlodel)	2.5-mg tablets	tid	Very slow increments; watch for a confusional state.
Chlorpromazine (Thorazine)	10-, 25-, and 50-mg tablets	tid	Hypotension; parkinsonism.
Clonazepam (Klonopin)	0.5-, 1.0-, and 2.0-mg tablets	tid	Begin with 0.5 mg tid; increase gradually to maintenance dosage of about 6 mg daily.
Clonidine (Catapres)	0.1-, 0.2-, and 0.3-mg tablets	bid	Be wary of hypotension.
Dantrolene sodium (Dantrium)	25-, 50-, and 100-mg capsules; injectable, 2 mg/vial	bid–qid	Watch for hepatotoxicity; half-life, 9 hr; start with 25 mg bid; slowly increase dosage.
Deanol acetamidobenzoate (Deaner)	25-, 100-, and 250-mg tablets	tid	Slowly increase dosage over 3 wk to maximum of 1 g.
Diazepam (Valium)	2-, 5-, and 10-mg tablets; injectable, 5 mg/ml	bid–qid	High dose needed for muscle relaxation.
L-Dopa (Dopar, Larodopa)	100-, 250-, and 500-mg capsules	qid or more	Half-life less than 2 hr; cumulative action; start with 250 mg tid after meals.
L-Dopa with benserazide (Prolopa)	100/25-mg capsules; 200/50-mg capsules	tid	May be less nausea than with Sinemet.

Drug	Available forms	Frequency	Comments
L-Dopa with carbidopa (Sinemet)	100/10-mg tablets; 100/25-mg tablets; 250/25-mg tablets; Sinemet CR 200/50	tid	Supplements of carbidopa or L-dopa may be needed.
Ethopropazine (Parsidol)	10-, 50-, and 100-mg tablets	tid or qid	Initial effect requires 24 hr; cumulative action; start with 10 mg tid.
Haloperidol (Haldol)	0.5, 1.0, 2.0, 5.0, and 10.0-mg tablets; injectable, 5 mg/ml	tid or qid	5-day half-life; hepatic toxicity; start with lowest dose.
Nadolol (Corgard)	40-, 80-, and 120-mg tablets	qid	Avoid use in asthmatics and patients with severe congestive heart failure or heart block.
Metoprolol (Lopressor)	50- and 100-mg tablets	bid	Avoid use in patients with heart block or severe heart failure.
D-Penicillamine (Cuprimine)	125- and 250-mg tablets	tid	Dose kept under 2 g to avoid toxicity.
Pergolide mesylate (Permax)	0.5-, 0.25-, 1.0-mg tablets	bid or tid	Use with L-dopa; potential for arrhythmias higher than bromocriptine.
Propranolol hydrochloride (Inderal)	10-, 20-, 40-, and 80-mg tablets; injectable, 1 mg/ml	tid–qid	Onset of effect within 30 min; half-life, 3 hr; hepatic toxicity; start with 20 mg tid.
Reserpine (Serpasil)	0.1-, 0.25-, and 1.0-mg tablets; 0.05 mg/ml elixir	qid	Several days for initial effect; start with 0.5 mg daily.
Selegiline (Eldepryl)	5-mg tablets	bid	1 tablet with breakfast and lunch; reduce L-dopa after 3 days.
Tetrabenazine (Nitoman)*	25-mg tablets	tid	Start with one-half tablet; MOA inhibitors contraindicated.
Trihexyphenidyl hydrochloride (Artane)	2.0- and 5.0-mg tablets; 0.4 mg/ml elixir, 5-mg sustained-release capsules	tid for tablets and elixir; qid or bid for sustained-release capsules	Initial effect requires 24 hr; half-life, 6–12 hr; cumulative action; start with 1 mg tid.

* Not yet available in the United States.

may be fatal. Toxic reactions are more common with dosages exceeding 2 g/day. Acute sensitivity reactions occur in one-third of patients. Reported side effects include nausea and vomiting, ageusia, rashes, adenopathy, arthralgia, leukopenia, and thrombocytopenia. The nephrotic syndrome and optic neuropathy have been reported following treatment with the D, L-isomer. Optic neuropathy may improve with pyridoxine, 100 mg daily. Acute sensitivity responses can be treated with corticosteroids. Ageusia may respond to zinc sulfate. A recently documented side effect is Good-pasture's syndrome. The drug is teratogenic in animals. Onset of benefit may be delayed for some months following institution of the drug.

(2) A **diet** low in copper (<1.5 mg/day) may decrease the requirement for penicillamine. Food such as shellfish, liver, mushroom, nuts, and chocolate should be avoided.

(3) Some authors have suggested that **zinc sulfate** or **acetate** containing 25 mg of elemental zinc administered q4h between meals and before bed is a useful, and essentially harmless, first-line therapy for Wilson's disease that reduces copper absorption and may delay the onset of the need to use drugs such as D-penicillamine. It is also used in conjunction with D-penicillamine and may be continued satisfactorily after D-penicillamine has been stopped because of side effects.

(4) Triethylenetetramine dihydrochloride (trientine) has been suggested for use in patients with serious toxic reactions to penicillamine. The dosage is 400–800 mg tid before meals.

(5) Ammonium tetrathiomolybdate is a promising new treatment for Wilson's disease that does not appear to be associated with initial worsening of the syndrome, as frequently seen with penicillamine.

(6) Treatment of metabolic acidosis may help the neurologic disease in those patients with renal tubular acidosis.

(7) Liver transplantation has been advocated on occasion for this disease.

(8) Symptomatic treatment of the movement disorder is outlined in sec. **IV.D.3.**

2. Calcification of the basal ganglia and dentate nucleus commonly occurs in the elderly and may account in part for the frequency of mild abnormal movements in that population. When calcium deposition is severe, a major progressive movement disorder may result that is manifested as either parkinsonism or choreoathetosis.

a. The **differential diagnosis** depends on the history and examination as well as on evaluation of the chemical data outlined in Table 15-7.

b. Treatment. In the presence of hypocalcemia (as in postsurgical hypoparathy-roidism, idiopathic hypoparathyroidism, or pseudohypoparathyroidism), the progress of the movement disorder appears to be arrested by restoring serum levels to the normal range through use of vitamin D (50,000–100,000 units/day) and calcium supplements. Serum chemistries should be monitored regularly to avoid vitamin D intoxication. Regression of the movement disorder is rare, except perhaps in idiopathic hypoparathyroidism. In striato-pallidodentate pseudocalcification (Fahr's disease), the serum chemistries are normal, and no treatment is available. Calcification also occurs rarely in hyperparathyroidism and pseudopseudohypoparathyroidism (normocalcemic pseudohypoparathyroidism).

3. In **Hallervorden-Spatz disease**, iron-containing pigments are deposited in the globus pallidus and pars reticularis of the substantia nigra. The disease is manifested in childhood as progressive parkinsonism or choreoathetosis, occasionally with other motor control system abnormalities. Iron-chelating agents are not useful in reversing the pigmentary deposits. The movement disorder is treated as outlined in sec. **IV.D.3.**

4. Ataxia-telangiectasia is a rare hereditary disease with variable elements of hyperkinesis, myoclonus, nystagmus and dystonia. The diagnostic clinical features are difficulty in generating horizontal eye movements and the conjunctival telangiectasia. This disease may occur in adults without immune deficiency and

Table 15-7. Differential diagnosis of calcification in the basal ganglia

Disease	Frequency of basal ganglia calcification	Chemical data			Urine cyclic AMP to PTH infusion	General
		Calcium	Phosphorus	PTH		
Hypoparathyroidism	Uncommon	→	↑	→	←	Postsurgical effects take 15 yr
Pseudohypoparathyroidism	Half of cases	→	↑	N or →	0	Characteristic facies, extremities, and stature
Pseudopseudohypoparathyroidism	Rare	N	N	N	←	Characteristic facies, extremities, and stature
Hyperparathyroidism	Very rare	←	→ or N	←		Chemistries vary with renal impairment
Fahr's disease	Always (required for diagnosis)	N	N	N		

Key: PTH = parathormone; AMP = adenosine monophosphate; ↑ = increased; → = decreased; N = normal; 0 = no response.

has a variable phenotype. Choreoacanthocytosis is another rare syndrome predominantly hyperkinetic in type.

5. Other diseases that may rarely be associated with parkinsonism or hyperkinesis include infections such as encephalitis, AIDS and syphilis, immunologic diseases such as systemic lupus erythematosus, and consequences of traumatic injury including subdural hematoma.

F. Hemiballismus. The flinging, rotatory movements of hemiballismus arise following lesions of the subthalamus, usually hemorrhage. Even without therapy, the symptoms often resolve to a considerable degree over a period of a few weeks. Initial pharmacologic approaches include **reserpine** or **tetrabenazine** for acute disability, then **phenothiazines** or **haloperidol**. The most effective treatment for chronic severe hemiballismus is probably ventrolateral thalamotomy.

G. Idiopathic dyskinesias and dystonias constitute a group of movement disorders that may be divided, for convenience, into generalized and segmental types. The former is 10 times more common, with a reported prevalence of 30/100,000. The prototype disorder in the generalized group is dystonia musculorum deformans, while other forms may be secondary to a variety of neurologic conditions including encephalitis, trauma, and poisons such as manganese. The segmental group consists of disorders such as torticollis, retrocollis, writer's cramp, Meige's facial dystonia, and blepharospasm.

1. **Treatment**

   a. **Medical treatment** of the idiopathic dyskinesias and dystonias, whether generalized or segmental, is generally unsatisfactory. Systemic drugs used include anticholinergics (especially high-dose **ethopropazine**), followed by **diazepam, haloperidol, tetrabenazine,** and **lithium.**

   b. **Botulinum toxin** type A (Botox) may be used to treat segmental dystonia. The dosage is site- and patient-dependent and should be administered by someone familiar with its use. Botulinum toxin acts by binding in a noncompetitive manner to presynaptic cholinergic terminals, thus leading to functional denervation and muscle weakness. It has been particularly effective for blepharospasm, spasmodic torticollis, hemifacial spasm, and spasmodic (adductor) dysphonia, with 90% success rates reported. Because of weakness, injection of zygomaticus should be avoided when injecting patients with hemifacial spasm. Weakness induced by botulinum toxin is reversible. Patients with apraxia of eye opening do poorly. Task-related dystonias such as writers' cramp respond less well. Botulinum toxin may also be of benefit in jaw-closing dystonia and patients with functional impairment due to spasticity rather than weakness from pathologies as diverse as head injury, stroke, and multiple sclerosis. Care must be taken only to inject symptomatic muscle with the minimum amount of toxin so as to preserve as much power as possible while dampening the dystonia. This may require electromyographic (EMG) control. The effect on the dystonia may not be apparent for several days, and it will recur in approximately 3 months, requiring reinjection. The activity of botulinum toxin varies in preparations from different sources. The preparation in the United States is approximately fivefold more active than that from the United Kingdom. The actual dose used varies from as low as 2 units for small intrinsic muscles of the hand and vocal adductor muscles to as much as 150 units for a large muscle such as tibialis posterior. A standard dose for blepharospasm might be 20 units. Treatment failure may lead to a second injection. Late treatment failure may be associated with increased antibody production. In this situation, botulinum F toxin may be helpful. Treatment failure may occur with or without weakness. Relative contraindications to its use include myasthenia gravis and concomitant administration of aminoglycosides.

   c. Some patients with dystonia may respond to closely applied **splints** (second skin) such as can be fashioned from Lycra garments.

   d. **Spinal cord stimulation** has recently been reported to be useful in some groups but must currently be considered experimental.

2. **Dystonia musculorum deformans** is a hereditary progressive dystonia seen most commonly in Jewish families. Treatment is generally not very effective, but

L-dopa has been used successfully in some patients. Ventrolateral thalamotomy is effective in a few selected patients. Orthoses may be useful.

3. **Spasmodic torticollis** is an example of an idiopathic segmental dystonia involving the musculature of the neck. It is usually a sporadic condition but has been reported in families. The anatomic substrate of the disorder is unknown. The movements may be brief and repetitive, as in a dyskinesia, or sustained, as in a dystonia.

   If medical therapy is unsuccessful, behavioral modification techniques may be used, including sensory and positional feedback therapy. Patients often learn that adoption of particular limb postures help control the movement even before that movement is fully executed. In the past, definitive treatment was a surgical lesion of the motor fibers involved, that is, section of the spinal accessory fibers and intradural section of C1–C3 anterior nerve roots. The spontaneous partial remission rate has been reported to be as high as 33% in 3 years.

4. Some **focal dystonias** occur following relatively minor injury. The pathogenesis is obscure.

5. **Paroxysmal choreoathetosis and dystonia** are rare clinical phenomena that may be familial, sporadic, or acquired.

   a. The familial phenotype is quite variable. Attacks may be induced by startle or movement. Choreoathetosis is usually asymmetric and generally lasts only a few seconds to minutes and responds to **carbamazepine** and **phenytoin** in its kinesogenic form.

   b. Paroxysmal nonkinesogenic dystonia may be precipitated by alcohol, emotion, or fatigue and may last for hours. It responds to treatment with **clonazepam**. In some cases it is a prelude to Parkinson's disease.

H. Tics

1. **Description.** Tics may be defined as quick, coordinated repetitive movements, in contrast to the irregular and nonrepetitive quasi-purposeful jerky movements of chorea. Tics may be defined as simple or multiple and as acute, subacute, and chronic.

   a. Five percent of **children** develop tics, the vast majority of which disappear by adolescence.

   b. The most dramatic tic is the multiple chronic tic syndrome known as **Gilles de la Tourette's syndrome.** In this disease, tics are first noted between the ages of 2 and 13 years and intermittently worsen during the life of the individual. It is more common in males. Patients develop involuntary grunts, whistles, and cough and may develop echolalia. In about half the cases, uncontrolled use of offensive language (coprolalia) develops. Tics may be voluntarily suppressed in early stages of the disease.

2. **Treatment**

   a. **Haloperidol** (Haldol) is the treatment of choice; however, success is limited by the frequent side effects of drug treatment. The starting dosage is 0.5 mg tid; the maximum dosage, determined by observation of the onset of side effects (e.g., sedation, hypotension, and parkinsonism), is usually between 8 and 16 mg qid. There have been rare reports of leukopenia.

   b. **Pimozide** (Orap), an oral dopamine-receptor blocking drug related to haloperidol, will sometimes be effective when haloperidol fails. The starting dosage is 1–2 mg daily, increasing gradually to 7–16 mg daily.

   c. **Clonidine** (Catapres), an alpha-2 adrenergic agonist, helps in half the patients on haloperidol with recurrence of the tics. Clonidine is started at 0.1 mg/day and gradually increased to as high as 2.0 mg/day. Maximum improvement may not be seen for 6 months. Behavioral symptoms are more responsive than tics. Sedation, fatigue, and postural hypotension are the main side effects. The drug should not be withdrawn rapidly because of the possibility of rebound hypertension.

   d. **Tetrabenazine** has been reported to be useful in young patients.

   e. The calcium channel blocking drugs **nifedipine, flunarazine,** and **verapamil** have also been used for this disorder.

   f. **Botulinum toxin A** (Botox) has been used for this disorder (see sec. **IV.G.1.b**).

V. Tremor

A. Description. Tremor may be defined as an involuntary, regular, and repetitive shaking of a body part around a fixed point. The anatomic substrate of most tremors is unknown, but progress has been made in physiologic classification.

B. Classification (Table 15-8). Tremors may be classified according to the following criteria: distribution, rate, amplitude, and relationship to voluntary movement. There may be tremor at rest (see sec. **IV**), tremor with sustained posture (action tremor), or intention tremor (see sec. **III**).

C. Action tremor

1. Description. The most common group of tremors to be managed are action tremors, which are usually of high frequency (7–12 cps) and low amplitude. They may be asymmetric. Action tremors may be induced in normal individuals under appropriate postural conditions, such as movements requiring extremes of precision or power (physiologic tremor). The tremor is increased in states of fatigue, anxiety, weakness, hypercapnia, drug withdrawal, and some metabolic and endocrine conditions (hypoglycemia, uremia, severe hepatic disease, thyrotoxicosis, and heavy-metal intoxication). Drugs that exaggerate the physiologic tremor include catecholamines (including amphetamine), theophylline, caffeine, lithium, tricyclic antidepressants, steroids, antipsychotic drugs, and sodium valproate. It may be **familial.** When it first appears in the elderly, it is known as **senile tremor.** Otherwise, if there is no demonstrable cause, it is known as **essential tremor.** The diagnosis of essential tremor does not preclude the later development of Parkinson's disease.

2. Mechanism. The anatomic substrate of action tremor is not clear. It appears that peripheral mechanisms are involved in the genesis of both physiologic tremor and that associated with thyrotoxicosis. In addition, central mechanisms are also involved in essential, familial, and senile tremors. Action tremors are usually synchronous on EMG analysis but may be alternating as seen in Parkinson's disease.

3. Treatment (see Table 15-3)

a. Tranquilizers may be used for anxiety-induced tremors. **Diazepam** (Valium), 6–15 mg in divided doses, would be appropriate.

b. A single dose of **alcohol** will reduce an action tremor for 3–4 hours; its therapeutic effect begins within 10 minutes of ingestion.

c. Beta-adrenergic antagonists

(1) Propranolol (Inderal), 40–240 mg daily in divided doses, will usually reduce action tremors within 48 hours of initiation of treatment. A useful starting dosage is 20 mg bid. Extensive first-pass metabolism occurs in the liver. Propranolol is **contraindicated** in asthma and insulin-dependent diabetes; side effects include congestive cardiac failure, intensification of atrioventricular heart block, and bradycardia. Other side effects include hypotension, nausea, diarrhea, insomnia, and hallucinations.

(2) For patients with asthma, **metoprolol** (Lopressor), a cardioselective beta blocker, is preferred. The starting dosage is 50 mg bid, increasing to 100 mg bid. This treatment is usually less effective than propranolol.

(3) When patient compliance is a problem, the water-soluble, long-acting, nonselective beta blocker **nadolol** (Corgard) may be used. Since it is long-acting, a single daily dose of 40–80 mg may be used, making it more convenient than the shorter-acting drugs. Because of its water solubility, nadolol crosses the blood-brain barrier poorly. In some patients, however, it reduces action tremor, thus indicating that the effects of beta blockade may be on the peripheral rather than the central nervous system.

d. Primidone (Mysoline), 25–500 mg PO in divided doses, may improve action tremors. Some now consider primidone to be the drug of first choice for treating these tremors. The mechanism of action is unknown. Acute toxicity with this drug may be severe. It should be introduced very slowly to avoid vomiting and ataxia.

e. Glutethimide in dosages between 250 and 1000 mg daily has been used for treating action tremor.

Table 15-8. Characteristics of major tremor syndromes

	Parkinsonism	Essential	Cerebellar	Rubral	Asterixis	Physiological
Clinical						
Rest	++ Pill-rolling	0	+	+	+	0
Sustained position	+	++	-	++ Sway	++ Irregular	+
Intention	+	+	++	++	+	0
Tremor during sleep	0	0	+	+	+	0
Electromyogram	Alternating agonist and antagonist contraction 3–7 cps Essential tremor also seen	Agonist and antagonist co-contraction	Agonist and antagonist contraction asynchronous and overlapping	Mixed pattern	Loss of activity	Alternating agonist and antagonist contraction 8–12 cps

      f. Botulinum toxin A (Botox) has been used as a method of last resort to treat essential tremor of the limbs and head (see sec. **IV.G**).

      g. Ventrolateral thalamotomy has been of benefit in severe action tremor and in congenital rubral and cerebellar intention tremor of the limbs, but not in head tremors.

  D. Orthostatic tremor is an unusual tremor variant manifested as unsteadiness while standing but steadiness while walking. Little is found on examination. However a rapid (16 cps) tremor of synchronous or, occasionally, alternating type is seen in the lower limbs when under conditions of load. Treatment consists of low-dose **clonazepam** (Klonopin), 0.5–1.0 mg/day.

VI. Asterixis may be considered a variant of tremor in which the rate of limb flexion and extension is irregular and usually slow. The EMG indicates that this disorder arises from temporary loss of tone in the outstretched limb. The anatomic substrate is unknown, although it has been seen in patients with focal lesions due to vascular disease. This disorder arises in metabolic diseases (renal, pulmonary, and hepatic), in Wilson's disease, and with some drugs including metoclopramide and anticonvulsants. Treatment is that of the underlying disorder.

VII. Myoclonus

  A. Description. The term *myoclonus* refers to the rapid, irregular, jerking movements commonly appreciated as "night start," which interrupts the steady drift into sleep. The anatomic substrate for myoclonus is not known, but aminergic mechanisms in the raphe nuclei have been implicated. Physiologically it often appears to be temporally related to an epileptiform slow wave on the EEG. The myoclonic jerk is followed by a transient inhibition of normal postural mechanisms. Myoclonus has many causes and is characterized by (1) brief, shocklike contractions, the EMG of which resembles but is often shorter than the EMG of a normal muscle contraction, and (2) the stimuli that induce the myoclonus. For example, intention myoclonus is found in patients with hypoxic brain damage; this type of myoclonus has brief, shocklike contractions.

  B. Treatment. Treatable causes of myoclonus include toxoplasmosis, neuroblastoma, thallium poisoning, uremia, hepatic encephalopathy, drug intoxications (imipramine, penicillin, L-dopa, MAO inhibitors, piperazines), and nocturnal myoclonus. Progressive myoclonic epilepsy is described in Chap. 6. Unfortunately, specific treatment of myoclonus is generally unsatisfactory. Occasionally effective drugs include the following:

    1. Clonazepam (Clonopin), 7–12 mg daily in divided doses, starting with 1.5 mg daily and increasing over 4 weeks.

    2. Valproic acid (Epilim) in gradually increasing doses (up to 1600 mg/day) has been useful in posthypoxic myoclonus.

    3. Piracetam, 18–24 g/day, has been reported as useful adjunctive therapy in myoclonus.

    4. 5-Hydroxytryptophan (5-HTP), 150–1600 mg PO daily divided into two to four doses, with and without carbidopa, has been used in the treatment of posthypoxic myoclonus with some success. A suggested protocol is 5-HTP, 100 mg, and carbidopa, 25 mg, increasing every second day to the maximum tolerated dose, usually around 3 g/day. Gastrointestinal upset is a common problem but often can be managed with antiemetics. Euphoria and mania may occur at higher doses. A scleroderma-like illness has been reported as a complication.

    5. Tetrabenazine has been shown to be useful in spinal myoclonus.

VIII. Restless legs syndrome is characterized by unusual sensations in the muscles and bones of the lower legs that occur at rest, most frequently at night, and that disappear on movement. The etiology and pathogenesis are usually unknown, although the syndrome may be seen in patients with chronic renal failure. Restless legs syndrome may also be seen in association with **periodic movements during sleep,** and the treatment of the two syndromes is the same. Both cause insomnia. Treatments have included anticonvulsants (**clonazepam** and **carbamazepine**), dopaminergic agents (**L-dopa** and **bromocriptine**), **clonidine,** and opioids (see Chap. 16, sec. **XVIII.H**).

Selected Readings

Fetal-tissue transplants in Parkinson's disease (editorial). *N. Engl. J. Med.* 327 (22): 1589, 1992.

Hoehn, M. M., and Yahr, M. D. Parkinsonism: Onset, progression, and mortality. *Neurology* 17:427, 1967.

Jankovic, J., and Tolosa, E. (eds). *Parkinson's Disease and Movement Disorders* (2nd ed.). Baltimore: Williams & Wilkins, 1993.

Penn, R. D. Medical and surgical treatment of spasticity. *Neurosurg. Clin. North Am.* 1 (3):719, 1990.

Weiner, W. J., and Singer, C. Parkinson's disease and nonpharmacologic treatment programs. *J. Am. Geriatr. Soc.* 37:359, 1989.

The Parkinsonian Study Group. Effects of tocopherol and deprenyl on the progression of disability in early Parkinson's disease. *N. Engl. J. Med.* 328:178, 1993.

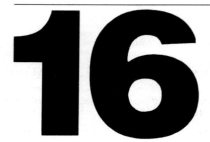

Diseases of Nerve and Muscle

Thomas M. Walshe III

Disorders of muscle, of the myoneural junction, of the peripheral nerve, or of the motor neuron often have specific therapy. When there is no specific therapy, however, the treatment is aimed at controlling symptoms, retarding progression, increasing the time of remission, and improving the quality of the patient's life. The management of these disorders requires the skills of physicians, physical therapists, social workers, and other providers. The severity and progression of the disorder dictates the complexity of the management plan.

I. **Electrophysiologic tests** are used to support the clinical diagnosis and to assess progression or improvement. There are four parts in the neurophysiologic evaluation of a patient with a neuromuscular disorder.

A. **Motor conduction velocity** in large myelinated fibers can be calculated by recording the time a standard current takes to produce a twitch when the distance between the stimulus and the reacting muscle is known. Nerves in the upper and lower extremities as well as the facial nerve can be tested.

Nerve conduction velocity may remain normal for up to 7 days following section of a nerve, and denervation changes may not appear for 10–21 days following section. Most patients with axonal neuropathies (e.g., nutritional) may have slightly reduced conduction velocity, but the reduction may be so slight that it is only in the low-normal range. Neuropathies that affect myelin early (and show segmental demyelination pathologically) reduce nerve conduction velocities. Acute inflammatory demyelinating polyneuropathy (AIDP), diptheria, Charcot-Marie-Tooth disease, metachromatic leukodystrophy, and entrapments often show definite slowing. When the nerve is completely degenerated, there is no way to measure nerve conduction velocity.

B. **Sensory conduction velocity** reflects the time it takes for an evoked potential to be recorded at a site that is distal along a nerve. In the upper extremity, the median, ulnar, and radial nerves can be tested easily. In the lower extremity, the sural, saphenous, deep peroneal, and lateral femoral cutaneous nerves are accessible. In addition, neural action potentials can be recorded by stimulating a mixed nerve. Changes in amplitude and conduction time of the neural action potential (whether from a sensory or mixed nerve) are useful in the evaluation of nerve entrapment syndromes, axonal neuropathies, or demyelinating neuropathies.

C. **Late responses**

1. The **Hoffman reflex (H reflex)** is an electrical equivalent to a deep tendon reflex that assesses both sensory and motor function. It can be elicited only from the soleus muscle in adults. A submaximal stimulus is applied to the tibial nerve, by which it follows the IA afferent fibers to the spinal cord, where it synapses with the motor neurons and causes a direct motor response and a delayed or H reflex response. The H reflex may be absent or prolonged in neuropathy when other conduction studies are normal. S1 radiculopathy also prolongs the H reflex. Patients with AIDP frequently have an abnormal H reflex.

2. The **F response** can be measured in both upper and lower extremities. It is elicited by supramaximal stimulation to a nerve, so the impulses travel antidromically in the efferent parts of the nerve. There is no synapse. In normal patients, the F response and the H reflex vary with the height of the patient. Abnormal late response latency may occur in neuropathy or radiculopathy even

when the other studies are in the normal range. The F response is not sensitive in identifying radiculopathy.

D. **Magnetic stimulation** can be used instead of electrical stimulation to study nerve conduction. The present technology does not provide adequate stimulus localization to warrant routine use, although it has been used in the diagnosis of radiculopathy.

E. **The electromyogram (EMG)** assesses the electrical characteristics of muscle. Signs of denervation include fibrillations, positive sharp waves, reduced interference pattern, and polyphasic units; such signs may support the suspicion of neurogenic disease. Primary muscle disorders have nonspecific and variable EMG patterns, usually with reduced amplitude. Myotonia and myasthenia gravis show distinct EMG patterns, which are described in sec. **VI** and sec. **XIII,** respectively.

II. **Muscle biopsy** is safe and may resolve a diagnostic problem, allowing correct diagnosis and treatment.

A. **Indications for muscle biopsy**

1. Progressive muscular atrophy.

2. Localized or diffuse inflammatory disease of muscle.

3. Systemic disease that is suspected to be vasculitis or collagen-vascular in nature.

4. Occasionally to determine the state of a muscle after injury to nerves and vessels of a limb.

5. To diagnose congenital and metabolic myopathies; histochemical stains are needed.

B. Ideally, the neuropathologist responsible for making the diagnosis should be present when the biopsy is done to ensure that the correct muscle is sampled and that the sample is handled correctly. The studies to be performed are set up in advance, and the specimen is fixed in the operating room. The specimen must be suitable for light and electron microscopy, and histochemical stains of frozen sections are needed. Muscle biopsies taken from an area tested with an EMG needle are often uninterpretable due to trauma.

III. **Nerve biopsy** is done when a specific etiology is suspected. However, the diagnosis can often be made by other means to prevent the painful dysesthesia that may occur after sural nerve biopsy.

A. Nerve biopsy may be **pathognomonic** in

1. Sarcoidosis.

2. Metachromatic leukodystrophy.

3. Amyloidosis.

4. Polyarteritis nodosa.

5. Leprosy.

6. Toxic and hereditary neuropathy.

B. In the majority of cases of neuromuscular disease, nerve biopsy yields nonspecific information and is of limited value. Electron microscopy is essential for separating axonal degeneration from segmental demyelination.

IV. **General principles on the chronic use of corticosteroids.** Corticosteroid therapy requires careful thought about its indications, and when it is started, it requires careful observation of the patient. The complications and adverse responses to corticosteroids are time- and dose-related. Therefore, long-term corticosteroid therapy is best avoided unless it produces a definite advantage.

As a general rule, other therapeutic agents are tried before corticosteroids are begun. In neuromuscular diseases, however, there are few choices, and a corticosteroid is often needed. When possible, less hazardous agents should be used to allow the lowest possible dose of corticosteroid.

A. **Complications during corticosteroid use.** Iatrogenic Cushing's syndrome, diabetes mellitus, osteoporosis, activation of tuberculosis, hypertension, psychosis, and increased susceptibility to infection are seen in some patients treated with corticosteroids. Also, some patients treated with high doses of corticosteroid for long periods have a tendency for gastric ulceration and bleeding.

B. **Considerations in stopping corticosteroid.** Three problems may arise when corticosteroids are stopped.

1. **Suppression** of the adrenal gland (hypothalamic-pituitary-adrenal axis) occurs regularly when the duration of therapy is longer than 1 week with dosages equivalent to prednisone, 20–30 mg/day in divided doses. Complete recovery may take up to 1 year. With doses closer to the physiologic level, suppression may not occur for a month.

Patients who have been treated with pharmacologic doses of corticosteroids usually need no replacement therapy, but they may require steroid coverage during acute illness or other stress.

2. Steroid **withdrawal symptoms** (anorexia, nausea, vomiting, lethargy, headache, fever, arthralgia, myalgia, or weight loss) may occur after chronic treatment is discontinued. Symptomatic treatment and small doses (10 mg) of cortisol for several weeks may help.

3. Acute **exacerbation** of the underlying disease is a major concern when steroids are stopped. Very gradual reduction of the dosage helps to prevent acute flare-ups.

C. **Choice of drugs**

1. **Prednisone** is the standard short-duration oral corticosteroid used in the treatment of neuromuscular disorders. Prednisone (and cortisone) are activated in the liver, and in severe liver failure, the active parenteral forms (prednisolone or cortisol) are given.

2. **Corticosteroids** are preferred to adrenocorticotropic hormone (ACTH) because they can be given PO and the dose is more precise. With corticosteroids, adrenal gland function does not determine the blood level of hormone, and there are fewer side effects. Although ACTH does not suppress the adrenal gland, neither does short-acting corticosteroid therapy used on alternate days.

D. **Treatment course**

1. Corresponding **dosages** of various corticosteroids are given in Table 16-1. Corticosteroids can be given in divided daily doses, a single morning dose, or a morning dose every other day. In short treatment courses of less than 1 month, the dosage schedule does not matter. In chronic treatment, divided daily doses produce iatrogenic Cushing's syndrome, adrenal suppression, and increased suceptibility to infection.

2. **Daily therapy.** The short-acting corticosteroids used chronically as a single morning dose produce less suppression of the adrenal gland, but they do not prevent iatrogenic Cushing's syndrome. The therapeutic effect of a single morning dose is the same as divided doses in most illnesses. Thus, when chronic daily therapy is required, the single-dose schedule is preferred.

3. **Alternate-day corticosteroid therapy** (twice the daily dose given on alternate days) helps to prevent suppression of adrenal function and iatrogenic Cushing's syndrome. There is some evidence that it also prevents increased susceptibility to infection.

Most neuromuscular diseases respond favorably to alternate-day therapy. In early-morning single-day therapy and alternate-day therapy, long-acting corticosteroids (e.g., dexamethasone) are not suitable because they do not allow a sufficient period of low steroid level in the blood to prevent side effects.

4. **To change from a daily dose to the alternate-day plan,** merely increase the dosage gradually on one day, while reducing the dosage by the same amount on the alternate day. At the same time, in the case of divided daily doses, the frequency of the dose is reduced until the whole dose is given in the morning.

Table 16-1. Common corticosteroid drugs

Generic name	Equivalent doses (mg)	Duration	Mineralocorticoid effect
Cortisol	20	Short	Yes
Prednisone	5	Short	Little
Dexamethasone	0.75	Long	No

V. Muscular dystrophy
A. Description
1. A **dystrophy** is a chronic inherited myopathy characterized by progressive muscular weakness and loss of muscle bulk. Pathologically, the number of muscle fibers is reduced, and the remaining fibers are variable in size. Loss of muscle bulk from defects in the nerve or motor neuron, usually called **atrophy,** shows a different pathologic change. There are several types of dystrophy (Table 16-2).
2. The **rate of progression** and the **severity** vary with both the type of dystrophy and the individual case. The Duchenne dystrophies are usually the most severe, and the majority of these patients die by the age of 20 years. Patients with other dystrophies survive into adulthood. Those with mild, restricted dystrophies may live a nearly normal life.
3. The **pathophysiology** of many of the muscular dystrophies remains unknown. However, recent investigations suggest that a defect in the muscle cell membrane is the underlying abnormality. A deletion mutation at the Xp21 locus (on the short arm of the X chromosome) is the cause of Duchenne or Becker's muscular dystrophy. The gene product, dystrophin, is absent in the muscle membrane of patients with Duchenne dystrophy and is reduced in amount or is of altered molecular weight in patients with Becker's dystrophy, a less severe variant. The pathophysiology of other types of dystrophy is not as well understood.

B. Diagnosis
1. The **history** and **signs** of muscle weakness and wasting in a child or young adult suggest the diagnosis. However, there are no absolute clinical criteria for separating neurogenic atrophy from dystrophy. Separation of the various dystrophies is made by the distribution of muscle involvement, speed of progression, and other clinical characteristics (see Table 16-2). Table 16-3 lists some differences that may be useful in distinguishing atrophy and dystrophy.
2. **Muscle biopsy** is helpful in diagnosing dystrophy and identifying certain benign myopathies (e.g., central core, nemaline) that may resemble dystrophy. The muscle biopsy is taken from an involved muscle, but not one that is severely weak. The deltoid or gastrocnemius is often used in patients with dystrophy, but the rectus abdominis may be a better choice because there is less problem with postoperative immobilization, which causes disuse weakness.
3. **DNA analysis** on blood by polymerase chain reaction may demonstrate a defect in up to 70% of patients with Duchenne or Becker's muscular dystrophy. The test can be done on cultured tissue from a fetus also. Dystrophin assay on muscle biopsy can distinguish the Duchenne and Becker's variants from each other and from other myopathies in which dystrophin is normal. Although the combination of the two tests is highly reliable in making the diagnosis, most clinicians omit the biopsy if a deletion is found on the blood test. Dystrophin analysis separates Duchenne from Becker types of dystrophy.

C. Treatment
1. **Mild cases** need no therapy early in the course. Careful motor assessment at 6- to 12-month intervals is usually enough.
2. In **severe cases,** especially in patients with Duchenne dystrophy, the family must be made aware of the natural history of the disease.
   a. Knowledge that faithful compliance with therapeutic directions helps to prolong the patient's independence should encourage the family to help. However, when the disease is obviously progressing, there often is disappointment. Thus, it is important to maintain a guarded hope for stabilization so the physical program will be maintained.
   b. Since many dystrophy patients are **children,** a treatment plan should include education and meeting social needs. For example, children can usually remain in normal schools until they cannot climb stairs easily. In Duchenne dystrophy, however, the intelligence quotient (IQ) is often reduced (many are below 90), and earlier transfer to special schools may be indicated.
   c. **The goal of therapy is more than keeping the patient ambulatory.** The patient who must spend most of the time concerned with the disease misses

Table 16-2. Types of muscular dystrophy*

Characteristic	Duchenne	Facioscapulohumeral	Limb-girdle	Myotonic dystrophy
Sex	Male	Both	Both	Both
Age at onset	Before 5 years	Adolescence	Adolescence	Childhood or later
Initial symptoms	Pelvic	Shoulder girdle	Either	Weakness and/or myotonia
Facial involvement	No	Always	No	Always
Pseudohypertrophy	Common	No	Rare	Never
Progression	Rapid	Slow	Slow	Slow
Inheritance	X-linked recessive	Autosomal dominant	Autosomal recessive	Autosomal dominant
Muscle enzymes	Very high	Normal	Normal or little increased	Normal
Abnormal ECG	Common	Rare	Occasional	Occasional
Myotonia	No	No	No	Yes

* Other forms of dystrophy are less common and include oculopharyngeal dystrophy, progressive dystrophic ophthalmoplegia, and late distal dystrophy of Welander.

Table 16-3. Separation of neurogenic from myopathic disorders

Sign	Neuropathy	Motor neuron disease	Myopathy
Weakness, wasting, decreased reflexes	Yes	Yes	Yes
Distribution	Distal	Distal	Proximal
Twitching	Yes	Yes	No
Hyperreflexia	No	Yes	No
Sensory loss	Yes	No	No
Nerve conduction	Slow	Normal	Normal
EMG	Fibrillations, decreased number of potentials	Fasciculations, giant motor units, fibrillations	Decreased amplitude and duration of potentials
Elevated CSF protein	Yes	No	No
Elevated muscle enzymes	No	Occasionally	Yes
Muscle biopsy	Group atrophy	Group atrophy	Degeneration

the purpose of therapy. The family and the patient should be encouraged to maintain as normal a life as possible for as long as possible.

3. **Prednisone** (0.75 mg/kg/day) can improve strength in Duchenne dystrophy, but potential risks outweigh benefits so routine treatment is not recommended. Steroid treatment should be considered in acute situations, such as sudden worsening of respiratory function due to pneumonia or atelectasis. Boys treated with steroid need to keep a low-fat, low-sodium diet to prevent weight gain. If exposed to chickenpox, the steroid-treated boy should receive zoster immune globulin.

4. **Physical treatment**
   a. Intensive physical therapy is begun early, and the family and patient are instructed in home exercises. Physical therapy is accepted better before contracture and deformity occur.
   b. Goals are to maintain good alignment in the weight-bearing joints and to prevent contractures. Flexion contractures are common around hips, ankles, and knees, since the flexors are often slightly less involved than the extensors.
   c. Range-of-motion exercises, instruction in proper positioning in bed and in a chair, frequent changes of position, and early use of splints, when necessary, help prevent contractures that make nursing care difficult and impede ambulation.
   d. There is no evidence that physical therapy retards the progression of muscular dystrophy. Independent ambulation can be maintained, however, for several years longer in patients who have it. The cost-effectiveness of physical therapy has not been studied.

5. **Respiratory care**
   a. **Swallowing and respiratory difficulty** occur in severe, generalized dystrophy and in pharyngeal dystrophy. Respiratory decompensation is usually a gradual process and occurs late in the course.
   b. **Pulmonary function tests** often are abnormal, even in patients with superficially normal respiratory reserve. Patients are encouraged to develop diaphragmatic breathing by using blow-bottles or playing wind instruments (e.g., harmonica). Breathing exercises, taught by a therapist, are also helpful.
   c. Later in the course of the disease, intermittent positive pressure breathing and postural drainage may become necessary.

d. A **rising CO_2** in patients without pulmonary infection is usually a bad prognostic sign in dystrophy because about 80% of severe muscular dystrophy patients die from respiratory causes. Muscular dystrophy patients are rarely intubated late in the course of illness.

6. Gait maintenance

a. Obesity is treated vigorously to improve the patient's ability to walk and to prevent hypoventilation.

b. Patients are asked to walk for a least 3 hours each day; if they are not ambulatory, they are instructed to stand for 3 hours in divided periods (30 minutes q3–4h)

c. As the disease progresses, independent ambulation can be maintained with crutches, braces, and surgical procedures. The wheelchair is avoided as the primary means of mobility until ambulation is impractical.

d. Patients may become weaker during acute illnesses, but bed rest usually is contraindicated, since weakness invariably follows prolonged bed rest, and it may become permanent.

7. Preventive therapy—genetic counseling. When the inheritance of a disease is known, it is often possible to predict the probability of the disease's occurring in offspring of affected parents. An important aspect in the care of muscular dystrophy is advising the family about recurrence rates in future generations.

a. Sex-linked recessive disorders (Duchenne dystrophy)

(1) Inheritance. A known carrier can be told that there is one chance in two of producing a dystrophic male or a carrier female. However, about one-third of patients have no prior family history.

(2) Carrier detection. The serum creatine kinase (CK) will be elevated in approximately one-half of obligate carriers. The enzymes should be checked at least 3 times, 10 days apart, since levels may fluctuate. It is best to avoid excessive exercise prior to the test, since this may result in confusion if the serum enzyme levels are elevated. A normal result does not exclude the possibility of the carrier state. Sixty to sixty-five percent of families have Duchenne muscular dystrophy/Becker muscular dystrophy mutations associated with intragenic deletions of the dystrophin gene. Once an affected male is diagnosed, the carrier status can be determined by detecting the same deletion in one of the two dystrophin alleles of a female at risk. In other cases, restriction fragment length polymorphism linkage analysis can be used. Carrier detection is accurate in 85–90% of girls tested.

(3) Prevention. Several choices are open to families who carry the abnormal gene:

(a) Voluntary sterilization or contraception.

(b) In utero determination of sex and of the disorder may allow abortion of all affected males.

(4) Spontaneous mutation occurs in one-third of Duchenne dystrophy patients. The more normal children a woman has before a dystrophic child is born, the smaller the probability that she is a carrier. If the mother of a dystrophic child is not a carrier, the chances of her having another dystrophic child are small.

b. Autosomal dominant disorders (facioscapulohumeral [FSH] dystrophy, myotonic dystrophy, and late distal dystrophy)

(1) Inheritance. Although the typical halting FSH dystrophy is usually an autosomal dominant trait, there are others that are similar clinically that may be autosomal recessive or sex-linked traits. The severity of the disease may vary. The affected person has one chance in two of having an affected offspring when there is autosomal dominant inheritance.

(2) There are no **carriers.**

(3) Prevention is by contraception. If the male partner is affected, artifical insemination may be used to produce normal offspring.

c. Autosomal recessive disorders (limb-girdle)

(1) Inheritance. Both parents must have the trait before the offspring are affected. If both parents are carriers, one in four children will have the disease, two out of four will be carriers, and one will not be affected at all.

    (2) Prevention. Contraception and avoidance of consanguineous marriage can help prevent these diseases.

VI. Myotonia and myotonic dystrophy

A. Description

1. Thinning of the muscles of the face and neck causes an expressionless countenance, with poor movement of the mouth. The patients have ptosis and the muscles of the hands and forearms are thinned.

2. On contraction and relaxation the muscles feel stiff. Percussion myotonia may be elicited in thenar muscles or the tongue. The myotonia usually is not severe.

3. The myotonia of myotonic dystrophy and congenital myotonia (Thomsen's disease) are treated with the same drugs. In congenital myotonia without dystrophy, the myotonia is usually much more severe. Myotonia is also seen in hyperkalemic periodic paralysis.

4. The EMG shows a decremental pattern without a plateau on repetitive stimulation as well as the characteristic myotonic irregular-pattern afterpotentials.

5. Hypogonadism, cataracts, mental retardation, and esophageal dysfunction are often associated problems.

6. The disease is usually an autosomal dominant trait, and it may appear from early infancy to adulthood.

B. Treatment

1. **Drugs** that act on the muscle cell membrane are used for myotonia.

    a. Phenytoin (Dilantin), 5 mg/kg/day PO, is effective and has fewer cardiac side effects than the other agents. It is the usual first choice.

    b. Procainamide, up to 50 mg/kg/day PO, divided into three or four doses.

    c. Quinine, 5–10 mg/kg/day PO, divided into six doses.

    d. Corticosteroids have been used in severe cases (see sec. **IV**).

    e. Diazepam (Valium) has no effect.

2. **Respiratory care.** Intercostal myotonia may interfere with regular breathing and present respiratory complications, even when there is little myotonia in the limbs. Patients with myotonic dystrophy often have oropharyngeal dysfunction and may develop aspiration pneumonia.

3. Treatment of the dystrophy depends on the severity. Usually the weakness is much more a problem than is the myotonia, and often the myotonia needs no therapy.

VII. Polymyositis

A. Description

1. **Polymyositis** is an inflammatory autoimmune muscle disease that causes weakness and fatigue. The natural history of the disease varies, relapsing and remitting when treated and occasionally improving spontaneously. Cancer, cardiac involvement, older age of onset, and delay of treatment are each associated with a poor prognosis. Other organ systems are also involved in polymyositis. Interstitial lung disease is one of the most frequent complications.

2. The **clinical features** of polymyositis are variable, but proximal muscle weakness is the rule. The disease is occasionally acute and may progress in weeks to complete disability. Some patients have a subacute course that evolves over several months; those with acute onset may have associated myoglobinuria. The face is often spared, and muscle atrophy is a late sign. Pharyngeal muscle involvement may produce dysphagia, but speech usually remains normal. Also, the posterior neck muscles are often weak. Some patients develop an erythematous skin eruption on the dorsum of the hands, proximal digits, knees, or elbows or a purple discoloration and edema of the eyelids. Some patients also develop sclerodactyly. Patients with skin involvement are said to have **dermatomyositis,** but the therapeutic approach is the same as for polymyositis. Cardiac involvement occurs in up to 30% of patients.

B. Diagnosis

1. **Muscle enzymes** (CK, transaminase, and aldolase) are usually elevated, but they may be normal in some cases.

2. The **erythrocyte sedimentation rate** does not correlate reliably with the activity of the disease.
3. The **EMG** is nonspecific, but it usually suggests a primary myopathic process with brief, small-amplitude polyphasic motor units. However, positive sharp waves, fibrillations, and high-frequency repetitive discharges are also frequently seen.
4. **Muscle biopsy** shows an inflammatory infiltrate and necrosis of muscle fibers in about 85–90% of patients. Often several biopsies must be taken to get a diagnostic specimen.
5. **Differential diagnosis**
   a. Other diseases that may be confused initially with polymyositis are
      (1) Paroxysmal myoglobinuria.
      (2) Parasitic myositis.
      (3) Polymyalgia rheumatica.
      (4) Muscular dystrophy.
      (5) Thyrotoxic and other endocrine myopathies.
      (6) Diabetic amyotrophy.
   b. Appropriate study and muscle biopsy usually distinguish these diseases from polymyositis.
6. **Relation to cancer.** Polymyositis has been linked to occult cancer, but recent reports have refuted the high incidence of occult cancer in patients with polymyositis. However, patients with true polymyositis, rather than muscle wasting from cachexia, have a 20% incidence of cancer. Patients with dermatomyositis and those who have evidence of denervation on EMG may have a higher incidence of cancer.

C. Treatment
1. **Corticosteroids**
   a. Corticosteroids have been found to benefit patients with polymyositis, although no controlled trials have been done. Mortality is not affected by corticosteroids, but remission is more rapid, and there is less morbidity when corticosteroids are used. Corticosteroids are usually used in combination with either methotrexate or azathioprine.
   b. Patients who have had disease of acute onset for a short time are most likely to benefit from corticosteroid therapy. However, those with chronic polymyositis and atrophy may not improve with steroid therapy. In chronic cases, when there is no improvement in 2 months, there will usually be no success with corticosteroids (see sec. **VII.C.2.b**).
   c. **Dosage**
      (1) The usual **beginning dosage** of prednisone is 60–100 mg PO every morning until improvement occurs; then the dosage may be reduced to 40 mg and maintained for several months.
      (2) **Dosage reduction.** After the initial treatment, the prednisone dosage is reduced slowly by 5–10 mg every 3–7 days to prevent flare-up of the disease. The dosage is kept at around two-thirds of the original dosage for several more months. As the dosage is reduced, each change represents a larger percent change. Therefore, as the dosage is decreased, longer intervals are needed to prevent a relapse. In 6–12 months, most patients can be dropped to a maintenance level (15–20 mg every morning) and kept there. If the disease remains quiescent, alternate-day corticosteroid therapy (30–40 mg every other day) is recommended for most patients. If exacerbation occurs, high dosages are resumed and maintained until signs of improvement occur. Response to therapy and relapse can be monitored in most cases by muscle enzyme determination.
      (3) Attempts at **steroid withdrawal** should be made after the first 24 months of therapy, since activity of the disease often subsides after 2 years. Most cases are quiescent after 8 years.
      (4) Low doses of corticosteroids are not useful in bringing active polymyositis into remission.
   d. **Steroid myopathy.** The occurrence of steroid-induced myopathy in patients with chronic polymyositis may complicate therapy. Steroid myopathy should

be suspected if the patient's weakness seems to increase while muscle enzymes and EMG remain unchanged. Increased type II muscle fiber atrophy on muscle biopsy is also suggestive of steroid-induced myopathy. Women with polymyositis seem to be more susceptible to steroid-induced myopathy, so lower doses of prednisone should be used when possible. Biopsy usually is not needed for confirming the diagnosis of steroid-induced myopathy; it is usually sufficient to reduce the dose of steroid, and if improvement follows, one can assume that the weakness was from the drug. Management requires reduction of steroids to a maintenance level and observation for a rise in muscle enzymes. If the enzymes rise and further deterioration occurs, high-dose corticosteroid therapy is restarted.

    e. Follow-up. The muscle enzymes (SGOT, CK, and aldolase) are useful indicators of disease activity, although in some cases all the enzymes or all but one may remain normal. The enzyme levels may fall for several weeks before clinical improvement is seen, and they may rise before weakness occurs in a relapse.

2. Immunotherapy

    a. Indications. Immunosuppressive drugs may be of benefit in chronic progressive polymyositis, in patients who are not improved by corticosteroid therapy, and in patients who have intolerable complications of steroid therapy.

    b. Immunosuppressive drugs may allow a smaller dosage of corticosteroid, or they may be effective if used alone.

        (1) Methotrexate

            (a) Dosage. Up to 75% of steroid-resistant patients respond when methotrexate is added to corticosteroid therapy. The drug must be given IV over 20–60 minutes. In patients with normal liver and kidney function, the starting dosage is 0.4 mg/kg/treatment, and it is increased to a maximum of 0.8 mg/kg/treatment in 2–3 weeks.

            (b) Frequency. Methotrexate is given weekly at the onset, and as improvement occurs, the frequency is reduced to biweekly and then triweekly. When improvement is maximal, monthly doses are given for 10–24 months. Corticosteroids may be reduced as improvement occurs.

            (c) Toxicity of methotrexate includes stomatitis and GI complaints, which usually subside with reduction of the dosage. Leukopenia and hepatic toxicity may occur and, when severe, require that the drug be stopped.

        (2) Azathioprine (Imuran), 1.5–2.0 mg/kg PO, is used in patients with polymyositis, either alone or with prednisone. Over the short term, there seems to be little benefit in adding azathioprine to prednisone. Azathioprine may be of use in long-term treatment, in patients who fail on prednisone, or in patients who do not tolerate prednisone. When used, the dosage is gradually increased until the WBC count becomes depressed, and that dosage is continued until remission of the myositis occurs. Major side effects are bone marrow suppression, anorexia, nausea, vomiting, and jaundice.

3. Other therapeutic measures

    a. Bed rest is essential in acute cases.

    b. As the patient improves, **physical therapy** is indicated for range-of-motion exercises.

    c. Patients with chronic weakness may benefit from **braces** and other physical measures.

VIII. Trichinosis

A. Description

    1. Incidence. In the United States, there are about 300 recorded cases/year of infestation with **Trichinella spiralis,** a nematode that affects skeletal muscle.

    2. The **clinical syndrome** varies as the parasite moves from the GI tract, through the lymphatics, to the bloodstream, and finally as it ends as an encapsulated embryo in the skeletal muscle. Nausea, vomiting, and diarrhea may occur acutely, with a low-grade fever. Fatigue and edema of the eyelids and face are common. Myalgia and muscle tenderness occur later. Occasionally, isolated muscle weakness may produce a focal sign (e.g., diplopia), but weakness is generalized and mild. Eosinophilia is present early, and muscle biopsy often demonstrates the parasite.

3. **Disease course.** Onset of the syndrome is usually within 2–3 days of ingestion of the parasite, and improvement begins at 4 weeks. By 2 months, symptoms are usually gone. The disease is seldom fatal, and its severity depends on the size of the inoculum.

4. **Etiology.** Undercooked pork is the most common source of infection (pigs are now rarely fed uncooked garbage, so there is less trichinosis in the pig population). Bear and walrus also have been implicated as sources of trichinosis.

B. **Treatment**

1. **Corticosteroids** can be used to improve the symptoms. Prednisone, 60 mg in the first 24–48 hours, may be given, with subsequent reduction to 20 mg/day for 7–10 days or until the patient improves.

2. **Thiabendazole,** 25 mg/kg bid PO for 10 days, may relieve the acute symptoms. Also, it acts to destroy the capsule of the *Trichinella* embryo. Side effects occur in about one-half of the patients treated with thiabendazole and include anorexia, nausea, vomiting, dizziness, lethargy, headache, and elevation of liver enzymes.

IX. **Rhabdomyolysis**

A. **Description.** Any process that disrupts the muscle cell may lead to the release of myoglobin and other muscle protein into the plasma. Major associated conditions include trauma, strenuous exercise, heat stroke, polymyositis, alcohol ingestion, licorice ingestion, McArdle's disease, diabetic acidosis, and hyperkalemia. There are also familial cases (Myer-Betz disease) in which myoglobinuria may follow exercise or infection. Three major complications of rhabdomyolysis may occur that require treatment:

1. **Respiratory distress** from weakness of respiratory muscles is a rare problem.

2. **Hyperkalemia** may occur because of the necrosis of muscles and may lead to lethal cardiac arrhythmia.

3. **Acute renal failure** occurs when plasma myoglobin concentration is high.

B. **Treatment** is strict bed rest, osmotic diuresis for preventing renal failure, and maintenance of electrolyte balance.

X. **Glycogen storage diseases**

A. **McArdle's disease (deficient muscle phosphorylase)**

1. **Description.** Pain and stiffness on physical exertion in young adults is the mark of the deficient muscle phosphorylase. Blood lactate does not rise following exercise, and weakness and wasting are rare. When the stiffness is severe, shortening of the muscles may occur. The EMG of the shortened muscles shows physiologic contracture with electrical silence; muscle glycogen is elevated on biopsy.

2. **Treatment**

a. The amount of **exercise is reduced** automatically by the patient, and that alone may provide relief in the early stages.

b. Ingestion of **glucose** or **fructose** (20–45 g tid) may increase exercise tolerance, but the treatment may lead to obesity.

c. **Drugs** that raise the concentration of free fatty acids may be used, including

(1) **Fenfluramine,** 20 mg bid.

(2) **Isoproterenol,** 10–20 mg daily.

d. **Glucagon** has been used to produce hyperglycemia, and it may increase tolerance in some patients.

B. **Pompe's disease (acid maltase deficiency)**

1. **Description.** Pompe's disease usually occurs in the first few months of life; it is associated with an enlarged heart from cardiomyopathy and hypotonia. Death usually occurs before 12 months, and diagnosis is made on muscle biopsy. An adult form exists.

2. **Treatment.** No definitive treatment is available, although there have been reports of improvement with a high-protein, high-fat diet. Some investigators have attempted bone marrow transplant to improve the disorder.

C. Phosphofructokinase deficiency
  1. Description. The clinical picture is very similar to McArdle's disease, but there is less pain associated with the stiffness. There are very few cases studied, but the inheritance seems to be autosomal recessive, since both parents generally leave low phosphofructokinase in muscle.
  2. Treatment. There is no accepted method of treatment.

XI. Carnitine deficiency
  A. Description. There are two primary genetic carnitine deficiency syndromes. Both are inherited in an autosomal recessive manner.
    1. The **systemic form** generally is manifest early in life as a recurrent illness similar to Reye's syndrome, with episodes of acute encephalopathy, hypoglycemia, hyperammonemia, elevated liver enzymes, and prolonged prothrombin time. These episodes may be precipitated by caloric deprivation, as may occur during an ordinary acute febrile illness. Patients with systemic carnitine deficiency have low levels of carnitine in liver, muscle, and serum, although the latter is variable.
    2. The **myopathic form** presents as a progressive myopathy with variable degrees of weakness. Encephalopathic episodes do not occur, and there is no liver involvement. Carnitine levels are normal in serum and liver but reduced in muscle.
  B. Treatment with carnitine (D, L-carnitine, 2 g/day PO) is indicated, but not all patients will respond favorably.

XII. Episodic muscle weakness
  A. Familial hypokalemic periodic paralysis
    1. Description
      a. Familial hypokalemic periodic paralysis is transmitted as an **autosomal dominant** trait. The disease is three times more common in males, and it usually appears in the late teens or early twenties.
      b. The **onset** is usually sudden with weakness of all four limbs. However, the muscles of respiration and swallowing usually are spared. The distribution of weakness may be asymmetric.
      c. The **attacks** often occur in the morning and, untreated, last from 1–36 hours. The muscles are weak and flaccid, and the deep tendon reflexes may be absent. Heavy carbohydrate ingestion or vigorous exercise followed by rest may precipitate attacks. Cold weather also may precipitate attacks.
      d. The **serum potassium** level is usually between 2 and 3 mEq/liter. Other laboratory tests are normal.
      e. The **EMG** shows decreased muscle excitability. Muscle biopsy during attacks may reveal large vacuoles in the affected muscle fibers.
      f. Hyperaldosteronism and **thyrotoxicosis** may be associated with episodic weakness and hypokalemia. Hyperthyroidism occurs with episodic weakness in Asians.
    2. Treatment
      a. Acute attack. High doses of **potassium** are given either PO (10–15 g of potassium chloride mixed in fluid) or IV in a potassium chloride solution (40–60 mEq in 500 ml of 5% D/W infused over several hours) to reverse the acute attack.
      b. Prophylaxis
        (1) High-potassium, low-carbohydrate, and low-sodium diet.
        (2) Spironolactone (Aldactone), 100 mg PO daily or bid.
        (3) Thiamine hydrochloride, 50–100 mg daily.
        (4) Treatment of **hyperthyroidism** when present.
        (5) Dichlorphenamide, 25–50 mg PO tid, or **acetazolamide** (Diamox), 250–500 mg PO q4–6h, to cause a mild metabolic acidosis.
  B. Familial hyperkalemic periodic paralysis
    1. Description
      a. Hyperkalemic periodic paralysis affects females and males equally, and it is transmitted as an autosomal dominant trait. Onset is usually during childhood.

    b. The **attacks** are milder and shorter (30–90 minutes) than in hypokalemic paralysis. Respiratory muscles are spared, but trunk and proximal limb muscles are involved. Mild myotonia may be present clinically in the tongue, hands, and eyelids.

    c. The **EMG** shows hyperirritability between attacks and myotonic-like discharges during attacks. Serum potassium level is either high or high normal.

  2. Treatment

    a. Acute attack

      (1) Most attacks are of short duration and require no specific therapy.

      (2) Attacks can be stopped with IV infusion of **10% calcium gluconate,** 10–20 ml.

    b. Prophylaxis

      (1) Acetazolamide, 250 mg PO qid, or **dichlorphenamide,** 25–50 mg tid.

      (2) Chlorothiazide, 50–100 mg PO daily.

XIII. Myasthenia gravis

  A. Description. Weakness and progressive fatigue with exercise are the hallmarks of generalized myasthenia gravis. However, diplopia may be the only symptom of ocular myasthenia, and the pupil is never involved. Muscle wasting may occur late, but it is not prominent. The course is variable and marked with remissions and exacerbations, which make evaluation of the therapy difficult. Most patients reach maximum severity of their disease within 1 year, but a few progress over several years. Classification into several general groups helps to predict the course and to determine the type of therapy.

    1. Group I. About 14% of patients have ocular myasthenia only.

    2. Group IIA. Mild generalized myasthenia with ocular signs.

    3. Group IIB. Moderately severe generalized myasthenia, with mild bulbar and ocular involvement.

    4. Group III. Acute severe myasthenia, with bulbar and respiratory complications. Tracheostomy is required.

    5. Group IV. Late severe myasthenia, usually developing from other groups within 2 years.

  B. Diagnostic tests

    1. Edrophonium (Tensilon) test

      a. Initial diagnosis. When there is a defect that is easily observed, such as grip strength, neck power, extraocular muscle function, ptosis, diplopia, swallowing, vital capacity, and occasionally on EMG, edrophonium chloride may cause transient improvement and support the diagnosis of myasthenia gravis. The edrophonium test is not used in patients with respiratory distress.

      (1) For best results a placebo control is used, and the trial is done double-blind. The placebo can be nicotinic acid (100 mg/10 ml of saline), which gives a systemic response, or saline alone. Atropine (0.4 mg) is often used both as a control and to protect against excessive muscarinic side effects, such as

        (a) Excessive sweating.

        (b) Excessive salivation.

        (c) Lacrimation.

        (d) Diarrhea.

        (e) Abdominal cramps and nausea.

        (f) Incontinence of stool and urine.

        (g) Bradycardia.

        (h) Hypotension.

        (i) Small pupils (< 2 mm).

      (2) Edrophonium, 10 mg, is used in the adult (0.2 mg/kg in children). To begin, 2 mg is infused into a secure IV line, and the patient is observed for excessive muscarinic side effects. If there are no severe effects, the remaining drug is infused in about 30 seconds.

      (3) The patient is observed for improvement. The duration of action is 2–20 minutes, but occasionally, in patients treated with prednisone, it may be longer (up to 2 hours). The clinical improvement should coincide with the drug's expected duration of action.

b. Smaller doses of edrophonium (1 mg) are used to diagnose **cholinergic crisis.** If there is no improvement, more drug is infused 1 mg at a time, up to 5 mg. Improvement is judged clinically, as in the diagnostic test. Respiratory function must be assessed carefully before the test, and if edrophonium causes apnea, facilities for tracheal intubation must be at hand.

c. Evaluation of oral anticholinesterase therapy can be done in some patients by infusing edrophonium, 2 mg, 1 hour after the last oral dose and watching for improvement and side effects. If there is improvement and there are no increased side effects, the oral dose is increased by 25–50%. If there is no change in the patient's power but there are mild side effects, the dose is kept the same. When the side effects are prominent and the patient's power is worse following the edrophonium, the oral dose is reduced by 25–50%.

2. Neostigmine test. If the duration of the action of edrophonium is too short to evaluate the patient's response, the anticholinesterase neostigmine (Prostigmin) may be used. Neostigmine, 0.04 mg/kg, is injected IM and reaches its maximum activity in 1–2 hours. The effect is gone at 3–4 hours. Pretreatment with atropine may prevent muscarinic side effects.

3. EMG. If a nerve is stimulated at 3–10 impulses/second repeatedly and an EMG is recorded, the amplitude of contraction is temporarily diminished in myasthenia gravis. When myasthenia patients are relaxed so that several muscles (at least one of which is proximal) are rested, 95% will show a pathognomonic EMG pattern. In myasthenia, a decrement in response is followed by a plateau or an increment, whereas in other disorders that may show a decrement (myotonia, poliomyelitis, amyotrophic lateral sclerosis, neuropathies, and McArdle's disease), the decrement is continuous. Single-fiber EMG recording often shows abnormalities characteristic of neuromuscular junction disease.

4. Acetylcholine receptor antibody assay is positive in 50% of patients with ocular myasthenia and in 80–90% of patients with generalized myasthenia. The antibody level reflects the severity of disease in untreated patients.

5. Evaluation of thymus

a. About three-fourths of patients with myasthenia gravis have abnormal thymus glands. The most common abnormality is hyperplasia, but 15% have thymoma.

b. CT scan of the mediastinum is highly reliable in identifying thymoma. CT scan is sometimes normal in patients with thymic hyperplasia.

C. Treatment

1. General measures

a. Patients with generalized myasthenia should be **hospitalized** and kept at rest while anticholinesterase medication is begun.

b. Contraindicated medications. Drugs that have mild neuromuscular blocking effects and sedatives, which may cause respiratory depression, are contraindicated. Common drugs of this type are

(1) Quinine.

(2) Quinidine.

(3) Procainamide.

(4) Propranolol.

(5) Lidocaine.

(6) Aminoglycoside antibiotics.

(7) Polymyxin.

(8) Viomycin.

(9) Colistin.

(10) Morphine.

(11) Barbiturates.

(12) Other tranquilizers.

c. The **goals of therapy** in myasthenia vary with the severity of the illness. Improvement in strength or increased time spent out of the hospital are goals in more severe cases. However, complete remission may occur with steroid therapy.

d. Thyroid abnormalities occur in association with myasthenia gravis, and antithyroid antibodies and antimuscle antibodies have been detected in some myasthenics. However, no clinical correlation between the abnormalities and these antibodies has been made. In thyrotoxic patients, thyrotoxic myopathy is more common than myasthenia gravis. However, in patients with myasthenia, thyrotoxicosis must be treated before the myasthenia gravis will improve.

    e. Ephedrine, 25 mg tid, or other stimulant drugs occasionally improve strength in patients on anticholinesterase therapy.

2. Respiratory care

    a. Acute generalized myasthenia is a medical emergency, and even when the patient appears to have normal respiratory function, decompensation can occur rapidly. Thus, myasthenics with generalized disease are kept under close observation in an intensive care unit until treatment is seen to be effective.

    b. Measurement of maximum voluntary ventilation (patient breathes as rapidly and as deeply as possible for 15 seconds while expired gases are collected and analyzed) gives the best indication of effects of myasthenia on respiratory muscles. Measurement of **vital capacity** with a hand spirometer is also a satisfactory way of following respiratory function.

    c. Ocular myasthenia (group I) is a benign illness. It is not associated with respiratory failure.

3. Anticholinesterase therapy remains the first choice in all cases of myasthenia. It is often used in conjunction with corticosteroid therapy.

    a. Pharmacology

        (1) Anticholinesterase drugs inhibit the destruction of acetylcholine and allow its accumulation at the synapse. Therefore, the effects of the drug are limited to the cholinergic synapse. The motor end-plate is the primary therapeutic target, but autonomic cholinergic synapses are also affected and produce side effects. The drugs used do not cross the blood-drain barrier, so there are insignificant central effects. The parasympathetic postganglionic effects predominate, since the ganglionic sites are less sensitive to inhibition. Both the dose of drug given and the level of activity at the synapse determine the degrees of the parasympathetic activity.

        (2) Side effects may be reduced by avoiding factors that increase parasympathetic activity (e.g., motion). Atropine, 0.4–0.8 mg PO, may be useful in reducing side effects in certain circumstances, but chronic use is usually not helpful because of atropine toxicity. However, patients should have atropine on hand for occasional use.

        (3) Smaller doses of anticholinesterase, taken more frequently, or doses taken with food to delay absorption may help to reduce side effects. The patient often becomes tolerant of the side effects with prolonged therapy.

        (4) The common anticholinesterase drugs are listed in Table 16-4.

    b. Administration

        (1) The **oral dosage** and frequency of administration depend on the severity of the disease and the patient's sensitivity to the drug. Therapy is by trial and error initially, but a usual starting dosage is **pyridostigmine** (Mestinon), 60 mg q4h, or its equivalent (see Table 16-4). The use of liquid dosage forms allows an individualized program.

            (a) If one anticholinesterase drug is ineffective, usually the others will be also. Side effects may be less bothersome with one preparation, but there is no way of determining which will be tolerated best.

            (b) Patients should be instructed to observe and record their response to the drug so adjustments can be made.

        (2) **Parenteral therapy** may be required during an acute attack, after surgery, or if dysphagia is a problem. Supplementary subcutaneous injection of anticholinesterase 1 hour before meals may improve dysphagia. The parenteral dose is one-thirtieth the oral dose for neostigmine and pyridostigmine.

Table 16-4. Anticholinesterase drugs commonly used for myasthenia gravis

Drug	Route	Adult dose	Child's dose[a]	Neonatal and infant dose	Frequency
Neostigmine bromide (Prostigmin)	PO	15 mg	10 mg	1–2 mg	q2–3h
Neostigmine methyl sulfate (Prostigmin injectable)	IM, IV	0.5 mg[b]	0.1 mg[a]	0.05 mg	q2–3h
Pyridostigmine bromide[c] (Mestinon)	PO IM, IV	60 mg 2 mg[b]	30 mg 0.5–1.5 mg/kg	4–10 mg 0.1–0.5 mg	q3–4h q3–4h
Mestinon/ Timespan	PO	180 mg			q8–10h
Ambenonium chloride (Mytelase)	PO	10 mg	0.3 mg/kg	0.3 mg/kg	q6–8h

[a] The dose in children varies so much that it must be determined for each case. Small amounts of the drug are given and increased as indicated by the clinical improvement.
[b] The parenteral dose is usually one-thirtieth of the oral dose.
[c] Also available as a liquid and as the chloride.

4. **Crisis** (acute weakening in a myasthenic)
   a. **Myasthenic crisis.** Changes in the absorption of medication or the natural worsening of the disease may cause increased weakness, requiring an increase of anticholinesterase drugs.
   b. **Cholinergic crisis**
      (1) Anticholinesterase drugs can occupy the same receptors as acetylcholine, and an excess of anticholinesterase will reduce neuromuscular transmission. The curarelike effect of anticholinesterase drugs gives them a bell-shaped dose-response curve and creates a serious hazard in therapy.
      (2) A slight decrease in neuromuscular transmission can produce severe weakness in the myasthenic patient. The clinical syndrome is much like that of a myasthenic crisis. Many patients may give a history of recent cholinergic side effects, suggesting excessive anticholinesterase therapy.
      (3) If the patient is treated with atropine, the warning side effects may not occur, and increased weakness will be the only sign of toxicity.
      (4) Chronic use of anticholinesterase medication damages the synapse, and some patients become refractory to the medication. Usually, after a time off the medication (often with respiratory support), the patient again responds to anticholinesterase medication.
   c. **Treatment of crisis**
      (1) Crisis is an emergency and requires intensive care. The patient's respiratory function must be maintained, and if respiratory (or swallowing) dysfunction is present, elective endotracheal intubation is done before emergency intubation is necessary. When the airway is secure, diagnosis of the type of crisis can continue.
      (2) The edrophonium test can be used in the nonapneic patient, and if unequivocal improvement occurs, the anticholinesterase dosage can be increased while the patient remains under close observation. In severe cases, the patient is unable to cooperate, so improvement with edrophonium is seldom consistent.
      (3) When there is doubt about the result of the edrophonium test, all anticholinesterase medications are stopped for 72 hours. The patient may

be followed with serial edrophonium tests until a definite improvement is seen. At that time, longer-acting drugs may be started.

(4) Often less medication is required following crisis because the patient is more sensitive to the drugs.

d. Patient education. Patients are taught not to increase the dosage of anticholinesterase in response to increased weakness. They should be aware that the smallest possible amount of drug is best and that full-strength dosage may be too much.

5. Immunotherapy background

a. Myasthenia gravis is an **autoimmune disease** in which circulating IgG antibody is activated against the acetylcholine receptor on the motor endplate. Animals immunized with purified acetylcholine receptor protein develop experimental myasthenia identical to the human disorder.

b. Myasthenia gravis seems to occur with high frequency in two separate **age groups.** The peak incidence in one group is at age 30, and women are more commonly affected. In the other group, peak incidence occurs at age 70, and both sexes are equally affected. Most of the younger patients have thymic germinal centers, whereas the older patients have atrophied thymuses or thymomas. The younger group responds better to treatment with anticholinesterase drugs and thymectomy but varies in response to corticosteroid. The older group often benefits from corticosteroid therapy and less commonly from anticholinesterase drugs or thymectomy.

6. Corticosteroid therapy

a. Indications

(1) Failure of anticholinesterase medication to allow an acceptable level of function without excessive side effects. Most patients with generalized myasthenia are treated with steroids unless there is a major contraindication.

(2) To improve the patient's strength preoperatively in preparation for thymectomy.

(3) Failure of remission following thymectomy.

(4) Rarely in pure ocular myasthenia when diplopia is disabling.

b. High-dose corticosteroid therapy

(1) Prednisone, 60–100 mg daily, may produce increased weakness about 5 days after onset of therapy. Anticholinesterase drugs or in severe cases plasmapheresis can be used to control steroid-induced exacerbation. Improvement begins at about 12 days. High-dose corticosteroids are as effective as ACTH, and with prolonged treatment, longer remissions can be obtained.

(2) High dosages are maintained until improvement is sustained (for about 2 weeks). There are seldom relapses after the first 2 weeks of therapy, and anticholinesterase drugs are gradually withdrawn over 1 month. About three-fourths of patients have a significant improvement following corticosteroid treatment.

(3) The corticosteroids are then gradually reduced to 5–15 mg daily (or the equivalent alternate-day dosage) over several months. Then the maintenance dosage is continued. Some patients may be able to stop the maintenance dosage without relapse.

(4) Care must be taken early in the treatment to protect the patient from **respiratory complications** or aspiration. The incidence of such problems is smaller in corticosteroid treatment than in treatment with ACTH.

(5) Dexamethasone, 20 mg daily for 10 days and then repeated for a second course, has been highly successful. Improvement or remission occurs in most patients and continues for 3 months or longer after the drug is stopped. Generally the higher the dosage of steroid used, the greater the remission rate. Dexamethasone is not often used as the first treatment, but it may be needed if prednisone treatment at lower dosages fails.

c. Low-dose corticosteroid therapy

(1) By starting with a low-dose alternate-day program (25 mg of prednisone on alternate days) and gradually increasing the dosage by 12.5 mg every third dose until the total dosage reaches 100 mg on alternate days, or until optimal results occur, the initial period of worsening is avoided.

(2) Improvement may not occur for 6–7 weeks of therapy with low-dose treatment, and therapy should be continued for 3 months before being abandoned.

(3) If relapse occurs after withdrawing or reducing the corticosteroids, the full dosage should be resumed.

7. **Other immunotherapy**
   a. **Plasmapheresis**
      (1) **Plasmapheresis** is directed toward removing the harmful antibody that causes myasthenia gravis. Patients with severe generalized myasthenia gravis who are resistant to other modes of therapy may improve transiently after plasmapheresis. The improvement following plasmapheresis may last for months in a few patients, but repeated exchanges are usually needed to maintain the improvement. The best results are achieved by using steroid, immunosuppressives, and plasmapheresis together.

      (2) Plasmapheresis is done using a blood component separator. The technique varies from center to center but usually begins with an initial exchange of 10–20 liters over several weeks. If the initial series is successful, it is followed by a chronic program in which 2 liters is exchanged weekly for several weeks, and then the exchanges are done as needed to continue the improvement.

      (3) The fluid removed during plasmapheresis is replaced with normal saline or, in large exchanges, with serum albumin or fresh-frozen plasma after removal of the cryoprecipitate factors.

      (4) Iron replacement usually is needed. The transient hypocalcemia that follows exchange is usually not clinically significant.

      (5) Plasmapheresis should be employed only in centers where adequate experience with the technique is available.

   b. **Azathioprine** (2.5 mg/kg) is added following plasma exchange to sustain improvement. Benefit appears in several months. The usual adult dosage is 50 mg tid. Some patients who fail to improve on steroids improve on azathioprine. The blood count and liver function need to be monitored frequently.

8. **Surgical therapy**
   a. **Patients without thymoma**
      (1) The thymus has been implicated in the etiology of myasthenia gravis. In 1939, a thymic cyst was removed from a patient, with coincidental improvement in the patient's myasthenia gravis. Since that time it has been found in young patients with generalized myasthenia that removal of the thymus often leads to a lasting remission. Also, as many as 90% of selected patients that have a thymectomy experience a remission or sustain improvement for 5 years. Many of these patients need less anticholinesterase medication, and some can discontinue it entirely.

      (2) With continued reduction of operative morbidity and mortality, many authorities advocate thymectomy in all young patients early in their course, especially when anticholinesterase medications do not produce optimum improvement with minimum side effects. Young patients who have the disease for a short time improve most rapidly, and pathologically, the thymus shows absent or few germinal centers. Patients with pure ocular myasthenia do not undergo thymectomy.

   b. **Patients with thymoma.** Mortality in patients with thymoma is much higher than in those without it, and removal of the thymoma may not improve myasthenia. Radiation therapy is used when the thymoma cannot be removed completely. About 30% of patients with thymoma have myasthenia, and 10% of myasthenic patients have thymoma.

   c. **Surgical approach.** There is some debate about the best approach for removal of the thymus.

(1) **Median sternotomy.** The classic approach is through a median sternotomy, and the method is safe in experienced hands.

(2) **Transcervical approach**

(a) The transcervical approach sacrifices the excellent exposure of the sternotomy, but it reduces the postoperative morbidity when successful.

(b) Hemorrhage, pneumothorax, and fragmentation of the gland with incomplete removal may complicate the transcervical approach and necessitate an unplanned open procedure.

(3) The procedure with which the surgeon is most comfortable is the best choice, but when uncomplicated, the transcervical approach results in the least morbidity.

9. **Postoperative treatment of the myasthenia patient**

a. **Tracheostomy** is performed by many surgeons if there is

(1) Oropharyngeal weakness.

(2) Previous myasthenic crisis.

(3) Previous history of respiratory complications.

(4) Vital capacity less than 2000 cc.

b. In patients without tracheostomy, the nasotracheal tube is left in place for 48 hours after surgery.

c. After thymectomy, the patient may show marked improvement for 12–24 hours.

(1) In the immediate postoperative period, no anticholinesterase drugs are given, and the patient is kept slightly underdosed to reduce excess secretions.

(2) The medication is changed from the parenteral to the oral form as soon as possible. It is increased to the optimal dosage level gradually (36–48 hours).

(3) Care must be taken not to overdose the patient, since previous doses of anticholinesterase drugs may be excessive after thymectomy.

d. **Sedatives and weak neuromuscular blockers must be used with extreme caution if the patient is not intubated.**

10. **Treatment of myasthenia in pregnancy**

a. During pregnancy, myasthenic patients may become worse, improve, or remain unchanged. When change occurs, it is usually in the first trimester or post partum.

b. **Abortion.** Therapeutic abortion is not indicated because it may cause worsening of the myasthenia. Spontaneous abortion is common during the first trimester in women with myasthenia gravis.

c. **Labor** in myasthenic mothers is usually shorter than in normal mothers. Intramuscular anticholinesterases are used during labor.

d. **Local or regional anesthetics** are preferred to general anesthesia, and caution is required with sedatives.

e. **Cesarean section** is done only for obstetric indications.

f. **Contraception.** The neurologist and obstetrician must help the myasthenic woman formulate plans for long-range family planning. Voluntary sterilization or contraception should be suggested when the myasthenia is severe.

11. **Neonatal myasthenia**

a. **Description.** Congenital myasthenia gravis is very rare, but neonatal myasthenia occurs in about 20% of babies born to myasthenic mothers. The condition is transitory and is usually gone in 24–36 hours. However, it may persist for weeks. Signs include masklike face, poor sucking, difficulty swallowing, regurgitation, and respiratory distress. Symptoms usually begin within 3 days of birth, but they sometimes do not appear for 10 days.

b. **Treatment.** Symptomatic treatment to prevent aspiration, provide nutrition, and maintain respiration is most important. Anticholinesterase drugs may be needed for a short time. **Neostigmine,** 1–2 mg PO (parenteral dose is one-thirtieth the oral dose) q4h, or **pyridostigmine,** 4–10 mg PO, is recommended for infants.

XIV. Lambert-Eaton myasthenic syndrome (LEMS)

A. Description. A myasthenia-like syndrome (LEMS) occurs with carcinoma (usually oat cell carcinoma of the lung). The syndrome is associated with generalized muscle weakness, but unlike that of myasthenia gravis, the weakness improves when the muscle is exercised. Patients with LEMS also often demonstrate autonomic symptoms, such as dry mouth, and neuropathic elements, such as absent reflexes, features that do not occur with myasthenia gravis. An EMG is helpful in differentiating the syndrome from true myasthenia gravis. It is now clear that many cases of LEMS occur without underlying carcinoma. The pathogenesis of LEMS involves an immune attack on the presynaptic aspect of the neuromuscular junction. There is a LEMS autoantibody test available.

B. Treatment

1. **Removal of the tumor,** when possible, may resolve the syndrome.

2. When the tumor is not resected or there is no improvement after removal, **guanidine hydrochloride** (35–40 mg/kg/day, divided into three or four doses) has been beneficial in some cases. Gastrointestinal upset is a frequent side effect and may require that the drug be stopped or the dosage reduced. Bone marrow suppression has resulted from guanidine therapy.

3. **3, 4-Diaminopyridine,** 18–25 mg PO qid, has been used to improve neuromuscular function in patients with LEMS.

4. **Plasmapheresis** used in conjunction with **prednisone** and **azathioprine** has been used to provide symptomatic improvement.

XV. Botulism

A. Description. Botulism is an intoxication caused by the exotoxin of *Clostridium botulinum,* an anaerobic, gram-positive, spore-forming rod that may contaminate foods.

1. As in tetanus, the toxin rather than the bacterial infection produces the illness. Botulinum toxin is a powerful presynaptic blocker of acetylcholine release. There are six antigenically distinct toxins (A, B, C, D, E, and F) but only A, B, and E are associated with human illness.

2. The **clinical syndrome** is one of progressive muscle weakness, often beginning in the extraocular or pharyngeal muscles and becoming generalized. Also, gastrointestinal complaints may be prominent. There are no sensory signs; dilated unreactive pupils are regularly seen, but the patient remains alert. Dry, erythematous mucous membranes are also common.

3. The **diagnosis** is confirmed when the disorder appears in a mouse injected either with serum from the patient or with an aliquot of the suspected food.

4. The **course** is usually rapid, with symptoms appearing within 18 hours of ingestion of the toxin. A more rapid onset is associated with more severe courses.

5. The **prognosis** in treated patients is about 80% survival. Patients whose cases are not generalized usually do very well. Those who are over 20 years old and those with type A toxin have a slightly higher mortality.

6. A syndrome of botulism occurs in **young infants** due to colonization of the gut by *Clostridium* with subsequent absorption of toxin. The course is subacute to chronic.

B. Treatment

1. **Antitoxin.** Therapy against the toxin is begun as soon as possible.

   a. Specific typing of the toxin can be done, but treatment is usually started with **trivalent (A, B, E) antitoxin.**

   b. The antitoxin is horse serum, so skin-testing and precautions for anaphylaxis are necessary; 10,000 units of antitoxin is administered IV in one dose.

   c. Approximately 15–20% of botulism patients will have minor **allergic reactions** to the antitoxin that may require treatment with antihistamines or corticosteroids. However, some patients have severe reactions, so provision for emergency endotracheal intubation should be made before the antitoxin is given.

2. **Emetics, cathartics,** and **enemas** are used with caution to eliminate any toxin that remains in the gastrointestinal tract.

3. **Guanidine hydrochloride,** an acetylcholine agonist, is useful in some patients to

counteract the presynaptic blockade caused by the toxin; 35–40 mg/kg/day is given PO q4h. The major side effect of guanidine is gastrointestinal upset, but suppression of blood counts has been observed in chronic treatment.

4. **Respiratory care.** Maintenance of respiratory function is the most important aspect in treating severe cases of botulism.

   a. Patients who appear to have mild symptoms (diplopia and mild weakness) may rapidly develop respiratory failure, so respiratory function must be monitored frequently in all patients until there are signs of improvement.

   b. If vital capacity falls to 1000 cc, elective intubation is considered. Severe dysphagia also requires nasogastric or endotracheal intubation to prevent aspiration.

XVI. Tetanus

A. **Description.** Tetanus is an intoxication that results from infection with *Clostridium tetani,* a gram-positive coccus that enters through a wound.

   1. An **exotoxin** causes the neuromuscular irritability and the syndrome of tetanus.

   2. **Clinical features.** The major presenting feature of generalized tetanus is muscle rigidity and discomfort in the jaws, neck, and lower back. The symptoms, which may be mild at the onset, progress over hours or days to a state of muscular hyperirritability and spasm that may involve the respiratory and pharyngeal muscles. Convulsive seizures are common.

   3. Tetanus may be localized to the area surrounding the wound rather than generalized. Often the jaw is involved early in both localized and generalized tetanus (lockjaw).

   4. The **prognosis** is good in localized tetanus, but mortality reaches 50% in patients with generalized disease, despite therapy.

B. **Treatment**

   1. **Treatment directed against the toxin.** The major emphasis is on the neutralization of the toxin. Some patients with tetanus may have no *C. tetani* in their wound cultures, and other (20%) may have no wound visible at the time of onset.

      a. **Human hyperimmune globulin** is the antitoxin of choice; 3000–10,000 units is given IM or IV, although lower doses may be effective. A single dose is adequate. Toxin already fixed in the neural tissues will not be eliminated by antitoxin, but circulating toxin will be neutralized by it.

      b. **Horse serum antitoxin** can be used, but prior skin tests for sensitivity are required. The usual dosage is 50,000 units IM followed by 50,000 units in a slow IV infusion. If surgical excision of the wound is impossible, a small amount of antitoxin may be injected locally.

   2. **Therapy directed against the bacteria**

      a. The **area of the wound** is surgically excised and drained.

      b. **Cultures of the wound** are taken, but they do not always grow the organisms.

      c. **Penicillin** is the antibiotic of choice: procaine penicillin, 1.2 million units IM or IV q6h for 10 days.

      d. For patients unable to take penicillin, **tetracycline,** 500 mg PO or IV q6h for 10 days, may be substituted.

   3. **General measures**

      a. The treatment of tetanus, as does that of any paralyzed patient, includes care of skin, bladder, bowel, fluid management, nutrition, and respiration. Prevention of aspiration pneumonia and pain is particularly important.

      b. Spasms of generalized tetanus are painful and interfere with respiration. A dark, quiet room will help reduce the spasms. Sedation is important in controlling the spasms, and the patient should be kept asleep. **Diazepam,** in dosages determined by the patient's response (2–10 mg IV q4–12h), is safe and effective. Meprobamate, barbiturates, and chlorpromazine have also been used with success. Diazepam may cause respiratory and **cardiac arrest** in a few patients if it is used with **barbiturates,** so the combination should be avoided.

      c. **Neuromuscular blockers** are helpful when the other methods fail to reduce the muscle spasm that interferes with swallowing or respiration. The patient must be artificially ventilated when neuromuscular blockers are used. It is not safe to try to give a dose of neuromuscular blocker to stop spasm in the extremities while preserving respiratory function. Pancuronium (Pavulon), succinylcholine, and other blocking agents may be useful when the patient is intubated. Sedation should be maintained or increased when blockers are used because it is extremely unpleasant for the patient to be awake and paralyzed. Intrathecal baclofen infusion has been used to control spasms.

d. Autonomic dysfunction (hypertension, hypotension, hyperpyrexia, and cardiac arrhythmia) is common. Treatment is directed at the symptoms.

4. Prophylaxis

a. All persons, beginning at 2 months of age, should be immunized against tetanus toxin. Initial immunization is **tetanus toxoid,** 0.5 ml in three injections 4 weeks apart. Booster injections are required every 10 years.

b. In **acute injuries,** thorough washing and debriding are necessary.

(1) In **fresh, clean wounds,** the toxoid course should be completed if it has not been completed already. If the initial immunization is complete, a booster dose of toxoid is given if the patient has not had one in the past 10 years.

(2) In **wounds that are dirty or infected,** toxoid booster is given if none has been received for 5 years. **Human antitoxin** (250 units IM), in addition to the toxoid, is given to patients who have not received earlier immunization. Contracting tetanus does not confer immunity, and the series of toxoid injections is required in these persons.

XVII. Malignant hyperthermia and neuroleptic malignant syndrome

A. Description. Exposure to various inhalation anesthetics, muscle relaxants (e.g., succinylcholine, curare, pancuronium), or stress alone may, in susceptible individuals, result in sudden release of calcium from the sarcoplasmic reticulum with resultant intense muscle contraction. Susceptibility is inherited as an autosomal dominant trait. The resultant clinical syndrome may begin during anesthesia or in the several hours thereafter. A similar syndrome may occur after exposure to certain neuroleptic drugs (neuroleptic malignant syndrome). If the syndrome is untreated, the mortality is nearly 100%. The common symptoms, in their usual order of appearance, are

1. Tachycardia.

2. Acidosis.

3. Tachypnea.

4. Cardiac arrhythmias.

5. Muscle stiffness.

6. Rise in body temperature.

B. Treatment. Early recognition is important. As soon as the characteristic clinical syndrome is noted:

1. Discontinue anesthesia or neuroleptic drugs.

2. Initiate **surface cooling** with ice packs applied to the body or immersion in ice or cold water.

3. Initiate **core cooling** with cool oral fluids and reestablish electrolyte balance with oral and intravenous fluids, 1–2 liters over 3–4 hours.

4. Administer **dantrolene,** 1 mg/kg, by rapid IV infusion, and repeat as necessary until symptoms subside (up to a maximum of 10 mg/kg). Dantrolene, 1–2 mg/kg PO qid, may be required for a few days thereafter to prevent recurrence. Dantrolene blocks the release of calcium from the sarcoplasmic reticulum, thus relieving the underlying pathologic alteration causing the syndrome. High intravenous doses of dantrolene may cause enough muscle weakness to precipitate respiratory failure.

C. Prophylaxis

1. In **patients with known propensity toward malignant hyperthermia,** inhalation anesthetics, neuroleptics, and muscle relaxants should be avoided if possible.

2. If possible, in **patients with a known family history of malignant hyperthermia,** anesthesia, neuroleptics, and muscle relaxants should not be administered until a muscle biopsy is performed to determine susceptibility. Muscle from susceptible people contracts in vitro on exposure to concentrations of caffeine, halothane, or suxamethonium that cause only minimal changes in normal muscle.

3. A history of anesthesia without an attack of malignant hyperthermia does not exclude susceptibility in patients with a positive family history. Such patients may suffer attacks of malignant hyperthermia on subsequent exposures to the known precipitating factors.

XVIII. Neuropathy

A. Description

1. Peripheral neuropathy of various types (polyneuropathy [PN], entrapment neuropathy [EN], mononeuritis multiplex [MNM]) is a symptom that may be associated with many **systemic disorders,** including the following:
   a. Multiple myeloma—PN.
   b. Carcinoma—PN.
   c. Myxedema—PN.
   d. Systemic lupus erythematosus—PN.
   e. Cryoglobulinemia—PN.
   f. Rheumatoid arthritis—PN, EN.
   g. Scleroderma—PN.
   h. Diptheria—PN (nerve conduction velocities greatly reduced).
   i. Hepatic failure—PN.
   j. Renal failure—PN.
   k. Diabetes mellitus—PN, MNM, EN.
   l. Porphyria—PN.
   m. Refsum's disease—PN.
   n. Tangier disease—PN.
   o. Metachromatic leukodystrophy—PN (nerve conduction velocities greatly reduced).
   p. Polyarteritis nodosa—MNM.
   q. Sarcoidosis—MNM.
   r. Tuberculosis—MNM.
   s. Waldenström's disease—MNM, PN.
   t. Acromegaly—EN.
   u. Amyloidosis—EN, PN.
   v. Monoclonal gammopathy—PN, MNM.
2. Certain **vitamin deficiencies** are associated with polyneuropathy, such as
   a. Thiamine.
   b. Pyridoxine.
   c. Pantothenic acid.
   d. Riboflavin.
   e. Vitamin B_{12}.
   f. Folic acid.
3. **Intoxication** from the following substances may cause polyneuropathy:
   a. Arsenic.
   b. Lead.
   c. Mercury.
   d. Thallium.
   e. Acrylamide.
   f. Carbon tetrachloride.
   g. Chlorinated hydrocarbons.
   h. Methyl butyl ketone.
   i. Triorthocresyl phosphate.
   j. Hexachlorophene.
   k. Plastic model glue.
4. Some commonly used **drugs** that may cause polyneuropathy are
   a. Chloroquine.
   b. Clioquinol (nonprescription antidiarrheal medicines).
   c. Dapsone.
   d. Phenytoin.
   e. Disulfiram.
   f. Glutethimide.
   g. Gold.

    h. Hydralazine.
    i. Isoniazid.
    j. Nitrofurantoin.
    k. Stilbamidine (facial numbness).
    l. Vincristine.
    m. Cisplatin.
    n. Immunization (rabies, typhoid, smallpox, rubella, pertussis).
5. There are also several **primary neurologic disorders** that affect peripheral nerves or roots (e.g., Landry-Guillain-Barré disease and Charcot-Marie Tooth disease). Thus, the first step in management of polyneuropathy is to diagnose the underlying disease. The details of therapy depend on the underlying illness, the severity of the neuropathy, and the rate of progression. Patients with acute progressive motor neuropathy require observation in the hospital, whereas those with chronic neuropathy can be treated as outpatients.
6. Polyneuropathy. Symmetric loss of sensory function, motor function, or both usually begins in the feet or fingertips in polyneuropathy. Deep tendon reflexes may be diminished early, especially in the ankles; later reflexes may be absent. Some neuropathies affect the proximal nerves early (diabetic amyotrophy), and these may be confused with myopathy.
7. Mononeuropathy is the asymmetric dysfunction of one or more large nerves. There is usually pain, and the cranial nerves may be affected. The cranial nerves may also be involved in polyneuropathies. The pathology of mononeuropathy and mononeuropathy multiplex is usually disruption of the vasa nervorum. In the polyneuropathies, the mechanism is often unknown; however, axonal degeneration occurs in some, and in others the myelin sheaths undergo segmental demyelination.

B. Diagnosis
1. The differentiation of chronic polyneuropathy from primary disease of muscle and other conditions that cause weakness is seldom a problem. However, identifying the cause of the neuropathy is difficult.
2. Muscle enzymes are normal in polyneuropathy.
3. Abnormal **nerve conduction studies** support the diagnosis of peripheral neuropathy, although normal studies do not exclude it. Mononeuropathy usually shows decreased conduction in the affected nerve, but other nerves are normal.

C. Acute idiopathic demyelinating polyradiculoneuritis (AIDP) (Landry-Guillain-Barré-Strohl syndrome)
1. Description
    a. Incidence. Persons of all ages are affected in AIDP, but the highest incidence is in persons between the ages of 50 and 74. The syndrome may follow a mild viral illness by 10–12 days or appear without prodrome.
    b. The **earliest signs** are motor weakness, paresthesias, and pain, progressing from lower extremities to upper extremities.
    c. The **cranial nerves** are affected in 75% of cases. The facial nerve is involved in half of those with cranial neuropathy, and of those with facial palsies, it is bilateral in about 80%.
    d. Autonomic disorders (cardiac arrhythmia, hypotension, hypertension, hyperpyrexia, and tachycardia) occur frequently and account for almost half the fatalities.
    e. Cerebrospinal fluid (CSF) protein is usually high. Cell counts in CSF are always below 70 lymphocytes/μm and usually lower than 20/μm.
    f. Nerve conduction velocities are reduced in 90% of patients.
2. Prognosis. Patients with normal nerve conduction studies have the best prognosis.
    a. The disease progresses over 7–21 days. Patients with more rapid progression usually need respiratory support. Improvement follows the progressive period by 10–14 days, and recovery continues for 6–36 months.
    b. Most patients recover enough to leave the hospital in 75 days or less. Atelectasis, aspiration, pneumonia, pulmonary abscess, venous thrombosis, and pulmonary embolus are serious complications of the paralysis. Despite

these complications, overall mortality is only 5% with modern intensive care.

c. Recovery is complete in about one-half of patients, and most of the remainder have only mild abnormalities. Severe disability occurs in about 10–15% of patients.

3. **Treatment.** The neuropathologic defect is an autoimmune inflammatory perivascular mononuclear infiltrate that may involve the entire peripheral nervous system. Both axonal degeneration and segmental demyelination occur. The major emphasis in management is supportive care to prevent complications, since given time most patients improve spontaneously.

a. **Plasma exchange** used within 7 days of onset seems to shorten the recovery time in about two-thirds of patients with severe Guillain-Barré syndrome. The usual course is three to five exchanges every other day.

b. **Intravenous immunoglobulin,** 0.4 g/kg, given in 1000 ml of saline over 6–8 hours, is used in patients in whom plasma exchange fails to provide benefit.

c. **Corticosteroids** are of little benefit in the acute disorder.

d. **Respiratory care.** The most important consideration is maintaining adequate respiration. Patients should be followed closely, with measurement of vital capacity, and endotracheal intubation is performed when the vital capacity drops to 25–30% of normal. (Normal vital capacity in males = 25 cc x height in centimeters; females = 20 cc x height in centimeters; children = 200 cc x age in years.) When bulbar muscles are involved, feeding is done by intravenous administration, nasogastric tube, or gastrostomy.

e. Prophylactic anticoagulation is indicated in paralyzed patients. Subcutaneous **heparin** in low doses (5000 units q12h) or warfarin helps to prevent thromboembolic complications of immobilization. Infants and small children need not be anticoagulated, since they can be easily mobilized.

f. Fecal impaction is a painful problem that occurs in bedridden patients. Thus, **suppositories** and **enemas** should be used from the outset, before problems arise.

g. **Physical therapy.** Bed rest is indicated in the acute phase of the illness until improvement begins.

(1) **Positioning.** Careful positioning of the patient in bed prevents bed sores and compression of nerves. A firm foundation or bedboard is necessary, and flexed positions are avoided for prolonged periods. Frequent (q2h) change of the patient's position is necessary to prevent pressure sores. A water mattress or "egg crate" mattress is useful in reducing pressure sores.

(2) **Prevention of contractures**

(a) Range-of-motion exercises prevent the connective tissues from shortening, which is a natural tendency. A short, passive range-of-motion program twice daily is started early in the course of the illness. However, as improvement occurs, most types of intensive physical therapy can be used.

(b) A footboard is necessary to prevent gastrocnemius and Achilles tendon contractures. Pillows under the shoulders should be avoided, since they may promote kyphosis. Allowing the patient periodically to lie face down helps to prevent flexion contractures of the hips.

(c) If contractures begin to form, stretching range-of-motion exercises may relieve them. Once contractures are fully formed, however, surgical release is necessary.

h. **Edema.** Paralyzed extremities lack the normal muscle tone that keeps edema from occurring. Edema makes the skin less resistant to pressure necrosis, infection, or mild trauma. Edema may be painful when it forms rapidly.

(1) Intermittent elevation of the extremities (above the level of the heart) may help to prevent edema and reduce edema that is already present.

(2) Intermittent compression of edematous extremities for 60–90 minutes twice daily, followed by massage and elevation, is useful.

(3) Ace bandages applied tightly to the trunk and unwrapped for 10–15 minutes 3 times a day or a pressure stocking can be used to prevent edema.

i. **Pain.** Myalgia and arthralgia are common in acute polyradiculoneuritis.
   (1) **Mild analgesics** are usually effective (aspirin, 600 mg q3–4h), but occasionally codeine (30–60 mg q4h) or morphine (5–10 mg IM) is needed.
   Narcotics cause respiratory depression and constipation.
   (2) **Heat** applied before range-of-motion exercises and warm baths (Hubbard
   tank) may reduce pain.
j. **Later phase of therapy.** Maximum development of residual function is the goal
   of late therapy.
   (1) **Restorative surgical procedures** may increase function.
   (2) A **brace** can be used to maintain the limb (often the foot) in good position,
   but it cannot overcome a fixed deformity. A brace must be strong enough
   to function but light enough to allow easy ambulation. The weight of the
   brace is especially important in the patient with weakness of hip flexion.
   A brace that allows controlled motion is usually more comfortable than
   one that allows no motion.
   (3) Management of **physical therapy** is done with the help of trained physical
   therapists and, if available, a competent physiatrist.
k. **Autonomic syndrome.** Occasionally, paroxysmal hypertension, headache,
   sweating, anxiety, and fever occur in patients with acute polyradiculoneuritis.
   Phenoxybenzamine (20–60 mg in divided doses) has been used to relieve this
   syndrome. Also, diabetes insipidus and the syndrome of inappropriate antidiuretic hormone secretion have been reported to occur in patients with acute
   polyradiculopathy. In these patients, observation of the urinary output, the
   state of hydration, and serum and urine electrolytes allows prompt therapy
   when needed.
D. **Chronic inflammatory demyelinating polyradiculoneuropathy (CIDP)** is similar to
   AIDP in its clinical features except that it has a relapsing remitting or progressive
   course lasting at least 2 months. Many patients do not recover fully.
   1. Some patients have **primarily motor dysfunction** with evidence of multifocal
   conduction block on electrophysiologic study. This entity, which is a demyelinating neuropathy, resembles motor neuron disease and sometimes has elevated
   antibody titers to gangliosides. The treatment with cyclophosphamide has
   improved some patients.
   2. There are several **diseases associated with a syndrome similar to CIDP.**
   Human immunodeficiency virus (HIV) infection, systemic lupus erythematosus,
   and plasma cell dyscrasia are only a few. Hereditary demyelinating neuropathies are also a consideration, especially in children.
   3. **Treatment** begins with a specific diagnosis and management of an underlying
   disorder if found. In the idiopathic cases, one can try corticosteroids, plasma
   exchange, and azathioprine. The plan depends on the severity of the disease and
   the availability of experienced plasma exchange technicians.
   a. **Corticosteroids.** Prednisone is started at 100 mg/day; this dosage is continued
   for 2–4 weeks and with improvement is gradually changed to 100 mg every
   other day. The dosage must be maintained for 3–6 months without improvement before steroid failure can be assumed. Most patients with CIDP who
   respond to steroid require maintenance dosages of 5–20 mg every other day
   for life.
   b. **Plasma exchange** (two exchanges per week for 3 weeks) is added to the
   corticosteroid if there is no improvement in the first week or two.
   c. **Azathioprine** (50 mg tid) is used in patients who do not respond to corticosteroids in the first 3–4 weeks and in patients who receive plasma exchange
   as initial treatment. It is also started concurrently with corticosteroids in
   severe progressive cases. Monitor liver function and blood counts.
   d. **Intravenous immunoglobulin treatment** has been effective in patients with
   refractory disease. Its use as the only treatment remains to be studied, but it
   has no serious side effects. The dosage is 0.4 g/kg given in 1000 ml of saline
   IV over 6–8 hours.
E. **Other chronic neuropathies.** The treatment of chronic neuropathy associated with
   a systemic disease begins with control or cure of the underlying disease or condition.

Management of the residual deficit is aimed at keeping patients functional and optimizing their motor and sensory function. Braces and splints help with the distal weakness. Sensory neuropathy interferes with gait subtly, causing a feeling of dizziness, which on questioning is a sense of imbalance, especially when other modalities of sense are also compromised.

1. **Neuropathy associated with deficiency diseases** (see sec. **XVIII.A.2**)
    a. **Alcoholic polyneuropathy** probably results from multiple vitamin deficiencies or from thiamine deficiency. Alcohol by itself is probably not responsible for the neuropathy. Adequate diet supplemented with multivitamins and **thiamine** (50–100 mg PO daily) is the usual method of treatment. Most patients improve in several months, but severe cases may take up to a year to improve.
    b. **Pyridoxine deficiency** occurs in patients treated with isoniazid. It may cause a mild sensorimotor neuropathy and optic neuritis. A preparation of isoniazid–vitamin B_6 combination prevents the neuropathy. Pyridoxine toxicity also causes a sensory neuropathy.
    c. **Folic acid deficiency** may occur with chronic phenytoin administration or in persons with a low folate intake. Folic acid, 1 mg every morning, prevents the neuropathy, but it may make the seizure disorder less responsive to phenytoin.
    d. **Niacin deficiency** by itself probably does not cause peripheral neuropathy, but pellagra patients with peripheral neuropathy have multiple vitamin deficiencies.

2. **Diabetes mellitus**
    a. **Polyneuropathy.** Diabetes mellitus is the most common cause of neuropathy in developed parts of the world. The polyneuropathy associated with diabetes is usually mixed but is often primarily sensory. Pain is common, and both legs and feet are involved.
        (1) Control of hyperglycemia may improve diabetic polyneuropathy. Treatment of the pain is difficult. Physical measures, such as warm compresses, massage, and whirlpool baths, may be temporarily helpful. Also, rest may help, and mild analgesics, such as aspirin, are often used.
        (2) Narcotics are not generally used for neuropathic pain because they are often ineffective and lead to addiction. **Phenytoin,** 300–400 mg daily, may help, but if improvement does not occur in 10–14 days, therapy should be stopped.
    b. **Autonomic neuropathy** is common in diabetes and causes decreased sweating, orthostatic hypertension, nocturnal diarrhea, fecal incontinence, constipation, urinary incontinence or retention, and impotency. Delayed gastric emptying may also occur, causing difficulty in controlling the blood sugar.
        (1) **Orthostatic hypotension** may improve with pressure stockings or mineralocorticoid (**Florinef,** 0.1 mg daily). **Ephedrine** (up to 25 mg tid) is also helpful in some patients.
        (2) Diarrhea may be intermittent and may resolve spontaneously. **Denatured tincture of opium,** 5–10 drops qid, or other antidiarrheals are often helpful.
        (3) When fecal incontinence is a problem, an **enema** each morning cleans the bowel and allows the patient relative safety, using only a pad.
        (4) Treatment of **urinary problems** is discussed in Chap. 14.
    c. **Mononeuritis.** The cranial nerves are frequently involved, particularly the oculomotor nerve. Diabetic oculomotor nerve palsy is usually painful. As a rule there is sparing of the pupil, a sign that helps to distinguish it from a posterior communicating artery aneurysm. Large peripheral nerves may also be involved, causing a pain syndrome. The pain is treated with analgesics, and often narcotics are required. This pain usually subsides spontaneously in a few days, and in the case of third-nerve palsy, the deficit improves in 1–4 months. An eye patch circumvents the diplopia until improvement is complete.

3. **Neuropathy associated with toxic diseases** (see sec. **XVIII.A.3**). Removal from exposure and, when possible, direct removal of the toxin are the treatment for all toxic conditions.

a. Chronic arsenic toxicity causes a painful mixed motor and sensory polyneuropathy.

  (1) The treatment is dimercaprol (BAL) oil suspension. However, dimercaprol is contraindicated in hepatic insufficiency, and acute renal failure may occur during therapy. Alkalinization of the urine helps to prevent breakdown of dimercaprol-metal complexes and protects the kidney. Other side effects are hypertension, nausea, vomiting, and headache. Reduction of dosage reduces the side effects.

  (2) For chronic arsenic poisoning, **dimercaprol**, 2.5 mg/kg, is given qid for 2 days, bid on the third day, and then daily by deep IM injection for 10 days. Dimercaprol therapy is thought to decrease the duration of the illness, but it has no effect on the recovery rate.

b. The sensorimotor neuropathy of **lead intoxication** is treated with ethylenediaminetetraacetic acid (EDTA). EDTA may cause renal failure, and daily urinalysis is indicated during therapy. If hematuria, proteinuria, or epithelial cell casts increase during treatment, the drug should be stopped.

  (1) EDTA is usually given IM, 0.04 g/kg bid. The prognosis depends on the amount of exposure and the degree of impairment. Early treatment results in the best prognosis.

  (2) Penicillamine, 25 mg/kg daily in divided doses, also has been used to remove lead from the body in chronic intoxication.

c. Mercury intoxication neuropathy is predominantly a motor disorder. It can also be treated with dimercaprol, but it is usually treated with **EDTA** (Calcium Disodium Versenate). Mercury poisoning causes dementia, which may not be reversible.

4. Neuropathy associated with drugs (see sec. **XVIII.A.4**)

a. Nitrofurantoin (Furadantin), 400 mg daily for 2 weeks, has produced decreased conduction velocities in all patients tested. The polyneuropathy is primarily sensory at the onset, with pain and paresthesias. However, the polyneuropathy is reversible when the drug is stopped.

b. Vincristine is consistently associated with peripheral polyneuropathy, and the neurotoxicity is the dose-limiting factor. Absent Achilles tendon reflex is the earliest sign that accompanies paresthesias in the fingers and toes. However, the cranial nerves may also be affected. The neuropathy usually improves within several months after the drug is stopped.

c. Phenytoin is occasionally associated with a mild polyneuropathy, which is thought to be related to folate deficiency.

d. Isoniazid causes vitamin B_6 (pyridoxine) deficiency with polyneuropathy.

5. Entrapment neuropathy

a. The carpal tunnel syndrome is the most common entrapment. It is the result of compression of the median nerve by the volar ligament.

  (1) Description. Pain and tingling in the hand are the usual early signs, and retrograde distribution of the pain may cause arm and shoulder pain in some patients. There may be no objective neurologic signs, and nerve conduction studies may be normal, but usually median nerve conduction is slowed across the wrist. Often, the earliest objective sign is failure to appreciate textures. Later, clear deficits of sensation with muscle wasting occur in the distribution of the median nerve.

  (2) Associated disease. A variety of diseases are associated with carpal tunnel syndrome (see sec. **XVIII.A.1**). Thus, before surgery is undertaken, underlying diseases that are treatable should be controlled.

  (3) Treatment

   (a) The treatment is usually **surgical release** at the site of entrapment.

   (b) When the symptoms are mild and there are no objective signs of nerve damage, conservative measures may be enough. For example, **splinting the wrist** at night may relieve carpal tunnel symptoms, especially in the transient syndrome seen in pregnancy.

   (c) Injection of corticosteroid into the volar ligament may relieve the symptoms temporarily. In some cases, remission may last for several years. If nerve conduction is slow, however, surgery is usually required.

b. **Pronator syndrome.** The median nerve may also be entrapped as it passes into the forearm between the two heads of the pronator teres muscle. Pain is reported in front of the elbow and at the wrist. Also, weakness in apposition of the thumb and hypesthesia on the radial side of the index finger have been reported. However, this condition is rare. Treatment is surgical release.

c. The **ulnar nerve** may be entrapped at the wrist or in the palm, but most commonly entrapment occurs at the elbow. Paresthesia of the fourth and fifth fingers is a common symptom. Weakness of the hand with atrophy of the first interosseous muscle and the hypothenar eminence is less common, and weakness of abduction of the fifth finger may be the only sign. When entrapment is at the elbow, therapy is surgical transposition of the nerve anteriorly.

d. The **radial nerve** is entrapped very rarely, and most isolated radial palsies are caused by direct trauma.

   (1) **Description.** Weakness of finger extension without weakness of wrist extension has been attributed to entrapment of the radial nerve at the level of the supinator muscle. The extensor carpi ulnaris is weak, but the extensor carpi radialis is normal, so weakness of finger extension occurs with radial deviation of the hand. Sparing of the extensor carpi radialis occurs because the branch of the radial nerve to the carpi radialis leaves proximal to the entrapment point.

   (2) The **onset** of entrapment is slow as opposed to the sudden onset seen in the common traumatic palsies.

   (3) **Treatment** is surgical release, but splints and physical therapy constitute the only therapy for traumatic lesions. Most patients with traumatic radial palsy recover in several months.

e. The lateral cutaneous nerve of the thigh may be entrapped between the two folds of the inguinal ligament. The syndrome produced is known as **meralgia paresthetica,** which is characterized by paresthesia, pain, or numbness in the lateral part of the thigh. There may be objective signs of decreased sensation in the region of numbness.

   (1) The **etiology** varies, but trauma, use of a corset or truss, and other external mechanical compressions around the waist have been implicated. Intrapelvic tumor and acute abdominal enlargement from ascites or pregnancy have also been implicated.

   (2) **Treatment** is unnecessary if there is no pain. Evaluation for a definite etiology must be done, and if pain is severe, injection of local anesthetic into the nerve at the anterior iliac spine may help. Resection of the nerve is rarely necessary.

f. The **posterior tibial** nerve may be entrapped under the flexor retinaculum, behind and inferior to the medial malleolus at the "tarsal tunnel." The patient complains of pain or numbness in the sole of the foot; walking and standing increase the pain. A tender tibial nerve may be found behind the medial malleolus, and dorsal extension and pronation of the foot may provoke pain. The syndrome is rare, but it may occur following previous trauma. Treatment is surgical release.

6. **Leprosy**

a. **Description.** In underdeveloped parts of the world, leprosy is a common cause of neuropathy. *Mycobacterium leprae,* an acid-fast rod, causes a predominantly sensory neuropathy.

   (1) **Lepromatous leprosy** is extensive, diffuse, and symmetric, involving skin and peripheral nerves.

   (2) **Tuberculoid leprosy** is less extensive, with fewer skin lesions that are sharply demarcated, but the neurologic involvement is more severe. The nerves are often enlarged.

b. **Treatment.** Free treatment and hospitalization are available at the United States Public Health hospitals at San Francisco, California; Carville, Louisiana; or Staten Island, New York. Most cases require less than 2 months of hospitalization.

(1) The drug of choice is **dapsone**, 50–100 mg PO daily for adults and 1 mg/kg for children. When there is no clinical evidence of activity and no acid-fast rods are seen on skin smears, treatment is continued for 18 months in tuberculoid leprosy and for 10 years in lepromatous leprosy. Patients who have features of both types are treated for lepromatous leprosy. Note that dapsone, by itself, may cause polyneuropathy.

(2) **Rifampin** is a more effective agent and is used in many parts of the world. However, it has not been released for use in leprosy by the Food and Drug Administration. Patients who relapse on dapsone alone are often given rifampin in addition.

(3) **Reactional states.** During therapy, tender inflamed subcutaneous nodules (erythema nodosum leprosum) may appear acutely. These nodules appear in groups and last 1 week or longer, and new groups occur as the older ones regress. Fever, myalgia, and other systemic symptoms also occur with these nodules. Treatment is with analgesics and antipyretics. Corticosteroids may be needed in some severe cases, and dapsone is continued.

(4) **Treatment of household contacts.** Dapsone, 50 mg twice weekly or 25 mg daily for 2–3 years, is recommended for close contacts.

7. Plasma cell dysplasia may be associated with a severe progressive sensory and/or motor neuropathy. The detection of a monoclonal spike on the serum protein electrophoresis of a patient with a neuropathy may lead to the diagnosis of multiple myeloma, amyloidosis, Waldenström's macroglobulinemia, cryoglobulinemia, lymphoma, or, most commonly, monoclonal gammopathy of undetermined significance (MGUS). In some patients with osteosclerotic myeloma, a characteristic syndrome of polyneuropathy, organomegaly, endocrinopathy, monoclonal gammopathy, and skin changes (POEMS) occurs. Even when the underlying disease cannot be treated (e.g., MGUS) the neuropathy may improve with plasma exchange or intravenous immunoglobulin.

F. Neuropathy in HIV infection. About 15% of patients with AIDS develop a distal symmetric axonal neuropathy. There is often pain and sensory loss in the feet. There is no response to immunotherapy, but the pain sometimes responds to carbamazepine, tricyclics, and nonnarcotic analgesics. HIV patients also have mononeuritis multiplex caused by nerve infarction. Treatment with antivirals (zidovudine, didanosine, dideoxycytidine) also causes axonal neuropathy. AIDP and CIDP in HIV infection often have a CSF pleocytosis greater than in idiopathic cases.

G. Idiopathic facial palsy (Bell's palsy)

1. Description. Acute idiopathic facial palsy is a mononeuropathy of the seventh cranial nerve.

a. Isolated unilateral facial weakness is the most common feature, but pain, hyperacusis, and ageusia may occur in some cases. In about 70% of patients the deficits improve completely, in 13% there is minimal deficit, and in 16% there is significant facial weakness.

b. In 85% of untreated patients who improve, the initial change appears within 3 weeks. The other 15% show signs of improvement within 3–6 months.

c. Patients older than 60 years of age, those with a complete lesion, and those with hypertension and diabetes mellitus are at risk of not recovering completely. When the EMG shows signs of denervation, the prognosis for complete recovery is worse.

2. Treatment. Corticosteroid therapy is recommended. Since most patients recover without treatment, however, there is some controversy about the necessity for therapy. **Prednisone**, 60 mg PO every morning for 5 days, then reduced gradually over 10–14 days, is standard and usually safe treatment. Evidence shows that the recovery time is shorter when steroids are used. If used, corticosteroids should be started as soon after the onset as possible, since the suspected effect of the drug is reduction of facial nerve edema.

3. Complications. Facial spasm is occasionally a late complication of Bell's palsy, and it is often refractory to medical treatment. Anxiety usually makes the twitches worse, and mild sedatives may help relieve them (**diazepam,** 5–10 mg qid, or **phenobarbital,** 30–60 mg tid). **Phenytoin** is occasionally helpful (300 mg PO every morning), but if no effect is seen in 10–14 days, the drug should be stopped.

H. Restless legs syndrome

1. **Description.** The restless legs syndrome is a rare condition in which an unpleasant creeping sensation occurs deep in the legs (and occasionally in the arms). The problem occurs when the patient is at rest, so it interferes with sleep. The person is compelled to move the legs around to avoid the unpleasant feeling. The calf and pretibial areas are the usual sites of discomfort, and it is often bilateral. It may be intermittent, lasting several minutes or hours, and there is no pain. The cause of the syndrome is unknown, but it has been associated with iron deficiency anemia, cancer, and pregnancy. It is found in some families as an autosomal dominant trait.

2. **Treatment**
   a. The underlying condition is treated.
   b. Clonazepam, 0.5 mg tid.
   c. Diazepam, 20–40 mg/day, helps occasionally.
   d. Carbamazepine, 200 mg tid.
   e. Clonidine, 0.1 mg tid.
   f. Sinemet, 10/100 mg tid.
   g. Bromocriptine, 2.5 mg tid.

XIX. Motor system disease

A. Description. Neuronal degeneration confined to the anterior horn cell and motor neurons in the cerebral cortex is called motor system disease. The course of motor system disease varies, depending on the age of the patient and the parts of the motor system that are involved. There are several distinct forms of motor system disease.

1. **Amyotrophic lateral sclerosis (ALS)** is the most common form of motor system disease. Its etiology is unknown, but it is easily recognized by atrophy, weakness, spasticity (from degeneration of upper motor neurons), and absolute lack of sensory signs. It usually occurs sporadically, but occasionally it may be found in families as a dominant trait. The gene for familial ALS codes for superoxide dysmutase (SOD), an important endogenous antioxidant, raising the possibility that oxidative stress may lead to anterior horn cell death in some forms of ALS. Males are affected more than females, and the onset is usually in middle age with rapid progression.

   Before making the diagnosis, treatable disease, such as spinal cord compression, must be sought. Myelography is necessary unless clear involvement of spinal and brainstem nuclei indicates a diffuse localization. Abdominal reflexes and bladder function are usually normal. The degenerative process may be localized only in the brainstem, in which case it is called **progressive bulbar palsy.** In Guam and the Kii Peninsula of Japan, an exceptionally high incidence of ALS has been reported.

2. **Progressive muscular atrophy** resembles ALS, but without involvement of the upper motor neurons. Tendon reflexes are almost always absent, although spinal cord and brainstem neurons may be involved. This is a very rare form of motor system disease, with an earlier onset and slower progression than ALS. Some forms of progressive muscular atrophy are hereditary, either as dominant or recessive traits. There is an infantile form, **Werdnig-Hoffman disease,** which is manifested as a "floppy infant." A juvenile variety with proximal distribution is called **Kugelberg-Welander disease.**

3. **Primary lateral sclerosis** is an extremely rare form of motor neuron disease, in which the spinal motor neurons are spared but the upper motor neurons degenerate, resulting in spasticity. The pathology of this disease is not fully known. The progression is slow, and it is usually not fatal. The disorder may be found in families, and the patient's kin may demonstrate other degenerative disorders.

4. **Multifocal motor neuropathy with conduction block** is an immune-mediated motor neuropathy that may mimic motor neuron diseases. Some patients have

demonstratable antibodies against gangliosides (e.g., anti-GM1 or anti-asialo-GM1), but the diagnosis depends on finding conduction block on nerve conduction studies. This disorder is important to recognize because it is treatable with intravenous immunoglobulin in 0.4 g/kg given in 1000 ml of saline over 6–8 hours, every 6–12 weeks.

B. Prognosis. Patients who have motor system disease with only spinal involvement usually die within 3–5 years. Those who have bulbar involvement (alone or with spinal disease) usually die within 2.5 years. Occasionally, the progression of this form of the disorder seems to slow down; some patients are reported to have lived 10–15 years with the spinal form of the disease. Thus, these cases may be cited when discussing the prognosis of the illness with patients and their family.

Physical disability is usually complete earlier in bulbar cases (several months) than in spinal cases (up to 4 years). However, progressive muscular atrophy and primary lateral sclerosis, as they progress, often develop into the complete syndrome of ALS. Patients with the juvenile form of progressive muscular atrophy (Kugelberg-Welander disease) may live for 20–40 years after diagnosis.

C. Treatment

  1. Emotional

    a. The psychological management of any terminal illness must be individualized. The general approach described for ALS can be modified to be of use in other terminal illnesses as well. When the mind is spared and patients can feel that they are becoming more disabled from one visit to another, there is a particularly severe sense of helplessness. Thus, frequently physicians will tend to avoid these patients and appear only during catastrophe, when certain tangible action can help. However, the management of ALS requires more availability and more support on the part of physicians than diseases that are directly treatable.

    b. When patients realize the severity of the illness, a massive reorganization of their life must be undertaken. Also, once they realize that death is inevitable, a variety of reactions will occur. For example, patients may become depressed, with a sense of uselessness and hopelessness, and increased dependence on the family and physician may follow. Self-pity and low self-esteem may also contribute to the depression. The physician can help in these situations by being appropriately available and by serving as a listener for patients to express their feelings. At times, antidepressant medication (amitriptyline hydrochloride [Elavil], 100–300 mg at bedtime) is useful, but it should not be used as a substitute for the doctor-patient relationship.

    Some patients react with denial of depression and present a front of pseudogaiety. In this case the physician can help by being receptive to the patient's underlying fears and anxieties and by not participating in the process of denial.

    c. Initial denial gives way to feelings related to job, family, religion, finances, self-esteem, physical incapacity, and emotional vulnerability. Dying patients have fear of pain and abandonment, as well as anxiety about desertion of their family and concern about other responsibilities. These are subjects about which patients may wish to talk with the physician. A psychiatric consultant or social worker may be needed if the neurologist is unable to provide enough time.

    d. In general, the physician should avoid offhand reassurances and superficial denial of the illness. It does not help to commiserate with patients, to grieve with them, or to provide false hopes. Instead, the physician should represent a warm, compassionate personal force, who is willing to help the patient.

    Patients should be included in all major discussions and decisions regarding the illness, and they are encouraged to remain as active as possible. Also, members of the patient's family need support and accurate information to allow them to adjust to the change in their lives with more ease.

    e. Patients with chronic progressive illness leave many questions unasked. The physician should provide opportunities for patients to acquire the knowledge they want and at the rate at which it is needed. It is best to tell the truth about the prognosis. Many answers need to be repeated and expanded as the illness progresses. Predicting the time of death is not possible and should be avoided, but patients should be advised to arrange their affairs "just in case." When direct questions about death are asked, pleading ignorance is not sufficient. Turn the question back to the patients and allow them to express their feelings about the condition.

   f. There is often a point in a chronic illness at which patients become angry. The anger may be directed at the family, physician, or hospital. The physician must allow patients to express this hostility and refrain from counterattack, thus maintaining the therapeutic alliance. The family and hospital staff must also be aware of the process behind the patient's anger.

2. Medical therapy. There is no medication that alters the course of motor system disease. Guanidine and snake venom are not used at present because they have not been effective in past trials. However, a number of treatment trials using neurotrophic factors (e.g., ciliary neurotrophic factor [CNTF], brain derived neurotrophic factor [BDNF]), glutamate receptor blockers (e.g., dextamorphan), or superoxide dismutase inhibitors are underway. In addition to their scientific benefit, participation in a drug trial may act as a sign to patients that an attempt is being made to help them. Early in treatment a tangible sign of help is useful to keep patients in the supportive program.

3. Treatment of weakness

   a. The treatment of weakness in ALS is purely mechanical. For example, a neck brace may help when neck muscles are too weak to hold the head up, and wrist splints occasionally improve grip in patients with weakness of wrist extension.

   b. Motorized and mechanical appliances (wheelchair, lifts, hospital beds) help to maintain maximal independence.

   c. Bracing is usually not done to preserve gait in ALS. However, in cases of juvenile motor neuron disease (Kugelberg-Welander disease), bracing may be indicated, since the progression is very slow.

   d. Physical therapy helps to minimize disuse atrophy and prevent contractures. Fatigue should be avoided, and strength should be used for necessary activities of daily living rather than in useless attempts to "build up" the muscles.

   e. Muscle cramps are common and may be prevented with **phenytoin,** 300 mg daily, or **diazepam,** 2–10 mg tid. Warmth and massage are helpful in releasing the cramps.

4. Most patients with motor system disease can be treated at home during most of their illness, with help from a visiting nurses association or other community agencies. It is expensive to keep these patients in acute care facilities. However, if the family is not able to manage the patient, placement in a chronic care facility for terminal care is necessary.

5. In following patients with motor system disease, body weight, ability to cough, vital capacity, and swallowing ability are evaluated to measure change and to anticipate problems.

6. Suicide is uncommon in these patients, perhaps because the weakness caused by the disorder renders them incapable of performing the act.

Selected Readings

GENERAL

Dalakas, M. Pharmacologic concerns of corticosteroids in the treatment of patients with immune-related neuromuscular diseases. *Neurol. Clin.* 8(1):93, 1990.

Kurtz, L. A., and Scull, S. A. Rehabilitation for developmental disabilities. *Pediatr. Clin. North Am.* 40(3):629, 1993.

McCabe, E. R. Genetic screening for the next decade: Application of present and new technologies. *Yale J. Biol. Med.* 64(1):9, 1991.

McGee, S. R. Muscle cramps. *Arch. Intern. Med.* 150(3):511, 1990.

Newsom-Davis, J., and Mills, K. R. Immunological associations of acquired neuromyotonia (Isaacs' syndrome): Report of five cases and literature review. *Brain* 116(Pt 2):453, 1993.

O'Donohue, W. J., et al. Respiratory failure in neuromuscular disease: Management in a respiratory intensive care unit. *J.A.M.A.* 235:733, 1976.

MUSCULAR DYSTROPHIES

Bieber, F. R., Hoffman, E. P., and Amos, J. A. Dystrophin analysis in Duchenne muscular dystrophy: Use in fetal diagnosis and in genetic counseling. *Am. J. Hum. Genet.* 45:362, 1989.

Fenichel, G. M., et al. Long term benefit from prednisone therapy in Duchenne muscular dystrophy. *Neurology* 41:1874, 1991.

Hardiman, O., et al. Neuropathic findings in oculopharyngeal muscular dystrophy: A report of seven cases and a review of the literature. *Arch. Neurol.* 50(5):481, 1993.

Harris, S. E., and Cherry, D. B. Childhood progressive muscular dystrophy and the role of physical therapy. *Phys. Ther.* 54:4, 1974.

Hook, R., Anderson, E. F., and Noto, P. Anesthetic management of a parturient with myotonia atrophica. *Anesthesiology* 43:689, 1975.

Iannaccone, S. T. Current status of Duchenne muscular dystrophy. *Pediatr. Clin. North Am.* 39(4):879, 1992.

Love, D. R., et al. Dystrophin and dystrophin-related proteins: A review of protein and RNA studies. *Neuromuscul. Disord.* 3(1):5, 1993.

Miller, G., and Wessel, H. B. Diagnosis of dystrophinopathies: Review for the clinician. *Pediatr. Neurol.* 9(1):3, 1993.

Sarnat, H. B., O'Connor, T., and Byrne, P. A. Clinical effects of myotonic dystrophy on pregnancy and the neonate. *Arch. Neurol.* 33:459, 1976.

Wessel, H. B. Dystrophin: A clinical perspective. *Pediatr. Neurol.* 6(1):3, 1990.

Zellweger, M. D., and Ionasecu, V. Myotonic dystrophy and its differential diagnosis. *Acta Neurol. Scand.* (Suppl. 55) 49:1, 1973.

POLYMYOSITIS

Barwick, D. D., and Walton, J. N. Polymyositis. *Am. J. Med.* 35:646, 1963.

Bromberg, M. B. The role of electrodiagnostic studies in the diagnosis and management of polymyositis. *Compr. Ther.* 18(4):17, 1992.

Bunch, T. W. Polymyositis: A case history approach to the differential diagnosis and treatment. *Mayo Clin. Proc.* 65(11):1480, 1990.

Bunch, T. W., et al. Azathioprine with prednisone for polymyositis: A controlled clinical trial. *Ann. Intern. Med.* 92:365, 1980.

Chwalinska-Sadowska, H., Maldykowa, H., and Madykowa, H. Polymyositis-dermatomyositis: 25 years of follow-up of 50 patients' disease course, treatment, prognostic factors. *Mater. Med. Pol.* 22(3):213, 1990.

Dalakas, M. C. Clinical, immunopathologic, and therapeutic considerations of inflammatory myopathies. *Clin. Neuropharmacol.* 15(5):327, 1992.

Devere, R., and Bradley, W. G., Polymyositis: Its presentation, morbidity, and mortality. *Brain* 98:637, 1975.

Targoff, I. N. Autoantibodies in polymyositis. *Rheum. Dis. Clin. North Am.* 18(2):455, 1992.

Walton, J. The inflammatory myopathies. *J. R. Soc. Med.* 76:998, 1983.

Winkleman, R. K., Mulder, D. W., and Lambert, E. H. Course of dermatomyositis-polymyositis: Comparison of untreated and cortisone-treated patients. *Mayo Clin. Proc.* 43:545, 1968.

PERIODIC PARALYSIS

Griggs, R. C., and Ptacek, L. J. The periodic paralyses. *Hosp. Pract.* (Off. Ed.) 27(11):123, 1992.

Gutmann, L., and Phillips, L. H. Myotonia congenita. *Semin. Neurol.* 11(3):244, 1991.

Resnick, J. S. Episodic muscle weakness. *Clin. Orthop.* 39:63, 1965.

Stedwell, R. E., Allen, K. M., and Binker, L. S. Hypokalemic paralyses: A review of the etiologies, pathophysiology, presentation, and therapy. *Am. J. Emerg. Med.* 10(2):143, 1992.

Vroom, F. O., Jarrell, X. X., and Maren, T. H. Acetazolamide treatment of hypokalemic periodic paralysis. *Arch. Neurol.* 32:385, 1975.

MYASTHENIA GRAVIS

Cooper, J. D. Current therapy for thymoma. *Chest* 103 (Suppl. 4):334S, 1993.

Dau, P. C., and Denys, E. H. Plasmapheresis and immunosuppressive drug therapy in the Eaton-Lambert syndrome. *Ann. Neurol.* 11:570, 1982.

Genkins, G., et al. Clinical experience in more than 2000 patients with myasthenia gravis. *Ann. N.Y. Acad. Sci.* 505:500, 1987.

Grob, D., et al. The course of myasthenia gravis and therapies affecting outcome. *Ann. N.Y. Acad. Sci.* 505:472, 1987.

Janssen, R. S., et al. Radiologic evaluation of the mediastinum in myasthenia gravis. *Neurology* 33:534, 1983.

Kelly, J. J., et al. The laboratory diagnosis of mild myasthenia gravis. *Ann. Neurol.* 12:238, 1982.

Kornfeld, P., et al. Plasmapheresis in refractory generalized myasthenia gravis. *Arch. Neurol.* 38:478, 1981.

Kuks, J. B., Djojoatmodjo, S., and Oosterhuis, H. J. Azathioprine in myasthenia gravis: Observations in 41 patients and a review of literature. *Neuromuscul. Disord.* 1(6):423, 1991.

Mann, J. D., Johns, T. R., and Campa, J. F. Long term administration of corticosteroids in myasthenia gravis. *Neurology* (Minneapolis) 26:729, 1976.

Mathew, P., Cuschieri, R. J., and Tankel, H. I. Outcome after thymectomy for myasthenia gravis: A retrospective review. *Scott. Med. J.* 37(4):103, 1992.

Mulder, D. G., et al. Thymectomy for myasthenia gravis. *Am. J. Surg.* 146:61, 1983.

Osserman, K. E., and Genkins, G. Critical reappraisal of the use of edrophonium chloride tests in myasthenia gravis and significance of clinical classification. *Ann. N.Y. Acad. Sci.* 135:312, 1966.

Pascuzzi, R. M., Coslett, H. B., and Johns, T. R. Long-term corticosteroid treatment of myasthenia gravis: Report of 116 patients. *Ann. Neurol.* 15:291, 1984.

Plauche, W. C. Myasthenia gravis in mothers and their newborns. *Clin. Obstet. Gynecol.* 34(1):82, 1991.

Roy, T. M., Walker, J. F., and Farrow, J. R. Respiratory failure associated with myasthenia gravis. *J. Ky. Med. Assoc.* 89(4):169, 1991.

Seybold, M. E., and Drachman, D. B. Gradually increasing dose of prednisone in myasthenia gravis. *N. Engl. J. Med.* 290:81, 1974.

Shah, A., and Lisak, R. P. Immunopharmacologic therapy in myasthenia gravis. *Clin. Neuropharmacol.* 16(2):97, 1993.

LAMBERT-EATON MYASTHENIC SYNDROME

McEvoy, K. M., et al. 3,4-Diaminopyridine in the treatment of Lambert-Eaton myasthenic syndrome. *N. Engl. J. Med.* 321:1567, 1989.

Pascuzzi, R. M., and Kim, Y. I. Lambert-Eaton syndrome. *Semin. Neurol.* 10(1):35, 1990.

TETANUS AND BOTULISM

Blake, P. A., Feldman, R. A., and Buchanan, T. M. Serologic therapy of tetanus in the United States, 1965–1971. *J.A.M.A.* 235:42, 1976.

Bleck, T. P. Tetanus: Pathophysiology, management, and prophylaxis. D. M. 37(9):545, 1991.

Dowell, V. R., Jr. Botulism and tetanus: Selected epidemiologic and microbiologic aspects. *Rev. Infect. Dis.* (Suppl. 1):S202, 1984.

Hambleton, P. *Clostridium botulinum* toxins: A general review of involvement in disease, structure, mode of action and preparation for clinical use. *J. Neurol.* 239(1):16, 1992.

Richardson, J. P. and Knight, A. L. The prevention of tetanus in the elderly. *Arch. Intern. Med.* 151(9):1712, 1991.

Schreiner, M. S., Field, E., and Ruddy, R. Infant botulism: A review of 12 years' experience at the Children's Hospital of Philadelphia. *Pediatrics* 87(2):159, 1991.

Sutton, D. N., et al. Management of autonomic dysfunction in severe tetanus: The use of magnesium sulphate and clonidine. *Intens. Care Med.* 16(2):75, 1990.

MALIGNANT HYPERTHERMIA AND NEUROLEPTIC MALIGNANT SYNDROME

Dantrolene for malignant hyperthermia during anesthesia. *Med. Lett. Drugs Ther.* 22:61, 1980.

Gronert, G. A. Malignant hyperthermia. *Anesthesiology* 5:395, 1980.

Morris, H., III, McCormick, W. F., and Reinarz, J. A. Neuroleptic malignant syndrome. *Arch. Neurol.* 37:362, 1980.

Wedel, D. J. Malignant hyperthermia and neuromuscular disease. *Neuromuscul. Disord.* 2(3):157, 1992.

FACIAL PARALYSIS

Adour, K. K., Medical management of idiopathic (Bell's) palsy. *Otolaryngol. Clin. North Am.* 24(3):663, 1991.

Adour, K. K., and Wingerd, J. Idiopathic facial paralysis (Bell's palsy): Factors affecting severity and outcome in 446 patients. *Neurology* (Minneapolis) 44:1112, 1974.

Collin, J. R., and Leatherbarrow, B. Ophthalmic management of seventh nerve palsy. *Aust. N. Z. J. Ophthalmol.* 18(3):267, 1990.

Murr, A. H., and Benecke, J. E., Jr. Association of facial paralysis with HIV positivity. *Am. J. Otol.* 12(6):450, 1991.

Peitersen, E. The natural history of Bell's palsy. *Am. J. Otol.* 4:107, 1982.

NEUROPATHY

Bosch, E. P., and Smith, B. E. Peripheral neuropathies associated with monoclonal proteins. *Med. Clin. North Am.* 77(1):125, 1993.

Dyck, P. J., et. al. Plasma exchange in polyneuropathy associated with monoclonal gammopathy of undetermined significance. *N. Engl. J. Med.* 325(21): 1482, 1991.

Gracey, D. R., et al. Respiratory failure in Guillain-Barré syndrome: A six-year experience. *Mayo Clin. Proc.* 57:742, 1982.

The Guillain-Barré Syndrome Study Group. Plasmapheresis and acute Guillain-Barré syndrome. *Neurology* 35:1096, 1985.

Jenkins, D., et al. Leprotic involvement of peripheral nerves in the absence of skin lesions: Case report and literature review. *J. Am. Acad. Dermatol.* 23 (5, Pt 2):1023, 1990.

Leneman, F. The Guillain-Barré syndrome: Definition, etiology, and review of 1100 cases. *Arch. Intern. Med.* 118:139, 1966.

Levinson, A. I. The use of IVIG in neurological disease. *Clin. Rev. Allergy* 10(1–2):119, 1992.

Mollman, J. E. Neuromuscular toxicity of therapy. *Curr. Opin. Oncol.* 4(3):540, 1992.

Pleasure, D. E., Lovelace, R. E., and Duvoisin, R. C. The prognosis of acute polyradiculoneuritis. *Neurology* (Minneapolis) 18:1143, 1968.

Shevell, M., et al. Congenital inflammatory myopathy. *Neurology* 40(7):1111, 1990.

Simpson, D. M., and Olney, R. K. Peripheral neuropathies associated with human immunodeficiency virus infection. *Neurol. Clin.* 10(3):685, 1992.

Soueidan, S. A., and Dalakas, M. C. Treatment of autoimmune neuromuscular diseases with high-dose intravenous immune globulin. *Pediatr. Res.* 33(Suppl. 1):S95, 1993.

Van der Meché, F. G. A., Schmitz, P. I. M., and the Dutch–Guillain-Barré Study Group. A randomized trial comparing intravenous immune globulin and plasma exchange in Guillain-Barré syndrome. *N. Engl. J. Med.* 326(17): 1123, 1992.

Yu, R. K., et al. Autoimmune mechanisms in peripheral neuropathies. *Ann. Neurol.* 27(Suppl.):S30, 1990.

MOTOR SYSTEM DISEASE

Agre, J. C., Rodriguez, A. A., and Tafel, J. A. Late effects of polio: Critical review of the literature on neuromuscular function. *Arch. Phys. Med. Rehabil.* 72(11):923, 1991.

Mackay, R. P. Course and prognosis in amyotrophic lateral sclerosis. *Arch. Neurol.* 8:117, 1963.

Parry, G. J., and Sumner, A. J. Multifocal motor neuropathy. *Neurol. Clin.* 10(3):671, 1992.

Smith, R. A., and Norris, F. H. Symptomatic care of patients with amyotrophic lateral sclerosis. *J.A.M.A.* 234:715, 1975.

Williams, D. B. Motor neuron disease (amyotrophic lateral sclerosis). *Mayo Clin. Proc.* 66:54, 1991.

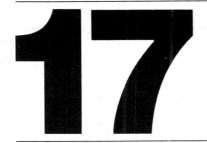

Problems Associated with Chronic Neurologic Disease

Thomas M. Walshe III and
Howard D. Weiss

Chronic neurologic disease may be stable or progressive. In mild stable cases, almost normal existence is possible with proper bracing or other rehabilitation. However, in disorders that cause severe deficits, management is aimed at maximizing the remaining function.

In progressive disorders, the treatment is adjusted to the tempo and severity of the illness. For example, malignant brain tumor or amyotrophic lateral sclerosis (ALS) becomes fatal rapidly, but an understanding of the prognosis and care of the symptoms provides a real benefit to patients and their family. The following sections describe the management of the ancillary problems seen in disabled neurologic patients. The guidelines discussed can be applied with slight modification regardless of the underlying neurologic process.

I. **Treatment of dysphagia.** Weakness, spasticity, or both of the pharynx and tongue cause dysphagia and a lethal tendency to aspirate secretions and foods.

A. Early use of a feeding tube, either through a **gastrostomy, cervical esophagostomy,** or **jejunostomy** is required. Nasogastric tubes can be used temporarily for feeding, but they are uncomfortable, cause pressure necrosis of the nares, and allow aspiration. If a nasogastric tube is used, the smallest possible diameter is best; the soft rubber pediatric tubes are large enough even for adults. The cervical esophagostomy may be useful in dysphagic patients who are ambulatory, since the tube can be inserted during feedings and the ostium can be covered with a dressing at other times. Patients with severe weakness are usually unable to feed themselves, so gastrostomy is the method of choice. However, multiple abdominal procedures, especially gastric operations, make gastrostomy more dangerous than cervical esophagostomy.

B. **Care of a gastrostomy** is simple: 10–14 days after the tube is inserted, a well-defined fistula is established, and the tube can be changed easily. A 22F or 24F Foley catheter or special gastrostomy tube may be used.

C. **Tube feedings** with commercial products (e.g., Sustacal or Sustagen) are calculated to deliver the desired amount of calories each day.

1. The caloric need is higher for active patients and ranges from 1200–2400 kcal/day. The liquid foods are usually concentrated to deliver 1 kcal/ml. If they cause diarrhea, they may need to be diluted. To avoid clogging of the tube, each feeding is followed with water.

2. Tube feeding is best started with about one-half the total desired calories diluted in water. A gradual increase in concentration (and calories) averts diarrhea and malabsorption. Before administering a feeding, the tube is aspirated to ensure that the previous feeding was absorbed. Small volumes are given at first at frequent intervals (q1–2h). The maximum volume given is about 200 ml (150 ml of food followed by 50 ml of water).

3. Large volumes may cause vomiting and aspiration, although larger individuals may require more volume. If the patient needs more water, small volumes may be given between feedings. Also, blended food mixed with milk or water may provide more bulk and prevent the feeling of hunger in patients with a gastrostomy. Some patients do best with continuous feeding at 60–70 ml/hour.

D. If **aspiration of saliva and nasal secretions** is a problem, a cuffed endotracheal tube is necessary. Anticholinergic drugs or tricyclic antidepressants may reduce salivation and prevent drooling, and in some cases the patient may be able to swallow th reduced volume of secretions safely. **Ligation** of the trachea above the tracheostom may be necessary to prevent chronic aspiration of secretions and food.

  E. The decision to undertake palliative surgery such as gastrostomy and tracheostom depends on the **general level of function** of the patient. Patients with progressiv illnesses are often not treated with tracheostomy late in the illness, when respira tory failure threatens. Patients with stable illnesses of brainstem or spinal cor often benefit from it.

II. Bladder dysfunction. Spinal cord trauma is the most common cause of sever

neurogenic bladder dysfunction, but other spinal cord conditions—such as multipl sclerosis, spinal cord tumor, ruptured disk, and tabes dorsalis—produce problems witl micturition. In addition, disorders of **peripheral nerves,** such as diabetes mellitus an herpes zoster, may cause hyporeflexive bladder. Neurologic disease affecting highe centers, such as Parkinson's disease, frontal lobe tumors, and cerebrovascular disease may also cause abnormal micturition. In each incidence, a cystometrogram is necessary to define the type of bladder dysfunction so that appropriate therapy can be attempted Early urologic consultation together with a cystometrogram is needed to defin structural abnormalities.

  A. Normal bladder function. The anatomy and physiology of the bladder are arrangec to allow storage of urine until it can be conveniently excreted.

  1. The majority of the detrusor muscle derives its **innervation** via parasympatheti fibers (S2–S4). The area of the trigone, however, is innervated by sympathetic fibers (T11–L2). (Ascending fibers provide appropriate feedback control.)

  a. Both somatic sensory fibers and parasympathetic ascending fibers leave the bladder to converge at the S2–S4 levels. There are also some ascending sympathetic fibers that synapse at the T9–L2 levels. The lateral spinotha lamic tracts and the fasciculus gracilis carry the ascending fibers to higher centers.

  b. The corticospinal tracts carry motor fibers to the external sphincter and pelvic floor muscles, which are under voluntary control. The primitive micturition reflex is at the S2–S4 level via parasympathetic efferent fibers.

  2. To maintain **continence of urine,** the urethral pressure must be higher than the vesical pressure. The muscles of the urogenital diaphragm and urethra may be flaccid or spastic. If they are flaccid there is little outflow obstruction, and incontinence is common even with low bladder pressure. If these muscles of the urogenital diaphragm and urethra are spastic, high bladder pressure is necessary to empty the bladder to avoid ureteral reflux and high volumes of residual urine. Optimal function requires a balance between the bladder and the urogenital musculature. In neurologic disease, the balance among urethral pressure at the bladder neck, external sphincter and pelvic muscle tension, and detrusor pressure is disturbed, which can cause incomplete or unexpected voiding.

  3. Micturition is the result of reflex and voluntary activity. In the normal bladder, a pressure of 30–40 cm H_2O causes reflex reduction of urethral pressure and consequent micturition. As the bladder fills, wall tension increases but intrave sicular pressure remains constant. At low volumes, a normal person feels the bladder filling, and when it reaches 100–200 ml, the urge to void occurs. Voluntary control of the external sphincter and pelvic floor muscles helps to maintain continence, but there is also reflex inhibition of the detrusor, so pressure is kept constant. In normal persons, the maximum bladder capacity is 400–450 ml, and at this point the detrusor contracts and all the urine is expelled. Initiation of micturition when the bladder is full is caused by reflex mostly. The latency between the decision to void and the initiation of flow is inversely related to the bladder volume.

  B. Goals for management of the neurogenic bladder

  1. Protect the kidneys from hydronephrosis and infection by reducing residual urine and reflux.

  2. Relieve incontinence.

  3. Maintain an acceptable functional capacity so voiding occurs only q4–6h.

  C. Hyperreflexive bladder management (lesions above S2–S4). The hyperreflexive bladder is characterized by many subthreshold, uninhibited detrusor contractions, reduced capacity, and spontaneous voiding with a strong stream. Chronic spinal cord lesions above S2–S4 cause a hyperreflexive bladder in which the patient has no sensation of bladder fullness. In these patients, the bladder empties by reflex action when a critical volume is reached. If the urogenital diaphragm muscles are coordinated with the reflex detrusor contraction, complete spontaneous voiding occurs. However, if the urethral pressure is too high, there is reflux into the ureters; and if the urethral pressure is too low, there is incontinence. In lesions that are higher (i.e., in the cortex, posterior hypothalamus, midbrain, or anterior pons), there may be a sensation of urgency and frequency without dysuria. Dyssynergy between the muscles of the urogenital diaphragm and the detrusor causes incontinence during small reflex contractions. In this case, instillation of ice water into the bladder will produce reflex micturition. Cystitis may cause bladder hyperreflexia because of irritation of nerves, and hyperactivity may occur in obstructive bladder disease, even without neurologic disease.

1. When a patient is incontinent with a hyperreflexic bladder or has an acute spinal cord injury with resolving spinal shock, **intermittent catheterization** is started. To avoid infection, an experienced person (or team) should perform the catheterization in the early stages.
   a. **Volume intake.** The patient is given large volumes of fluid either PO, through a nasogastric tube, or IV, and the bladder is drained q2–4h. High volume intake reduces the risk of infection and calculus formation.
   b. **Bladder training** is begun (see sec. II.C.2), and as the patient begins to void on his or her own (usually by reflex), the frequency of catheterization is reduced until the patient voids by reflex and carries an acceptable residual volume (i.e., < 100 ml). It usually takes less than 90 days for most patients with a complete spinal cord lesion to become catheter-free. Approximately 10–20% fail to improve because of either a very small bladder capacity or excessive bladder hyperreflexia. If intermittent catheterization fails, an indwelling catheter is placed or other methods are used to maintain continence.
   c. **Incomplete spinal cord lesions** have the most rapid and complete return of reflex micturition. Some patients may require chronic intermittent catheterization in addition to reflex voiding.
2. **Bladder training.** Intermittent catheterization prevents excess bladder distention. Bladder training helps to prevent bladder contracture, conditions a regulated reflex pattern, and causes the patient to take notice of bladder function.
   a. **Regular attempts** at initiating the voiding reflex should be made. In patients with a complete sensory level below the waist, the best means of beginning the reflex varies. Squeezing the glans penis, scratching the scrotum, pulling the pubic hair, tapping over the bladder, and (most often successful) deep digital stimulation of the rectum are useful methods.
   b. High **volume intake** keeps the urine dilute and helps prevent infection. However, once a patient is trained, fluid volume must be adjusted so voiding is not too frequent.
   c. Observance of intake and output ensures **fluid balance.**
   d. **External compression of the bladder** (Credé's maneuver) helps reduce residual volume and, with triple voiding, increases the total amount voided.
   e. **Alternation of the patient's position** increases the total volume voided.
3. **Drug therapy.** The use of drugs is limited because chronic use causes toxicity.
   a. **Bethanechol chloride** (Urecholine), a cholinergic agonist, may increase detrusor function and facilitate reflex activity. The dosage is 10–50 mg q4–6h PO or 5–10 mg q4–6h SC.
   b. A similar drug, **methacholine chloride** (Mecholyl), is used in dosages of 200–400 mg q4–6h PO or 10–20 mg q4–6h SC. Methacholine chloride is used to lower threshold for reflex voiding when the reflex is not adequate to empty the bladder and early in spinal cord trauma to promote reflex activity.
   c. When small bladder volumes cause excessive reflex activity, reduction in reflex may increase the time between voidings.
      (1) Useful drugs are **methantheline bromide** (Banthīne) and **propantheline**

bromide (Pro-Banthīne), which are anticholinergic agents that reduce detrusor reflex activity in dosages of 50 mg PO qid (Banthīne) or 15 mg PO qid (Pro-Banthīne). Anticholinergic drugs such as these are most useful in partial spinal cord or higher lesions to reduce urgency and frequency. The anticholinergic drugs may, however, increase residual volume and paradoxically cause more frequency because of reduced functional capacity. Increased residual volume also increases the risk of infection, which may lead to chronic cystitis or even pyelonephritis. Thus, these drugs are discontinued if the residual volume is increased to more than 15% of the voided volume.

   (2) Tricyclic antidepressants (150 mg at bedtime) may act to increase bladder capacity through their anticholinergic activity.

  d. Phenoxybenzamine, an alpha-adrenergic blocking agent, acts on the proximal urethra and reduces urethra pressure. Residual volume may be reduced when phenoxybenzamine, is given in dosages of 20–40 mg tid. Also, bladder neck resection may be averted when alpha blockers are effective.

  e. Propranolol (Inderal), a beta-adrenergic blocker, increases urethral resistance and may be helpful when incontinence is caused by uninhibited contractions that overcome the urethral pressure. Usual doses are 20–40 mg qid or more.

  f. Drugs to reduce spasticity of the pelvic floor may reduce residual volume and allow more complete voiding. **Dantrolene sodium** (Dantrium) has not been systematically tested, but **baclofen** (Lioresal), used for bladder training, has been reported to reduce residual urine volume.

4. Surgical therapy

  a. When medical measures fail to allow reflex voiding or there is high bladder pressure with reflux of urine into the ureters, causing hydronephrosis, **bladder neck resection** or **external sphincterotomy** will reduce both resistance to flow and bladder pressure. Removal of prostate or urethral valve **obstruction** also may be necessary to allow adequate reflex voiding.

  b. Other procedures are available to increase the voiding pressure, reduce capacity, increase capacity, or divert the urinary stream. Urologic consultation is needed in all these cases.

  c. When a hyperreflexive bladder is severe and contracted so there is low functional capacity, **alcohol block of the cauda equina** or anterior and posterior **rhizotomy** of T12–S5 will cause it to become hypotonic. However, these procedures can only be done in paraplegics, and they often cause impotence. The major consideration is to spare the kidneys from hydronephrosis.

D. Hyporeflexive bladder management. The hyporeflexive bladder is characterized by very low pressure, no contractions, high capacity, high residual volume, and poor stream. There is absent or decreased sensation of fullness. It is associated with lesions at either the S2–S4 level or on the peripheral nerves and roots. Transient urinary retention may follow lumbar puncture or, more commonly, lumbar myelography. Men with prostate enlargement are particularly susceptible to retention. Intermittent catheterization q4–6h will keep the bladder drained, but occasionally bethanechol chloride (10–25 mg PO q6–8h) is needed. The retention usually resolves spontaneously in 24–48 hours.

1. Chronic intermittent catheterization done by the patient on a timed schedule is effective in keeping the bladder empty. Also, it can be done, if necessary, using nonsterile technique without danger of serious infection. Patients can carry the catheter with them in a pocket or purse. Patients with ataxia, upper extremity weakness, excessive adduction spasticity in the legs, or dementia are often not able to catheterize themselves.

2. The use of **external bladder compression** (Credé's maneuver) and contraction of abdominal muscles may allow the patient to void sufficiently to reduce residual urine to an acceptable volume (usually < 15% of voided volume). Since the patient may not perceive bladder fullness, regular attempts at voiding at specific times are important. In patients with weak abdominal muscles, a lumbosacral corset helps to increase intra-abdominal pressure.

3. Drug therapy

a. Incomplete lesions in which there is diminished reflex activity may improve with **bethanechol chloride,** 10–25 mg PO q8h. If the oral dose is ineffective, subcutaneous injection may be useful.

b. Phenoxybenzamine may reduce urethral pressure so that voiding is more complete (20–40 mg tid).

4. Surgical therapy

a. Bladder neck resection reduces physiologic obstruction and allows more complete emptying of the bladder.

b. Relief of obstruction from prostate or urethral valves may also reduce residual volume.

E. Incontinence. Overflow incontinence occurs in hypotonic bladders, and higher-volume reflex incontinence occurs in hyperreflexive bladders. The easiest method to control incontinence is to keep the bladder empty by voiding every hour or at a rate that prevents either overflow or urgency. The patient starts at a frequent rate and determines what rate is adequate.

1. Incontinence in the **female** is difficult to treat if the volume is great, as in a hyperreflexic bladder, and an indwelling catheter may be necessary. If the volume is small and the patient can use intermittent catheterization, a pad may be sufficient between catheterizations.

2. For the incontinent **male,** several **appliances** are available.

a. The **condom collecting device** is useful for both temporary and chronic use. The device is attached around the shaft of the penis with cement or tape, and it can be left in place for up to 12 hours. A reservoir bag can be strapped to the leg and be hidden by clothing. Many males with bladder dysfunction use a condom device when they are in public. Frequent changes of the condom (q6–8h) and local care usually prevent local complications. However, if ulceration or maceration of the skin of the penis occurs, the device should be removed, the area kept dry, and a bland ointment used to help with healing. In hospitalized patients, a diaper can be used instead of the device to allow the penis to heal. Condom devices promote urinary tract infection in bedridden patients, especially if the condom becomes obstructed and urine remains in the condom.

b. The **Cunningham clamp** is a device designed to occlude the urethra mechanically by external compression of the penis. However, the clamp should be released frequently to prevent pressure necrosis of the penis or urethra. This old-fashioned device should not be used in patients who do not have tactile sensation of the penis.

3. Surgically implanted prosthetic devices to provide sphincteric effect are available. These devices are useful in patients with hyporeflexive and hyperreflexive bladders.

4. Electrodes placed in the S2-S4 area of the spinal cord have produced detrusor contraction in some cases of hyporeflexive bladder.

5. Chronic indwelling catheters should be avoided if possible.

a. The **catheter** is inserted, using strict aseptic technique.

(1) Teflon catheters have less chance of accumulating mineral deposits; therefore, they can be changed less frequently.

(2) The **standard rubber catheter** is changed every 7–10 days.

(3) A Foley balloon-type catheter is less desirable for chronic use because the balloon may cause bladder irritation and pressure damage. In women, the Foley catheter is usually necessary, since there is no effective way of securing a straight catheter. In males, a straight catheter taped to the penis can be substituted for the balloon type.

b. In all cases, the **drainage system** should remain closed, and the **reservoir** should never be raised above the bladder to prevent reflux into the bladder. A disinfectant may be added to the reservoir.

    c. Irrigation of the bladder is done through a double-lumen catheter perfused qid or tid with a volume that is equal to the bladder capacity. Any sterile solution is suitable. A citric acid solution (e.g., Renacidin) helps to prevent calcium salts from aggregating on the catheter, and solutions of acetic acid or neomycin are also available. When the patient is ambulatory, continuous irrigation may be stopped by clamping the inflow tube.

    d. Catheter size. A 16F catheter or smaller is optimal. Large catheters are associated with urethral abscess in men, but in women the urethra will dilate if larger catheters are used. If a balloon catheter is used, 5-ml volume in the balloon is sufficient. In males, the catheter should be taped to the abdomen to prevent extreme angulation, causing pressure necrosis at the penoscrotal junction.

    e. Drainage of the upper urinary tracts is facilitated by:

      (1) Early ambulation or wheelchair activity.

      (2) Frequent changes of position.

      (3) Elevation of the head of the bed.

    f. High **fluid intake** helps to prevent infection and calculus formation. Intake of 3000–4000 ml of fluid each day is indicated for persons with indwelling catheters in place, unless there is a strong medical contraindication to this fluid load.

F. Stone prevention

    1. Chronically bedridden patients have a high incidence of renal calculi. Good **nutrition** and high **fluid volume** are important to prevent stones. If hypercalciuria is present, a reduction in the amount of dietary calcium may help to prevent stone formation.

    2. Acidification of the urine helps to prevent infection as well as to keep mineral salts in solution. Thus, most patients with bladder dysfunction, especially those with indwelling catheters, should have their urine acidified to prevent precipitation of mineral deposits and help prevent infection.

      a. Cranberry juice lowers the pH irregularly and is not as useful as other agents; 250 ml tid has been used in selected cases.

      b. Ascorbic acid, 250 mg PO qid, will lower urine pH if there is no infection present. **Methenamine mandelate** (Mandelamine), 1 g PO qid, will lower urine pH if there is no infection present; 1 g PO qid, used with ascorbic acid, is useful in keeping urine acidified when infection is present. It also has bactericidal action.

G. Urine infection

    1. It is not necessary to treat **asymptomatic,** chronic urinary infection rigorously while a catheter is in place. Acidification of the urine and use of suppressive agents, such as **methenamine mandelate,** 1 g qid, **methenamine hippurate** (Hiprex), 1 g bid, or **sulfisoxazole** (Gantrisin), 1 g qid, are sufficient to keep the bacterial count as low as possible. Prevention of reflux is critical to protect the upper tracts from infection.

    2. When **acute infection** occurs or the patient becomes **febrile,** specific therapy is necessary. If the patient is on intermittent catheterization, a Teflon catheter is inserted and kept in place until the infection is under control. If the patient is on continuous drainage, the old catheter is replaced and specific antibiotics are used. However, frequent aseptic change of the catheter may be necessary.

      Although the urine may never become sterile, the goal of therapy is to eradicate the bacteria in the tissue and upper tracts. Bladder urine may remain infected.

III. Bowel dysfunction

A. Fecal impaction occurs in patients with a variety of illnesses, but it is especially common with neurologic disease. Adequate investigation for ostruction is necessary in persistent cases.

    1. Predisposition

      a. Bedridden patients.

      b. Elderly patients, especially those with a history of fecal impaction or constipation.

    c. Patients with abdominal weakness from neuromuscular, neuropathic, spinal cord, or other disorders.

    d. Patients receiving narcotics or other drugs that reduce bowel motility (anticholinergics).

    e. Dehydrated patients (e.g., those on glycerol, mannitol, or alumina gels).

  2. Signs and symptoms

    a. The urge to defecate but the inability to do so is a common complaint in fecal impaction.

    b. Frequent watery stools.

    c. Crampy abdominal pain.

    d. Bowel obstruction with air-fluid levels seen on abdominal x rays.

    e. A hard mass in the rectum or an abdominal mass that moves easily with palpation.

  3. Treatment

    a. Adequate **hydration** softens the stool and prevents impaction.

    b. **Natural laxatives** (e.g., whole bran and prunes) in the diet are useful to keep the stool soft.

    c. Drugs, such as **dioctyl sulfosuccinate** (Colace), also increase stool water and soften stools.

    d. **Digital removal** of the impaction or removal through a sigmoidoscope is often necessary.

    e. **Oral mineral oil,** 30 ml PO daily or bid for several days, also helps to move impactions.

B. Fecal retention and incontinence

  1. Paralyzed patients often have no problem with fecal incontinence or constipation, even when bladder dysfunction is severe.

  2. Diarrhea may precipitate fecal incontinence in an otherwise controlled patient. When diarrhea is controlled, the bowel is often continent.

  3. Bowel training is necessary in some patients.

    a. Regular **enemas** or a **suppository** is utilized each day until a bowel pattern is established.

    b. **Regular attempts at defecation** should be made, using an abdominal corset if necessary. Attempts to open the bowel after meals involve use of the gastrocolic reflex to improve evacuation.

    c. **Maintenance of a soft stool,** using adequate hydration, prunes, bran cereals, and stool softeners (dioctyl sulfosuccinate, 100 mg tid), helps to promote bowel function.

    d. An **abdominal corset** may help to increase intra-abdominal pressure in patients with weak abdominal muscles.

    e. In **severe idiopathic polyradiculitis** (Landry-Guillain-Barré syndrome), regular enemas and suppositories are often necessary until the patient can contract the abdominal muscles. Vacuetts suppositories are very useful when the stool is soft; they release carbon dioxide, increase pressure in the lumen of the bowel, and help stimulate reflex defecation.

    f. **Avoid constipating medications,** such as narcotics.

  4. Patients with **chronic fecal incontinence** (e.g., diabetics) can be helped occasionally.

    a. Use of denatured **tincture of opium** (5–10 drops bid) may reduce motility of the bowel.

    b. A regular morning **enema** to cleanse the bowel may allow the patient to go through the day with only a pad, with little risk of an unexpected loss of stool.

    c. **Biofeedback techniques** have been used to train some patients to use the external sphincter and the other voluntary muscles to maintain fecal continence.

IV. Management of tracheostomy

  A. Placement

    1. Acute respiratory distress is managed by endotracheal intubation. Tracheostomy can be done as an elective procedure if improvement is not expected to occur within 7–10 days.

2. **Indications.** Patients with neuromuscular, motor system, or brainstem lesions often require tracheostomy to
    a. Maintain airway.
    b. Prevent aspiration.
    c. Permit deep suctioning.
    d. Reduce dead space and reduce the work of breathing.
B. **Complications**
    1. Overall mortality is 1.6% in adults and 1.4% in children. Hemorrhage and a displaced tube are the most common causes of death. Death rarely occurs as a late complication unless there is obstruction or detachment of the tube from the ventilator.
    2. **Causes of obstruction**
        a. **Secretions** harden and occlude the lumen of the tube, especially when inadequate humidity is administered or the tube is not changed frequently.
        b. In metal tubes, the **cuff** is separate from the tube, and it may slip down and occlude the lumen.
        c. If the tracheostomy is low in the neck, the **cannula** may obstruct at the carina. If a tube is used that is too long, it may intubate only a single bronchus. Postintubation auscultation and chest x ray will identify this complication.
        d. **Trauma.** Injured mucosa causes collection of tissue debris and granulation at the lumen of the tube, which may obstruct it.
    3. **Hemorrhage**
        a. Acute postoperative hemorrhage around the wound may be life-threatening.
        b. Later, hemorrhage caused by erosion of the mucosa or erosion into an artery or vein, causing massive hemorrhage, may be fatal because of aspiration or exsanguination.
    4. **Subcutaneous or mediastinal emphysema** usually needs no treatment, but, if excessive, change of the tube position and repair of the rent may be indicated. At times pneumothorax may follow subcutaneous emphysema, and appropriate x rays of the chest should be obtained in all patients with subcutaneous or mediastinal air.
    5. **Infection**
        a. **Wound** infections.
        b. **Chronic tracheitis.** Culture of bacteria in the secretions of a tracheotomized patient is not enough to diagnose infection. Most patients with tracheostomies harbor a number of potential pathogens.
C. **Choice of tube**
    1. **Metal tubes** usually have an outer cannula that remains in the trachea and an inner cannula that can be removed and cleaned. Metal tubes have no built-in cuff, but one can be added. These tubes are used for permanent tracheostomies. Patients with chronic tracheostomies can be instructed in self-management of these tubes at home if they have arm function.
    2. **Valved tubes** are also metal. They are used so the patient can speak. At night a nonvalved inner cannula can be inserted.
    3. **Plastic tubes** are becoming more popular and are used for tracheostomy when a cuff is necessary. However, the whole tube must be changed when secretions accumulate. Most neurologic patients require a cuff, since protection against aspiration is an important consideration.
D. **Management of the cuffed tube**
    1. Choice of a low-pressure, high-volume cuff helps to prevent pressure necrosis of the trachea.
    2. The cuff is never inflated with an arbitrary volume. The volume is determined by leakage of air around the cuff. When positive pressure ventilation is used, the cuff is inflated until no leakage is heard around the cuff, and then several milliliters are withdrawn until there is a slight leak.
    3. The cuff will cause pressure necrosis unless it is deflated for 5–10 minutes q1–2h. Also, if a high-volume, low-pressure cuff is used, there is less chance of necrosis. When aspiration is a problem, the patient is placed in the Trendelenburg

position, or at least supine, when the cuff is deflated. Note that suctioning above the cuff is necessary before it is deflated.

4. The patient requires adequate fluid intake, and when a plastic cuffed tube is used, hydration in the form of aerosol is necessary to keep the patient's secretion thin. Room humidity should be kept high and the room temperature warm. A tracheostomy mask is useful to deliver warm humidified air to the patient.

5. Frequent suction of secretions keeps the accumulation on the tube to a minimum. Instillation of 5–10 ml of sterile saline may help when secretions are very thick.

6. Postural drainage helps to remove secretions from the bronchi.

7. Speech is possible with any tracheostomy if the tube is occluded and the cuff is deflated.

8. Tracheostomy wounds close spontaneously in several days when the tube is removed. If healing is slow, taping the edges of the wound together or using a bandage with petroleum jelly to make an airtight seal will speed healing. In a few cases, the tracheostomy must be closed surgically.

9. Once artificial respiration is not necessary, the tracheostomy can be allowed to close unless aspiration or prophylactic use (as in severe myasthenia) requires continuation. Occlusion of the tracheostomy, breathing through the mouth for several minutes, increasing to hours, tests the need for a tracheostomy. In many cases, patient comfort without the tracheostomy is basis enough to remove it, despite the blood gases and other parameters.

10. In chronic aspiration, the upper trachea can be ligated and the tube is left in place. Then the patient can take fluid and food by mouth.

11. Otolaryngology consultation is helpful in management of a chronic tracheostomy.

E. **Changing the tracheostomy tube**

1. Plastic tubes must be changed every 5–10 days. Metal tubes can be cleaned daily and changed less frequently.

2. The orifice at the neck communicates with the trachea and is well formed after about 3–5 days postoperatively. If the tube is changed earlier, a surgeon should do it.

3. Gentle, firm pressure slips the tube into place and usually causes a cough reflex.

4. It is best to use the same size tube with each change. There is a tendency for staff members to use a smaller tube at each change, because the larger tubes are not as easily inserted. However, if progressively smaller tubes are used there will be a point at which the orifice is not adequate and surgical dilatation is needed.

V. **Decubitus ulcer**

A. **Prevention**

1. Neurologic patients who are paralyzed and those with sensory deficits are highly susceptible to pressure necrosis of the skin. The most important preventive measures are **frequent turning of the patient** and **frequent changing of the patient's posture**. In quadriplegic patients, the Stryker frame is useful, and the patient can be rotated easily q1–2h. Careful turning and positioning will prevent decubitus ulcer in these patients. Thus, prevention of decubitus ulcer depends on the quality of nursing care.

2. **Protection of bony prominences** (e.g., heels, ischial tuberosities, and sacral areas) from trauma is necessary. In infants with chronic compensated hydrocephalus, care must be taken to shift the enlarged head and keep it protected; otherwise decubitus ulcer will occur.

3. Sheepskin, water mattress, and other soft material help to protect the skin. However, cushions in donut shape may cause ischemia of the central area and actually **promote** decubitus ulcer formation.

4. The patient's **skin** should be kept dry, and urinary incontinence must be controlled. A diaper can be used to keep the patient dry without using an indwelling catheter.

5. Use of bland **ointment,** such as petroleum jelly, in areas exposed to dampness may help to prevent maceration of the skin.

6. Good **nutrition** is important to maintain healthy skin.

7. If **edema** forms, the skin becomes thin and vascularity decreases. Aggressive

treatment of dependent edema in a paralyzed limb and special protection of it will help to prevent skin breakdown.

B. Treatment of established pressure sores

1. Pressure must be removed from the area of the skin that is involved. As long as pressure is maintained, the ulcer will fail to heal and may progress. The area of the ulcer is gently scrubbed with saline or hydrogen peroxide and mechanically debrided if there is necrotic tissue present. Wet-to-dry dressings are useful for large necrotic ulcers until there is a fresh area of granulation tissue. Also, **lytic enzyme ointment** (e.g., Biozyme, Elase, Penafil, and Travase) can be applied to the ulcer or in solution with a wet-to-dry dressing, which may be enough to debride the lesion. The enzyme is applied bid or tid, and the ulcer is washed before application. Large ulcers usually require surgical debridement. After debridement the area is kept dry, using a light 4- x 4-in. dressing or other lightly applied bandage.

2. **Petroleum jelly** or **zinc oxide** can be used as an occlusive dressing. A paste of magnesium aluminum gel can be made by pouring off the supernatant liquid of a bottle of antacid. This paste can be applied to the ulcer and will dry, forming a crust that protects the area. Application tid is adequate.

3. **Capillary circulation** is thought to be defective in patients with pressure sores. A moist environment and gentle massage around the ulcer may improve circulation and promote healing.

4. Patients with poor **nutrition** or anemia have more difficulty healing.

5. In **severe deep ulcers with undermined edges,** surgical debridement and skin grafting may be necessary.

6. **Infection** in decubitis ulcer is usually not a contributing cause of the ulcer, but in severe undermined ulcers, septicemia and death can occur. Topical antibiotics are not useful in these cases.

7. **Op-Site** is a synthetic material that is permeable to both oxygen and water. It has been used as a film to cover decubitus ulcers and seems to increase the healing rate. The film is applied over the ulcer and left in place until there is fluid leakage through it. Initially, changes are needed frequently, but, as healing progresses, changes may be weekly. Cellulitis is a very rare complication.

VI. Sexual dysfunction. Sexual performance and enjoyment depend on a complex interplay of psychological, neurologic, endocrine, vascular, and anatomic factors. The evaluation and treatment of patients with sexual dysfunction require expertise in several disciplines of medicine.

A. Initial evaluation

1. **History.** Many patients and physicians are reluctant to discuss sexual difficulties. The nature and duration of the patient's problem must be clarified. The strength of the patient's sexual desire must be assessed. Severely reduced sexual drive is a common manifestation of chronic physical illness but it may also reflect depression, medication effects, alcohol or drug abuse, endocrine disturbances, sexual inhibition, or lack of an appropriate partner. The partner's sexual functioning and expectations must also be assessed to gain accurate insight into the patient's problem.

2. **Examination.** General physical examination, urologic or gynecologic examination, neurologic examination, vascular examination, and psychological assessment are all imperative in the evaluation of the patient with sexual dysfunction.

B. Impotence is the inability to have an erection that is sufficient for sexual intercourse.

1. **Physiology of penile erection.** Penile erection is a segmental reflex involving autonomic centers in the lower spinal cord. The stimuli that activate the erection reflex include psychic sexual arousal, local stimulation of the genital region, and interoceptive signals arising from the bowel or bladder. Psychological stimuli can also activate inhibitory pathways to suppress the erection reflex. The efferent impulses of the erection reflex travel through sacral parasympathetic fibers from segments S2–S4. These signals trigger increased arterial blood flow into the sinusoidal erectile tissues of the penis. The expanded sinusoids compress the draining veins to reduce outflow and further trap blood within the penis.

Eventually a steady state is reached, where the rate of arterial inflow and venous outflow is equal, and the penis stops enlarging but remains rigid.

2. **Psychogenic impotence.** It was once thought that the majority of impotent men were suffering from emotional disturbances that inhibited the erection reflex. Recent studies reveal that most impotent men have an "organic" disorder, although emotional problems commonly exacerbate the physical condition.

   a. **Description.** Depression, anxiety, phobias, and partner problems are common causes of impotence. Although psychological factors can inhibit the erection reflex, erections may still occur under specific circumstances. Thus, the patient may report that he awakens in the morning with a full erection, is potent with some sexual partners but not others, or is able to obtain a full erection by masturbation.

   b. **Diagnosis.** Psychogenic impotence is a diagnosis by exclusion. In uncertain cases, a nocturnal penile tumescence study can be helpful. During the night most men experience several erections associated with rapid eye movement (REM) sleep. The test involves attaching an apparatus to the penis that can measure penile circumference (and with more sophisticated devices, penile rigidity) during a night's sleep. The test is not infallible. There are some patients with neurogenic erectile dysfunction who will have normal nocturnal erections. Therefore, a normal nocturnal penile tumescence study is highly suspicious, but does not unequivocally prove, that impotence is psychogenic.

   c. **Psychotherapy** must be directed at the specific factors that impair the patient's sexual performance (e.g., stress management, depression, performance anxiety, marital discord). The specific experience and personal style of the therapist are the most important predictors of successful psychotherapy.

   d. **Drug therapy.** The most important medical treatment for psychogenic or organic impotence consists of withdrawing drugs rather than giving them. Medications and alcohol contribute to 25% or more cases of impotence.

      (1) **Androgens.** There is little rationale for the administration of androgens to men with psychogenic impotence. Testosterone is unlikely to be more effective than a placebo and carries the risks of many side effects (e.g., aggravation of prostatic cancer, fluid retention, hypercalcemia).

      (2) **Yohimbine,** an herbal alkaloid with alpha-adrenergic blocking properties, dilates smooth muscle in blood vessels and may promote erection. It is unclear whether this drug is of any clinical benefit. The usual dosage is 5.4 mg tid–qid. Side effects are minimal.

3. **Neurogenic causes of impotence**

   a. **Autonomic neuropathies** are a common cause of impotence. Diabetes mellitus is often associated with autonomic neuropathy, with impotence occurring in 10–25% of young diabetics and over 50% of older diabetics. There is a strong correlation between neurogenic bladder abnormalities (as demonstrated on cystometrogram) and impotence. Other disorders of the autonomic nervous system commonly associated with impotence include alcoholic polyneuropathy, primary amyloidosis, Shy-Drager syndrome, familial dysautonomia, and acute pandysautonomia.

   b. **Multiple sclerosis** (MS). Neurogenic impotence is common in patients with MS and does not necessarily correlate with the severity of general neurologic disability. In a recent study of 29 men with erectile dysfunction and MS, only 3 were found to have a purely psychogenic cause.

   c. **Spinal cord trauma**

      (1) **Description.** Disorders of sexual function have been carefully studied in patients with spinal cord injuries. The level and degree of spinal trauma are important in determining residual sexual function. Most men with transection of the cervical or thoracic cord will retain the ability to have erections. These erections can occur spontaneously during a flexor spasm or at other inappropriate times, but not in response to psychic stimuli unless the cord lesion is incomplete. Men with lesions of the lumbosacral cord or cauda equina are less likely to have erections.

      (2) **Treatment.** Counseling by physicians familiar with the problems of sexual

activity in paraplegics and tetraplegics enables some of these patients to resume intercourse. Fertility is usually impaired in severely spinal-injured men, but it is possible to obtain semen from these patients for artificial insemination.

d. Brain disorders

(1) There have been reports of impotence associated with temporal lobe tumors or trauma. Some patients with temporal lobe epilepsy are described as "hyposexual," and the relation between psychogenic factors and impotence is not clear in these cases. However, successful treatment of temporal lobe seizures may reverse the hyposexuality.

(2) Since the introduction of L-dopa, many previously impotent men with **Parkinson's disease** have been able to resume sexual activity. On rare occasions, L-dopa or dopamine agonist therapy results in elderly men becoming hypersexual.

e. Endocrine impotence. In general, the endocrine disorders that affect potency do so by impairing sexual drive rather than causing a direct effect on the erection reflex. Addison's disease, hypothyroidism, hypopituitarism, Cushing's syndrome, acromegaly, hypogonadism, Klinefelter's syndrome, and myotonic dystrophy have all been associated with decreased libido and potency. Men with prolactin-secreting pituitary adenomas often present with impotence. In large series of men with erectile dysfunction, the number of patients whose impotence is due to endocrine disorder is quite small.

f. Vascular impotence. Adequate blood flow to the penis is necessary to initiate and maintain erection. Thus, atheromatous narrowing of the abdominal aorta or iliac arteries can lead to impotence. Bruits, intermittent claudication, and diminished pulses are often found in these patients. Measuring the ratio of penile systolic blood pressure to brachial systolic blood pressure is helpful in diagnosing arterial insufficiency as a cause of impotence (but a normal ratio does not completely exclude the possibility). If the underlying vascular problem cannot be corrected, these patients may be candidates for intracavernous injections or penile prostheses.

g. Venous leakage from the penis is an uncommon, but surgically correctable, cause of impotence.

4. Treatment. The underlying neurologic disorder may not be correctable, but several treatment modalities are available to enable the patient to resume sexual intercourse.

a. Intracavernous injections. Injection of vasoactive drugs, such as **papaverine** or **prostaglandin E₁,** directly into the corpus cavernosum of the penis is being used to produce erections. Unilateral injection produces bilateral engorgement due to cross-circulation. The injections are made with a very fine needle and are nearly painless. Erection begins 5–10 minutes after injection and lasts 30 minutes to 2 hours, with partial detumescence after ejaculation. The dose of papaverine has to be individually titrated. Priapism, usually after the first injection, has been the most serious complication and requires emergency treatment. Penile scarring and infection due to multiple injections have not been common problems. Prostaglandin E₁ may be better tolerated than papaverine but is not generally available.

b. Vacuum devices have been manufactured to draw blood into the penis. When an adequate erection has been produced, it can be maintained by putting a constricting band around the penis.

c. A variety of **surgical implants** directly into the corpora cavernosa have been devised, including permanently rigid and inflatable penile prostheses. Sensation and ejaculation are not adversely affected by the implant. The best candidate for an implant is a relatively healthy patient with organic impotence that cannot be palliated by other means. Patient satisfaction rates have been over 90% in several recent series of men with penile implants.

C. Medication and drug-induced sexual dysfunction. Many commonly used drugs can interfere with sexual function in men and women, resulting in loss of libido, impotence, or impaired orgasm. It is appropriate to discontinue medications whenever possible in evaluating patients with sexual dysfunction.

1. **Antihypertensive medications,** including thiazide diuretics, sympatholytics (e.g., clonidine, methyldopa), and beta blockers (e.g., propranolol, metoprolol, pindolol) are common causes of sexual dysfunction. Angiotensin-converting enzyme inhibitors (e.g., captopril, enalapril) and calcium channel blockers (e.g., verapamil) are antihypertensive medications that have not been associated with sexual dysfunction.

2. The **H$_2$-receptor antagonists** cimetidine and ranitidine increase prolactin secretion and can cause loss of libido and impotence. Famotidine is a new drug in this category that may not affect sexual function.

3. **Antipsychotic drugs** (e.g., haloperidol, chlorpromazine, perphenazine, thiothixene) and **tricyclic antidepressants** (e.g., amitriptyline, imipramine, desipramine, nortriptyline) may impair sexual function due to their anticholinergic and sympatholytic activity. The antidepressant trazodone can cause priapism.

4. **Monoamine oxidase inhibitors** (e.g., phenelzine) can cause anorgasmia in men and women.

5. **Central nervous system depressants,** including sedatives, antianxiety drugs, marijuana, alcohol, and heroin can all decrease libido, impair erection, and inhibit ejaculation.

D. **Disorders of ejaculation and orgasm**

1. Physiologically, ejaculation is a spinal reflex mediated by pathways in the thoracolumbar segments. Sympathetic nerve stimuli provoke release of semen from the seminal vesicles, and the presence of semen in the posterior urethra causes reflex contraction of the periurethral muscles, resulting in ejaculation. Supraspinal connections can modify the ejaculation reflex, but they are not necessary for ejaculation to occur.

2. **Orgasm** is a cortical sensory experience accompanied by contractions of the voluntary perineal muscles and smooth muscles of the internal sex organs. Brain mechanisms are important for the subjective experience of orgasm, as it can occur as part of an epileptic seizure and "phantom orgasms" have been reported in paraplegics.

3. **Premature ejaculation**

   a. **Definition.** Premature ejaculation must be judged relative to the man's performance wishes and the woman's sexual desires. Thus, a man with an average vaginal containment time of 5–10 minutes may label himself as premature or normal, depending on his partner's sexual response. These patients, who consider their vaginal containment time inadequate, can be classified as suffering from the sexual dysfunction "premature ejaculation."

   b. **Differential diagnosis.** Ejaculatory control is an acquired skill. It tends to be minimal during adolescence, at the onset of sexual activity, and improves considerably with intercourse experience. Also, a man might not be motivated to develop ejaculatory control because he views his partner's responsiveness as unimportant or impossible. Other psychological factors, such as performance anxiety, relationship deterioration, or hostility may also underlie premature ejaculation. Only rarely can premature ejaculation be attributed to organic causes, such as spinal cord diseases (e.g., multiple sclerosis, spinal tumors) or urologic disorders.

   c. **Treatment.** Premature ejaculation is frequently a treatable sexual dysfunction. The patient should be reassured about the possibilities for significant improvement. Discussion of the underlying psychic problems may provide the patient with helpful insights, and emphasis should be placed on the importance of the man's relaxation while receiving sexual pleasure. Some commonly used remedies include masturbation before intercourse, attempts at more than one orgasm per sexual encounter, use of a condom, or use of a self- or partner-applied penile squeeze before ejaculation.

4. **Inability to ejaculate or achieve orgasm**

   a. **Description.** The inability to ejaculate or achieve orgasm may be selective (e.g., inability to ejaculate under some circumstances but not others) or global (e.g., inability to ejaculate during either masturbation or intercourse).

b. Differential diagnosis. A variety of organic disorders can cause a global inability to ejaculate or reach orgasm.

(1) Conditions that **interfere with the sympathetic nerve supply** to the pelvis such as sympathectomy or radical surgery, can prevent ejaculation Women with diabetes mellitus may be unable to achieve orgasm due to diabetic autonomic neuropathy.

(2) Spinal cord trauma can result in inability to ejaculate even when potency is not lost.

(3) Drugs that deplete sympathetic neurotransmitter stores, such as guanethidine, monoamine oxidase inhibitors, and alpha methyldopa sometimes impair ejaculation and orgasm.

(4) Aging may be associated with increasing ejaculatory control and, ultimately, with an intermittent inability to ejaculate. The pathophysiology of this change is uncertain. Patients who are unable to ejaculate intravaginally or with a particular partner are likely suffering from a psychogenic disorder (e.g., fear of impregnating the partner, relationship deterioration).

5. Retrograde ejaculation

a. Description. Retrograde ejaculation occurs when the internal vesical sphincter fails to close as the seminal secretions are discharged into the urethra. The patient may have an orgasm without producing an ejaculate, only later to find semen in the urine.

b. Differential diagnosis. Retrograde ejaculation is caused by disorders that interfere with the sympathetic nerve supply or anatomic integrity of the bladder neck. For example, retrograde ejaculation may be an early sign of diabetic autonomic neuropathy. Some patients with impotence secondary to autonomic neuropathy give a prior history of retrograde ejaculation. Postganglionic sympathetic blocking agents, such as guanethidine, bilateral sympathectomies, and transurethral resections of the prostate or bladder neck may also cause retrograde ejaculation.

E. Professional and general literature as well as other services are available from the local chapters of the various neurologic disease charities. To locate the nearest office, just write or call the national office listed in the Appendix. Most of the charitable organizations will help if the disease is similar to the one of their major interest, even if it is not exactly the same.

Selected Readings

FECAL INCONTINENCE

Engel, B. T., Nikoomanesh, P., and Schuster, M. M. Operant conditioning of rectosphincteric responses in the treatment of fecal incontinence. *N. Engl. J. Med.* 290:646, 1974.

Smith, R. G. Fecal incontinence. *J. Am. Geriatr. Soc.* 31:394, 1983.

TRACHEOSTOMY

Applebaum, E. L., and Bruce, D. L. *Tracheal Intubation.* Philadelphia: Saunders, 1976.

Egan, D. G. *Fundamentals of Respiratory Therapy.* St. Louis: Mosby, 1973.

Montgomery, W. *Surgery of the Upper Respiratory System.* Philadelphia: Lea & Febiger, 1973. Pp. 315–368.

DECUBITUS ULCER

Guttmann, L. *Spinal Cord Injuries: Comprehensive Management and Research.* Oxford, England: Blackwell, 1973. P. 484.

NEUROGENIC BLADDER DYSFUNCTION

Bors, E., and Comarr, A. E. *Neurological Urology: Physiology of Micturition, Its Neurological Disorders and Sequelae.* Baltimore: University Park Press, 1971.

Boyarsky, S. (ed.). *Neurogenic Bladder: A Symposium.* Baltimore: William & Wilkins, 1967.

Bradley, W. E., et al. Neurology of micturition. *J. Urol.* 115:481, 1976.

Firlit, C. F., et al. Experience with intermittent catheterization in chronic spinal cord injury patients. *J. Urol.* 114:234, 1975.

Krane, R. J., and Olsson, C. Phenoxybenzamine in neurogenic bladder dysfunction: II. Clinical considerations. *J. Urol.* 110:653, 1973.

Orikasa, S., et al. Experience with nonsterile intermittent self-catheterization. *J. Urol.* 115:141, 1976.

Perkash, I. Intermittent catheterization and bladder rehabilitation in spinal cord injury patients. *J. Urol.* 114:230, 1975.

Scott, F. B., Bradley, E., and Timm, G. W. Treatment of urinary incontinence by an implantable prosthetic urinary sphincter. *J. Urol.* 112:74, 1974.

SEXUAL DYSFUNCTION

Drugs that cause sexual dysfunction. *Med. Lett.* 29:65, 1987.

Kirkeby, H. J., et al. Erectile dysfunction in multiple sclerosis. *Neurology* 38:1366, 1988.

Masters, W. H., and Johnson, V. E. *Human Sexual Response.* Boston: Little, Brown, 1966.

Masters, W. H., and Johnson, V. E. *Human Sexual Inadequacy.* Boston: Little, Brown, 1970.

Mooney, T. O., et al. *Sexual Options for Paraplegics and Quadriplegics.* Boston: Little, Brown, 1975.

Sidi, A. A., et al. Intracavernous drug induced erections in management of male erectile dysfunction. *J. Urol.* 135:704, 1986.

Weiss, H. D. The physiology of human penile erection. *Ann Intern. Med.* 76:793, 1972.

Yeates, W. K. Ejaculation and its disorders. *Arch. Ital. Urol. Nefrol. Androl.* 62(1):137, 1990.

Patient Information Guide

Acoustic Neuroma

Acoustic Neuroma Association
P. O. Box 398
Carlisle, PA 17013
(717) 249-4783

Alzheimer's Disease

Alzheimer's Disease and Related
  Disorders Association
70 East Lake Street
Chicago, IL 60601
(312) 853-3060

National Institute on Aging
9000 Rockville Pike
Bethesda, MD 20205
(301) 496-9265

The Alzheimer's Foundation
8177 South Harvard
M/C-114
Tulsa, OK 74137
(918) 631-3665

Amyotrophic Lateral Sclerosis (ALS)

ALS and Neuromuscular Research
  Foundation
Pacific Presbyterian Medical Center
2351 Clay Street #416
San Francisco, CA 94115
(415) 923-3604

ALS Research Foundation
Pacific Medical Center
P. O. Box 7999
San Francisco, CA 94120
(415) 923-3604

The ALS Association
21021 Ventura Boulevard #321
Woodland Hills, CA 91364
(818) 340-7500

National Institute of Neurological
  Disorders and Stroke (NINDS)
National Institutes of Health
Building 31, Room 8A-16
Bethesda, MD 20205
(410) 496-5751

Ataxia

National Ataxia Foundation
600 Twelve Oaks Center
15500 Wayzata Blvd.
Wayzata, MN 55391
(612) 473-7666

Autism

Autism Society of America
1234 Massachusetts Ave. NW
Suite 1017
Washington, DC 20005

Benign Essential Blepharospasm

Benign Essential Blepharospasm
  Research Foundation, Inc.
755 Howell Street
Beaumont, TX 77706
(409) 832-0788

Birth Defects

March of Dimes Birth Defects
  Foundation
1275 Mamaroneck Avenue
White Plains, NY 10605
(914) 428-7100

Brain Tumors

Association for Brain Tumor Research
2720 River Road, Suite 146
Des Plaines, IL 60018
(708) 827-9910

Cerebral Palsy

American Academy for Cerebral Palsy
and Developmental Medicine
(708) 698-1635

Charcot-Marie-Tooth Disease (CMT)

Charcot-Marie-Tooth Disease
Peroneal Muscular Atrophy Int'l
Assoc. Inc.
One Springbank Drive
St. Catharines, Ontario
CANADA L2S 2K1

Down Syndrome

Down Syndrome Congress
1605 Chantilly Drive, Suite 250
Atlanta, GA 30324
1-800-232-6372

Dysautonomia

Dysautonomia Foundation
20 East 46th Street
Room 302
New York, NY 10017
(212) 949-6644

Dystonia

Dystonia Medical Research Foundation
8383 Wilshire Boulevard
Suite 800
Beverly Hills, CA 90211
(213) 852-1630

EEG/Evoked Potentials

American Society of
Electroneurodiagnostic Techs.
6th Street at Quint
Carroll, IA 51401

Epilepsy

Epilepsy Foundation of America
4351 Garden City Drive
Landover, MD 20785
(301) 459-3700

Friedreich's Ataxia

Friedreich's Ataxia Group in America,
Inc.
P.O. Box 11116
Oakland, CA 94611
(415) 655-0833

Guillain-Barré Syndrome

Guillain-Barré Syndrome Foundation
International
P.O. Box 262
Wynnewood, PA 19096
(215) 667-0131

Headache

National Headache Foundation
5252 North Western Avenue
Chicago, IL 60625

Head Injury

The National Head Injury Foundation
333 Turnpike Road
Southboro, MA 01772
(617) 485-9950

Hereditary Diseases

Hereditary Disease Foundation
1427 7th Street
Suite 2
Santa Monica, CA 90401
(213) 458-4183

Huntington's Disease

Huntington's Disease Society of
America
140 West 22nd St.
6th Floor
New York, NY 10011-2420
(212) 242-1968

Huntington Society of Canada
Box 333
Cambridge, Ontario
CANADA N1R 5T8

Hydrocephalus

National Hydrocephalus Foundation
Rt. 1, Box 210A
River Road
Joliet, IL 60436

Joseph Disease

International Joseph Disease
Foundation
P.O. Box 2550
Livermore, CA 94550

Leukodystrophy

United Leukodystrophy Foundation, Inc.
2304 Highland Drive
Sycamore, IL 60178
(815) 896-3211

Mental Retardation

Learning Disabilities Association of America
4156 Library Road
Pittsburgh, PA 15234
(412) 341-1515

Migraine

National Migraine Foundation
5252 North Western Avenue
Chicago, IL 60625
(312) 878-7715

Multiple Sclerosis (MS)

National Multiple Sclerosis Society
205 East 42nd Street
New York, NY 10017-5706
(212) 986-3240

Muscular Dystrophy

Muscular Dystrophy Association
810 Seventh Ave.
New York, NY 10019
(212) 586-0808

Myasthenia Gravis

The Myasthenia Gravis Foundation
National Office
52 West Jackson Blvd.
Suite 909
Chicago, IL 60604
(312) 427-6252

Myoclonus

Myoclonus Research Fund
220 Hardenburgh Avenue
Demarest, NJ 07627
(201) 767-3784

Myotonic Dystrophy

Muscular Dystrophy Association
810 Seventh Ave.
New York, NY 10019
(212) 586-0808

Narcolepsy

American Narcolepsy Association
P.O. Box 1187
San Carlos, CA 94070
(415) 591-7979

National Institute of Neurological Disorders and Stroke

NINDS
Building 31, Room 8A-16
Bethesda, MD 20205
(301) 496-5751

National Organization for Rare Disorders (NORD)

NORD
P.O. Box 8923
New Fairfield, CT 06812
(203) 746-6518

Neurofibromatosis

National Neurofibromatosis Foundation
141-5th Avenue
Suite 7-S
New York, NY 10010
(212) 460-8980

Pain

Chronic Pain Outreach
822 Wycliff Court
Manassas, VA 22110
(703) 368-7357

National Chronic Pain Outreach Assoc., Inc.
4922 Hampden Lane
Bethesda, MD 20814
(301) 652-4948

Parkinson's Disease

American Parkinson Disease Association
116 John Street
Suite 417
New York, NY 10038

National Parkinson Foundation
1501 NW Ninth Ave.
Miami, FL 33136

Parkinson's Disease Foundation
Wm. Black Medical Building
640 West 168th Street
New York, NY 10032

Parkinson's Educational Program
1800 Park Newport #302
Newport Beach, CA 92660
(714) 640-0218

United Parkinson Foundation
360 West Superior Street
Chicago, IL 60610
(312) 664-2344

Rett's Syndrome

International Rett Syndrome
  Association
8511 Rose Marie Drive
Ft. Washington, MD 20744
(301) 248-7031

Reye's Syndrome

National Reye's Syndrome Foundation
426 North Lewis Street
Bryon, OH 43506
(419) 636-2679

Sexual Dysfunction

Sexual Dysfunction Program
Univ. of MN School of Medicine
2630 University Ave. SE
Minneapolis, MN 55414
(612) 627-4360

Spasmodic Torticollis

National Spasmodic Torticollis
  Association, Inc.
P.O. Box 873
Royal Oak, MI 48068
(313) 647-2280

Spina Bifida

Spina Bifida Association of America
1700 Rockville Pike
Suite 540
Rockville, MD 20853
(800) 621-3141

Spinal Injuries

American Paralysis Association
500 Morris Avenue
Springfield, NJ 07081
(800) 225-0292

National Spinal Cord Injury Assoc.
600 West Cummings Park
Suite 2000
Woburn, MA 01801

Paralyzed Veterans of America
801 18th Street NW
Washington, DC 20006
(202) 872-1300

Spinal Cord Society
Wendell Road
Fergus Falls, MN 56537
(218) 739-5252

Stroke

American Heart Association
7320 Greenville Avenue
Dallas, TX 75231
(214) 750-5300

American Occupational Therapy
  Association
1383 Piccard Drive
Box 1725
Rockville, MD 20850

National Stroke Association
300 East Hampden Ave., Suite 240
Englewood, CO 80110-2622
(303) 762-9922

Sturge-Weber Syndrome

The Sturge-Weber Foundation
P.O. Box 460931
Aurora, CO 80015
(800) 627-5482

Tardive Dyskinesia

Tardive Dyskinesia/Tardive Dystonia
  National Association
4244 University Way, Northeast
Post Office Box 45732
Seattle, WA 98145-0732
(206) 522-3166

Tardive Dystonia

Tardive Dyskinesia/Tardive Dystonia
  National Association
4244 University Way, Northeast
Post Office Box 45732
Seattle, WA 98145-0732
(206) 522-3166

Tay-Sachs

National Tay-Sachs and Allied
  Diseases Association Inc.
385 Elliot Street
Newton, MA 02164
(617) 964-5508

Tinnitus

American Tinnitus Assoc.
P.O. Box 5
Portland, OR 97297
(503) 248-9985

Tourette Syndrome

Tourette Syndrome Association
42-40 Bell Boulevard
Bayside, NY 11361
1-800-237-0717

Tourette Syndrome
  Foundation of Canada
173 Owen Boulevard
Willowdale, Ontario
CANADA M2P 1GB

Tremor

International Tremor Foundation
360 West Superior Street
Chicago, IL 60610
(312) 664-2344

Tuberous Sclerosis

National Tuberous Sclerosis
  Association, Inc.
4351 Garden City Drive
Suite 660
Landover, MD 20785
1-800-225-NTSA

Vestibular Disorders and Dizziness

Vestibular Disorders Association
(formerly Dizziness and Balance
  Disorders Association of America)
1015 N.W. 22nd Ave.
Portland, OR 97210-3079
(503) 229-7705

Index

Index